The Collected Works
of
Arthur Hill Grimmer
M.D.

Edited by

Ahmed N. Currim

Ph.D., M.D.

D1720195

Hahnemann International Institute
for Homeopathic Documentation

The Collected Works of Arthur Hill Grimmer, M.D.
Edited by Ahmed N. Currim, Ph. D., M.D.
Norwalk, Connecticut, USA & Greifenberg, Germany:
Hahnemann International Institute for Homeopathic Documentation

ISBN 3-929271-05-2

Layout: Reinhard Rosé und Peter Vint

Printed by: EOS Verlag, Erzabtei St. Ottilien (Germany)

This book is dedicated to:

HAZUR MAHRAJ KIRPAL SINGH JI
who is forever guiding me

NOORUDDIN AND MALAIK
my father and mother
for their constant love

ARTHUR HILL GRIMMER
for his inspiration through
his work and dedication
to our Homeopathic Principles

AUDREY GRIMMER WINTHERS
who entrusted me with the treasures
so that Dr. Grimmer's (her father's)
last wishes could be fulfilled

Ahmed Noorrudin Currim
(Editor)

Acknowledgements

The Editor is *JOYOUS* in the collaboration between himself,
Reinhard Rosé and Peter Vint, the trio forming the
Hahnemann International Institute
for Homeopathic Documentation.

Reinhard Rosé has worked a labor
of love to meticulously prepare the
manuscript in its present form.

Peter Vint prepared the
Index and Table of contents.

The Editor feels a great privilage to work with
Reinhard Rosé and Peter Vint
and is deeply grateful to them
for their wonderful work.

Ahmed Noorrudin Currim
(Editor)

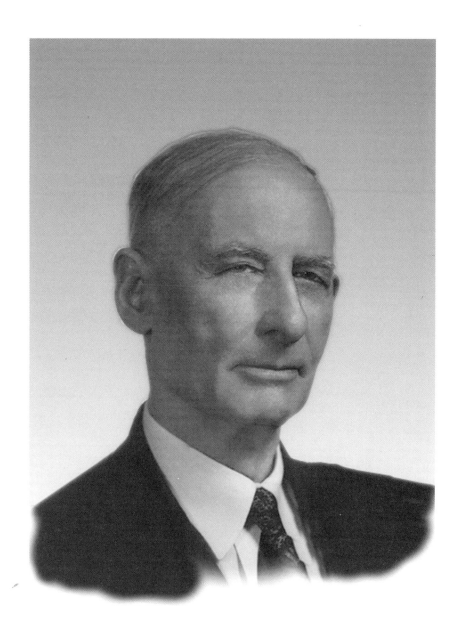

Arthur Hill Grimmer, M. D.
August 29, 1874 - March 5, 1967

Preface

The Collected Works of Arthur Hill Grimmer. M.D.

Edited by: Ahmed N. Currim, Ph.D., M.D.

I heard the name of Arthur Hill Grimmer (when I was about eight years old) from a relative who had been cured of a chronic eczema by Dr. Grimmer. The story was that this relative, a student in America in 1947, had visited the good doctor in Chicago in his office on State Street (which once was also the office of James Tyler Kent). Dr. Grimmer did a good history and exam and prescribed one dose of the indicated remedy Kali-s. in the CM potency. A wonderful cure followed after an initial aggravation of the itching for a few days. The eczema of some 12 years duration was gone within ten days (with only this one dose), never to return.

However, this story was forgotten, but in 1966 when I had become interested in Homeopathy, the name of Grimmer came into my consciousness and I tried to find him. It was through the kindness of Roger Ehrhart, one of the founders of Ehrhart and Karl, Homeopathic Pharmacists and publisher of Kent's Repertory, that I learned (in 1969) of the whereabouts of Dr. Grimmer. Dr. Gimmer had passed on about two years previously but his daughter was alive and well and I was successful in locating her.

In December 1972 during the Christmas vacation, I was able to journey to Florida to seek the company of my spiritual teacher, Kirpal Singh. Whether luck would have it or whether the guiding spirit of Dr. Grimmer and that of Kirpal Singh so willed I do not know, but I met with Audrey Grimmer Winthers, Dr. Grimmer's daughter. With the first knock on her door (from an unknown and peculiar math professor of foreign origin) there began a spirit of cooperation and love.

Audrey opened up to my idea of collecting her father's work both published and unpublished and bringing it to the Homeopathic Profession.

Audrey had many handwritten manuscripts of her father. and there was a large collection of them with Dr. Ruth Rogers (who had been a student of Dr. Grimmer). So I collected the manuscripts from both these sources. Thanks to the graciousness and trust of Audrey Winthers, I was able to collect all the manuscripts and arrived back at the university to continue my teaching.

I opened the three boxes of papers, many of them brown with time and storage, and looked at them with disbelief and wonderment and anxiety about my abilities to assemble from such a mass a work that could do justice to such a man who lived and practiced Homeopathy for over 57 years. How could I, at most a mathematician, without medical training do such a task. What had I undertaken to do?

Gradually, however, I calmed myself down and started the work. At first it involved only seeing the titles of the various papers and gradually I formed a plan to classify the various papers into various categories--Philosophy, Essays, Materia Medica, Special Diseases, Clinical Cases, Homeopathic Prophylaxis, Cancer and Electronic Reactions.

Then, in September 1973, I had the opportunity to enter medical school and so started the study of medicine at the University of Brussels. Every summer I would return to America for clinical rotations and during that time for three to four months I worked on these manuscripts. The manuscripts were classified, then a search would be made in the literature to see where that article had been published, then the hand written article would be compared word by word with what was printed. The errors in the journals were corrected using the original manuscripts. Each article was retyped. Audrey helped in the typing and other people who helped were paid by barter (their typing and my treatment of their chronic illness). Somehow the spirits of Dr. Grimmer and the Provider of all good and my Spiritual Teacher provided so that this work could get done. After six summers in 1978, the work was more or less complete with all the articles classified, verified, and a table of contents made.

We were all excited and were now eager to find a publisher. Audrey and I had mutually encouraged each other. The literature had been searched quite well and with my acquired knowledge of medicine I had been able to interact well with the material. I also felt free to add references to the main text. In one paper I included a clinical case of James Tyler Kent (not in the original paper) to further show the use of CADM-s. in a case of cancer of the stomach. Appropriate rubrics from Kent's repertory (not included in the original papers of Dr. Grimmer) were included in some of the papers to make them more complete.

During my six years of study in medical school in Brussels there were many times I had "to endure privations, loneliness, hardships, temptations, despair, and the black form of fear in its numerous aspects. I learned to replace fear with faith and despair with courage and to develop a will that defied obstacles and frustrations." I must have read and reread Dr. Grimmer's farewell address, "Fifty-Seven Years in the Practice of Homeopathic Medicine" at least 100 times, as it would give me faith, courage, and inspiration during the dark days of medical school.

Just before my final exams for obtaining the M.D. degree in June of 1979, I attended the LIGA Congress in Hamburg and brought a copy of the manuscript to show it to various possible publishers. But my efforts in that regard were met with resistance. Most of the German and French Homeopaths had not even heard of Grimmer and were definitely not interested. A well known English publisher told me he "dare not have anything to do with cancer." And besides, "this manuscript was too long." I knew then that the time to send out the light of Homeopathic Healing from Dr. Grimmer was not yet and I would have to wait.

I returned to America to do my medical internship and hospital training from 1979 to 1983.

Towards the end of my residency in October 1983, I had the opportunity to speak to a group of Naturopathic physicians and students at the Naturopathic College in Portland, Oregon, of my Homeopathic clinical experiences in the (allopathic) hospitals where I did my internship and residency. A possibility of publishing Dr. Grimmer's work through the NCNM in Portland arose, but the effort ended in disappointment. Instead an unauthorised copy of the whole Cancer section was published without permission of Mrs. Audrey Winthers or myself, with all my additions and editorial comments, without any reference of where the material was obtained, with many changes of Dr. Grimmer's own words - thereby resulting in an inaccurate work of questionable scientific value. Some of the older Homeopathic physicians in America are aware of this. We were able to bear on this person to stop his illegal publishing.

The time for this work really came in 1993 when Reinhard Rosé and Peter Vint of the Hahnemann International Institute for Homeopathic Documentation (HIIHD) visited me in Fairfield. I had been telling them of the Grimmer project and how we need to bring forth this work to the Homeopathic profession. Whereas in 1979 there was ignorance about Dr. Grimmer and even a resistance to publishing this work by English Homeopathic publishers, there now was a keen interest.

In August 1994, the Hahnemann International Institute for Homeopathic Documentation had a memorable meeting in Florida with Mrs.

Audrey Grimmer Winthers and an agreement was reached to publish these incredible writings.

It took 22 years from the time I first met Audrey Grimmer Winthers in December 1972 to August 1994 for the fruit to be ripe.

The work comprises of several sections - Electronic Reactions of Albert Abrams, Homeopathic Philosophy, Essays, Homeopathic Prophylaxis, Treatment of Special Diseases, Materia Medica, Clinical Cases, and Cancer. It should be read and studied as a whole. The articles in Homeopathic Philosophy bring out in an inimitable way the principles of Homeopathy as expounded by Hahnemann, but with the spirit of Dr. Grimmer; thereby helping us to understand further what the Master taught us. The section on Essays gives us the lores between 1900 and 1967 and gives us insight of the Homeopathy practiced in that glorious age when such Masters as Kent, Grimmer, Hering, Allen, Lippe, and Boger practiced in America and took Homeopathy to such heights, especially in the treatment of very serious chronic diseases. The Essays entitled, "An Autobiography" and "Fifty-Seven Years in the Practice of Homeopathic Medicine" are truly inspirational and should be read and reread by every Homeopathic physician many times throughout his lifetime. The essay on James Tyler Kent shows how Dr. Grimmer was influenced by this great master. The next section teaches us that the Law of Similars applies not only to curing diseases but also to prophylaxis and thereby gives Homeopathy an additional power in preventing illness (especially epidemics). In Special Diseases we learn of Dr. Grimmer's experience in treating alcoholism, cardiac disease, arthritis, and many other chronic diseases. The Materia Medica section is Dr. Grimmer's views of our remedies and gives another facet of our well-known remedies and introduces us to some new ones that he had first introduced into Homeopathy. The section on Clinical Cases is a sample of the incredible work Dr. Grimmer did in such complex diseases as cancer, arthritis, heart disease, etc. and further illuminates the power of the similimum. The section on Cancer is an expose of Dr. Grimmer's special expertise and gives us indications to find the road ahead in this serious problem confronting us today. The section on the Electronic Reactions of Abrams was Dr. Grimmer's research into applying the work of Dr. Albert Abrams to an expansion of Homeopathic Philosopy and in particular using these reactions in choosing more accurately the remedy for those especially difficult chronic advanced cases. It is, as far as I know, completely new in our science and is unique to Dr. Grimmer. He tried to pass on this unique knowledge and technique and it is really a pity that nobody made use of these achievements so that much of the knowledge is lost. So today we have Dr. Grimmer's writings and clinical cases showing this new idea; but unfortunately no operational instructions to either make similar machines or use them effectively in choosing the remedies or further understanding the cases. However the editor has taken great pains at reconstructing all that was left in Dr. Grimmer's manuscripts with the hope that one day some one will be found who will be able to reconstruct what is missing.

a) I give the source for every article whenever it was published.

b) For all other cases I used the handwritten manuscripts in my possession, including an approximate date whenever possible.

c) I introduced international abbreviations for the remedies (exept in the articles The Polarity of Remedies in Relation to the Polarity of Disease and List of Remedies According to their Polarity (Magnetic))

d) There is an index of all the remedies mentioned in the book at the end of the book.

LIFE SKETCH OF ARTHUR HILL GRIMMER

Born August 29, 1874, in San Jose, California, the oldest of nine children, of poor but thrifty and industrious parents. His childhood and playtime were brief in span and broken at intervals in the performance of certain chores in the household of every large family not financially able to hire servants. After his sixth birthday the family moved to San Francisco where he attended his first public school. When he was not in school mornings and evenings he sold papers to help swell the family budget. In pursuing the sale of papers, he covered much of San Francisco, in saloons, restaurants, and other public places, and on trolley and cable cars as well; he plied his trade energetically and untiringly with all the enthusiasm of impetous youth. Two years later the family moved to Oakland, California, where he spent the happiest years of his youth. There he completed all the primary schooling he was destined to have. When he was 12 years of age his father decided to locate on a 160-acre piece of government land in the mountains of Northern California in Lake County, where the quicksilver mines are found.

"The 12 years that followed were rugged and adventuresome and beset with many difficulties and tribulations. Money and rations were scant and poor, but game was abundant and wild fruits and berries were plentiful. With a little flour, corn meal, coffee, and sugar we were able to survive the first few years of real hardship and privation and were able to procure some chickens and other poultry together with a few hogs and cattle. We learned to cope with the elements and vicissitudes of the changing seasons."

"The second year after our arrival my father suffered severe injuries from a fall and he was left an invalid for the rest of his life. This unhappy event added new responsibilities on my shoulders. I was 14 years old and had to leave my mother and younger brothers to care for the home and go in search of work in order to get a little cash to buy the bare necessities needed. My first job was on a large ranch, and after eight months of dissatisfaction, I became a mucker - shoveling the rock and earth dug loose by the miners for $8 per month, with board, which sufficed to help meet the needs at home. From this time on things became brighter for the Grimmer family, and in a few years three of my younger brothers were able to obtain similar employment, thus enabling us to add improvements and other comforts to the home."

"My father was a highly educated man and his most prized possession was his library which was made up of a wonderful collection of books on science and literature, together with ancient and modern history. I had free access to these books and made the most of the opportunity they presented for acquiring more knowledge. I read long hours every night, averaging five hours sleep from my 14th birthday up until my 34th year. This reading, together with my father's tutoring, enabled me to pass a successful high school examination.

"My father treated our family with homeopathic remedies by following Johnson's Family Guide, an excellent work. He had 60 polychrests, a good selection for many homeopathic physicians. By the time I was seven, I knew most of the indications of those 60 remedies by heart and at that early age I had the urge to be a homeopathic doctor." (Dr. Grimmer actually cured several people at the age of eight years).

"After we had lived six or eight years in the mountains, I met Dr. J.E. Hoffman of Healdsburgh, California. Dr. Hoffman was my real preceptor and never let up telling me I must go to Hering Medical College, Chicago and enroll under the teaching of Dr. J.T. Kent. He also fired my mother with ambition for me by telling her I was an unusual prospect for a successful homeopathic prescriber. He used to say physicians, like poets, were born, not made; but how he could visualize a great physician in the raw, uncouth youth from the mountains has always been a mystery to me. In early September 1902, a gangling, uncouth youth left his mountain habitat in California, on horseback, to begin the study of medicine. No visions of grandeur, or dreams of wealth or worldly fame disturbed the even tenure of his way; only a burning desire to qualify for the privilege of becoming a homeopathic physician and serve as a humble healer of the sick and needy inspired his every thought and effort. No sacrifice of time or worldly possessions, which were meager indeed, was too much to give to attain this precious goal set by a longing heart.

Well, he came and saw and conquered, in the language of the great Roman warrior, Julius Caesar. He conquered, not an empire or destroyed armies with their spoils of victory, but he conquered self by the grace of God, to endure privations, loneliness, hardships, temptations, despair, and the black form of fear in its numerous aspects; he learned to replace fear with faith and despair with courage, and to develop a Will that defied obstacles and frustrations. He cultivated the God-sent light of reason and intelligence to lead him on life's stormy highway in preparation for his life's work, the practice of medicine.

Four tedious, painful, but exciting years glided by and graduation day came, and the fledgling doctor, with many of his colleagues, was born and dedicated to the healing arts.

In June 1906, at high noon, he hung out his shingle, A.H. Grimmer, M.D., at 29th and Groveland Avenue, Chicago, to embark on a new career, the practice of medicine. From miner and lumberjack and farmer and "Jack of all trades", laborer, etc. came the sudden, startling transformation to a Doctor of Medicine, this coveted degree was a prize whose worth was priceless; yes, it meant opportunity and prestige and eventual wealth, but it really meant much more, a chance to serve, to comfort, and instruct in the restoration of lives from pain, sickness, and sorrow, to states of health and happiness. With these desirable boons came a deep sense of responsibility for the custodianship of other lives coming for help and healing and guidance. Many questions loomed, with but vague answers. Was he really prepared to meet the challenges and obligations imposed? Did he have the patience and equipment needed to successfully cope with the numerous trying situations coming up in this work? Only if the love of the work and its uses was strong enough could he be sure of success and happiness in its performance.

"Forty-seven years of homeopathic practice had made my life replete with much joy and few regrets, for the outstanding miracles of cure and deep satisfaction far outweigh the relatively few disappointments that come to those who really follow the law of faith, because faith in the law implies faith in God. Without faith the healer will fail, and without faith the sick will succumb."

CONCLUSION

The editor is deeply grateful to Audrey Grimmer Winthers for her wonderful colloboration and trust in allowing this work to be published by entrusting me with the precious manuscripts, trusting even during those trying and difficult moments these many years. He also is appreciative of the support of her husband William Winthers, her sister June Grimmer Bayler and her son Don Bayler and the whole family for their trust and support during these 23 years to the end of this project.

In conclusion we Reinhard Rosé, Peter Vint and the editor Ahmed Nooruddin Currim of the Hahnemann International Institute for Homeopathic Documentation are joyous and proud to bring this work of this great homeopathic master, Arthur Hill Grimmer, to the homeopathic profession, and pray for the blessing of his spirit that it go forth and bring the light of Homeopathic Healing to all the nations of our planet as was so earnestly the wish of Dr. Grimmer.

Ahmed Nooruddin Currim

Editor

November 20, 1996

TABLE OF CONTENTS

Occult Causes and Material Effects 238
Heredity, Environment, Homeopathy 242
The Sphere of the Repertory in the Practice of Medicine 243
Repertory Study 246
Object and Need for a Repertory Compendium 250
Astro-physics and Homeopathy 254
Observations Relative to the Curative Action of Remedies 258
Review of Homeopathic Philosophy 262
Case Taking 265
The Essentials for a Homeopathic Prescription 270
The Relative Value of Symptoms 273
After the First Prescription 276
The Value of Mental Symptoms in Homeopathic Prescribing 281
    Happy Surprise 283
    Complaints after Laughing 284
    Fright and Fear 285
    Shock of Injury 288
    Homesickness, Nostalgia 289
    Love Pangs 290
    Jealousy 290
    Grief and Sorrow 291
    Conclusion 292
Things that Interfere with the Homeopathic Prescription 293
Things that Prevent the Curative Action of Well Selected
    Remedies 297
Interference and Disappointments 303
Hindrances to the Homeopathic Prescription 306
Materia Medica Study 308
The Relation of Surgery to Homeopathy 312
The Law of Similars 316
The Law of Similars and Empiricism 319
    First 321
    Mentals 321
    Generals 321
    Particulars 321
    Second 322
    Third 322

Materia Medica

ANTIMONIUM TARTARICUM, TEUCRIUM SCORODINA AND HELIX TOSTA[1]

This remedy is deep enough and broad enough in its sick-making power to include all the chronic miasmata of Hahnemann. It must be strongly scycotic, as Hering states, in order that warts on the dorsum of the penis have been observed. Clarke verified this statement with a cure of the same condition. It has also cured gonorrheal opthalmia.

About the most pronounced general feature of ANT-T. is the state of weakness prevading throughout its entire proving.

Another prominent characteristic is the tendency to produce catarrhal conditions everywhere throughout the economy. While no mucous membrane is exempt to the action of the drug, the bronchial tubes and lungs are more marked and more frequently affected than are those of other parts.

The characteristic discharges and exudates are copious, white, viscid and are frequently expelled from the body with difficulty. This is especially true of the expectoration; the bronchial tubes and lungs may be loaded with a loose rattling expectoration that, owing both to the viscid nature of the mucous and to the insufficient expulsive power of the lungs, can be dislodged with extreme difficulty, if at all, and then in only scanty amounts.

This remedy affects the vitality so profoundly that the reactive powers of the body are depleted and weak, causing a feeble response to the action of the curative remedies. Perhaps for this reason, we find it frequently a needed remedy for both extremes of life, infancy and old age.

The next most important center affected is the gastro-intestinal tract. Nausea, gagging and retching is a strong characteristic; vomiting of copious ropy white mucous, sometimes mixed with bile or blood. The digestion like the general organism is weak, especially sensitive to acid fruits, which may be the only thing desired. Most food is repugnant, even the attempt to eat, or the sight or thought of food cannot be tolerated; milk the natural food of the infants cannot be taken or used, even cold water which at times may be desired will irritate and upset the highly sensitive stomach. Inflammations of mucous membranes slowly go on to ulceration which are equally slow to repair.

With the weakness already mentioned there is an accompanying coldness. And cold wet weather brings on or aggravates all complaints

---

1. THE HOMEOPATHIC RECORDER, Vol. XLVII, No. 12, Dec. 1932, p. 918.

the catarrhal affections of the respiratory tract, and the symptoms of the stomach and bowels, also the rheumatic and gouty states that make up the third important center to be involved.

The pains of the limbs and back are severe and constant and associated with great weakness and heaviness, even going on to a paralytic weakness.

The fourth point of note is a copious sweat that does not relieve the other symptoms (MERC. and HEP.); the patient sweats without relief. And with this weakness and coldness and sweating the patient is mentally irritable and sensitive to a high degree.

Complaints especially of children are often brought on by becoming angry, like CHAM., COLOC., and STAPH.[1]

Another therapeutic symptom of real value, frequently met with, is a febrile state occurring with no accompanying thirst.

Next in importance is the action of the remedy on the skin. Eruptions of various kinds are produced by this remedy; herpetic, pustular and ulcerative and they are slow to heal.

From this brief sketch of the general aspects of the remedy, we may gleam somewhat of the conditions requiring it homeopathic use.

A novice in the application of the homeopathic law, would know that lung and respiratory conditions of a serious nature might require this medicant. The pneumonias of the aged, weak, cold with broken constitutions who have suffered from chronic catarrhal troubles and weak impaired digestion or those affected by gouty and arthritic conditions aggravates by every change to cold wet weather. The inability to expectorate the load of mucous that rattles and chokes him until he becomes cyanotic, cold and sinking. The bronchial pneumonias of infants of a sickly weak constitution, who have been unable to assimilate their food because of a faulty digestive tract. The child needing this medicine is desperately ill, because of its weakness and poor reaction to remedies. IP., (the nearest analogue to ANT-T.) likely has failed or only palliated for a time, then it is, this medicine may save a life. In a typical ANT-T. picture where the remedy acts only feebly or slowly, a dose of SULPH. will wonderfully strengthen and hasten curative action in these infantile pneumonias.

Another place for this remedy is the newborn. Where cyanosed and asphyxiated as a result of pressure and delay incident to a difficult birth,

---

1. and ARS. - Editor.

life can sometimes be saved (after all other methods fail) by giving this remedy.[1]

It also acts as a great palliative and comfort in many cases of late tuberculosis, when the exhausted and partly destroyed lungs can function no longer, yet the patient continues to live and suffer. ANT-T. will give such a patient, a painless death if it does not prolong his life.

Also it will serve you well in the pneumonias of high bred dogs, especially the short-necked blooded bulls, that inevitably die after a few days under other forms of treatment. ANT-T. is almost a specific for the pneumonia of dogs. And experimentally the dog has proven highly susceptible to its action, taking on the pathological findings of pneumonia, from its administration in so-called physiologic doses. It is surprising how happy you can make your patients by saving their pets; that is why this feature of the remedy is mentioned.

Certain forms of bronchial asthma are intractable and chronic and resistant to all kinds of treatment. Those catarrhal cases loaded with mucous, that cannot be expectorated; it lays in the bronchial tubes and rattles and chokes and gags the patient and produces a more or less irritating cough, which only brings up a little mucous with difficulty. And all these conditions are worse in cold wet weather and are met with in those of weakened, broken states.

The stomach symptoms have led to its use in the complaints of old drunkards, those who have ruined their stomachs with excessive indulgence in alcoholic drinks, where symptoms of ulcerative irritability supervene. They become so weak that nothing is tolerated and there is gaging and vomiting of viscid mucous, blood and bile.

This remedy has proven of great use in the treatment of smallpox and even prophylactic properties are claimed for it. There is a stronger thing about this drug that might be suggested. If you scarify a small area on the skin and rub in a little tartar emetic, in the 1x triturate, you can produce a typical vaccination scar, one that will satisfy the most bigoted health officer anywhere. The pustular eruptions, the dreadful back and limb pains, the disturbed digestive symptoms and the great weakness, all could well make it a splendid medicine for certain cases of small pox. Clarke says ANT-T. develops the small-pox pustule and that THUJ. dries it up.

---

1. This remedy is of capital value in helping restore premature lungs and Hyaline Membrane Disease - Editor.

Kent says that the sufferings and symptoms of the ANT-T. patient shows on the face, which may be dusky[1] pale and even cyanosed; a marked symptom is the flapping of the wings of the nose like LYC., to which it must be compared in some cases of late pneumonia.

The infant is very fretful and wants to be left alone, even does not want to be looked at or touched, and convulsions at times come on from anger. Much of this looks like CHAM. and CINA. Another feature that is quite marked is a drowsiness that may be part of the weakness. At times this lapses into almost a stupor in children, this aspect will lead you to compare AETH., especially in the intestinal conditions.

Such a paper as this cannot do justice to this wonderful remedy; an attempt to bring out the general features and highlights is all that we expect to do, so that interest might be awakened for further and deeper study of it.

A summary reveals a few cardinal symptoms and states that will prove helpful to the busy practician:

First, is the marked weakness everywhere.

Second, is the general coldness and the aggravation from becoming cold and from cold wet weather. There is also an aggravation from external heat and from the heat of a closed room, especially the respiratory symptoms.

The extremely weak and irritable digestive tract presents symptoms of nausea, retching and vomiting. Thirstless during the fever. Copious sweat without relief of symptoms.

Rattling of much mucous that comes up with difficulty and only in small amounts. Flapping of the alae nasi in respiratory complaints. Pallor and cyanosis complete a fairly full list of important symptoms of this drug.

A few of the most marked modalities will serve to complete our too brief study of a great medicine.

The cough is agg. from warm drinks, also becoming warm while lying in bed. Also agg. from cold and dampness. ANT-T. has agg. sitting down, and on rising from a seat, sitting bent forward, (yet sitting erect amel.), agg. lying on affected side, agg. motion and on every effort to move.

A characteristic of ANT-T. in lung affections is: lies with head back.

---

1. dark - Editor.

Clarke says there is not the amel. from rest which is apparent in many symptoms of Ant-c. ANT.-T. headaches are aggravated by rest, also earache and respiration.

Cough agg. at 4 a.m. amel by eructation. Clarke recommends this remedy as being one of the best for cases of lumbago.

TEUCR-S. is mentioned because, it has cured a case with strong ANT-T. symptoms on a tubercular base, where ANT-T. was given without relief of the constant rattling cough or of the emaciation and general weakness present. In TEUCR-S., the cervical glands of the neck are more pronounced than is generally found under ANT-T. TEUCR-S. has cured a case of advanced tuberculosis with a cavity of the left lung. A case of chronic periodical headache very severe, occurring at the menstrual period of a young unmarried woman, who also suffered from very profuse flow and almost unbearable cramps all at the same time, yielded promptly and permanently to this remedy given in potencies of the 10M and 50M, each dose at long intervals apart. This remedy needs a proving as its empirical applications shows great possibilities in curative energy, that can only be developed by a good proving.

HELX., is another lung remedy of undoubted power; tubercular cases with hemorrhage may find this the needed remedy. Cough with blood spitting, continuous hoarseness, and a cough at night which prevents sleep. Dyspnea, agg. ascending stairs.

Two cases mentioned by Clarke cured with the CM potency: First case: A man had frequent attacks of hemoptysis, continuous hoarseness, dry tickling cough agg. night preventing sleep, dyspnea agg. climbing stairs. He had had all the usual remedies, HELX. CM three powders given. There was no more hemorrhage. A few weeks later a return was feared and a few more doses given. Four months later the patient was greatly improved in health and remained well. Second case: A lady of tubercular diathesis, developed the disease after confinement. Several well-indicated remedies failed to check its progress. At length hemorrhage set in. Helix was given as in the other case with prompt effect; hemorrhage ceased, cough and expectoration gradually improved, and in eight months the patient was well and remained so. These cases quoted from Clarke, indicate the value of this remedy and the need of a proving of it, that we may better apply another weapon in our fight against the great "white plague". The key as we see the remedy now is the hemorrhagic tendency it has cured, and remedies that are valuable for this phase of tuberculosis are especially desirable because, such cases are noted for the difficulty in curing them.

BOMHENIA[1]

A new and valuable remedy especially efficient in the uterine hemorrhages of women at or around the time of the climacteric. The hemorrhage is dark red to dark with few if any clots, with or without pain and
at times profuse and alarming. There is a marked tendency to ulceration
and malignancy of the cervix, a condition in which a number of
patients suffering from it have with this medicine been cured.

This wonderful remedy is prepared from the beautiful flowering tree,
Bomhenia, whose numerous blossoms resemble the delicacy and coloring of the orchid, but unlike the orchid it is not parasitic. This tree is a
native of Brazil, but it also grows in Florida. A fresh portion of the
leaves, twigs and blooms of the plant were sent to Ehrhart and Karl,
and they made a tincture and potencies ranging from the lower to the
CM. My cures were effected by potencies from the two hundred to the
CM.

The question may be asked how was the knowledge of the healing
powers of this tree obtained and what were the indications for its application to the needs of the sick? All things in nature, animate and inanimate, have electro-magnetic polarity. Be they crude or in potentized
form, the polarity does not change. All matter and all energy have specific rates of vibration for each different substance or energy in the Cosmos. A remedy in its crudest state or form has the same polarity as it
has when run up to the highest potency. The process of potentization
does not change the specific rate of vibration of a substance but its electronic structure is so altered; there is a great increase in the electronic
power because of the greater space between the electrons to vibrate in.
Before this remedy was extracted from its natural habitat, the growing
tree, and made into the healing remedy that it is, the leaves, stems and
flowers were tested to ascertain its polarity. After the polarity was
found, tests for vibratory rates of disease were searched for and tabulated.

The doctrine of correspondences throughout the whole realm of
nature is wonderfully illustrated here and is another aspect of the
unbroken unity operating throughout the Cosmos. Every plant, mineral or chemical substance throughout all nature, of the earth, or the
oceans, or the gases of the air have medicinal properties to heal the ills
and infirmities of man and beast because they contain similar vibratory

---

1. JOURNAL OF THE AMERICAN INSTITUTE OF HOMEOPATHY, Vol. 49, No. 5, June 1956, p. 151.

and polarity forces to the disease vibrations and polarities that sicken and kill creatures of the animal and plant worlds. No clearer action of similia can be found anywhere else in nature than this proven fact of two similar forces, one in the plant and one in the animal body, nullifying each other when they meet in that animal organism. It is possible by vibratory analysis to know the disease-making properties contained in every substance in nature. Such being the case, it is relatively easy to predict the conditions and states of sickness that a plant or a mineral substance can cure when the polarity and the disease vibratory rates are found and known.[1]

Of course, this knowledge is only preliminary and far from complete, but when it is confirmed by cures, it becomes more valuable and reliable. Only when a complete proving in accordance with the Hahnemannian technique is made and added to this knowledge can we get the best and widest and most certain results from a remedy.

This remedy now needs such a thorough proving on healthy humans that we may learn the mental and emotional states it can produce on the healthy and cure in the sick. Its nature corresponds to the acute destructive *aspects of chronic malignant disease*, and too few of even our well-proven remedies have such properties.

---

1. See "Recent Concepts and New Formulas in Medicine" p. 679 and "Importance of Electronic Reactions to Future Medicine" p. 683. - Editor.

Cadmium sulphuricum[1]

This is one of the deepest and most terrible medicines of the materia medica, affecting the blood elements and nervous system profoundly.

Though its provings are meager, there have been many cures made with it of serious sickness that did not respond to other remedies. In its native habitat it is found closely associated with ZINC., and symptomatically it has many states in common with that metal. Kent places it symptomatically between ARS. and BRY., but in some of its nerve manifestations it resembles ZINC. and PHOS., especially in its tendency to produce paralysis of single muscles or groups of muscles as in facial paralysis, etc.

The tendency to produce necrosis and gangrene with profound blood changes brings it into competition with ARS. and the snake poisons. Wherever inflammatory processes start in the body under CADM-S., there soon follows death of cellular tissues. Many cases of gastric and intestinal ulcer have been cured with this remedy; even cancerous conditions have been greatly mitigated and life prolonged.

According to Clarke, apoplexy, boils, chilblains, cholera infantum, corneal opacity, other eye affections, facial paralysis, indigestion, meningitis, nasal polypus, oceana and yellow fever have been cured by this remedy.

The CADM-S. patient is very chilly, lacking in vital heat to a marked degree; icy coldness even when near a fire; horripilation, after drinking, with hot hands. Sweat in axilla like HEP. Bad effects of checked perspiration from exposure to a draft of cold air. Itching of the skin when cold < by sunshine. Many symptoms are < in the morning and after sleep; < walking, ascending stairs. In fact, any exertion or motion aggravates this patient and his symptoms (BRY.).

The wearing effects of grief may need this medicine; also the bad effects following anger may call for it.

One of our best remedies for the complaints and weakness of chronic drunkards. The nausea and vomiting - even the coffee-ground type of vomiting - has been cured.

The array of skin symptoms: intense itching at night in bed; when touched; when cold; which is > scratching, causing a voluptuous feeling. Skin blue; yellow; scaly, cracking, damp, suppurating herpes; chilblains - all stamp this remedy as an anti-psoric of the highest rank.

---

1. From the handwritten manuscript of Dr. Grimmer, exact date unknown. - Editor.

The character of the pains is burning, cutting and lancinating. There is tendency to spasm and constriction of many parts, but especially the throat often associated with painful difficult swallowing. The nasal symptoms and conditions are pronounced and striking. Nasal polypus with blocked nostrils and severe types of eczema have been repeatedly cured.

Great irritability of mind is found in the CADM-S. patient. Also there is a horror of solitude and of work. These symptoms are compatible with the extreme physical weakness and anemia common to this patient. The appearance of the CADM-S. patient is sad to behold: cachexic thin, anxious expression with a greyish sallowness and blue circles around puffed lachrymose eyes. Such patients have the mark of deep illness stamped upon them. Blood disorders and other changes in vital organs have long been at work and have ultimated, or soon will, in cancer or some other chronic degenerative disease.

In the head there are keen sufferings: constriction; stitches; pulsation; hammering in the head followed by vomiting; headache with restlessness and icy coldness of the body with epistaxis, constriction of throat, thirst, nausea, vomiting. Headache comes on awaking, in open air, of from a draft of air in the sun. Herpes of scalp is frequently found.

The eyes come in for many troubles: cannot read small type; night blindness; scrofulous inflammation; opacity of cornea; hot tears and swelling of the lids; hollow deep-sunken eyes with blue circles around them.

Ear noises which echo in the head.

The nose emits an ulcerative or cancerous odor - Ozena. Tightness at root of nose with tension inside. Obstruction of nose with swelling and from the presence of polypus. Numbness of the nose, erysipelas and boils on the nose. Caries of the nasal bones. Ulceration of the nostrils.

Spasmodic movements of the upper lip, facial paralysis from exposure to cold air - like CAUST. and KALI-P. Crawling sensations on the face, chronic eruption on forehead, nose and around the mouth; swelling of the lips. Salivation with a sweetish taste at first followed by bitter or burning. Fetid breath; ulcers; dryness and itching, burning constriction in throat - dysphagia.

In the gastro-intestinal tract there are many sufferings and symptoms. Nausea referred to the mouth, chest and abdomen with vomiting of acid yellow substances accompanied by cold perspiration and great weakness with inability to move as all symptoms are < by the least motion (BRY.). Salty or rancid belching with cold sweat on the face.

Aggravated cases of sickness have the black vomit that occurs in the late stages of yellow fever or coffee-ground vomit occurring in cancer cases. Burning and cutting pains in the stomach. Gastric symptoms < after drinking beer and there is < in the forenoon; during the pregnant state; the nausea of drunkards, especially the chronic broken-down individuals with pathological changes present.

Severe pain with vomiting comes in the abdomen; cutting pains in the bowels and kidneys. Lancinations in the left hypochondrium. Symptoms of stomach and hypochondria < by walking or carrying burdens. Stools almost gelatinous, yellowish-green, semi-fluid (cholera infantum). Severe cutting in region of the kidneys; urine suppressed, or scanty or bloody. Extreme weakness of the male sexual organs manifested by too frequent seminal emissions - cured or checked by the remedy. (Clarke) In the female, the remedy acts well during pregnancy. Erysipelas of the mammae; inflamed nipples.

The chest feels dilated. Feeling as if the lungs adhered to the chest. Cough with loss of consciousness, agitation, red face, pain in the stomach or vomiting of bile. Interrupted breathing during sleep. Chest symptoms < squatting. Brown spots on the chest. Swelling of external chest. Suppuration of the axillary glands. In fact, the glands everywhere tend to enlarge and break down.

Brown spot on elbow. Boils on the buttocks. Restlessness of the limbs; jactitations, startings.

The sleep symptoms are as troubled and broken as are those found under Lach. or Op. Sleeps with eyes open; stops breathing on going to sleep; wakes up suffocating. Symptoms < after sleep; annoying protracted sleeplessness.

Remedies to compare are Zinc. in nervous conditions. Ars. is the nearest analogue, especially in the chronic - gastric and intestinal conditions with weakness and burning pains and deathly nausea, Ip. and Tab. for the extreme nausea and collapse symptoms; but these remedies correspond to the more acute and short-lasting complaints. Ip. has nausea with a clean tongue as a characteristic. Lach. may be compared in the constrictions of the throat and other parts, also the aggravation coming on during and after sleep.

DIFFERENTIATING SYMPTOMS OF SOME OF THE CADMIUM SALTS[1]

CADMIUM SULPHURICUM

CADM-S. presents some striking features that run through all the other cadmiums. First of all the Cadmium patient is cold, always freezing, and complaints are all made worse from becoming cold, or from cold changes in the weather. Another thing about CADM-S. is the weakness it produces; so weak and tired. Examine this weakness a little closer and you find it is accompanied with a cachectic state that simulates the cachexia of advanced cancer or pernicious anemia.

Mentally there is a marked increase in irritability with a horror of solitude and of work.

There are some uncommon sleep symptoms that resemble the carbons and the snake poisons. Sleeps with eyes wide open, stops breathing on going to sleep. Wakens up suffocationg. Symptoms worse after sleep. Annoying protracted sleeplessness; insomnia.

CADM-S. acts most intensely on the gastro-intestinal tract, causing nausea aggravated by motion; later there is vomiting of acid or yellow substances. With these symptoms the face is bathed with cold perspiration and there are cutting pains in the abdomen. Black vomit like that occurring in the severe types of zymotic diseases. This remedy competes with ARS. in the ulcerations of the stomach of drunkards. Beer aggravates the gastric complaints.

Salivation with bitter burning in the mouth and throat; fetid breath.

Ulcers with dryness and burning constriction of the throat. This remedy should be a splendid one for those cases of the vomiting of pregnancy that fail to respond to the usual remedies; pernicious forms of vomiting of black blood from chronic ulcers or cancer of the stomach. Coffee ground vomit.

Such, in brief, is a general view of CADM-S. Our proving of this remedy is still far too meager, a wider knowledge of its symptomatology would enable us to cure sever types of intestinal disease that many times fail to respond to our ordinary remedies.

CADMIUM METALICUM

A study of the best proved of the cadmiums viz: CADM-S. must give us a basis for comparison until the proving of CADM-MET. is completed when we shall have more symptoms and a fuller data to prescribe on.

---

1. From the handwritten manuscript of Dr. Grimmer, exact date unknown. - Editor.

CADMIUM METALICUM ...

During my work with CADM-MET. in the last two years I have gathered a number of cured symptoms and some symptoms produced on sensitive subjects during its primary action when the so called aggravations so often occur.

CADM-MET. produces an impulsive irritability going to the verge of insanity in its violence alternating with a deep depression of the mind. Loathing of life, hopeless and apathetic all joy is gone. Unable to concentrate, saying and doing the wrong things such as putting salt in her tea instead of sugar. Vivid unhappy dreams of sickness, causing worry after awakening. Averse to people, to certain kinds of music; to noise. Odors and unpleasant things produce nausea, even when thinking of them.

Vertigo while looking at moving pictures accompanied with sensation of something taking the breath away, objects recede and return.

Extreme constant neuralgic headaches, maddening pressing pains through whole head extending to eyes and ears.

Old ear discharge with ear pain returned after many years with improvement in hearing. Hearing had been gradually getting fainter for years; suddenly improved with ear discharge.

Sore pressing pains in the liver and spleen. Violent vomiting attack with headache; alternating of heat and coldness. Vomiting bile and acid.

Diarrhea of black mushy stools with intestinal pains, this was followed by improvement in an inveterate constipation of years standing. Stools clay colored later.

Breasts felt enlarged and sore, this occurred in several patients. Intense squeezing pain in region of the heart with a sense of weakness.

More frequent urination, discoloring the vessel brownish or deep lemon color, very hard to wash off the vessel. Hemorrhages from the bladder and the rectum has been cured many times, commonly dark colored with small clots, but several bright red hemorrhages were cured.

Pains severe in all the joints. Numbness of feet and hands while sitting.

Severe neuralgic pains in the face with plugged sinuses followed by facial paralysis after large doses of quinine and aspirin cured with one dose of CADM-MET. 10M.

Cadmium metalicum ...

This remedy, together with Cadm-o., is the best antidote to aluminum posioning especially the subtle form that comes gradually from the prolonged intake of foods prepared in alumina cooking utensils.

Cadmium iodatum

Cadm-i. is a great gland remedy: the cervical glands of the neck, the tonsils, the thyroid, the mammary glands, the lymphatics everywhere, the testicles of the male, and the ovaries of the female. The liver, the spleen and the pancreas are all sooner or later involved under the influence of this remedy.

One distinctive mental symptom is hatred. Hates everybody and everything. Atheistic and hateful with a high degree of self pity. As these symptoms, together with an ulceration of the transverse colon cleared up and got well, a patient under Cadm-i. lost his hates and became quite humane and kind, and gained greatly in weight.

This is a powerful antisyphilitic as well as antipsoric and antisycotic, in fact all the cadmiums may be classed in the three miasms of Hahnemann.

Cadm-i. at times has an aggravation from extreme heat as well as extreme cold. As a rule the patient is less chilly than in the other Cadmiums.

Only a glimpse of the possibilities is here shown of these wonderful medicines. More complete provings will add greatly to the power and use of our glorious Materia Medica.

Cadmium oxidatum[1]

Among the most useful of our new remedies is Cadm-o. which is the most active of the Cadmiums and has a wide range of action in chronic and intractable conditions of cancer, degenerative diseases of heart and kidneys and many forms of arthritic and nerve inflamations all most resistant to ordinary remedial measured.

This remedy is indispensable and unequalled as an antidote to the alumina toxins afflicting humanity at the present time and which stem from the use of aluminum cooking utensils, as well as from the toxins resulting from water softeners in which aluminum chloride is used. Those who use the water treated with aluminum chloride for cooking

---

1. This remedy originally was included in the article "New Remedies and New Aspects of Old Remedies" p. 112, from where it was deleted. - Editor.

and drinking purposes are sure to suffer from the ill effects of aluminum poisoning and when so affected will not respond to curative remedies until this pernicious toxin is antidoted and eradicated completely from the system. This poison acts like one of the basic miasms of Hahnemann as the patient will not get well until it is entirely removed.

A case in point: A patient suffering from chronic asthma having excellent homeopathic treatment over a long period of time with only short acting palliation of the asthmatic attacks, which gradually became more intense and wearing. The patient was greatly reduced in weight and strength with an ever increasing dyspnea which made him very depressed with despair of recovery. Then it was discovered that he was poisoned with chronic aluminum from using aluminum cooking ware for a long time. A dose of CADM-O. 30 and later a 200 brought quick relief which was superseded by an attack of what appeared to be the symptoms of a virus flu. In this condition a perfect picture of HEP. was presented. Chill, fever and copious sweat, must be covered in all stages, no relief from sweat. HEP. 30 has brought complete relief of the asthma for several weeks without a break and the patient is rapidly regaining weight and strength.

CADM-O. is magnetically negative and the symptoms for its indication may be found in the other CADMIUMS, notably CADM-MET. and CADM-S.

CARBO VEGETABILIS[1]

In presenting this brief sketch of this wonderful remedy, my object is to bring out an image of sickness that will not tax the memory with a few scattered symptoms however valuable they may be. A long painful list of symptoms must fail to hold interest, for such a list can easily be obtained in any of our many works on materia medica as the need may arise for it. In such a group of symptoms there is a lack of continuity and spirit that relegates it to the category of dead inanimate things.

When pictures of sick individuals are presented to our mind's eye, living, breathing although suffering, and clotted in the aspects of death, there is that subtle indefinable force that grasps and impresses our consciousness with a lasting imprint; no effort of memory is required to recall the needed remedy of a sick individual when we have absorbed the spiritual, mental and physical aspects of each medicine as an entity. Materia Medica then becomes an intensely fascinating passtime and ceases to be a difficult and laborious pursuit.

CARB-V. is one of our many-sided remedies of broad range, corresponding to both acute and chronic states of disease and indicated alike in the complaints of the infant, the child, the adult and the aged, a consolation and a boon to the suffering along life's highway from the cradle to the grave.

Often in the delayed or hindered respiration of the newborn, where there is just weakness and cyanosis present rather than excessive mucous which occurs when ANT-T. is needed, CARB-V. will be the magic touch to start the tides of life pulsating on in the rhythm of health.

And in the early marches of life's battle, when acute disease or food disagreements have weakened the nutritive side of the organism or the sequela of acute disease, especially whooping cough, then CARB-V. is the most likely remedy to raise the vital tides to health.

Then later when the adult has fallen victim to his appetite and dissipation has weakened the body stamina so that every little strain, every little indiscretion in eating and drinking fills him with suffering and weakness, he becomes sensitive to his environment and cannot adjust his nervous mechanism to even the slightest changes, this remedy has the power to rehabilitate that broken constitution and bring back warmth, strength and hope.

1. THE HOMEOPATHIC RECORDER, Vol. LI, No. 1, January 1936, p. 43.

And at the end of life's journey, when racked with suffering and anguish, cold, pulseless, blue and gasping for breath; wants to be fanned that more of the life sustaining oxygen may be wafted to his air-hungry tissues, what a comfort and power is released in the administration of this remedy.

Even the most desperate state of sickness at the brink of the grave may be restored, surgical shock, loss of vital fluids, exhausting debilitating diseases, protracted fevers with exhaustion, pneumonia with gangrene of the lungs, prune juice expectoration, cold sweat, cyanosis, complete exhaustion, almost pulseless and wants to be fanned, is a picture of one of the worst aspects of CARB-V.; yet this picture of terror often is magically changed to one of hope and health by this wonderful remedy.

It is an antidote for many poisoning conditions. Food poisonings from tainted foods, especially fish tainted; with extreme burning pains, flatulence, extreme distension, weakness, cold sweats, weakened pulse and blueness yet craves the air and is relieved by fanning.

Gas poisoning and noxious fumes of all kinds are likely to need this remedy. The patient may be unconscious, pulseless and blue, and still CARB-V. can save.

The CARB-V. patient is sensitive to even a very little alcohol, becomes dizzy and flushed with burning at the stomach, and later weak and depressed from only a small amount of wine. This is one of the remedies for patients having very feeble re-active power. Their weakness is such they cannot respond to remedy action.

CARB-V. must be thought of along with OP. for the effects of shock and fright and with PSOR. in the sequela and weakness of long-lasting chronic or sub-acute illness. It also may be compared with ARN. and RHUS-T. from the ill effects of injuries, strains and bruises. CUPR., CAMPH. and VERAT. in cholera-like conditions, all are to be compared with CARB-V. and CHIN. for the weakness that follows hemorrhage and the loss of other vital fluids, with SEP. where the woman has never been well since the birth of her child.

The chronic aspect of CARB-V. is very distinctive. An individual slowed down mentally and physically; sleepy and tired, even to a state of exhaustion, a venous patient with engorged capillaries giving the face a dark flush, or even a purplish hue. One who is sensitive to the two extremes of temperature, whose feet and knees are icy cold and whose head and face hot except perhaps the nose, which may be cold and dark red with engorged capillaries showing. Kent calls the CARB-V. patient a venous patient. Varicosities with burning pains is a marked feature. And as one might expect, the heart of the CARB-V. subject is weak and irregular in function, the flabby heart muscles may go on to dilatation either acute or chronic. Acute dilatation following acute digestive troubles with great flatulence and distension with weakness, collapse and even unconsciousness and death may close the scene if this remedy is not recognized and give soon enough.

There are some striking mental symptoms. Timidity, especially the fear of darkness, is very marked. Darkness also aggravates some of the physical states as the difficult breathing. We have mentioned the mental sluggishness and memory weakness. Fixed ideas, fear of ghosts, especially in the dark. Some of the general aspects of this remedy will remind us of the snake poisons, of OP. and AM-C., especially the sleep aggravations; awakens out of sleep, suffocating and frightened.

The afore going synopsis of this truly wonderful remedy is designed only to stimulate study and research into the materia medica. Such study will be amply rewarded, because this medicine is not used as frequently as it should be by the average prescriber.

Chlorum[1]

This element has been proved in the form of "Chlorine water" and tested clinically. Clarke says, "It produces spasms and convulsions, coryza, and catarrh." Its most specific action is on the larynx producing great difficulty in exhaling. Inspiration is easy, but the air cannot be exhaled; is the likeness of a typical chlorine attack.

Clinically this remedy has cured severe cases of aphthae, asthma of a specific type, catarrh, chlorosis, colds, convulsions, croup, complaints of dentition, diptheria, gastritis, haemoptysis, impotence, laryngismus, phthisis, pleurisy, sore throat, typhus, and ulcers.

Rapid emaciation is a general condition observed in the provings. Also, a change in the character and number of the red blood cells is produced. Convulsive attacks while cutting the eye teeth; inflammation of mouth and gums rapidly going to ulceration is a feature. Acute rheumatic pains have been cured. Extreme sensitiveness of the skin with various forms of eruptions, inflammations and even ulcerations are produced and cured with this remedy. Malignant pustule, carbuncle, nettle rash with fever; skin becomes dry, yellow, and shrivelled. Catarrhal inflammations everywhere but especially in the respiratory tract is a strong characteristic of the remedy.

MIND: Some striking mental states have been noted. Fears he will go crazy; or that he will be unable to earn a living; cannot remember names of people he sees, or if he sees the names, cannot remember the persons to whom they belong. Apprehension and irritability to anger. Weakness and restlessness are marked symptoms in the more serious cases of sickness; also coma and fainting with cold viscous sweats.

HEAD: Painful aching of the head in the vertex and down left side with inclination to lie down. Warm sweat breaks out on forehead while coughing.

EYES: Lacrymation < in the open air. Suddenly numerous fantastic images appeared before the eyes, disappearing with lightning-like rapidity.

NOSE: Coryza with headache, violent sneezing in the morning, nose smoky or sooty, corrosive feeling in corners of nose. Sudden running from nose in drops of sharp corroding fluid, with tears in the eyes, with dry tongue, palate and fauces; or thin coryza soon changing to yellow, copious mucous; loss of smell. These local symptoms with weakness

---

1. From the handwritten manuscript of Dr. Grimmer, exact date unknown. - Editor.

and coldness, followed by burning heat, might easily place this in our group of flu remedies.

FACE: The face is swollen with protruding eyes. This symptom taken with the increased action of the heart might suggest its use in certain cases of exophthalmic goiter. Also the face may take on a greenish color.

TEETH: The teeth become black and are very sensitive as if injured by acids; enamel becomes thin and even disappears leaving the teeth black and sensitive.

MOUTH: Tongue is black and feels as if burnt; very acid saliva; aphthae; putrid odor from mouth.

THROAT: Throat dry; sore from uvula to bronchi; choking sensation; inability to swallow.

STOMACH: Acid stomach and other gastric troubles (in workmen exposed to the fumes of chlorine and who eat chalk for it). Desire to vomit without nausea, when coughing.

STOOL: Diarrhea in the morning, with dry mouth, after the eruption appears in typhus; stools of bright blood; hemorrhage in typhus, blood black, coagulated, or thin and smelling like carrion.

MALE SEXUAL ORGANS: Sudden impotence and aversion to sexual intercourse in the male.

RESPIRATORY ORGANS: In the respiratory organs are found the most profound and striking symptoms produced by this remedy. Aphonia, especially from damp air; great difficulty in articulating or breathing. Spasms of the glottis; air enters easily but cannot be expelled. Feeling as if the rima glottidis were stiff, as if composed of an iron band or ring. Sudden tightness of chest. Any attempt to cough brings on spasm of the glottis. Desire to cough from tickling and sensation of rawness behind the thyroid cartilage, but the cough is abortive, as he cannot expel the air from the chest. A continuous little dry cough; at each cough a spot in chest (region of right bronchus) feels sore, as if the cough jarred and hurt it. Phlegm raised with difficulty; soon collects again. Cough with spitting of blood and with pleuritic pains. Sensation of warmth in respiratory organs; sensation in lower and inner third of right lung as if it were ruptured and as if air escaped from lung into the pleural cavity at each inspiration.[1] Rales frequent, sibulent, and loud. Heart's action much increased.

---

1. This remedy should be considered for pneumo-thorax, because this is what actually happens in pneumo-thorax. - Editor.

FEVER: Chilliness and crawls, 10 a.m. to 2 p.m. Burning dry heat with anxiety and raving. Genial glow all over with night sweat. Cold sweat; viscous sweat in typhus.

GENERAL: The symptoms of the remedy are worse from midnight to 7 a.m., especially the spasm of the glottis. Lying down < nasal complaints, yet inclined to lie down with the headaches. Restless, yet < walking up and down. Sitting with the sun shining on back causes shuddering. Open air relieves the chest symptoms but aggravates and causes lachrymation; damp weather aggravates loss of voice.

RELATIONS: This remedy is an antidote to HYDR-AC. and SUL-H. and in turn is antidoted by SUL-H. and ALUMN. LYC. antidotes the state of impotency produced by it. PLB-AC., the blood spitting and pleurisy. It follows PHOS. well.

Such is the fragmentary homeopathic proving of this searching element.

Like the other halogens, this is a valuable croup and diptheria remedy in the gravest cases after other apparently well indicated remedies fail. In the middle West where much alkali dust at times permeates the air, in severe cases of croup, SPONG. will frequently fail, but this remedy will save life if given in a potency not too low. It is a banner remedy in the laryngeal types of diptheria a condition wherein we have developed by far too few remedies to meet such a serious condition.

The provers did not note any urinary symptoms but times when our water supply was heavily charged with chlorine gas, many doctors reported numerous cases of cystitis, many quite severe with blood and albumen in the urine.

The marked increase in heart and kidney disease that has been coincident with the almost universal use of chlorine in the water supply of our country, suggests that this highly irritating substance might be a big factor in this increase of kidney and heart conditions noted by the various boards of vital statistics. And our old school friends who at one time lauded this substance as a splendid germicide and disinfectant against all forms of disease have concluded that its efficacy as a germicide in unsatisfactory, because, if used in sufficient strength to make it effective, it is dangerous and deliterious to those subjected to its influence. Hence at present it is rarely if ever used either as a disinfectant or remedy.

I have observed a few things in my practice during the period when water chlorinization was carried on in an intense way in Chicago that may be helpful to other physicians. Cases of asthma, heart, kidney, and gastrointestinal disease will respond very slowly if at all to treatment until you substitute distilled or spring water in their drink and diet for the chlorianted water they are ordinarily compelled to use.

While some acute conditions of disease may have been mitigated by chlorinization of water, it has indisputably increased to an alarming degree many forms of chronic sickness including the more alarming and difficult conditions such as Bright's disease and cancer. For proof of the aforementioned statement we need only cite the reports of the various boards of vital statistics, state and federal, showing the alarming increase of those diseases during the period of chlorination of the country's water supply. Any substance that changes the vital processes and brings about even blood and tissue changes in a relatively short time even when taken in very minute, even infinitesmal doses, if given over longer periods in more material dosage, must necessarily produce serious harm in a large majority of those using such a substance.

The system may become immune to a degree to a poison if given in small graduated doses so that immediate death or even much inconvenience may not be noted, but such apparent immunity is purchased at the price of weakened body resistance and damaged vital organs.

DIFFERENTIATION OF DIPHTHERITIC POLYCRESTS[1]

The remedies are listed according to the frequency of their indication.

MERCURIUS CYANATUS

MERC-CY. comes nearer to being a specific for diphtheria than any one of our proven remedies. For all non-descript cases I would sooner trust to its use than to that of any other known agent. Its poisonous effects produce states and pathological aspects so closely simulating the worst types of diphtheria that physicians have treated poison cases for diphtheria before finding out the cause of sickness toxic poisoning by MERC-CY.

In my practice I have found it a perfect prophylactic never having seen a single case develop in any member of a family where I have given it after exposure to the disease. According to Dr. Dewey this remedy given in a routine way in the most malignant epidemics in Europe cured above 95% of cases. The concensus of testimony favors its use in potencies ranging above the 6th. (The use of the lower potencies are said to tend to produce heart failure and weakness.) Dr. Villiers of St. Petersberg treated 200 cases of all sorts of severity with this remedy without a single death. There is nothing in the history of medicine to approach such results.

Its indications are striking and highly characteristic. Extreme weakness, even from the onset; symptoms of collapse may manifest. Cyanosis is an early and persistent symptom with marked coldness of the body and extremities. The exudation is white at first soon becoming dark and even of a gangrenous condition. There may be edema of the soft palate (like APIS and KALI-BI.) There is likewise a thick tenacious, even a gristle-like exudate on the tonsils. Profuse nose-bleed with cynotic flushed face, later pale and wan. Eyes sunken; fixed dilated injested pupils. Great difficulty of swallowing with much redness and swelling of fauces; salivation fetid breath; teeth painful, gums swollen and covered with white adherent layers under which is found a violet border. But the rapid prostration, cynosis and coldness are the surest guides in any color or type of membrane presented.

Aversion to food is soon marked. Intense thirst but drinks are speedily vomited; cannot endure soup or hot drinks. Violent retching from

---

1. From the handwritten manuscript of Dr. Grimmer, exact date unknown. - Editor.

merely thinking of sweetened water; milk relieves the gastric symptoms. On the kidney there is marked action; urination is albuminous, retained or suppressed. The stools are offensive, slimy or green, often bloody stools, or scanty stool preceded by colic in abdomen and followed by tenesmus. Violent and abrupt beating of the heart; strong palpitations. Repeated fainting. Skin moist and cold.

DIPHTHERINUM

Called by H. C. Allen, the homeopathic antitoxin. It is another remedy whose symptoms correspond to some of the worst cases. Patients with weak or exhausted vitality when the attack from the onset tend to malignancy. A differentiation point from MERC-CY. is the painlessness that runs through this patient. No pain in the throat, no complaints of body pain. Just a weak exhausted individual apathetic and too weak to complain. Much like the typhoid states of ARN. and BAPT. the patient soon goes into sopor or even stupor but easily aroused when spoken to. Dark red dusky swelling of tonsils and palatine arches; parotid and cervical glands greatly swollen. Breath and discharges from throat, nose and mouth very offensive. Tongue swollen and very red; little coating.

FERRUM IODATUM[1]

This is a wide deep-acting remedy corresponding to many forms of chronic disease.

The blood and glandular systems are markedly affected, especially the thyroid gland; the liver and spleen; all present many symptoms and pathologic changes, such as inflammation and enlargements with drastic disfunction of these organs.

The lung and respiratory system is another center influenced greatly by this drug; even tubercular complaints have been cured with it.

Enlargement of spleen and liver as a result of the combined effects of malaria, suppressed by quinine, have yielded to the curative power of this remedy.

Reported cures of cancerous tumor of the breast, exophthalmic goiter, scrofulous inflammation of the eyes, ovarian dropsy, kidney afflictions, periostitis, plethora, pneumonia, gonorrhea and scoliosis are pathologic conditions listed as cured by *Clarke* in *The Dictionary of Practical Materia Medica*.

From this we see that the female genital system is another center that this remedy has a strong affinity for.

Quoting Clarke, he states that: FERR-I. corresponds more particularly to scrofulous affections, which translated into more modern terms is the **tubercular miasm** or type, for this inherited toxin is present today in a large number of sick people suffering from many forms of chronic disease with an underlying inherited tubercular soil condition. It is very subtle, only discernible by means of the electronic blood tests.

Some day our allopathic friends will come up with a tubercular virus, something not yet found; but FERR-I. does in a most decided way correspond to the drastic forms of tuberculosis and malignant types of blood and gland diseases which become more prevalent with each passing year.

Our provings are fragmentary and inadequate for successful prescribing purposes, but there are some peculiar symptoms and conditions garnered from clinical observations that are suggestive for possible curative use.

---

1. THE HOMEOPATHIC RECORDER, Vol. LXIII, Nos. 7-9, Jan., Feb., and March, 1958, p.75. It is primarily the whole text of FERR-I. from Clarce's DICTIONARY OF PRACTICAL MATERIA MEDICA - Editor.

HEAD: Headache with confused sensation and heaviness, < in a warm room, by smoking, wearing hats, reading, writing, motion; > in open air, sitting or standing in a draught. Sharp pain from below eye up through head to vertex, cutting from bridge of nose through the occiput.

EYES: Purulent inflammation of eyes and photophobia; glands swollen; exophthalmus after suppressed menses; trachoma; painful lancination in eyes and ears.

EARS: Roaring in ears.

NOSE: Nose stopped, freer toward noon; thick nose of scrofula, nose swollen with ulcers and crusts. Profuse discharge of mucous from nose and frequent expectoration of mucous from larynx and trachea. Chronic nasal catarrh becomes worse. Discharge usually in the mornings now lasts all day. Blowing nose gives no relief, discharge thick yellow or green.

MOUTH: Taste: metallic, bitter, flat, insipid, inky, pasty, sharp, biting, bad in the morning, like peppermint. Tongue, thick yellow coat. Burning of tongue and mouth; mucous membranes of mouth and throat uniform red, or dotted with fine dense. Bright red papular eruption. Burning pain and prickling and swelling of mucous membrane. Dryness of mouth and throat.

THROAT: Violent tickling and scraping in throat with a sensation as though he would suffocate. Hawking of mucous and cough; rattling of mucous. Food seems to come up to throat as if it had not been swallowed.

STOMACH: No appetite, no relish for smoking. Great thirst, sour bitter taste rising from stomach. Rising up in throat of greasy, acrid, tinging taste. Eructations; nausea and vomiting.

ABDOMEN: Tenderness at epigastrum, at the same time pinching in back over spine directly behind epigastrum. Fullness even after a little food as if she had eaten too much, a sort of upward pressure; stuffed feeling, as if she could not lean forward. Stomach full of wind, every breath gives pain as from a weight in epigastrium. On rising, or at night when turning in bed, heart beats violently, with pains in epigastrium or lower end of sternum. Dull pain under short ribs. Abdomen swollen; bloated after food or drink; pushed up; food soon satisfies. Rumbling with slight colic before stool. Abdomen when pressed feels like a rubber ball. Feeling as of a cord drawn connecting anus and navel, with cutting pain on straightening up from bent position. Abdominal walls numb; if pinched feels sore long after. Inguinal pain extending across hypogastrium; sides feel stiff as if after a strain. Feeling in sides, low down, as if needles were pricking her; < raising arms or walking.

STOOL AND ANUS: Bowels not moved for a week, then stools loose; may have two movements, first costive, second sudden and loose. Pain as from constriction of anus on passage of feces through it. Thin light yellow stools preceeded by griping; small hard stool with sticking and pain as from constriction in anus; constricting as if worms were in it; stool easy and painless. Peculiar feeling in rectum and anus as if something twisted and turned about in a circle and something like drops of water flowed down and as if a screw were boring upward and downward. Urging to stool with much pain in abdomen drawing from above navel down right side, followed by small, yellowish brown, somewhat hard stool in the morning. Frequent ineffectual urging to stool.

URINARY ORGANS: Pain in both kidneys especially left; feeling in the fossa navicularis as if water remained in it and could not be forced out any farther in the morning. Urine dark colored depositing thick white sediment; urine scalds; frequent profuse emission of light colored urine having a sweetish smell and slight milky sediment. Albuminuria with edema in hard drinkers.

MALE SEXUAL ORGANS: Erections at night, with violent pain and burning in urethra; unable to urinate; tenesmus in neck of bladder. Prickling itching in urethra, especially forepart, with frequent urging to urinate; but very little flow; crawling tickling in urethra and rectum.

FEMALE SEXUAL ORGANS: Hysterical attacks, great debility; leucorrhea, anorexia, finally dropsy of right ovary; menses scanty preceeded by pain in right breast and followed by profuse leucorrhea. Three weeks after beginning treatment, sudden loss of consciousness and discharge of two quarts of yellowish fluid from vagina, after which swelling subsided and health was entirely restored. Constant bearing down as if something was coming away; when sitting feels as if pushing something up. Retroversio uteri; sensation of pressure and protrusion of rectum on standing. Prolapse; inversion, antiversion; amenorrhea; itching; soreness and swelling at vulva and vagina; leucorrhea like boiled starch; when bowels move, the discharge is stringy.

RESPIRATORY ORGANS: shortness of breath; obliged to take a deep breath, with sensation of oppression of chest, and a pressure beneath sternum. Short, hacking cough, with yellowish white and rather thick expectoration and at times a pain in chest. Expectoration of greyish white, rather tenacious mucous drawn in threads. Hemoptysis.

CHEST: Sudden sharp sticking pain extenting from left nipple outward to arm, < by pressure. Frequently returns during afternoon and evening. Scirrhous tumor near right nipple, small and painless at first, increasing with sharp lancinating pains from breast to axilla, sensitive to touch (cured).

HEART: Many symptoms involving heart are found under this remedy. Running upstairs cause violent palpitation and pain on top of head. Heart beat so violent it awoke her from sleep, throbbing all over. Heart beats quickly and seems to force the blood violently through the whole body. Blood vessels throb all over even when quiet.

NECK AND BACK: The sides of the neck are sore when touched or on moving. Small of back as if broken; felt only at night; as if lying in a cramped position. Dull pains on each side about six inches above kidneys, extending through chest. Painful sensation in back and kidneys and lower portion of spine starting from lumbar vertebra.

LIMBS: In all the limbs there is weakness and bruised sensation with aversion to moving about; periostitis of fingers and toes. Painful drawings in tendons of back of right hand and left foot. Rheumatic bruised, paralysed feeling in right upper arm and shoulder; right arm weary and as if paralysed. Has to stop writing in the evening because of pain. Rheumatic pain extending upward from back of foot to pelvis in the evening; right tibia painful.

SKIN: On the skin there is short lasting eruption like urticaria, eczema and lichen.

SLEEP: The sleep is restless with frequent waking; many dreams of long-past events. Easy erection. Frequent waking with excessive urging to stool and pain on micturition. Dreams of thieves and fighting with them. Dreams that he has grown very large, thirty feet high, and everything about is small and insignificant. Frequent starting in sleep and waking with a feeling as though paralysed.

GENERALITIES: Coldness in a warm room about noon, heat 3 to 4 p.m.

CONCLUSION

The scope, range and pace of action of this remedy with its tendency to produce pathologic changes in the economy and its marked affinity to act on important vital organs and centers stamp it as a curative agent of great value. Because of all these features, which are shown with even the meager provings that have been made, a sufficient interest should be awakened in the homeopathic profession to make a more thorough and more complete proving of this powerful curative agent and in that way give us a finished implement for the cure of cases of chronic sickness which this medicine alone is destined by law to subdue.

Gnaphalium[1]

Gnaph. is a remedy with but a fragmentary proving. Its sphere of action is wide in painful states and its power effective. It stands high in the group of remedies for pain. Therefore it should be studied and compared with Coloc., its nearest analogue in periodical intermitent nerve pains or in gastro-intestinal pains and in diarrheic conditions. Coloc. is relieved by pressure, Gnaph. is not. Coloc. has a 4 p.m. aggravation like Lyc. and Hell. which has never been observed with Gnaph. with exception of the headaches which may occur at 3 - 4 p.m.

Cham. must be compared in painful states because of the marked irritability occuring in both remedies. Both Cham. and Gnaph. have numbness with the pains, Gnaph. more often has numbness alternating with the pain. Cham. is relieved by walking or is compelled to walk with great irritability and anger. Many of the pains, especially, toothache are aggravated by applied heat. Gnaph. is better sitting in a chair with painful leg drawn up, and its headache is better by cold bathing or applications. In both of these remedies the nerve pains are aggravated at night.

The Mercuries, especially Merc-c. in dysenteric conditions should be studied and compared. Mag-p., has intermittent severe neuralgic pains which are better by heat and pressure and rest. Rhus-t. must be thought of in painful conditions where motion and pressure relieve; it too has numbness with its pain. Clarke mentions other remedies for comparative study: Caul., Ip., Lyc., Merc., Puls., Xan.

Another remedy to think of for comparison is Nux-v.

MIND: Gnaph.'s most marked mental characteristic is irritability; especially coming on several days after a diarrhea and during the severe attacks of neuralgic pain.

HEAD: Vertigo may be present while rising from the bed. There is fullness about the temples; also a dull continuous pain in the occiput with shooting pains in the eyeballs. The headache comes on or is worse at 3 to 4 p.m. or on waking, it is relieved by washing in cold water or bathing the head with bay rum.

FACE: The face presents a dull heavy bloated appearance. Intermittent neuralgic pain in both upper maxillary bones.

---

1. The Homeopathic Recorder, Vol. LXVI, No. 4, October 1950, p. 101

MOUTH: There is a flat sweetish sickening taste and the tongue covered with long white fur which can be removed by thorough washing with cold water. Mouth feels parched and tastes badly.

STOMACH AND ABDOMEN: The stomach and abdomen are distended with much flatus and there is nausea, windy eructations and hiccough; colicky pains in various parts with sensitive caecum. Borborygmi with emission of much flatus. Rumbling in bowels with stool before breakfast (NAT-S.). Looseness of bowels with passage of pale colored feces. Diarrheic discharge in the morning and during the day with irritable temper, pains in bowels of children; dark colored, liquid offensive stool in morning followed by pain in bowels all day. Vomiting and purging like cholera morbus in the night and all next day.

URINARY ORGANS: Pain in the kidneys with frequent slight pain in prostate gland; sensation of pain and fullness in bladder even when just emptied.

MALE SEXUAL ORGANS: In the male the provings brought out an increased sexual passion with an irritation of the prostate gland. A frequent characteristic symptom is pain extending along cord to testicles.

FEMALE SEXUAL ORGANS: In the female dysmenorrhea; menses scant and very painful the first day. Sensation of weight in the pelvis, or of fullness in the pelvis.

NECK AND BACK: Numbness of lower part of back with lumbago is a strong characteristic, pains often extending down over gluteal regions and along the course of the sciatic nerve to the foot.

UPPER LIMBS: In the upper limbs feeling of weakness as if unable to lift the slightest weight. Rheumatic pains in the elbows and shoulders.

LOWER LIMBS: In the lower limbs the pains are first dull then darting or cutting from the right hip joint extending positively downward to the foot. Worse lying down, from motion, by stepping. Relieved sitting in a chair with painful limb drawn up. Intense pain along the sciatic nerve causing the patient to toss and roll and cry out in great agony. Numbness at times alternates with, or takes the place of the pain. Exercise is very fatiguing. Cramps in calves or feet, at night in bed. Gouty pains in the large toes This remedy has cured severe sciatica after RHUS-T., COLOC. and SULPH. failed. It likewise has affinity for the anterior crural nerve. The nerve and rheumatic symptoms are worse in cold damp weather, from exertion and strain, at night and the early morning; better sitting in a chair with painful limb drawn up. The headaches are relieved by cold bathing.

FEVER: Fever and night sweats.

There are two reasons for bringing this fragmentary sketch to your attention. First because it is one of the greatest medicines not only for relief of pain, but for its cure as well. Second it is a far deeper remedy than most homeopathic physicans suspect it to be because it has cured very chronic and obstinate cases of arthritis after the failure of some of our best proven and sucessful polycrests.

INDIGO[1]

Quoting Dr. Clarke of London: "This is an oxidation product from the juices of several plants chiefly Indigofera tinctoria; belonging to the natural order of leguminosae; it is a trituration. Clinically it has been useful in acne, amenorrhea, prolapsus ani, brachial neuralgia, constipation, cough, diarrhea, epilepsy, epistaxis, face pimples, headaches, hysteria, renal colic, sciatica, skin affections, toothache, urethral stricture, worms."

"It was introduced into medicine as a remedy for epilepsy. It has been extensively proved by homeopaths, and observations have also been made of its effects on epileptic patients who were receiving large doses from old-school practitioners".

The provings establish its strong affinity for the nerve trunks of the arms and lower limbs. Catarrhal conditions are next in prominence catarrh of the bladder and of the respiratory tract, and of the gastro-intestinal canal are well brought out.

A peculiar thing about the neuralgias is the marked aggravation after every meal, and they are < while sitting or come on during rest and are > by moving about.

Symptoms in general are < by rest and when sitting, > by motion, rising, walking; > by pressure, by rubbing; < in the afternoon, and in the evening. The vertigo with headache is > in the evening and < in open air. Warmth rushes to the head on entering a warm room, after walking in the cold air. All symptoms are worse after eating and after the evening meal. This remedy causes sensitiveness to the two extremes of temperature; chilliness accompanies many complaints especially coldness of the extremities with the violent headache, with a constant desire to urinate. The urine is turbid containing much mucous, or there may be frequent emissions of small amounts with pain and contracture of the urethra. Stricture of the urethra after gonorrhea. Frequently great heat in the face with increased secretion of urine.

In the epileptic attacks needing this remedy, great heat of the face arising from the solar plexus has been noted. In the epilepsy the mental states of depression are in evidence. Great melancholy before the attacks; the patient seeks to hide his depression and sadness, spending many nights crying alone. Or there may be a furious excitable state before the attacks and mild and timid after. The attacks are sudden and

---

1. From the handwritten manuscript of Dr. Grimmer, exact date unknown. - Editor.

apparently come from the solar plexus from which flushes of heat arise to the head. Undulating sensation in the brain with obscured vision with the spasms.

HEAD: Excessive vertigo with the headache. Rush of blood to the head; congestion, sensation as if the head were enlarged or as if the head were tightly bandaged around the forehead. Pressure deep in the brain; shooting and tearing pains deep in the brain. Sensation of weight or pressure in the vertex; noise and throbbings in the head; heat and bubbling in the occiput as if caused by boiling water. Headache with sensation as if head were frozen with anorexia; sensation in the crown as if a bunch of hair were being torn out.

EYES: Convulsive twitching and quivering of the eyelids impeding sight; pressure in the ball of the eye; inflammation of the meibomian glands on the lower lids.

EARS: Tearing in and behind the ears as well as in the lower jaw; pressure and roaring in the ears.

NOSE: Epistaxis with vanishing of sight in the afternoon, and with the cough; excessive continued violent sneezing succeeded by violent bleeding of the nose; tearing and incisive pains in the bones and cartilage of the nose.

FACE: Tearing, piercing, gnawing pains in the bones of the face especially the lower jaw extending to the teeth.

TEETH: Drawing, gnawing, tearing pains of the teeth with increase of saliva and sweat of the right half of the head, and general sweat in the evening in bed. Teeth pains worse by warmth, relieved by motion, momentarily relieved by cold air; pulsation in the whole lower jaw which was relieved by NUX-v., but it returned succeeding days and became paroxysmal.

MOUTH: Numbness of interior of mouth in the morning after waking. Sensation of burning on the tongue and in the bottom of the palate. Vesicles on tip of tongue; metallic taste with contracted feeling in the pharynx. Spitting of bloody saliva.

STOMACH: Risings from the stomach tasting like milk or sweetish risings retching and vomiting of watery fluid; vomiting of glue-like mucous; tingling pains in pit of stomach. Sensation of hunger or weakness in stomach.

ABDOMEN: Maybe loose evacuations with pinchings in the abdomen and urgent desire for stool.

RECTUM: Dull sticking in rectum; emission of an excessive amount of flatulence. Creeping over the skin and hands and colic. Obstinate constipation; stool scanty hard retained; itching at anus; pin worms; prolapsus ani after each stool.

URINARY ORGANS: Renal colic with frequent desire to urinate with burning in the fundus of the bladder.

MALE SEXUAL ORGANS: In the male, depressed sexual desire with itching of the urethra; glans and scrotum.

FEMALE SEXUAL ORGANS: In the woman, menses too early; has been used to produce abortion; stinging in the mammae and burning in the mammae during menses.

RESPIRATORY ORGANS: Violent cough inducing vomiting with bleeding of the nose; might well be thought of in whooping cough. Suffocating cough exciting vomiting in the evening, before and after lying down.

CHEST: Rumbling and grumbling in the chest with every inspiration; shooting pains in and around the mammae.

EXTREMITIES: Weakness in upper limbs; drawing in the muscles, in the deltoid; pains extending down arms from lower part of neck; extending from right shoulder joint down whole arm to below joint of thumb, where it ended in the bone with a jerking while sitting; relieved moving about. Veins of hands red, inflammed and tense. Aching, stinging bruised pain in sciatic nerve, boring in knee joint, aggravated sitting, ameliorated moving. Indescribable pain from middle of thigh to knee in the bone.

Bone pains are a marked feature of the proving running through out; face, arms, lower limbs, back, chest.

SKIN: Face and whole body covered by pimples, boils and itching skin.

SLEEP: Sleepiness in the evening, anxious dreams, disturbed sleep at night; children aroused at night with horrible itching at anus; ascarides.

Indium[1]

One of the rare metals receiving its name from the *indigo* blue line in the spectrum through which its presence was discovered in zinc-blende.

It is similar in action to SEL. and TITAN., especially as related to the male sexual symptoms and aspects. Diminished power and control; frequent nocturnal emissions, sexual dreams of perversion of which Clarke observes should render it serviceable in some cases of sexual psycopathy.

MIND: Mental depression as in INDG., but with it is a weariness unfitting him for work; in fact, mental effort makes him feel almost crazed, with headache on attempting to study. Unable to concentrate or fix thoughts on anything; feels stupid and careless. Restless, cannot sit still, must walk about.

VERTIGO: Vertigo on rising from a seat; after retiring with nausea; when sitting and stooping slightly; between 3 and 4 a.m., < on turning and on rising, cannot sit up.

HEAD: Beating throbbing pain in head with much heat and a stupid, cross feeling; > washing in cold water; head very hot, face red with clammy hands; afterwards bruised feeling of brain in vertex, better in the cold air. Headache in the morning on rising, > by eating; an hour afterwards headache returns and lasts until noon. Severe itching of scalp on vertex lasting several days, > in the morning.

EYES: The eyes are much disturbed in the proving of this drug; people and things look ghastly pale or saffron colored. Mist before the eye in the evening; sharp pain in eyeball from before backward, on turning or moving the eyes. Irritation of left eye, as if heavy with sleep, coming and going, not affected by daylight, worse from artificial light and from closing eye, with a desire to close it; in the evening the right eye affected in the same way. Spasmodic twitching at outer angle of left eye.

EARS: Throbbing in ears in evening; bright redness of whole right ear with a row of very sore pimples on the helix.

NOSE: Violent attacks of sneezing; epistaxis; nose bleeds whenever blown or touched; nasal discharge green; bloody, then watery; thin and yellowish.

FACE: Very painful red suppurating pimples appear on the face; pain in them as if pierced with a needle. Sore pustules all over face, burning

---

1. From the handwritten manuscript of Dr. Grimmer, exact date unknown. The majority of this work is taken from Clarke: DICTIONARY OF PRACTICAL MATERIA MEDICA. - Editor.

stinging; face red and hot during headache; complexion sallow. Fiery red patches about an inch long over left eye. Patches of small vesicles on mucous membrane of lower lip; vesicles containing a colorless limpid fluid. Corners of mouth cracked and very sore.

THROAT: Many symptoms of the throat are brought out by this medicine. Uvula greatly enlarged, back part of pharynx covered with a thick yellow mucous very tough and hard to remove (like KALI-BI.). Destructive ulceration of uvula, soft palate and tonsils with thich yellow secretion in the ulcers. Left tonsil swollen; pain and difficulty in swallowing; throat sore on right side. Tickling in the throat inducing continual swallowing. Dryness, throbbing, stinging soreness; swallowing painful; throat worse in evening, better eating and drinking cold water. After eating lobster, taste of iodide of potash. Post-pharyngeal catarrh with tough leathery streak of yellow mucous down back of throat.

STOMACH: Qualmishness, Nausea: with headache; during breakfast, with faintness at 11 a.m. and on rising; after retiring with dizziness, and pain in the liver. Sick feeling at stomach for two days; felt as if vomiting would relieve.

ABDOMEN: Stitches in region of the liver, Colic: gripping; from umbilicus downward; as if diarrhea would set in.

STOOL AND ANUS: Stool pasty, brownish-yellow, fetid with particles of undigested food, preceeded by colic; involuntary, slight, when urinating; small, hard, afterward pappy; hard stool with blood. Diarrhea worse drinking beer; with headache on the right side. Burning tenesmus and pain in the anus after stool. VIOLENT PAIN IN HEAD WHEN STRAINING AT STOOL.

URINARY ORGANS: Painful urination; when urinating loss of power over sphincter ani. Horribly offensive smell of urine after it stands for a short time.

MALE SEXUAL ORGANS: In the male, sexual desire and power diminished, emission too soon, thrill deficient; or there may be an increased desire with weakness. Emissions twice the same night; four nights in succession. Itching of glans penis. Severe pain in right testicle. Testicles tumified and very tender to touch; drawing pains along spermatic cords, worse left side.

FEMALE SEXUAL ORGANS: In the female, menses two weeks too soon, bearing-down pains with cross temper and weeping mood; face very red.

RESPIRATORY ORGANS: Hoarseness on rising, with sore throat. Habitual bronchial expectoration freer, but a little blood appeared in the mucous. Frequent desire to take a deep breath when lying down, worse lying on left side, better lying on back.

CHEST: Severe pain behind lower right portion of sternum; sharp pains through upper part of chest; burning pain in left side of chest near sternum, which feels as if drawn towards back. Dull pain in left pectoral and axilla regions.

NECK AND BACK: Stiffness of the neck and shoulders. Drawing through side of head down neck to clavicle, first right side, next day left side. Pain worse on beginning to move. Pains under either scapula. Rheumatic drawing across shoulders up to head, worse moving. Constant pain in left shoulder as if bruised with soreness extending down left arm, at times so severe as to disable the arm.

EXTREMITIES: Shooting pains in the fingers. Muscles of left arm and shoulder flabby and soft, with no power in the arm. Severe lancinating pains in left biceps with paralytic weakness. Palms of hands sweat continually with itching. Weakness of lower limbs; tired weak sensation. Drawing, strained feeling of muscles of inside the thigh; legs from knees down feel heavy as if loaded. Peculiar hot tingling in the legs. Dull, boring pain in left great toe joint, almost unbearable, must move foot to relieve it, for three evenings worse from 8 to 9. Burning and intense itching of all the toes the whole day. Profuse foot sweat; cold sweat of feet.

SLEEP: Sleepiness with headache and nausea. Dreams, lascivious, amorous of having unsuccessful intercourse with men; vivid dreams of what had occupied his mind during the day; annoying dreams of being in foreign countries, of being chased by mad bulls or of being lost in the mountains. Nightmare from lying on the back; very stupid on awakening.

FEVER: Sensitive to cold; high fever with chilliness on moving, great weakness, sore throat, violent headache and backache. Fever with nausea after eating, better out of doors, easy perspiration.

GENERALS: In general this cold weak patient is < from motion and exertion, physical or mental; < from 3 to 4 a.m. < in a warm room. He is better in the open air and from eating, especially the headache. Though this patient's symptoms are all < from exertion, yet he is restless and must move about.

CHARACTERISTICS AND DIFFERENTIATIONS OF THE KALI SALTS[1]

Potash is widely distributed and is formed in the feldspar and silicates and chlorides of the earth' s crust. By the process of oxidation and hydration it becomes one of the most important ingredients of the soil for the sustenance and growth of plant life. When soils become deficient in potash, plant life languishes and becomes infected with destructive fungi which end its existence. This is especially true in the growth and production of corn. And from observations made, it has been found that the sap channels of the stalk were clogged with iron deposits as a result of a lack of potash. When these potash exhausted soils were supplied with potassium sulphate in sufficient quantities healthy corn would grow, flourish and mature free of fungi and disease.

But potash is equally essential to animal life and when it is deficient either from lack of supply or from faulty potassium metabolism the animal weakens and takes on many forms of disease which end in death. Even as the corn stalk sap channels becomes clogged and useless to distribute the life giving juices to the plant organism, so does the lymphatic system of the animal be come impaired and blocked leaving the tissues wasting and non-resisitant to infective organisms, because the nourishing lymph is checked in its journey of repair if the normal potassium content is not present.

Clarke says that the potassium salts have more specific relation to the solid tissues than the fluids of the body; to the blood corpuscles rather than to the blood plasma. The fibrous tissues such as the ligaments and joints of the back and the ligaments of the uterus are all particularly affected. He also cites KALI-C. and CAUST. as the two preparations that are most typical and profound in action and expression symptomatically of the potash group.

The potassium patient is anemic and weak, always tired and lacking stamina. His muscles are weak and easily strained. Potassium is found more abundantly in the red blood cells than in the blood plasma and its presence is essential to the hemoglobin balance in the red corpuscles; if the potassium is deficient there, hemoglobin breaks down and its iron content is released and oxidized and deposited in lymph channels and glands with impairment of function in these tissues. Without potassium the heartbeat would fail, small amounts stimulate, but large

---

1. From the handwritten manuscript of Dr. Grimmer, exact date unknown. The majority of this paper is taken from Clarke: DICTIONARY OF PRACTICAL MATERIA MEDICA. - Editor.

amounts weaken and inhibit. Potassium and the other alkaline minerals act in the maintenance of the alkali-acid balance of the organism. Also potassium is essential in the mechanism controlling the blood pressure and, still more important, it is one of the essential factors in the oxidation, that basic function of life where the interchange of gases take place in the body organism to produce and use all the multitudinous energies needed in the physiologic activities of repair and growth.

Such is a brief sketch of the physiologic chemistry of potassium and important and useful as this knowledge is, it is inadequate[1] to obtain truly curative results against the ravages of disease. Only the homeopathic concept of life, of sickness, and the needed remedial agents are sufficient to meet the needs of each individual case with its individual remedy properly attuned to harmonize disturbed life forces and restore weakened tissues. And potassium, when properly prepared and intelligently applied and directed under unfailing law, is frought with almost infinite possibilies of cure far behond the visability of the chemical plane. Volumes would be required to impart the full provings of the potassium remedies and for that reason we will attempt only to give some of the important highlights of the homeopathic symptomatology of the potassium salts.

KALI ACETICUM

This well known diurectic and cathartic has cured diabetes, dropsy, hemorrhoids and alkaline urine. In material doses this remedy has been palliative in cases of ascites and hydrothorax. Clarke says it is quite possible that this action may be specific (i.e. homeopathic). The few provings made with this remedy show that most of the symptoms produced involved the abdomen, and the urinary tract: Griping; diarrhea; bleeding hemorrhoids; increased flow of urine which is watery and alkaline. Weakness; trembling; profuse perspiration especially about the head. (CALC.).

Symptoms generally worse in the morning but headache came at 4 p.m. (LYC.). The urine is very much increased in amount and watery with increase of solids and urea and strongly alkaline.

---

1. This article was originally written at a time when the physiological chemistry of potassium was hardly known. The inaccuracy of this knowledge in no way affects the (homeopathic) administration of the Kalis on the basis of symptoms. - Editor

KALI ARSENICOSUM

Fowler's Solution has been curative in Bright's disease, cancer, deafness, diarrhea, dropsy, eczema, epithelioma, exophthalmos, eye affections, herpes zoster, jealousy, measels, melancholy, milliary rash, neuralgia, neurasthenia, psoriasis, skin affections, neuralgia of the tongue, varicose veins, ulcers.

MENTALS: The mental symptoms are: Scolding, morose, retired, quarrelsome and discontented, jealous, indifferent to everything; scarely answered questions addressed to her, or replied to them in a peevish tone. Eyes had a fixed look, face appeared frightened and anxious; worse every third day. Great nervousness.

HEAD feels larger. Headache in left parietal bone as if it were sore and pressed upon by a hand; behaves like a crazy person. Crusta lactea.

EYES: have a startled look, protruding, brilliant with pale face and sunken cheeks. Eyes red. Heat and itchiness of the lids followed by swelling and tenderness. Conjunctivitis. Eyes sensitive to light; dark discoloration around the orbit; protrusion of eyeballs. Whites of eyes look thick and yellow, jaundice. The blue iris becomes more grey. Conjunctiva glassy with dyspnea; eye balls fixed. Right eye weaker, watery as after weeping.

FACE: Nodular eruption on face; boils; face pale, complexion muddy looks older. Furfuraceous eruption on beard.

MOUTH: Gums swoolen and tender. Tongue clear, red like raw beef. Neuralgia of the tonge. Tongue swollen, felt too large in the mouth. Burning and numbness of tongue.

THROAT: Sensation in throat and larynx as if forced asunder. Throat dry and sore or constricted with copious flow of saliva.

STOMACH: Appetite lost, with intense thirst. Constant pain in stomach with nausea after food; frequent vomiting of ingesta. For several hours repeated every five or ten minutes sensation as of a ball rising from pit of stomach to larynx threatening suffocation, relieved by loud belching. Sinking at epigastrium with faintness.

RECTUM: Violent diarrhea; stools white, watery, frothy. Sensation as of a red hot iron in anus.

FEMALE GENITALIA: Cauliflower excrecence of os uteri with flying pains; pressure below os pubis and stinking discharge; menses absent; milk entirely arrested.

KALI ARSENICOSUM ...

LARYNX: Sore gastric cough; and frequent raking of throat and fauces of a muco-purulent secretion mixed with specks of blood. Complete aphonia following skin affection.

HEART: Pulse weak and contracted, pulse small scarcely perceptible, rapid.

BACK: Much tenderness and pain down spine.

EXTREMITIES: Palms and soles spreckled with corns. Aching pain in right shoulder and elbow followed by herpetic eruption. Knees bent up so he could not move his feet. Varicose veins of legs. Crampy feeling of lower extremities with partial loss of motion and sensation, livid in places tending to slough.

GENERALITIES: So weak she cannot sit up in bed. A loud or sudden noise, or unexpected motion causes her whole body to tremble. Emaciation; tremor; faintness; phagadenic ulcers deep base with turned up edges. Rheumatic, gouty or syphilitic pains; gouty nodosities.

SKIN: Dry wilted skin; emaciated to a skeleton. Erysipelas invading whole face ending in desquamation. Acne: appearance of the early stages of variola. Severe attacks of shingles, covering entire body except scalp. Shingles on r. side of chest. Intolerable itching; stinging and burning of skin at night especially on undressing. Many chronic forms of skin troubles including epithelioma and psoriasis have followed the prolonged use of this drug in allopahtic hands.

SOME PECULIAR SYMPTOMS: Head feels larger; protrusion of eyeballs as in exopthalmus; burning numbness of tongue, tongue feels too large. Sensation of a ball rising from pit of stomach to larynx causing suffocation; feels as if a red hot iron were in the anus. Periodicity as marked as in ARS. Symptoms < every other day, mental symptoms < every third day. Symptoms, especially those of the skin, herpes worse on the right side. KALI-I. is said to be antidotal. This remedy has cured a case of ascites and extensive edema in a child whose whoe body resembled a great toad as a result of a severe case of diffuse nephritis. The urine in the test tube was almost solid.

KALI BICHROMICUM

This remedy is said to be especially suitable to fair haired fat people, especially fat children, the general weakness of the other Kali salts is marked. Shifting, wandering pains or pains in small spots are a feature. "Alternating complaints" is peculiar, such as rheumatic conditions alter-

KALI BICHROMICUM ...

nating with intestinal troubles. Though a cold patient lacking vital heat many complaints come on in hot weather, many seemingly contradictory symptoms. Open air > symptoms generally, especially vertigo. Eruptions < warm weather; gastric symptoms and chilliness < in open air. Uncovering <, wrapping up >. Warmth > the cough; undressing < cough. Many symptoms < by eating; touch < most symptoms but pressure > except pressure on sciatic nerve which <; moving the affected part > the pain, most symptoms < at rest and > by motion. Stooping and sitting <.

The discharges of this salt are very characteristic, tough and stringy or viscid, thick and jelly-like. Many complaints of syphilitic origin have been cured.

Eyelids burning red and swollen. Large acute granulations. Large polypus springing from conjunctiva; rheumatic sclero iritis with excessive pain and photophobia. Syphilitic iritis and its sequelae. Ulcers and pustules of cornea with no photophobia and no redness. Ulcers everywhere, eye, stomach or limbs tend to perforate rather than spread laterally; punched out ulcers. Thickening and induration of the coats of the eyes after inflammations and too drastic local treatment especially after abuse of the silver preparation such as silver nitrate and argyrol.

The whole respiratory tract is the seat of much trouble when this remedy is needed, and the characteristic stringy viscid difficult discharges are guiding; expectoration of tough mucus or fibrous elastic plugs (in croup, membranous or croupous bronchitis); violent rattling cough with gagging and vomiting.

Wandering rheumatic pains but there is a left sided sciatic pain better by motion.

KALI BROMATUM

Most of our knowledge of this drug comes from the drastic doses of the allopaths for epilepsy, although there have been some incomplete provings.

This remedy disturbs the mental and emotional spheres more profoundly than the other Kali salts. In the stage of excitement there is fearful deleriums with delusions and hallucinations, frightful imaginings at night in pregnant women and in children night terrors. Fear of being alone, of being poisoned, or that he is pursued. Delerium tremens, with flushed face and red eyes. Purperal mania with congestion

KALI BROMATUM ...

of blood vessels of the brain. These are followed by profound depression with fits of uncontrolable weeping and profound melancholic delusions. Nervous anxiety, religious delusions. Later still comes marked impairment of memory even absolutely destroyed. Inability to express himself, writing almost unintelligable.

The sexual and emotional sphere of both sexes are greatly disturbed and many symptoms come on, or are aggravated by coition. Sensual lascivious fancies; satyriasis and nymphomania ending in impotence and wasting of the sexual organs.

This might be a valuable remedy for youth troubled with erections and sexual excitement.

In old school hands this drug has been much abused in the treatment of epilepsy for large material doses were given over long periods.

Clarke states that the only cases of epilepsy that might be homeopathically cured are those associated with sexual abuses and excesses. Epileptic convulsions at the new moon is a strong indication.

Asthma of a marked and persistant nature follow the prolonged use of this drug hence it will cure this stubborn condition in suitable cases.

KALI CARBONICUM

It is the central and typical homeopathic preparation of the Kali group and a complete study of its symptomatology will aid in a knowledge of the other Kalis.

This patient is cold anemic and of weakened muscular and fibrous development.

MIND: Exertion of mind and body is difficult and aggravates most of the symptoms, the asthma, the pains in back and limbs, the heart weakness etc. The pains are sharp and shifting. Mentally the patient is excitable, fearful and anxious especially about his health. Great depression of mind with much weeping. Often the patient breaks into tears and weeps while relating her symptoms to the physician. This is like PULS., and there often is a complementary relation between these remedies. Changeable moods at one time mild, at another time full of passion and rage. Easily startled and alarmed; sensitive to touch, especially the soles of the feet. The memory is weak or lost and there is a tendency to misapply words or syllables.

HEAD: Many symptoms relating to the head, confusion and vertigo; sudden attacks of unconsciousness. Violent headaches worse stopping

KALI CARBONICUM ...

and moving. Congestive (semilateral headaches with vomiting), aggravated by the slightest motion. Many of the head complaints as well as nausea come from riding in a carriage or cars. There is a strong tendency to catch cold in the head especially on being exposed to a draft after overheating.

EYE: Many inflammatory and other eye symptoms belong to this remedy, but a peculiar one is the swelling of the upper lids. Extreme photophobia.

EARS: Pains, swelling and discharge of yellow pus from the ears; ulcer in ears; excoriation and suppuration behind the ears. There may be either an unusual acuteness of hearing or a dullness of hearing with singing, buzzing and cracking in ears.

NOSE: Nose swollen red with burning heat or red and covered with pimples. Fluent coryza with excessive sneezing. Epistaxis in a.m. While washing the face (AM-C., PHOS.). Many symptoms of chronic catarrh with offensive nasal discharges.

FACE: Haggard exausted appearance of the face with sunken eyes surrounded by a livid circle.

TEETH: The teeth are much affected and sensitive to touch and pains are excited by eating or drinking with hot or cold things; teeth pain with soreness of the bones of the face. Offensive smell from teeth.

THROAT: Sore lancinating splinter-like pains with deglutition because of inertia of muscles of the gullet. The food decends very slowly in the esophagus and small particles of food easily get into the wind pipe. Copious amounts of mucus in the throat, difficult to hawk up or swallow with a sensation of a lump of mucus in throat.

STOMACH: There is much digestive trouble; frequent risings. Bad taste; disgust for brown bread with great desire for sugar or acids. Milk and warm food are unsuitable. Sensation of a lump in stomach. Nausea and faintness. Nausea so intense as to cause unconsciousness. Nausea of pregnancy. Vomiting of food and acid with great prostration. Nocturnal vomiting of food. Often shock or a start from sudden noise will be referred directly to the epigastrium.

ABDOMEN: Much flatulence and sensitiveness to whole abdomen. Pain in liver region as if it were wrenched. Inertia and coldness in abdomen. Incarceration of flatulence.

RECTUM: There are many sufferings relating to the anus. Constipation with constricition of intestines with difficult evacuation of large

Kali carbonicum ...

hard faeces. Obstruction from inactivity of bowels, lacks peristaltic action. Hemorrhoids with protrusion during stool followed by blood and white mucus. Hemorrhoids dating from birth of child. Hemorrhoidal pimples in rectum, painful bleeing with shooting pains. Sensation of a red hot poker being thrust up rectum temporarily relieved by sitting in cold water. Excoriation and pustulous eruptions in anus.

URINARY ORGANS: Frequent urination day and night; urine scanty, burning or slowly discharging urine. Discharge of prostatic fluid after urination. Incissive pains in bladder.

GENITALIA: The male sexual organs are affected, the glans penis has much tension and pulling. Itching and pain as from a bruise in scrotum. Hot swelling of testes and spermatic cord. Excessive increase of desire for intercourse, later an absense of desire with impotence. After coition and pollutions weakness of body, but especially of the eyes.

In the woman there is repugnance to coition. During coition pinching and pain as of excoriation in the vagina. Constant sensation of bearing down. (SEP.) Burning pain and shooting in vulva. Erosion, itching and gnawing genital parts. Difficult first menses. Catamenia premature or too weak. Suppression of menses with anasarca and ascites. Hemorrhages of pregnant women with clotted blood. Gastric disturbance during menses, morning headache. Leucorrhea sometimes with violent pains up the loins and pains like those of labor extending from back to uterus. Yellow leucorrhea with itching and burning in vulva. Uterine cancer with pain around loins extending down right thigh to knee. The breasts are often painful, swollen or hard before and during the menses, sometimes with a flow of milk. Protracted hemorrhages after labor, hemorrhoids, peritonitis. Chills after delivery, puerperal fever with intense thirst.

RESPIRATORY ORGANS: This is a great lung remedy. Hoarseness; aphonia with violent sneezing; sensation as of a plug in larynx. Cough dry and often painful 2 to 4 a.m. Difficult respiration on walking or exertion. Spasmodic asthma in early morning better sitting up in bed and bending forward. Oppression of chest as from hydrothorax. Sensation in chest as if heart was compressed. Suppuration of lung after pneumonia, Tuberculosis: one of our best remedies; Hahnemann said of it that many of the tubercular could not get well without this deep acting antipsotic remedy.

KALI CARBONICUM ...

HEART: The heart is much disturbed, palpitation with anguish with intermittent heart beats. Palpitation when hungry. Burning crampy and sticking pains in region of heart. Sensation as if heart was hanging by tightly drawn bands, aggravted on deep inspiration and cough, not affected by motion of body. On lying on right side heart feels attached to and suspended from left ribs. Feels pulse over whole body to tips of toes. This is one of our best remedies in many forms of heart disease.

BACK AND LIMBS: In the back and limbs there are many sufferings and pains of a sharp drawing, tearing nature, sometimes relieved by heat applied. But pains that wander and shift from joint to joint are characteristic of this and most of the other Kali salts.

But the deep general symptoms and states are the guide for selection. The weak, anemic, cold, extremely sensitive patient whose resistance is feeble with more or less bad inheritance.

KALI CHLORICUM

The chlorate is not to be confused with the chloride, although Hering amalgamated the symptoms of both salts, but there are some distinct shades of difference.

MIND: Liveliness followed by ill humor. Ill-humored anxious tension in precordial region relieved by nose bleed. Sudden loss of consciousness after a glass of wine.

HEAD: Much vertigo especially after violent motion. Congestion of the brain with one half of head, face and nose feeling paralysed. Crusta lactea of children.

EYES: Many eye conditions, conjunctivitis, keratitis.

FACE: Swollen face in a.m. Pale bluish livid suffering expression. Drawing pains in face, cheeks and gums.

MOUTH: Teeth aching as in the other Kalis. Tongue coated white with ulcers on mouth, cheeks, gums. Stomatitis ulcerative and follicular.

THROAT: Submaxillary glands swollen, throat painful, red and edematous. Violent cough as from sulphur fumes.

STOMACH: Much stomachache and intestinal disturbance, flatulence and pain and colic.

RECTUM: External piles with constipation, congestions and obstruction to portal system and liver. Painful diarrhea and dysentsry with blood and slime. Green stools or light colored stools.

KALI CHLORICUM ...

URINARY ORGANS: Nephritis with frequent urging, scanty black albuminous and casts.

GENITALIA: Violent frequent erections with itching scrotum. Frequent emissions with lascivious dreams.

RESPIRATORY ORGANS: Respiratory organs much irritated; hoarsness and cough.

HEART: Precordial anxiety with palpitation as in KALI-C. Much disturbance of pulse rate with the characteristic weakness of KALI-C.

SKIN: Cynosis of lips and extremities

The pains of the back, limbs and generalities are similar to KALI-C.

KALI CHLOROSUM

Has been curative in aphonia, asthma, coryza and diptheria. The poisonous effects produce watery eyes, pale puffy face, constriciton of throat and chest.

KALI CITRICUM

Has been useful in Bright's disease. Material doses, given to a patient suffering from suppressed kidney action after influenza produced, three days later, the following symptoms: kidneys acted freely; tympanites; contant flow of mucus from anus; awful gastric and abdominal pains; flatus constant in great amounts. Intestines and stomach felt skinned inside.

KALI CYANATUM[1]

Has produced symptoms of apoplexy, asthma, cancer espcially of the tongue, Cheyne-stokes breathing. Ciliary neuralgia, epilepsy, headache, rheumatism, speech lost. Much of our knowledge of this remedy comes from cases of poisoning. The irritability and weakness of potassium present combined with the profound and rapid action of the cyanogen element.

Loss of consciousness and obscuration of vision with marked convulsive symptoms; later staggering, uncertain gait and agonizing attacks of ciliary and maxillary neuralgia.

Face pale or of livid and bloated, marked cyanosis.

Copious vomiting followed by a return of consciousness.

---

1. This remedy is dealt with in more detail on p. 62. See also the footnote there. - Editor.

Kali cyanatum ...

Voice hoarse after attack. Loud mucus rattlling. Slow and difficult respiration. Anxious feeling in chest stitches in heart and lungs; palpitation. Limbs rigid and convulsed, fingers stretched out and spasmodically contracted, marked weakness of lumbar region. Surface of body moist and cold.[1]

Kali ferro-cyanatum

Has been useful in chlorosis, debility, dysmenorrhea, dyspesia, fatty degneration of heart, leucorrhea, menorrhagia, rheumatism.

Sad tearful anticipates death yet irritable, easily vexed.

Vertigo, coldness, numbness, sensation of gastric sinking sometimes with universal tremor.

In the male too easy emissions and little pleasure. Nocturnal emissions with indistinct amourous dreams.

Menses too frequent and profuse or late. Metrorrhagia. Passive, painless flow causing much debility. Leucorrhoea like pus, yellow creamy, copious with pain in small of back.

Fatty heart, weak irregular pulse. Hypertrophy, dilation.

Debility; pale lips, gums and skin; cold hands and feet, frequent profuse watery urine sometimes with traces of clotted blood. Wandering neuralgic pains.

Kali iodatum

One of the great antisyphilitics as well as antipsoric, it has been useful in actinomycosis, aneurism, anhidrosis, Bright's disease, bubo, bunion, cancer, caries, condylomata, consumption, cough, croup, debility, dropsy, ear conditions, emaciation, erythema nodosum, eye affections, fibroma, glandular swellings, gonorrhea, gout, gumma, hemorrhages, hay fever, house maid's knee, influenza, joint affections, laryngitis, liver diseases, locomotor ataxy, lumbago, hepatisiation of lungs, oedema of lungs, menstrual disorders, neuralgia, nodes, ear noises, nystagmus, odor of body abnormal, edema glottidis, pancreatitis, paralysis, pleurisy, prostate affections, rheumatisim, rickets, rupia, sciatica, scrofula, small pox, spinal curvature, spleen, syphilis, tic douloureux, neuralgia of tongue, tumors, ulcers, wens. All of these conditions of disease and many more will yield to the power of this remarkable remedy when strictly indicated by the characteristic symptoms of the drug.

---

1. This is an important remedy in bone metastasis of prostate cancer. - Editor.

KALI IODATUM ...

It has all the irritability and weakness of the other Kalis but there are some very distinguishing features peculiar to this remedy alone. It is sensitive to both extremes of temperature and one marked feature is the extreme restlessness and relief by continued motion of most of the symptoms except those of the heart: endocarditis; rheumatic or syphilitic with oppression, faintness and exaustion; tumultuous, violent intermittant and irregular action of heart and pulse.

This patient while chilly craves the open air, and the head and nasal symptoms are relieved therein, and though weak emaciated and exausted he is so restless he cannot remain in bed. Nightly aggravations are characteristic. Loquacity is as strong as in LACH. Chronic lung conditions dating from an imperfectly cured pneumonia will often clear up under this remedy and it has cured cases of tuberculosis.

KALI MURIATICUM

One of Schüssler's tissue remedies and claimed by him to be related chemically to fibrin. Disturbances of its molecular action cause fibrinous exudations. This salt is found in the blood corpuscles, muscles, nerve and brain cells as well as in the intercellular fluids.

KALI-M. corresponds to the second stage of inflamation of serous membranes when the exudation is of a plastic character, and may be useful in croupous or diptheritic exudations. Discharges of a thick white fibrinous slime or phlegm from any mucus membrane or flour like scaling of the skin.

Patient imagines he must starve.

Sick headache with white coated tongue, vomiting of white phlegm arising from sluggish liver. Crusta lactea, dandruff, copious white scales.

Many eye symptoms but blisters on the cornea. Parenchymatous keratitis and cataract.

Chronic catarahal inflamation of the ears with impaired hearing. Closed Eustachian tube.

White ulcers in mouth. Aphthae thrush in the mouths of little children. Tonsils excessively swoolen with stringy tough *white* mucous in throat. (KALI-BI. tough *yellow* mucous).

Many skin symptoms, acne, erythsma, eczema, and vesicular eruptions containing thick white contents. Schüssler's specific or chief rem-

KALI MURIATICUM ...

edy in epilepsy, especially if occuring with or after suppression of eczema.

It has the weakness and disturbed cardiac states, palpitation, weakness etc. of the other Kali salts.

KALI NITRICUM

Asthma, chest pains, colic, diabetes insipidus, dysentary, dysmenorrhea, enuresis, gastritis, headache, heart affections, herpes preputialis, Meniere's disease, pleurisy, pneumonia, polypus, rheumatism, vertigo.

Excitement after a glass of wine, anxiety and agitation, discouragement and fear of death.

Confusion and vertigo, fainting fits with vertigo in the morning on standing, relieved sitting down.

The pains everywhere are sharp and stabbing.

The male experiences increased erections with increased desire and pleasure. After unsatisfied desire violent drawing tension and pressure in both testicles extending along cords into abdomen lasting some hours; testicles very painful.

Menses too early and profuse, of blood black as ink. Menses retarded or suppressed, violent pains in abdomen and sacrum before menses. White serous leucorrhea which stiffens the linen and is discharged during sacral pains.

Heart and pulse disturbed and violently palpitating which awakens him from sleep. The weakness of potassium is present but with the sharp pains there is a numbness in the affected part, feet as if made of wood.

KALI OXALICUM

Only cases of poisoning have been observed producing violent irritation, convulsions, violent continued vomiting, cramps severe pain in back coldness and collapse. One patient became insane. Throbbing in head with great thirst; nails and fingers blue as in cholera; great weakness of lower limbs with cramps; great muscular weakness; falls and utters loud cries; coldness followed by burning heat; marked tendency to faint. We need a proving of this remedy.

KALI PERMANGANICUM

Has been used in cough, diptheria, gastritis, ozaena, sore throat, swollen uvula, warts.

KALI PERMANGANICUM ...

An aqueous solution 2 grains to the pint of water antidoted a case of opium poisoning promptly and efficiently.

Mouth and throat are the most prominent tissues affected by this salt; swollen painful throat with ulcerated spots with profuse flow of saliva. Hawked up mucus streaked with blood, obstinate constipation. Legs so weak he could scarcely stand.

KALI PHOSPHORICUM

"KALI-P. is a constituent of all animal fluids and tissues notably of the brain, nerves, muscles and blood cells. All tissue forming substances retain it with the greatest obstincy, all nutritious fluids contain it, hence we may conclude that it is indispensible to the formation of tissues. We know also that the oxidation processes, the exchange of gases in the respiration and other chemical transformations in the blood, as well as the saponifying of the fat and its further oxidation are brought about by the presence of alkalis and chiefly by the presence of KALI-P. This alkaline reaction is essential to a large number of vital processes taking place in the interior, and is present without exception in all animal fluids which are actually contained in the circulation system, or in the closed cavities of the body. (Dalton)"

It is found that the nerves retain their vital properties for a long time and very completely in a solution of this salt. By the diminution of the excretion of Kali phos in the urine conditions are produced within the organism which may present many sided resistance to the typhus decomposing element, as well as to the extension of the typhus process. (Grauvogl).

KALI-P. is an antiseptic and hinders the decay of tissues. Adynamia and decay are the characteristic states of KALI-P. (from Dewey' s Twelve Tissue Remedies.)

This is a valuable remedy in the weak irritable sensitive depressed individuals of tubercular constitutions. Extreme lassitude and depression. Physical and mental effort exaust.

The headaches are many and severe and often occur in over worked students or exhausted business men especially those who suffer from the evil effects of sexual excesses.

In the male passion at first increased, priapism in the morning; later sexual instinct depressed and impotency. Utter prostration and weak

KALI PHOSPHORICUM ...

vision after coition. Emissions without erections, express the sexual weakness that may come on.

In the female, the menses are early, scanty with dragging pain in lower jaw; or they may be irregular, scanty almost black and thick the first day. During menses sharp bearing down pains, sensation of being bloated to bursting. Chronic abscess discharging periodically through vagina and rectum, copious orange colored fluid. Vomiting of blood with palpitation, palpitation from the slightest motion. Pains and stiffness through back and all the limbs.

The particular symptoms are too many to relate in a paper of this nature.

KALI PICRICUM

Weakness, jaundice, diarrhea, pain in pit of stomach, violent eructations, colic, urine brownish red not from bile but from large amounts of urate of ammonia. This salt acts powerfully on the liver.

KALI SULPHURATUM

Violently effects the gastro-intestinal tract with redness of the face. Vomiting at first ineffective later convulsive. Great chilliness at first followed tardily by fever and sweat with burning skin and very strong rapid pulse.

KALI SULPHURICUM[1]

Another Schüssler salt which is the function remedy of the epidermis and of the epithelium. A deficiency of this cell salt causes a yellow slimy deposit on the tongue. Slimy, thin or decidedly yellow or greenish discharge and secretion of watery matter from any of the mucous membranes.

KALI-S. plays an important role in oxygen carrying function in the blood. The oxygen taken up by the iron contained in the blood corpuscles is carried to every cell in the organism by the reciprocal action of KALI-S. and iron. Every cell requires, for its growth and development, the vitalizing influence of oxygen.

This salt belongs to the hot group of patients who crave the fresh open air and whose complaints are relieved by the cool air and aggra-

---

1. This remedy is dealt with in detail in the article "Kali sulphuricum" p. 66. Editor.

Kali sulphuricum ...

vated in a hot closed room like Puls.; in fact this is the chronic of Puls. and often compliments it in chronic cases. The yellow discharges are characteristic and the shifing wandering pains also.

Kali tartaricum

Brown dry tongue, vomiting of blackish green fluid, feces like coffee grounds and pain in umbilical region with great thirst, pulse feeble, thighs and legs paralysed. Emaciation and extreme weakness, can scarcely walk.

Kali telluricum

Breath offensive, salivation and swelling of tongue, garlic like odor from mouth, oppression in cardiac region.

Kali carbonicum[1]

This element is essential to all plant life and is hardly less important to the welfare and existence of animals including humans, since so much of nutrition comes from the plant world. As a food, it is indispensible; as a medicine equally so.

It is a remedy of wide range of action useful both in acute and chronic manifestations of disease. It contains the vibratory rates corresponding to all the chronic miasms; but is most often useful in the cure of respiratory and tubercular diseases. One of its early effects is its action on the blood,producing anemias and dropsical conditions.

MIND: Its action on the mental and nervous sphere is striking; producing nervous fears and numerous worries, apprehensions, anxiety and unquitetude, irresolution and timidity as well as irritability and impatience. Changeable humor, at one time mild and tranquil, at another time passion and rage prevail; again extreme sensitiveness to noise, touch, etc. Sadness, gloom and tears with fear of disease, undefined harm. The KALI-C. patient weeps when relating her symptoms, and the rational mind may be impaired causing shrieking from imaginary appearances. Easily startled; starts when touched; especially the feet are extremely sensitive and ticklish. Loss of memory, misapplying words and syllables. Confusion of the head; sudden attacks of unconsciousness. Confused stupid feeling, or a sense of dullness in the head.

VERTIGO: Vertigo as if the ears were stopped up, with darkness before the eyes. Vertigo in the morning or evening, or after a meal as well as on turning the head or body quickly. Vertigo with tottering, vertigo preceeding from the stomach.

HEAD: Many severe headaches of various descriptions and types may be cured by this remedy. Headache caused from the motion of a carriage or from sneezing or coughing. Morning headaches; semi-lateral headache with nausea and vomiting, dreadfully aggravated by the slightest motion. (Migraine type). Violent headache across the eye; pressive headache in the occiput (eye strain); headache with photophobia. Lancinating pains in the head especially around the temples and forehead, worse from stooping or moving head, eyes and lower jaw; relieved when raising head and from applied heat. Congestion of the head with throbbing and buzzing. Trembling in the head and sensation as if it contained something movable. Constant sensation of something

---

1.   From the handwritten manuscript of Dr. Grimmer, exact date unknown. The majority of this paper is taken from Clarke: DICTIONARY OF PRACTICAL MATERIA MEDICA. - Editor.

loose in the head, turning and twisting toward the forehead. The headaches are relieved by pressing the forehead. Vertigo with the headache is common. Strong tendency to take cold in the head, especially if exposed to a draught after being heated. Painful and purulent tumors on the scalp beginning like blood boils. Falling off and dryness of the hair more around the temples. Wens and scabby eruptions of the scalp; even the eyebrows and beard become dry and fall away. Violent burning, itching eruptions in the morning and evening which ooze serum if scratched.

EYES: The eyes of the KALI-C. patient present many symptoms and sufferings; pressive and tearing pains, shooting, biting, smarting and burning with lachrymation. Redness and inflammation of the eyes, with pain on reading by candle or artificial light. Swelling of eyes and lids, with difficulty of opening them. Swelling like a bag of water between the upper eyelids and eyebrows. Capillaries injected; agglutination of eyelids in the morning; eyes red and painfully inflammed. Spots: green and dazzling in the field of vision; photophobia; vivid painful brightness before the eyes.

EARS: Inflammation and shooting pains in the ears, with yellow pus or liquid cerumen discharge. Redness, heat and violent itching of the external ear. Excoriation and suppuration behind the ears. Inflammation and swelling of parotids. Excessive acuteness of hearing or dullness of hearing or weak confused hearing; tingling, buzzing, singing, cracking sounds in the ear.

NOSE: Swelling and redness of the nose covered with pimples; ulceration of internal membranes of nose. Epistaxis in the morning, when washing the face (AM-C.). Dull smell. Coryza and stoppage of nose sometime with secretion of yellow green mucous and constant want of air. Fluent coryza; sneezing; extreme dryness of nasal passages with blood-streaked mucous. Sore scurfy nostrils.

FACE: Exhausted haggard look to the face, with a yellow or sickly aspect; lifeless expression. Great redness of face alternating with palor. Flushes of the face; bloated appearance; tearing pains in bones of face. Warts on face (CAUST.). Lips thick and ulcerated, cracked and exfoliating; cramp-like sensation of the lips. Cramps in the jaws; swelling of lower jaws and submaxillary glands; cracking of jaw joints.

TEETH: The teeth are sensitive and painful, excited by cold things in the mouth; drawing, tearing; lancinating pains in the teeth and bones of the face; especially in the evening in bed. Looseness of teeth with bad odor; inflammatory swelling and ulceration of the gums.

MOUTH: Bitter taste and fetid exhalation from mouth. Swelling of tongue with small painful vesicles; painful pimple on tip of tongue. Bitter acid taste or putrid sweetish taste or of blood in the mouth as if it came from the stomach derangement.

THROAT: Sore throat with cutting, sticking pain on swallowing. Deglutition impeded by inertia of muscles of the gullet. The food descends very slowly in the esophagus, and small particles of food easily get into the wind pipe. Copious accumulation of mucous on palate and in throat; difficult to hawk up or swallow with sensation as if a lump of mucous were in the throat. Hawking up mucous; dryness of posterior part of throat.

STOMACH: Strong desire for sugar or acids. Disgust for brown bread, which lies heavily on stomach. Milk and warm food are unsuitable; sleepiness during a meal: After a meal; drowsiness; paleness of face; shivering; headache and ill humor; nausea; sour risings and pyrosis; colic inflammation; inflammation of abdomen and flatulency worse after hot food. Frequent sour risings and regurgitation. Burning acidity, acidity rising from stomach with spasmodic constriction. Feeling in stomach as if cut to pieces. Constant feeling as if stomach were full of water, wobbling on motion. Lump sensation in stomach. Pryosis and nausea from emotional disturbances. Nausea as if he would faint with anxiety. Nausea during pregnancy. Nausea with loss of consciousness; sometimes during a meal, or after mental and emotional upsets. Retching in the evening with vomiting of food and acid water with prostration.

ABDOMEN: Pressure at epigastrium with extreme sensitiveness there. Pain in the liver region as if it were wrenched. Burning, aching and shooting pains in the liver; spasmodic contractive abdomenal pain with severe colic, worse after eating. Great flatulence. Sensation of cold fluid passing through intestine. Colic, like labor pain, sometimes extending to loins. Dropsical swelling of abdomen.

STOOL AND ANUS: Constipation worse at the menstrual period. Difficult retarded large stools, with inactivity of rectum. Intestinal inertia. Obstruction from paralytic weakness of the bowels. Lack of peristaltic action of bowels. Hemorrhoids painful, large, worse after labor. Discharge of mucous or blood during evacuation; stools may be like sheep's dung. Discharge of teniae and lumbrici. Anxiety before stool with burning pain after. Protrusion and distention of hemorrhoids during stool or during micturition. Sensation as of a red hot poker being thrust up rectum, temporarily relieved by sitting in cold water.

URINARAY ORGANS: Frequent scanty emission of fiery urine, slow urination; after urination, discharge of prostatic fluid; urine pale greenish, turbid. Burning in urethra during and after voiding urine.

MALE SEXUAL ORGANS: Tension, tearing and pulling in glans and penis. Hot swelling of testes and spermatic cord. Excessive increase or absence of sexual desire. Repugnance to coition. Lack of erections, or erections too frequent and painful. Absence of or immoderate pollutions; pollutions with voluptuous dreams. After coition and pollutions, weakness of the body but especially the eyes.

FEMALE SEXUAL ORGANS: Repugnance to coition in women; during coition pinching and pain as of excoriation in vagina. Constant sensation of bearing down. Erosion, itching and gnawing in genital parts. Difficult first menstruation; catamenia premature or too weak; suppression of flow with anasarca and ascites. Hemorrhages in pregnant women with clots of coagulated blood. Corrosive menstrual flux, acrid flow excoriating the inner thighs. During menses: agitated and anxious sleep; gastric symptoms and morning headache; cutting pains in back and loins; severe abdominal cramping. Leucorrhea at times with violent pains in loins like the pains of labor extending from back to uterus; yellow, itching, burning leucorrhea. Uterine cancer, with pain I around the loins extending down right thigh to knee. Tearing stitches in breasts on flow of the milk. During pregnancy, sickness only during a walk, without vomiting but with a feeling as if she could lie down and die; pulsations of arteries even down to tips of toes; hollow feeling in the whole body. Only with the greatest effort can any exertion be made. Back aches so badly while walking she could lie down in the street; pressing forcing pains in small of back as if heavy weight came into pelvis low down; also stitching, pressing proctalgia. Impending abortion with pain from back into buttocks and thighs; discharge of clots second and third months. Weakness after abortion; labor pains insufficient, violent backache, wants back pressed which relieves. False pains, sharp cutting pains across loins or passing off down buttocks hindering labor; pulse weak; pains stitching or shooting. Chills after delivery, puerperal fever, intense thirst. After confinement hemorrhage, hemorrhoids, peritonitis.

RESPIRATORY ORGANS: In the respiratory organs, chest and heart there is much suffering and numerous symptoms of a characteristic nature belonging to this remedy. Hoarseness and roughness in throat with violent sneezing. Aphonia with violent sneezing. Easy choking; sensation of a plug in larynx.

COUGH: from motion of arms and from any exertion; excited by a tickling in throat. Dry cough especially at night, in morning with expectoration. Cough worse from 3 to 4 a.m. Cough with inclination to gag and vomit. Expectoration difficult or small round lumps fly out without effort. Whooping cough or pneumonia with bag-like swelling between upper eyelids and eyebrows. Cough with sour tasting expectoration.

RESPIRATION: Difficult respiration on walking quickly. Stitches in sternum and sides of chest through to back on inspiration. Spasmodic asthma relieved by sitting up.[1]

CHEST: Oppression in chest as from hydrothorax. Pain in chest when speaking, sensation as if heart were compressed in the chest. Inflammation of lungs and liver with stitches in right chest. The breasts become swollen and sore and painful; nodules form in them before and during menses. Suppuration of lungs, abcessed lungs with weakness and faintness in chest from walking fast. Tuberculosis in all stages. This was Hahnemann's frequently used remedy in tubercular complaints, and he said such sufferers could hardly get well without this antipsoric. The tubercle bacilli became calcified and encysted under the action of this remedy.

Hard swelling of axillary glands. The lymphatic glands everywhere are affected by soreness, swelling and inflammation. Most of the pains are worse from exertion and coldness, relieved by rest and warmth. The special time of aggravation at 3 to 4 a.m. holds good here as with many other KALI-C. complaints, such as asthmatic attacks; the coughs and even the nervous states of fear and wakefulness come on or are worse at that time.

HEART: The heart is greatly disturbed under KALI-C. Palpatation with anguish especially in the morning on waking with ebullition of blood. Frequent violent palpitation with anxiety. Palpitation when he becomes hungry. Intermittent weak heart beats, burning and cramping pain in region of the heart. Pinching pain in or by heart; as if heart were hanging by tightly drawn bands; worse on deep inspiration or on coughing. On lying on right side, heart feels suspended to the left ribs. Feels pulse over whole body to tips of toes. Pulse slow, weak, intermittent.[2]

BACK: In the neck, back and limbs are found a multiplicity of symptoms and conditions. Stitching, tearing, shooting, burning, bruised,

---

1. Orthopnea of CHF, also PND. - Editor.
2. A great remedy in chronic congestive heart failure - when the symptoms agree - Editor.

sore and drawing pains with stiffness and tension of muscles and tendons.

EXTREMITIES: The right deltoid and shoulder is a frequent point of trouble; while in the lower limbs and back are the sites of great weakness and suffering. Acute rheumatic pains at night in joints, bones of hip, leg, feet and toes. Numbness; a great inclination of the whole right limb to fall asleep and tingle.

SLEEP: The sleep symptoms are often guiding and significant. Drowsiness and yawning; falls asleep while eating; half asleep at night. During sleep shuddering, tears, talking and starting in fright. Gnashing of teeth while asleep. Agitated sleep, with frequent anxious frightful dreams. Dreams of robbers, death, danger, serpents, sickness, devils, etc. Fits of anguish at night; gastric sufferings, pains in stomach and precordial region. Colic flatulency, diarrhea, frequent erections and pollutions, asthmatic sufferings; nightmare and cramps in calves of the legs. Wakens suffocating, wakens too early about 3 to 4 in the morning.

The blood corpuscles, the glandular system, the muscular and fibrous tissues and the bones are markedly affected. Extreme weakness, even to exhaustion; faintness and unconsciousness are often met with in the KALI-C. diseases. The ailments of the heart, lungs and sex organs are centers that frequently require this medicine.

Clarke says, "Among the grand characteristics of KALI-C. three stand out above the rest: stitching lancinating pains also called jerking pains < during rest, < lying on affected side; early morning aggravations, 2 to 4 a.m.; the occurrence of bag-like swellings over the eyes between upper eyelids and eye brows."

It is suited to persons of soft tissues with a tendency to be fat. Easy copious perspiration is found throughout the proving and occurring with most of the sufferings. Anemia and great debility; skin watery and white; muscles weakened especially the heart. Weak intermittent pulse. Shiverings immediately after the pains. Remaining in the open air greatly aggravates many of the symptoms. Nocturnal epileptic fits, tendency to suffer easy strain in the muscles of the loins.

KALI-C. may be summed up in a few general characteristics, that when found in any sickness will make the physician think of it strongly: great weakness, great coldness, great anxiety, great tendency to sweat, full of fear especially of being alone. Extremely sensitive to all impressions and uncontrollably tearful. Add the sharp sticking shifting pains, generally better by heat and worse from cold, aggravations of most complaints at menstrual period with the 2 to 4 a.m. aggravations, and you have a brief summary of this mighty implement of cure.

Kali cyanatum[1]

Much of our knowledge of this drug comes from its poisonous effects observed on those subjected to its influence either accidently or intentionally. There has been a fragmentary proving made by Lembke and others.

Suddenness, violence, and intensity of action constitute its pace. It smites with all the suddenness and certainty of the deadliest venom of the serpent; in fact so sudden at times as to preclude the possibility of pain paralyzing the cardiac and respiratory centers and bringing instant death. In this respect it is more like an electric bolt.

It produces apolectic and epileptic states, much like those of hydrocyanic acid. Loss of consciousness and vision occur and as vision returns with consciousness it is double. Strong tetanic convulsions fingers stretched out and spasmodically contracted. Sec. has stretching out of fingers with convulsions and might need to be compared.

Cyanosis is a pronounced feature. Such symptoms are among the more violent of the acute states observed. It has a chronic side very useful and instructive to the homeopath. There are severe pains in the head and gastric regions with great muscular weakness, in some cases going on to complete paralysis. Impairment of speech which is long lasting is a marked condition often found. Agonizing attacks of neuralgic pains in head and face with screaming and loss of sensibility.

Clinically it has proven curative in epithelioma of the tongue, apoplexy epileptic conditions, respiratory disorders, rheumatism of the joints and violent neuralgia. Daily attacks of neuralgia beginning at 4 a.m. (many Kalis have this time aggravation) gradual rise and decline of pain as in Stann. and Plat. Cedr. and Chinin-s. have a daily periodic pain beginning at the same hour, generally 9 to 10 a.m. It is related to and should be compared with Hydr-ac., Amyg., Camph. and Laur.

It may look like Op. in apoplexy but the eye symptoms alone will serve to differentiate. The closed eyes will reveal on opening the lids, instead of the pin point pupils of Op., widely distended pupils insensible to light and the eyeballs will be in interrupted by convulsive motion. The eyes may be fixed with dilated pupils in alternation with spasmodic shutting and closing of the eyelids; eyeballs staring in differ-

---

1. From the handwritten manuscript of Dr. Grimmer, exact date unknown. A large part of this article is taken from Clarke: Dictionary of Practical Materia Medica, Vol. II. pgs. 122 ff. - Editor.

ent directions every few seconds. The general symptoms of these two drugs in the convulsive and apoplectic states are very similar. OP. is worse by heat. A hot bath or immersion frequently kills the child whose symptoms call for OP.

A poison case of KALI-CY. reported by Clarke was restored to consciousness after all the other measures had failed by placing the patient in a hot sitz-bath and pouring ice water over the head and nape. Each time the cold water was poured over the patient it caused him to take a deep inspiration growing deeper with each application until normal respiration and consciousness was obtained. From this experience we might infer that cold applications ameliorates and heat aggravates KALI-CY. states

In my early practice I saw a sad illustration of the OP. aggravation from a hot immersion. A child about eight months of age while cutting its first teeth developed convulsions of a typical OP. nature; there was cyanosis, hot sweat and pin point pupils that were fixed and insensible to light together with an obstinate constipation, with stools of round black balls. This was such a classical picture of the drug that I warned the parents in the event of another convulsion not to immerse the child in hot water as it might prove fatal. Sure enough another convulsion did follow in less than twelve hours and the first thing the excited father did was to dash the babe, clothes and all into a dish pan of hot water with the result of almost instant death. The child grew deathly pale, gasped and died. This warning has been given by many of the old masters yet still many physicians and, I am sorry to say, many homeopathic doctors order such a proceeding not knowing the danger.

MENTAL: There has been some unusual mental states produced. Almost uncontrollable crossness on entering the room while cold open air produces good spirits. Disposition gentle especially in the cold open air. Inability to recollect certain words, aphasia for several days. Deep stupor and insensibility.

VERTIGO: Intense vertigo so that all objects seemed to be moving around him.

HEAD: Head drawn backwards. Unable to tolerate any covering on head because it caused the frightful headache for months after the attack. Gnawing pains across the temple. Sharp pains in the occiput. Soreness of scalp over parietal region.

EYES: We have mentioned the eye symptoms while comparing Opium.

EARS: Rushing sounds in the ears.

NOSE: Bleeding from nose; inside of nose feeling parched, hot and dry; blood drying in nose very quickly.

FACE: Pallor at first, later lined and bloated, turned blue in the face. Torturing neuralgic pains in orbital and supra maxillary regions, recurring darts at the same hour with much flushing of that side of face; twitching of muscles of face. Lips white almost immediately covered the nose.

There was noticed slight twitching of mouth when patient was spoken to in a loud tone as though a sense of hearing was awakened though stupor still continued. Some difficulty in using the lower jaw in act of speaking.

Patient lay in a frightful tetanic cramp, jaws so tightly closed that it was impossible to open them, eye drawn completely back into orbits, face distorted, nose pointed, mouth drawn outward, pulse imperceptible, and hands frequently attacked with muscular twitches.

MOUTH: No remedy presents a more terrifying aspect, a picture of sickness in its worst and most destroying form. A peculiar astringent taste as of alum or green vitrol; cancerous ulceration of right side of tongue, power of speech lost with intelligence preserved, long lasting impediment of speech.

THROAT: Astringent sensation in throat with nausea lasting until after midnight. Feeling of constriciton about the fauces with muscular tremors about throat, great stiffness of throat. Patient unable to swallow as soon as much fluid filled the pharynx; after every swallow, the whole body was seized with convulsive tremors and flushes of redness overspreading face; had no sensation of act of swallowing, (peculiar).[1]

STOMACH: Copious vomiting followed by return of consciousness. Sharp gastric pains; pain at epigastrium of a gripping intermittant character. Epigastrium prominent almost immediately; severe burning in stomach. Great sensitiveness of epigastric region. Involuntary stool; later obstinate constipation.

BLADDER: Bladder distended by a large amount of urine which had to be taken by a catheter. Involuntary urination.

PROSTATE:[2]

LARYNX AND TRACHEA: Voice hoarse after attack. Loud mucus rattle.

RESPIRATION: Repiration superficial. Slow difficult breathing; respiration very slow, seven per minute, expiratory act prolonged. Respira-

---

1. Gag reflex - Editor.

tion nearly suspended, but thorax convulsively raised at irregular intervals.

CHEST: Anxious feeling in chest, oppression. Stitches in heart and lungs. Jerking stitches in heart on respiration; palpitation of heart; pulse at times fifteen beats slower than usual - compare (DIG.).

BACK: Marked weakness in lumbar region, with dull pain in both iliac regions while walking.

EXTREMITIES: Limbs rigid and convulsed. Tetanic spasms of muscles of arms and legs. Limbs flaccid with occasional slight convulsions more like a shuddering. Fingers stretched out and spasmodically contracted. Gait unsteady.

GENERALITIES: General convulsions, sudden convulsive action of whole body about ten minutes after the heart ceased to beat.

Sphincters rigidly contracted. Took some weak milk punch and smoked in afternoon, after which all symptoms vanished and the effects of the medicine seemed to have been cut short by this slight irregularity.

SLEEP: Sleepiness by day, Restless dreamful sleeps all night. Could not lie on one side very long. Dreams lively or horrid and exciting with partial waking and turning from side to side, feeling of great fatigue during sleep.

CHILL, FEVER AND PERSPIRATION: Surface of whole body cold and moist. Shivering, coldness of extremities which were pendulous and without muscular power. Icy coldness of extremities almost immediately. On awaking from cat-naps has a chill which wakes him before he can get soundly asleep, followed by a slight sweat. Awoke about 6 a.m. with heat and disagreeable feverish perspiration over whole body, except legs below knees, with flushed face. Hands and face bathed in cold perspiration. The patient is icy cold yet heat aggravates many symptoms and states and cold douche restored consciousness and declining respiration.

---

2. Prostate: It has proved a wonderful palliative in metastasis of prostate to bone. This remedy started in 6x with increasing potencies completely relieved pain. Morphine was no longer needed and the patient died four months later. HOMEOPATHIC RECORDER Vol. LXXIII Nos. 10 - 12, Cookingham, Franklin. This article has been reproduced in the section on Cancer in this book. See also the remarks of the editor in regard to prostate cancer and bladder symptoms - Editor.

Kali sulphuricum [1]

Much of our knowledge of this remedy comes from Schüssler, it being one of his tissue remedies. There is no homeopathic proving, but Dr. John Clarke of London has gathered a number of observed symptoms of the drug's action, which with the indications given for its use by Schüssler, together with the clinical cures from its application to the sick all mark it as a medicine of deep action and splendid value.[2]

It is said that KALI-s., in reciprocal action with iron, effects the transfer of inhaled oxygen to all the cells and that it is contained in all the cells containing iron. Hence, it is highly important in oxidation processes. And oxidation, according to Crile of Cleveland[3], is the fundamental process in the modus operandi of life itself, because it is through oxidation that all electric energy in the body organism is manufactured and maintained to perform its intricate and multitudinous functions.

A deficiency of this substance in the body causes a sensation of heaviness and weariness, vertigo, chilliness, palpitation of the heart anxiety, sadness, toothache, headache, pain in the limbs. These symptoms are < in a warm room and on becoming warm and towards evening; > in open cool air.

Clinically this remedy has accomplished its most marked work in diseases of the skin and mucous membranes, disease of the antrum of Highmore and other sinus conditions of a chronic nature, asthma, cataract, catarrh, chorea, dandruff, dyspepsia, eczema, epithelioma, eustachian catarrh, gleet, gonorrhea, itch, diseased nails, nettle rash, ozena, polypus, psoriasis, rheumatism, rhus poisoning, vertigo and whooping cough. Now the afore-mentioned conditions of disease that respond to this medicine must occur in individuals of certain types and whose symptoms are modified by very definite circumstances and conditions.

The KALI-s. patient is typically warm blooded and suffers from a slight excess of heat; his complaints are definitely worse in a warm

---

1. THE HOMEOPATHIC RECORDER, Vol. LVII, No. 11, May, 1942, p. 536. A large part of it is from Clarke: Dictionary of Practical Materia Medica vol. II pg. 159 ff.
2. Kent in his LECTURES ON HOMEOPATHIC MATERIA MEDICA has painstakingly gathered symptoms from reported cures for many years. The reader is invited to carefully study Kent's lecture which brings out many points of the remedy. - Editor.
3. Crile, George W.: THE BIPOLAR THEORY OF LIVING PROCESSES. MacMillan Company New York 1926

room or place and better in the cool open air. This strong general modality by temperature is strongly like PULS. and strange that KALI-S. is one of the chemical ingredients of PULSATILLA. The time of aggravation of this remedy is in the evening - another similarity to PULS. Also the characteristic yellow or yellow-green discharges from mucous membranes and the shifting wandering rheumatic pains are common to both these remedies. Many cases only palliated by PULS. will be cured by KALI-S. KALI-S. is therefore said to be complimentary to PULS. and often follows it satisfactorily in chronic states to complete the cure.

W. A. Dewey says, of its general action, "This remedy is applicable to the third stage of inflammation or to its stage of retrogression, the sulphates being characteristic products of the oxidation of tissue and the potassium having its special sphere in the solids, and the resulting salt becomes a prominent constituent of their ashes, whence we can infer its homeopathicity to the same stage."

Ailments accompanied by profuse desquamation of epidermis. Yellow mucous discharges. Rise in temperature at night producing an evening aggravation. Another characteristic indication is amelioration in the cool open air.

Diseases caused by a retrocession of eruptions (suppressions).

MIND: Dewey mentions fear of falling as a mental state belonging to this remedy.

VERTIGO: There is marked vertigo < by rising from lying or standing or when looking up.

HEAD: Great pain on moving head from side to side or backwards; can move it forward without pain. Yellow dandruff moist sticky. Bald spot on left side of head; also falling of the beard after gonorrhea.

EYES: Purulent or yellow mucous in eye diseases, yellow crusts, yellow discharge. Opthalmia neonatorum, catarrh.

EARS: Catarrhal deafness; swollen eustachian tubes, discharge watery thin yellow sticky, brown, offensive with stinking polypus.

NOSE: Smell and taste lost, ozena. Nasal discharge yellow offensive, alternating with watery, < left side, thick dark brown semi-fluid, fetid, from antrum of Highmore. Yellow viscous old catarrh.

FACE: Faceache, < warm room and at evening, > cool or open air. Epithelioma right cheek, right side of nose has been cured. Lips blistered and swollen.

TEETH: Toothache worse in warm room, better in open air.

MOUTH: Taste insipid, pappy or lost. Tongue coated with yellow mucous, yellow slimy, sometimes with whitish edge.

STOMACH: Faint sensation at stomach and befogged feeling in head; fears to loose her reason, pressure as of a load, fullness with yellow mucous coat on tongue. Gastro duodenal catarrh, jaundice.

ABDOMEN: Hard tympanitic abdomen in whooping cough.

RECTUM: Diarrhea, stools yellow slimy, watery, watery thin, offensive; constipation, hemorrhoids with yellow tongue.

MALE GENITALIA: Gonorrhea of yellow or greenish discharge; orchitis from suppressed discharge, gleet.

FEMALE GENITALIA: Menses too late and scanty, with weight and fullness in abdomen, or menses every three weeks with ozena and headache. Menorrhagia; leucorrhea yellowish or watery, matter.

RESPIRATORY ORGANS: Hoarseness from cold; bronchitis; asthma; whooping cough; pneumonia with yellow slimy skin or watery mattery and profuse expectoration easily expelled.

NECK AND BACK: Stiff neck, head inclined to left, shoulder raised; periodical pains in back, nape or limbs worse in warm room, better in cool air. Acute wandering rheumatism of joints from chill when overheated.

SKIN: Eruption on left axilla, on neck, and on back of hands (Rhus poisoning). Scaly eruption most on arms, better from hot water. Jaundice. Suppressed rash of measles etc. Abundant scaling of epidermis; burning, itching, papular eruption exuding pus-like moisture. Fine pimples, running together. Scurfs, scaling, chapping; sores with yellow sticky secretions. Epithelial cancer; eczema; itch; intertrigo; nails diseased.

SLEEP: Sleep with very vivid dreams.

FEVER: intermittent with characteristic yellow coated tongue.

CONCLUSION

This union of SULPH., the great antipsoric, and Potassium, the essential ingredient of all plant and animal life, is truly one of our fundamental constitutional remedies capable of over- coming inherited diseased soil conditions and establishing normal healthy states of mind and body. Electro-magnetically, it belongs to the *neutral group* of remedies and corresponds to the tubercular and sycotic miasma; hence it is curative in very grave conditions.

An epitome of characteristics of this medicine will aid the prescriber in remembering its place and use in our homeopathic armementarium. Fundamentally a hot-blooded patient, sensitive to heat and whose complaints are worse in the day, heat and better in the cool open air. Most complaints are worse in the evening. Yellow color to the mucous discharge, yellow coating on the tongue and even the oozing eruptions ooze yellow serum,and yellow scales are formed and thrown off the eruptions on the skin. The skin has a yellow color in chronic cases. The rheumatic pains are sharp and wandering like KALI-BI. and KALI-C. and the other Kali preparations.

This wonderful remedy needs a complete homeopathic proving to bring it to its true place in the realm of healing.

Lycopodium[1]

The club moss from which this amazing remedial agent comes was one of the first plants emerging from the sea to appear on the earth's cooling crust. Coming down from that early time when the world was young and its foundations were becoming stabilized, this medicine presents a strange correspondence for its use to the needs of early human life. It is also one of our fundamental constitutional remedies occupying a sphere of action both broad and deep in the human economy.

Clarke in his DICTIONARY OF PRACTICAL MATERIA MEDICA calls it one of the "pivotal remedies of the materia medica" and further adds that "an intimate acquaintance with its properties and relations is essential to a proper understanding of the materia medica as a whole, because it ranks with SULPH. and CALC. in the central trio around which all the rest of the materia medica can be grouped."

Often in chronic and obstinate cases of disease, resulting from the mixed miasms many of the old masters gave in sequential order SULPH., CALC. and LYC. to effect and complete cures which had proved resistant to the single remedy even in a series of potencies.

APPETITE: Among the marked and important spheres of LYC. is its action on the nutritive system; hence its vast influence in growth and development. Loss of appetite with clammy or bitter taste especially in the morning with nausea. Nausea referred to the pharynx and stomach; nausea in the morning and when riding in a carriage (in modern times the automobile has proven to be equally unpleasant); and this might be a good remedy even for the sickness of airplane if the totality of symptoms are present. There is much sourness of the mouth and stomach, or sour taste of the food. Often a loss of appetite with the first mouthful; sudden satiety or immoderate hunger; bulimy; aversion to cooked or warm food, rye bread, meat, coffee, tobacco smoke. Craves sweet things; inability to digest heavy food; it ferments and quickly bloats and distresses the patient.

After a meal hepatic pains, oppression and fullness in chest and abdomen with nausea, heat in head, redness of face, pulsation and trembling over the whole body, hands hot, palpation of heart, colic, etc; sourness and diarrhea after taking milk; and because of this fact it

---

1. The major part of this article is taken from Clarke: DICTIONARY OF PRACTICAL MATERIA MEDICA, Vol II, p. 329 - 348.

frequently is a good remedy for the marasmas of infants. Cabbage, onions and other green vegetables frequently aggravate the LYC. digestive tract and great flatulence and acute distress follow their intake.

STOMACH: The thirst of LYC. varies with time, circumstance and condition. Thirstless in chronic states often with a dry mouth; there may be nocturnal thirst, absence of thirst or burning thirst.

Burning sour or greasy bitter risings are common features, sour regurgitations of food especially milk. Nausea in a warm room going away in the open air; heartburn; cancer of the stomach; vomiting of food and bile especially at night; vomiting after a meal or at night; vomiting at the menstrual period; or between the heat and chill in intermittant fever. Vomiting of blood. Gnawing griping pains in region of stomach, slow digestion; pains in stomach after drinking wine; pains relieved by heat of bed, applied heat and hot drinks sometimes relieve; most of the other Lycopodium complaints and pains are < by heat.

ABDOMEN: There is much pain and distress in liver region, pain when walking in upper part of right hypchondrium as if the superior ligament of the liver would tear. Violent gall-stone colic, sharp in dorsal hepatic region and in right shoulder and arm; inflamation and induration of the liver, dropsical swelling of abdomen, incarcerated flatus with great distension and pain with imperfect expulsion of gas. Rumbling and noisy flatulence through whole abdomen with so much impaired function of the gastro-intestinal tract and the liver. Right sided hernia in infants has been cured with LYC.

RECTUM: We need not be surprised to find long-standing constipation, hard stool with ineffectual urging to evacuate; desire for stool followed by painful constriction of anus; hemorrhage from rectum even after a soft stool. Grey light colored stools. The pains and distress often end in syncope; constipation or diarrhea of pregnant women. Feces pale and of a putrid odor; thin brown or pale green mixed with hard lumps, thin yellow or reddish yellow fluid, shaggy reddish mucous, dysentary or green stringy odorless mucous, lumbrici, hemorrhoidal excresences in rectum with prolapsus. Itching eruption in anus.

MIND: The LYC. patient is a sensitive irritable, high strung individual often melancholic and deeply despondent. Sensitive to noise, light, jar and vibrations and impressions. Inability to concentrate; confusion and unable to perform even simple mental labor, without confusion and exhaustion. Many fears and dreads; fears darkness; fears solitude, yet dreads men and desires to be alone; bad effects from anger or excitement, tearful yet sympathy <; wants to cry and laugh at the same time.

Memory weak and extreme fatigue from mental labor; unable to express himself correctly; misplaces words and syllables, confused speech. Confusion about everyday things but rational talking on abstract subjects. Inability to remember what is read, stupefaction and dullness. A peculiar state of this remedy is the dread of appearing in public for fear of failure, but on getting started he goes along to success. Silica has much the same condition but the latter belongs to the decidedly cold group of remedies while Lyc. is sensitive to heat in all of its general states.

Lycopodium in some disease conditions presents a lack of vital heat but at the same time is sensitive to any excess of warmth. It especially craves the cool open air like Puls. and Arg-n. The Lyc. patient is restless and hurried and impatient, again as in Arg-n.; these remedies run parallel in their symptomatology a long way and in only some of their particular symptoms do they differ; one is the Arg-n. patient craves cold things in the stomach which relieve and the Lyc. patient is better by warm or hot drinks.

Many symptoms and disturbances referred to the head, eyes, ears, nose and throat are caused and cured by this medicine.

HEAD: Dizziness as if intoxicated, on seeing objects whirl about she feels as if her body were turning about. Whirling vertigo, especially when stooping or in a warm room, with inclination to vomit.

Headaches from vexation. Headache with disposition to faint. Fainting is a strong tendency in this remedy from pains anywhere in a warm room, while at stool, at the menstrual period. Semilateral headaches are a marked feature, generally right-sided or traveling from right to left. Headaches < by jar, noise, anger, excitement and mental exertion, throbbing with every paroxysm of cough; aching as if the brain were swashing to and fro, could not work or scarcely step without vertigo. Headaches < lying down and at night in bed, > walking slowly in open air; > from cold and uncovering the head; pressive headaches as if a nail were driven into the head. Headaches < in afternoon and evening, especially coming on from 4 to 8 p.m. Marked tendency to take cold in head especially after becoming overheated. Eruption on scalp and behind and around their ears and fetid suppuration sometimes with obstruction of glands of neck. Premature graying of the hair is a noted symptom also found under Ph-ac. Gray hair after abdominal disease or after parturition with violent burning and itching of scalp, < becoming warm. Scurf over whole scalp, the child scratches it raw at night until it bleeds. Hair falls from the scalp but increases on other parts of the body.

EYES: Many LYC. symptoms are found in the eyes, inflamatory conditions, styes, etc. Double vision or half vision, intense photophobia and night blindness.

EARS: In the ears there is impaired hearing following inflamatory and catarrhal states. Noise and buzzing and roaring in ears. Blocked eustachian tubes. Eruptions with yellow crusts around and behind the ears, sticky eruptions, like those of GRAPH.

NOSE: Many severe nasal symptoms and sufferings are inflicted on the LYC. patient. The snuffles of infants may often be cured by this remedy, blocked nasal passages from adenoids, swollen turbinates and polypoid growths. Chronic catarrhal and sinus infections even blocked sinus often following local nasal packs of argerol and other powerful antiseptics. The discharges are yellow, grayish, green and often blood streaked, catarrhal ulcers with tendency to bleed after the removal of crusts from the nasal cavities. Fanlike motion of the nostrils in pneumonia is a strong indication for LYC. (compare ANT-T.). Coryza with acrid discharge excoriating the upper lip. All kinds of coryza; dry coryza with obstruction of the nose. Dryness of posterior nares with obstruction of nostrils at night when mouth is open (LACH., OP., AM-C.).

MOUTH: The mouth and throat have numerous symptoms but the great dryness throughout is a cardinal feature; often dry mouth without thirst is a peculiar characteristic. Tongue foul and coated, at times studded with small pin point ulcers. Scalded feeling in tongue. In typhoid states the tongue is heavy and parched with a heavy brown coating with indistinct speech; stiffness of tongue, convulsions of the tongue; tongue black and cracked; tongue distended, giving patient silly expression in angina or diptheria.

THROAT: In the throat constriction with difficult deglutition; burning pains in throat, sensation in throat as if a ball were ascending from pit of stomach. Inflammation of throat and palate; swelling and suppuration of the tonsils commonly beginning on right side and going to the left. Pains in throat, better swallowing warm or hot drinks, < swallowing cold.

URINARY ORGANS: Many symptoms and distresses associated with the urinary tract come under LYC. but the more characteristic symptoms are greasy pellicle on the urine, red sand in the urine, clear urine depositing a heavy red crystalized sediment in the vessel. A very severe pain in the back every time before urination is felt causing patient to cry out; retention; must wait for urine to start; the pain in the back ceases when the urine flows. Children often cry out with pain before urinating. Turbid milky urine with an offensive purulent sediment, dull pressure in region of bladder and abdomen, disposition to form calculi; cystitis; haematuria from gravel or chronic catarrh; renal calculi and gravel; emission of blood instead of urine, sometimes with paralysis of the legs and constipation. Incontinence of urine with burning, smarting and itching in the urethra; urine burning hot like molten lead.

MALE SEXUAL ORGANS: LYC. affects the sexual system in both sexes profoundly. In the male, there is shooting drawing incisive pain in the glans, bastard gonorrhea with a deep red and smarting pustule behind the glans; excoriation between the scrotum and the inner thigh, dropsical swelling of the genitals; immoderate excitement or absence of sexual desire. Repugnance to coition or disposed to be too easily excited to it; impotence of long standing; weakness or total absence of erections; penis small, cold, relaxed; excessive pollutions, emission too speedy or too tardy during coition; falling asleep during coition; lassitude after coition or pollutions; flow of prostatic fluid without an erection. Nash recommends LYC. as the remedy par excellance for old men who marry young women and find themselves inadequate to perform their family duty.

FEMALE SEXUAL ORGANS: In the female there is nymphomania with terrible teasing desire in external organs; itching, burning and gnawing in vulva; expulsion of wind from vagina; chronic dryness of vagina; excoriation between the thighs; burning pain in vagina during and after coition. Catamenia too early, too profuse and too long lasting; catamenia easily suppressed by fright and other emotions. Before menses: shivering, sadness and melancholy; bloated abdomen. During menses delirium with tears, headache, sourness of mouth, pain in loins and swelling of the feet, fainting, vomiting of sour material, cutting colic and back pains; flow partly black, clotted, partly bright red or partly serum. May find females at the change of life with one side of the body greatly hypertrophied; metrorrhagia, at the menopause, dark blood with large clots pours from her. Foetus appears to be turning somersaults. Leucorrhea, milky yellowish, reddish, corrosive. Varices of the genitals. Disposition to miscarriages (SEP.); swelling of the breasts with nodosities; excoriation and moist scabs of the nipples.

RESPIRATORY ORGANS: In the chest, respiratory organs and heart many symptoms are manifested; many nondescript coughs, obstinate dry cough in the morning or nocturnal cough < before sunrise, which effects the head, diaphragm and stomach; cough as if produced by the vapor of sulphur; or from deep inspiration; generally with a yellowish gray salty expectoration. Cough with expectoration during the day or without expectoration at night with expectoration of fetid pus streaked with blood; cough < 4 to 6 p.m. or on alternate days; < exertion. Continued oppression of chest with shortness of breath. Hepatisation of lungs, paralysis of lungs; Hydrothorax. In delayed or slow resolution of pneumonias (SULPH.).

HEART: Much heart disturbance associated with digestive troubles. Palpitation and trembling with anxiety, accelerated pulse with cold feet and hands. Palpitation of the heart with flapping of alae-nasi; enlargement of the heart, cramp, constriction and dyspnoea; sharp pains shooting into the heart with fright and cold sweat, pulse quick and unsteady, (angina pectoris). Dyspnoea, cyanosis, hasty eating and drinking in heart disease. Beating of temporal arteries and carotids, heart sounds heard loudly at night when lying in bed, keeping patient awake. Hypertrophy; aneurism; hydropericardium.

Many sufferings of a rheumatic nature; neuritis and arthritis of back, neck and limbs; paralysis and numbness of the limbs, but these symptoms are best met by prescribing for the patient on his general and characteristic indications.

Clarke gives a great array of clinical conditions and diseases cured by this remedy; but these are of little value as an aid in the selection of this remedy. So definite and characteristic is the symptomology of this remedy for its use in sickness that whenever met with regardless of diagnosis or pathology, it can be given with certainty of curative results.

A comparatively brief summary of characteristic symptoms or key notes will enable the prescriber to use this broad, deep remedy with certainty and satisfaction, regardless of diagnostic and pathologic conditions found. A restless, sensitive, timid individual, sensitive to both extremes of temperature but much more sensitive to extreme heat. The direction of symptoms going from right to left or markedly right-sided complaints, predominating or upper right and lower left. Extreme dryness of mucous membranes, general aggravation of complaints from 4 to 8 p.m. Red sand in urine, severe back pain > by urination. One foot cold the other hot; emaciation of neck, arms and upper parts of body. Easy satiety, a few mouthfuls fill up, even when extremely hungry. Thirstless more often than great thirst and then a preference to warm drinks. Inability to assimilate milk. Easy fainting from pain, fright and fatigue. Flapping of the wings of the nose in respiratory affections. Child sleeps with eyes half open. Inordinate craving for sweets.

MEDORRHINUM[1]

Because of the wide-spread infection of the sycotic disease together with the suppressive measures employed in its treatment, this nosode is a remedy of great importance.

Many cases of obscure and chronic sickness need this medicine to effect a cure, and no doubt we all fail to make cures because of neglect or lack of sufficient knowledge of this subtle and far-reaching poison.

Failure to elicit a history of infection in the individual or his family should not prevent the study and use of this remedy in any case of obscure or difficult disease if the symptoms of this remedy are presented.

A study of this nosode and its clinical application and related cures by many practitioners described by Dr. John Clarke of London in his wonderful DICTIONARY OF PRACTICAL HOMEOPATHIC MATERIA MEDICA will reward one immensely for the time spent and enhance his knowledge of the possibility of cure residing in this universal solvent, for I doubt if any have escaped some taint of this everspreading insidious disease, made more subtle and illusive by measures of suppression employed in the treatment of its victims i.e., directing treatment of a local nature to the stopping of the discharge with substances consisting of injections of powerful astringent metals, silver and zinc salts called antiseptics which deprive the local cells and tissues of their natural germicidal resistance and at the same time drive the infection to deeper and more vital parts of the economy. At present massive injections of penicillin are used to suppress local symptoms viz, the discharge, which they do for a time but with the sequence of much more serious symptoms to follow later, involving deeper structures, even the brain and nervous system being involved.

Clarke states that this nosode has cured asthma, chronic spasms, corns, diabetes, dysmenorrhea, epilepsy, eye inflammations, favus, gleet, suppressed gonorrhea, gonorrheal rheumatism, headache, neuralgia, polyp, priapism, psoriasis, ptosis, renal colic, rheumatism, sciatica, shoulder pains, stricture, urticaria and warts.

This imposing array of clinical cures does not embrace all the possibilities of this remedy, for it has cured many neurotic and even serious

---

1. From the handwritten manuscript of Dr. Grimmer, exact date unknown. The major part of this article is taken from: Hering, Constantine: THE GUIDING SYMPTOMS OF OUR MATERIA MEDICA, Vol. VII, pgs. 292 ff., American Homeopathic Publishing Company, Philadelphia, 1881. Most of it is also reproduced in Clarke: Dictionary vol. II, pgs. 409 ff. - Editor.

mental afflictions. In fact, the mental states furnish us with some of our best indications for the application of the remedy.

MIND: Forgetfulness of names, of words and initial letter; time moves too slowly; dazed feeling; a far-off sensation, as though things done today occurred a week ago. Constantly loses the thread of her talks; seem to herself to make wrong statements because she does not know what to say next, begins all right but does not know how to finish; weight on vertex which seems to affect the mind. Difficulty in concentrating his thoughts on abstract subjects. Could not read or use mind at all from pain in head. Thinks someone is behind her, hears whispering; sees faces that peer at her from behind bed and furniture. Saw large people in the room; large rats running; felt a delicate hand smoothing her head from front to back. Is sure she is going to die. Sensation as if all life is unreal, like a dream. Cannot speak without crying; suicidal. Is in a great hurry; when doing anything is in such a hurry that she gets fatigued; spirits are in the depths, weighted down with heavy solid gloom relieved by torrents of tears. Is always anticipating; feels most matters sensitively before they occur and generally correctly (clairvoyance). Dread of saying the wrong thing when she has a headache. Apprehensive, fear of the dark. Feeling as if she had committed the unpardonable sin and was going to hell. Irritated at little things, very impatient; great selfishness.

VERTIGO: Vertigo when stooping, slightly relieved lying, aggravated on movement. Sensation of tightness in head causing intensive vertigo.

HEAD: Frontal headache: with nausea; feeling of a tight band across the forehead, < leaning head forward; as if skin were drawn tightly; with fluent coryza, with pressure back of the eyes as if they would be forced out: extending over brain to neck. Brain seems weary; slightest sound annoys and fatigues her. Wakes with headache over eyes and temples, < from sunlight. Pain in center of brain; in evening sharp pain through temples; pains commence and cease suddenly (NIT-AC.). Brain exceedingly tender, and all mental work is irksome. Pain in left parietal bone when wind blows on it. Pain circling through head and around crown. Terrible pains all through head in every direction, with continuous and violent vomiting, followed by aching in sacrum and down back of legs to feet. Intense headache for three days with inflammation of eye. Intense cerebral suffering, causing continual rubbing of head in pillow, with rolling from side to side (HELL.). Tensive pains in head as if she would go crazy; could not read or use her mind. Aching pain at base of brain, with swelling of cords of neck. Head heavy and drawn backwards; Pain in back of head and right eye.

Hair lusterless, dry and crispy, electrical; intense itching of scalp; quantities of dandruff.

EYES: When eyes were shut, felt as if pulling out of head to one side or other; when open all things seemed to flicker; blurring visions, black or brown spots dance over page when reading; sees objects double; things appear very small; sees imaginary objects. Neuralgic pains in eye balls when pressing lids together. Feeling of pain and irritation, and sensation of sticks in eyes, sensation of a cold wind blowing in eyes. Ptosis of outer rim of both upper lids, difficult to open them. Hardness of upper lid as if it had a cartilage in it.

EAR: Nearly total deafness of both ears, with every little noise; had to use a trumpet. Partial or transient deafness; pulsation in ears. Singular sensation of deafness from one ear to the other, as if a tube went through head while yet there was an overacuteness of hearing. When whistling, the sound in ears is double, with peculiar vibrations as when two persons whistle thirds. Quick darting pains in right ear from without inward; pains follow each other in quick succession.

NOSE: Intense itching of nose. Coldness of end of nose. Entire loss of smell for several days. Epistaxis. Nose swollen and inflamed. Obstruction in posterior nares > hawking of thick greyish mucous, followed by bloody mucous.

FACE: Greenish shining appearance. Blotches on skin. Flushes of heat in face and neck. Fever blisters around mouth, very sore. Neuralgia of right upper and lower jaws extending to temple. Face covered with acne, dry herpes, freckles. Tendency to stiffness of jaws and tongue.

TEETH: Teeth have serrated edges or are chalky and decay. Feel sore and soft; yellowness of teeth.

MOUTH: Taste is coppery, disagreeable and bad on arising in the morning. Tongue heavily coated brown, thick, white at base, the rest is red. Tongue blistered. Small sores, pustules, canker sores very painful. Mouth feels dry and burnt.

THROAT: Throat sore with much mucous dropping from posterior nares.

STOMACH: Appetite ravenous immediately after eating, thirst enormous for liquor. Craves salt, sweets, hard green fruits, ice, sour things, oranges and ale.

Many stomach and intestinal symptoms are noted under this remedy. Nausea: with frontal headache, after drinking water; after dinner.

Violent retching and vomiting for forty-eight hours; first glairy mucous, then frothy and watery and later like coffee-ground substance; accompanied by intense headache with great despondency and sensation of impending death; during paroxysm was continually praying (STRAM.). Vomiting thick mucous and bile, black bile without nausea, tasting bitter and sour with considerable mucous.

Sensation of a pin in pit of stomach forcing through the flesh. Sick gnawing not relieved by eating. Trembling, burning in stomach. Feeling of lump after eating. Cramps and clawing, worse drawing up knees. Intense pain in stomach and upper abdomen with a sensation of tightness. Sensation of sinking and agonizing sickness at stomach with a desire to tear something away.

This is a wonderful remedy for marasmic babies when other well-indicated remedies fail or relieve but a short while, with or without a sycotic history in the parents.

ABDOMEN: Terrible pains in liver, thought she would die they were so acute. Grasping pain in liver and spleen.

Intense agonizing pain in the solar plexus, surface cold; eructations tasting of sulphurated hydrogen and, after eating, vomiting of ingesta. Applied right hand to pit of stomach and left hand over lumbar region. Tensive pain in right side of abdomen, as of a hard, biconvex, body; with heat and gnawing aching pain, continued a short while. Cutting in right lower abdomen running into right spermatic cord; right testicles very tender. Testicles enormously swollen, hot and extremely painful, has been rapidly cured with the recurrance of the suppressed gonorrheal flow after a single dose of this nosode.

ANUS AND STOOL: The stools are often a bilious diarrhea, verging on dysentary, with mucous stools. Pains of the most intense kind (threatening cramps) in the upper abdomen (darting and tearing) pains coming on at stool; stool diarrheic, thin and hot but not copious; after stool profound weakness (ARS., LYC., CON.) and cramp in left leg. Profuse bloody discharges from rectum sometimes in large clotted masses, followed by shivering. Black stool or white diarrheic stools; tenacious, clay-like, sluggish, cannot be forced because of sensation of prolapsus of rectum. Can only pass stool by leaning far back; very painful, as if there was a lump on posterior surface of sphincter; so painful as to cause tears. Constriction and inertia of bowels with ball-like stools. Child of fifteen months brought on a pillow to clinic, apparently dead; eyes glassy, set; pulse could not be found but felt heart beat; running from anus a greenish yellow, thin, horrible offensive stool. Oozing of moisture from anus, fetid like fish brine (cured by MED.).

URINARY ORGANS: In the urinary organs there is much suffering. Intense renal colic; severe pains in ureters, with sensation as of passage of calculus; during kidney attack great craving for ice. Dull pinching pain in region of supra renal capsules at 11 a.m.; fingers cold at the same time; great pressure in bladder, greater than the amount of urine warrants; urine scanty and high colored; strong smelling, covered with thick greasy pellicle, intensely yellow, slow flow cutting across root of penis transversely just as last drops are voided, intermittant flow; syncope after urination.

Many cases of diabetes have been cured with this remedy. In those cases of enlarged, inflamed prostates of men with a history of suppressed gonorrhea ("a gonorrhea that has been cured!") by the application of injections will often find this remedy re-establishes the gonorrheal discharge with complete relief and eventual cure of all their troubles.

MALE GENITALIA: In the male there are emissions during sleep, watery and causing no stiffness of linen; transparent, consistence of gum arabic mucilage, too thick to pour and voided with difficulty; thick, with threads of white, opaque substance. Impotence, or intense and frequent erections day and night. Drawing, burning pains along urethra while urinating in suppressed gonorrhea.

FEMALE GENITALIA: Many symptoms and sufferings are found in the female; great sexual desires after menses in a single woman. A great deal of pain in left ovary, with a sensation as if a sac was distended and if pressed would burst; sensation as if something was pulling it down, causing it to be sore; pain when walking passed to left groin, as if leg pushed something, with great amount of heat. Intense excruiating neuralgic pains in whole pelvic region extending downwards through ovarian region to uterus; cutting like knives forcing tears and groans. Profuse menstrual flow; dark and clotted, stains difficult to wash out, also bright blood with faintness and pain. Intense menstrual colic, causing drawing up of knees with terrible bearing down labor-like pains, with pressing of feet against support, as in labor. A burning pain in lower part of back and hips during menses. After very profuse menses neuralgia in paroxysms in head, with twitching and drawing in of limbs and cords of neck, which were like wires; pain in lower abdomen with profuse, yellowish leucorrhea. Itching of labia and vagina, thinking of it makes it worse. Small chancres on edge of right labia (had no sexual intercourse for three years and never had venereal disease). Short, shooting pains, passing outwards, chiefly in breasts. Breasts as cold as ice especially the nipples (during menses), rest of body warm. Coldness of single parts, tip of nose, nipples and fingers is a peculiar feature of this remedy. Large but not painful swelling of left breast. Breasts and nipples very tender to touch and inflamed. Soreness of nipples with a gummy secretion drying on orifice; when picked off nipples bleed freely.

RESPIRATORY ORGANS: The respiratory organs are powerfully affected under this remedy. Hoarseness while reading aloud with loss of voice at times. Choking caused by weakness or spasm of the epiglottis, could not tell which. Larynx stopped so that air could not enter, only better by lying on face and protruding tongue. Dryness of glottis very annoying with tenacious mucous in larynx. Sensation of a lump in the larynx, soreness as if ulcerated, pain during deglutition; great hoarseness. Bronchial catarrh spreading into larynx, swelling of tonsils and glands of throat extending into ears causing transient deafness.

RESPIRATION: Great oppression of breathing every afternoon about 5 p.m., sense of constriction, breathing difficult. Has to fill lungs but no power to eject the air (CHLOR.). Breath hot, feels hot even when breathing through nose.

COUGH AND EXPECTORATION: Cough from tickling under upper part of sternum. Incessant dry cough, worst at night; wakes just as she is falling to sleep (LACH.); worse from sweet things. Terrible, painful cough, as if larynx would be torn to pieces and as if the mucous membrane was torn off with profuse discharge of viscid, greyish mucous mixed with blood. Cough, worse on lying, relieved lying on stomach (CINA). Expectoration white albuminous or little green bitter balls, ropy and difficult to raise (KALI-BI.), as if flecked with infinitesimal dark spots.

CHEST: Chest sore to touch, at times burning extends over whole chest; cold seems to aggravate it; a piece of ice seems to cool it for an instant; then it is hotter; lungs feel as if beaten or bruised. Constricted sensation at bottom of both lungs. Incipient consumption; sensation of abscess between the pectoral muscles.

HEART: Heart palpitation after slight exertion. With heat in chest, heart felt very hot, beat very fast and felt large, accompanied by a bursting sensation. Feeling of a cavity where heart ought to be. Pain in heart acute, sharp and quick. Intense pain in heart radiates to left chest; worse least movement. Burning in heart went through the back and down left arm. This remedy will cure some cases of Angina pectoris.

BACK AND EXTREMITIES: In the neck, back and limbs there are burning, drawing, stabbing pains with intense soreness and often stiffness and contractures of muscles and tendons. Almost entire loss of nervous force in legs and arms, numbness, burning and soreness along the whole back bone.

Burning in the soles of the feet, must uncover them (SULPH.) wants them fanned.

GENERALITIES: Gangrene, trembling spasms, epileptiform spasms, foaming at mouth, opisthotonos, risus sardonicus, collapse. Much disturbance in sleep, many symptoms worse during or following sleep like OP. and the snake poisons.

This unique remedy has given many cures of nocturnal enuresis after the failure of other well indicated remedies.

In summarizing the symptoms and states of this remedy, we can see a wide range for its use in the field of sickness. In its nature it seems to blend much that is found in the other nosodes; evidently the economy while under the influence of this poison strained out as it were the toxins of psora, tuberculosis and congenital lues to give us a complex and unique antidote against the blend of these many constitutional poisons merged into one.

The above observations may explain some of the brilliant cures obtained by this remedy after the failure of other apparently well indicated remedies. This medicine seems endowed with power to reach and activate the deepest sources of vital energy, thereby restoring seemingly hopeless cases of disease to a state of health.

From this fact we may be justified in giving to many a cancer patient somewhere in the course of treatment a dose of MED. as an intercurrent and complimentary remedy to other deep constitutional remedies. For cancer is the sum total of constitutional evils made more virulent and vicious by drug and serum suppressions.

In these times no one remedy is needed as much as this one is because the regular medical profession has only suppressed and held back a universal poison in the race that, like the hydra headed monster of old, keeps returning to prey with unconquered energy and venom, to plague and afflict the race down through the generations.

All those chronic diseases that are leaders in the cause of death today, heart, kidney disease, cancer and many forms of mental and nervous conditions are in their incipency amenable to cure through this and other far-reaching constitutional remedies in the homeopathic fund of healing knowledge.

This is only one of the important reasons for the existence of the homeopathic schools. From the first cry of the new-born infant carrying in its innocent body the inherited toxins engendered of violated law, to the tottering steps of the aged and repentant sinner going down under the lash of his own misdeed there is need for this medicine. It is indeed the balm of Gilead in a world of sin and suffering. We have been told that 80% of operations on married women were made necessary by this subtle poison given them as a marriage dowry from their husbands, who before marriage, were told they were free of venereal poisons and fit for marriage. Because we have in the archives of homeopathic knowledge such subtle and deep, long-acting instruments as this and many other remedies for the eradication of constitutional and inherited toxins as well as the acquired ones, the need for Homeopathy in the world is imperative for the very salvation of universally sick humanity. With each passing year it becomes even more necessary that the Hahnemannian doctrine be taught, promulgated and practiced in all its purity and efficiency.

Because of these things, the homeopathic physician is privileged to perform cures and uses no other therapeutist can. Great as he may be in the field of cure, he can be potentially greater in the realm of disease prevention because nothing else except Homeopathy has been discovered that can lift the heavy burden of inherited disease from the race. Because Homeopathy has such far-reaching powers for good, it is the one hope for the health and well being of the future of the race, and for that reason we can rejoice in strengthened faith because our efforts move in unison with the universal law of the cosmos. Though our numbers decline, we need have no fear because our glorious philosophy of healing is born of the everlasting truth and will abide to serve the sick and afflicted even in a world of sordid commercialism.

Again let us salute the memory of the great Hahnemann whose genius, special courage and tireless efforts under God gave us and, all the future as well, the benign balm of Homeopathy. Hahnemann, the instrumentality of Divine Providence for the healing of the nations, brought to earth not only a law of healing but with that law the magic touch of love and universal peace. For men and women of every creed and from every clime and nation of the earth have been fired with a desire to serve sick humanity regardless of race, creed or station, and in doing so many have made sacrifices for the privilege. Homeopathy begets love and understanding and vanishes prejudice and ignorance.

CHARACTERISTICS AND DIFFERENTIATIONS OF THE NATRUM REMEDIES[1]

Sodium is found in nature in enormous quantities and is widely distributed. It is a constituent of countless silicates and as a result of rock decay gets into the soil whence it enters the plants and finally reaches the animal organism. The nitrate is known as Chile Salpete; the crystalite, (ice stone) or Greenland is a sodium aluminum fluoride. Common salt constitutes the main part of the saline matter in sea water. The Dead Sea of Palestine and the great Salt Lake in Utah are almost saturated solutions of common salt.

In the human economy, sodium together with potassium and calcium are the chief alkali metals in the maintenance of the acid base balance of the body fluids. Droy says that sodium in the form the chloride is a constituent of every liquid and solid part of the body. Its function is to regulate the degree of moisture within the cells.

Quoting Clarke in the Dictionary of Practical Materia Medica, "NAT-C. is the typical salt of the Natrum group (as KALI-C. is of the kalis). NAT-M. is by far the most important. In power and range it stands in the first rank of homeopathic remedies, but has an additional significance in that it exemplifies the power of attenuation in a remarkable way. The problems involved in NAT-M. may be regarded in a sense as the pons asinorium of homeopathy.

NATRUM ARSENICOSUM

This remedy has not been extensively proved but given good results in several conditions. Diptheria and asthma.

MIND: Nervous, restless patient. Depressed. Cannot concentrate; dull, listless and forgetful.

HEAD: Vacant feeling in the whole head. Wavering, floating sensation on turning head quickly. Full feeling in head; numbness in the evening. Dull feeling in forehead extending to root of nose; on awaking in the morning. It has the restlessness and chilliness of ARS. Complications from exposure to cold.

EARS: Pain in ears with dull pain. Rushing noise synchronizes with the pulse.

NOSE: Smell defective or lost; nose stuffed, worse night. Breathes at night through mouth. Nasal discharge yellow and tough pieces of hard-

---

1. From the handwritten manuscript of Dr. Grimmer, exact date unknown. - Editor.

NATRUM ARSENICOSUM ...

ened bluish mucus flow from nose, leaving mucus membrane raw. Nasal mucus membrane thickened, can inhale but not exhale easily.

FACE: Face flushed and hot; feels puffed. Malar bone feels large, as if swollen. Face swollen, edemateous; especially in orbital region; worse morning on awaking. Corners of mouth fissured and indurated. Muscles of mastication stiff and painful on moving jaw.

MOUTH: Teeth and gums tender. Tongue furred coated yellow; deep red, corrugated, fissured; large moist flabby. Ulcer in mouth very sore.

THROAT: Fauces and pharynx red and glossy or purplish and edemateous; patched with yellow mucus; diptheria.

STOMACH: Drinks often but little at a time (like ARS.). Very thirsty but worse by water. Vomits large amounts of sour water, worse after eating. Warm things cause sensation of burning.

ABDOMEN: There is much flatulence gas forming rapidly.

STOOL AND ANUS: Alternate diarrhea and constipation. Soft dark, thin stool leaving a burning in rectum; yellowish copious; hurries patient out of bed in the morning; stool preceded by colic, > after.

URINARY ORGANS: Dull aching in the kidneys with profuse uring.

MALE SEXUAL ORGANS: Dull cutting pain along the Pompart's ligaments followed by a sickening sensation in left testicle, as after a blow. Emission during sleep.

RESPIRATORY ORGANS: Dark slate colored scanty mucus in larynx detached with difficulty. Oppressed or stifled sensation from larynx to bottom of sternum. Lungs feel dry, as though smoke had been inhaled. Exertion aggravates the oppression in chest.

HEART AND PULSE: Oppression about the heart from least exertion. Pulse irregular, slower than usual.

NECK AND BACK: Neck stiff and sore extending down to top of dorsal vertebras. Severe pain between the scapula, worse inspiring. Lumbar pain.

LIMBS: In the limbs frequent neuralgic pains. Lower limbs feel heavy, weary, and bruised.

GENERALITIES: This is a chilly restless patient subject to squamous eruptions with thin white scales.

NATRUM CACODYLICUM

Has been of clinical use in phithisis. Poisoning symptoms are heavy vomiting; tongue like a piece of raw beef; conjunctiva inflamed; eyelids

Natrum cacodylicum ...

edematous, breath of gangrenous odor. Peripheral neuritis; wrist drop; paralysis of left leg.

Natrum carbonicum

The typical Natrum salt a deep aching antipsoric remedy.

Mind: Alternating states. At one time marked degree of gaiety, joyous talkativeness, inclination to sing. Again sadness and depression with tears and unquietude regarding the future. Fits of anguish especially during a storm or when engaged in intellectual labor. Sensitive to noise, to music, to certain individuals. Estrangement from individuals and from society. Irritable with spite and malice. Disposition to be angry and to fly into fits of passion. Difficulty of comprehension; unable to concentrate; makes mistakes in writing. Unfitness for intellectual effort or meditation which fatigue the head.

Head: Vertigo especially after drinking wine. Sun headaches; chronic heat headache after sunstroke. Congestive headaches with heat.

Eyes: Many eye symptoms, inflammation and photophobia. Ulcers on cornea. Abscess in lachrymal gland.

Ears: Otalgia with sharp shooting pains. Hardness of hearing. Deafness with ozena and amenorrhea in light haired girls. Deafness with skin eruptions after typhoid or other infectious diseases with recurring earache.

Nose: Nose red with white pimples on it. Dryness heat and obstruction in nose with catarrhal conditions.

Face: Face bloated and hot or yellow color of face. Ulcers, eruptions and tetters around the mouth and lips.

Teeth: Toothache with boring digging pains after and while eating. Extreme sensitiveness of lower teeth.

Mouth and Throat: Throat and mouth dry and rough with burning about tip of tongue. Much thick mucus requiring violent effort to hawk up.

Stomach: Incessant thirst for cold water which aggravates the stomach. Extreme, voracious hunger. Repugnance to milk and diarrhea comes on after drinking it. Great weakness of digestion with peevishness and hypochondriacal humor after a meal. Distension, heaviness and weakness of stomach after a meal.

NATRUM CARBONICUM ...

ABDOMEN: Chronic liver inflammation, violent stitches in hepatic and splenic regions. Swelling of the glands of groin and axilla; generally painful.

STOOL AND ANUS: Ineffectual urging to stool, hard and difficult evacuation or diarrhea from milk. Diarrhea during a thunderstorm.

URINARY ORGANS. Enuresis. Involuntary urination with mucus in urine. Urine smells like the urine of horses. (NIT-AC.)

MALE SEXUAL ORGANS: Increases sexual desire in the male with continued and painful erections and pollutions. Incomplete coition. Emissions without erections. Discharge of prostatic fluid when urinating or during a hard evacuation. Great tendency to perspire after coition.

FEMALE SEXUAL ORGANS: In the woman bearing down toward the genitals as if the womb would protrude. Deficient menstruation in adults. Metrorrhagia. Deformed cervix uteri. Excoriation at vulva, and between thighs. Discharge of mucus from vagina after coition, causing sterility. Profuse thick yellow fetid leucorrhea. Labor pains weak or accompanied by anguish and sweat with desire to be rubbed.

RESPIRATORY ORGANS: Catarrh of the chest with rattling of much mucus. Cough with expectoration of blood.

CHEST AND HEART: Shortness of breath. Violent anxious palpitation especially on climbing stairs, or at night lying on left side. Painful cracking in heart region.

BACK: Stiffness of nape; cracking in cervical vertebrae.

LIMBS: Drawing rheumatic pains in limbs and back. Weakness of ankles is a marked feature of this remedy. Coldness of feet with chronic ulcers of the heel; black ulcerations on heel. Cracks and excoriation between the toes. Boring drawing shooting in corns.

NATRUM HYPOCHLOROSUM

In some ways this remedy resembles NAT-M. to which it is chemically related. It is more toxic and violent in its action causing rapid emaciation, weakness to exhaustion and fainting.

MIND: Mind is much distressed, laughs, cries, talks in sleep. Very low spirited cries all day and keeps her husband awake all night.

HEAD: Constant vertigo with aching across forehead. Paralyzed feeling in the brain, in all the limbs, and in the fingertips. Extreme tenderness of scalp. Throbbing headache soon after midday meal, better after drinking tea. Pain right side of head, from behind the mastoid to the

Natrum hypochlorosum ...

upper part of orbit across the eye causes eye to be weak and stiff, better after sleep, but constant day and night.

EARS: Pain under right ear when swallowing with tenderness, and swelling up right side of head, with a painful gathering which broke and discharged copiously.

NOSE: Influenza with much nasal discharge with soreness inside cheek. Epistaxis dark colored blood comes away in clots day and night in a pregnant woman.

FACE: Face pain severe shooting day and night; left-sided neuralgia. Recurring gum boils. Pains of face; worse warmth and by worry, better cold applications.

MOUTH: Teeth get loose and tongue swollen, lower jaw sore; difficult to chew.

THROAT: Sore throat with difficult swallowing. Flat ulcer on tongue for back.

STOMACH: Nausea and weight in the stomach; with aching in vertex after each dose.

ABDOMEN: Swelling in abdomen going up to chest causing dyspepsia, worse after eating, with much flatus. Fearful pain in whole lower abdomen which settled in right hip joint and spread over whole abdomen; voiding "white gravel" with great pain.

RECTUM: Cutting pain in rectum between 6 - 7 p.m. passes off during night. Constipation; large hard offensive stool after three days. Great exhaustion before stool, better after forceful stool.

URINARY ORGANS: Within 24 hours diffuse nephritis; urine scanty, smoke colored, then black containing blood, much albumen and casts. Vomiting, diarrhea and headache. Coma (man died on fourth day after drinking ten drachms). Scalding when urinating, with itching and smarting of vagina. Red sand in urine. White gravel (cured).

MALE SEXUAL ORGANS: Male sexual desire almost unconquerable after each dose with priapism.

FEMALE SEXUAL ORGANS: Very marked action on the female genitalia. Opening and shutting sensation in the womb. Uterine bearing down; severe backache and headache. Uterus congested, enlarged, sensitive; constant oozing of blood, worse exertion. Violent metrorrhagia. Menses clotted; black blood; early; severe backaches. Ovarian affection with pain in right hip. Water-logged uterus. Subinvolution. Feels as if womb were pressed when she sits down.

Natrum hypochlorosum ...

Respiratory Organs: Cough and much distress in chest.

Chest: Tightness, weight, dyspepsia; gnawing sensation in front of chest. Many chest pains especially in the left, better lying down. Pain under heart with catching inspiration.

Back: Much back pain in lumbar regions.

Limbs: Aching limbs, feels bereft of power.

Natrum iodatum

This improved sodium preparation has been extensively used by French physicians in cardiac cases, in rheumatism, asthma, chronic bronchitis, scrofula, tertiary syphilis. It has been curative in hayfever, laryngitis, pharyngitis.

Natrum lacticum

Not proven but has been used with success. Gout and gouty congestions; rheumatic complaints; vomiting from large doses. Abnormal sense of fatigue, yawning, and sleepiness.

Natrum muriaticum

One of the greatest of our polycrests as the following list of disease conditions to which it has been successfully applied will show. (Compiled by Clarke): Addison's disease. Anemia. Aphlexea. Atrophy. Brain-fag. Catarrh. Chorea. Constipation. Cough. Cracks in skin. Debility. Depression. Diabetes. Dispareunia. Dropsy. Dyspepsia. Epilepsy. Erysipelas. Eye affections. Eye strain. Face, unhealthy complexion. Gleet. Glossopharyngea Paralysis. Goiter. Gonorrhea. Gout. Headache. Heart affections. Hemiopia. Hernia. Herpes. Hiccough. Hodgkins disease. Hypochondriasis. Intermittent fever. Leucocythemia. Leuchorrhea. Lips, eruptions around. Lungs, edema of. Menstruation disorders. Mouth inflammations. Nettle rash, Pediculosis. Ranula. Seborrhea. Self abuse. Somnambulism. Speech, embarrassed. Spermatorrhea. Spinal irritation. Spleen, enlarged. Sterility. Stomatitis. Sunstroke. Taste, lost or disordered. Tongue, blistered, white coated, heavy. Trifacial nerve paralysis. Ulcers. Varices. Vaginismus. Vertigo. Warts. Whooping cough. Worms. Yawning.

No remedy in our Materia Medica so forcefully exhibits the power of potency over crude drugs. We need but recall the fact that while taking the crude material in our food daily, such startling and specific symptoms are produced on the healthy and cured in the sick by the adminis-

NATRUM MURIATICUM ...

tration of this same drug in potentized form. Other inert substances such as sand, charcoal, iron, and the other metals all have the same inherent quality of increased power and activity in the transforming influence of the Hahnemann process of potentization, but they are not common articles of food.

It would require a small volume to relate the extensive symptomalogy of this remedy and to go into the minute symptoms of all the anatomical parts with all their modalities; therefore, we will only give the broad characteristics of this wonderful remedy which will well repay a close and painstaking study of the Materia Medica.

MIND: Melancholy sadness, which induces a constant recurrence to unpleasant recollections, and much weeping that is aggravated from consolation. Tired of life. Joyless, tactiturn. Hurried and easily startled. Anxiety, with fluttering of the heart. Averse to company, prefers solitude. Anguish, sometimes during a storm. Anxious about the future. Irritability increased, irrasibility, and rage. Hatred to those who formerly gave offense. Alternate gaiety and ill humor. Absense of mind, weakness of memory. Brain fag with sleepiness gloomy forbodings; makes mistakes in reading and writing.

HEAD: The headaches are severe periodical, chronic of a migraine nature.

STOMACH: Great craving for salt things, for acids and bitters. Thirst extreme for water, not too cold; thirst during the chill stage in intermittent fever.

GENERALITIES: This patient is sensitive to both extremes of temperature; suffers from the effects of chronic suppressed malaria; malaria suppressed by quinine. The chills have long ceased to come but the patient is weak, emaciated (while eating well) anemic, nervous, and exhausted. Often chronic liver and spleen troubles supervene. The bad effects of fright often leave a chorea. The muscles and ligaments are weak and easily strained; tendons tend to contract like in CAUST. Bad effects of grief and especially disappointment in love. The symptoms are renewed or come on while lying in bed, especially at night and in the morning.

SLEEP: Great sleepiness during the day and impaired broken or retarded sleep at night. Distressing dreams especially of thieves.

Natrum nitricum

Nat-n. or Chile Salpetre has not been extensively proved, but has been used in anemia, constipation, debility, distension, flatulence, otalgia, otitis. Anemic and exhausted with coldness of left foot. Coldness through upper part of body. Symptoms worse exertion. Nat-n. was Rademacher's Acon. He used it in inflammations of all kinds especially laryngo-tracheitis and croup, acute pneumonia, acute rheumatism, and heart affections and purpura, hemorrhages, inflammation of the eyes, exopthalmic goiter.

Natrum nitrosum

Clinical: Angina pectoris. Apoplexy. Cyanosis. Fainting. Gastroenteritis. Giddy with sensation as would lose consciousness. Staring and livid lips. Thought she would die. Face, lips, hands turned blue. All strength gone with trembling sensation over whole body. Rash like roseola syphilitica on chest, measly, spreading to abdomen and thighs, gradually covering whole body except face. Violent perspiration.

Natrum phosphoricum

Another Schüssler remedy for which he states that it is contained in the blood corpuscles, muscle cells and the cells of the brain, and nerve tissues as well as in the intercellular fluids. In the presence of Nat-p., lactic acid is decomposed into carbonic acid and water, hence, it is the remedy for those diseases which are caused by an excess of lactic acid and therefore is useful in the complaints of infants. Sour eructations, vomiting of sour cheesy masses, yellowish green, so called hacked diarrhea. Colic and spasms with acidity. Uric acid is dissolved in the blood by its warmth in the presence of Nat-p.

This remedy is sensitive to thunderstorms like the Natrums and Phos.

Besides the acid indigestion caused by sugar and milk it has a marked effect on the sexual spheres of both sexes. The man suffers from nightly erections and copious emissions followed by lame back and weak knees.

The woman has early menses with weakness and trembling of heart, severe headache with heavy leucorrhea: honey-colored, creamy, sour smelling, acrid and watery.

Natrum salicylicum

Meniere's disease.

Paeonia[1]

The provings of this drug (even though fragmentary) and the clinical application of it over a period of many years stamps it on my mind as a remedy of great power in a rather specific way. Its herbal relations are the ACONITES, the ACTAEAS and the HELLEBORES, in fine the family of the RANUNCULACEAE. The medicine is prepared from the fresh root dug up in springtime, it is said to be inert in the autumn.

The clinical uses given by Clarke in his Dictionary of Practical Materia Medica has been abundantly confirmed by actual practice and observation. It is as follows: Anus, fissure of; fistula of, affectations of. Bed sores. Breast; ulceration of. Ciliary neuralgia. Coccyx, ulcer on. Hemorrhoids. Headache. Head, rush of blood to. Nightmares. Perineum; ulcer on. Sternum; pain in. Ulcers. Varicose veins. Vertigo. This paragraph of clinical uses is an epitome of the drug's sphere of action and curative use.

Mentally and physically the PAEON. patient is supersensitive to bad news and unpleasant happenings, and physically to the severe pains this remedy is noted for; and these emotional upsets, and attacks of physical suffering both prostrate and weaken the patient to a great degree. Hence, the PAEON. subject is delicate and weak and often completely broken in health and spirit.

Peonia manifests on the veneous side of circulation; producing engorged veins, and varicosities which tend to ulcerate. Ulceration on skin and mucus membranes is a dominate factor in this remedy's action. Bedsores are readily formed and soon become ulcerous; the pressure or rubbing of a shoe readily produces an ulcer. Hemorrhoids tend to take on ulceration accompanied with the most excruciating, sharp burning pains. Varicosities on the leg take on the same tendency to break down and ulcerate. Ulcers at the site of abscesses of the breast that never healed; abscesses, ulcers in old scars might find its best remedy here.

Peonia affects profoundly the nerves and the nerve sheaves - hence the intensity and predominance of pain wherever symptoms manifest. Neuralgias are a prominent feature of the remedy.

---

1. From the handwritten manuscript of Dr. Grimmer, exact date unknown. The major part of this article was taken from Clarke: DICTIONARY OF PRACTICAL MATERIA MEDICA Vol. II, pg. 707 ff. - Editor.

Vertigo, faintness and weakness are also noted. This sensitive weak patient, over anxious and fearful presents many of the general aspects of ARS., but the latter is broader in its sphere of action and less specific than is PAEON.

The sharp pains in ulcers reminds us of NIT-AC. and HEP.; SIL.; in toe ulcers compare M-AUST.

HEAD: Many head compaints are found in the proving of this remedy. Vertigo is marked, worse from every motion and in a warm room, with constant reeling and staggering. Fullness and heat in head with syncope and cold sweat. Rush of blood to head; Pains and confusion in head. Pain with roaring in ears and flickering before eyes. Gnawing headaches. Headaches with pressure pain in left side after a meal. Pain in the forehead morning and evening and in the orbits and above the left brow with sticking, jerking, tearing in right temple extending into the head. Boring outward in right temple. Pain in occiput and nape. Heaviness in occiput.

EYES: The eyes of the PAEON. patient is a point of suffering and weakness. Eyes red and watery; pains severe tearing or sticking with redness, photophobia and lachrymation; or the eyes may be smarting dry, and difficult to open. Burning dryness itching of eyes and lids. Violent tearing around right eye. Conjunctivitis with lachrymation and contracted pupil. Sensation and pain as of a grain of sand under the upper lid.

EARS: Jerking in cartilages of the ears, sticking outward in right ear. Pinching behind the right ear. One ear cold the other hot at 3 p.m. Itching in concha. Ringing in ears.

NOSE: Stoppage of nose in evening and morning with dryness, crawling in tip of nose.

FACE: Face red and puffy with burning heat; pains in face, crawling in upper lip. Pain extending from articular fossa of lower jaw through inner ear, relieved keeping jaws open for a long time and when drinking; worse pressing them together.

THROAT: There is biting posteriorly in palate in evening. Hawking caused by tenacious mucus in throat, with scanty expectoration. Sensation as if an acid burning vapor ascended throat. Heat in fauces extending to pharynx, throat and esophagus, worse hawking. Swallowing difficult.

STOMACH: The appetite is lost, and nausea comes on entering a warm room, after a moderate walk, with seething in head; vanishing or obscuration of senses and attacks of faintness. Vomiting with painful diarrhea. Anxious aching (pressing in epigastrium). Periodical sticking upward from middle of epigastric region. Buring in epigastric region, at night.

ABDOMEN: Borborygmi. Griping pain in forenoon preceeded and followed by anxiety trembling of limbs and arms, as if frightened, and apprehensious when any one spoke to him. Unpleasant news affected him exceedingly. Pinching in abdominal muscles Cutting in umbilical region. Colic with diarrhea transversely across upper abdomen. Sensitiveness worse along transverse colon and epigastric region that were hard and retracted. Crawling in abdomen.

RECTUM: In the rectum and lower bowel we find the most intense suffering; the large red engorged hemorrrhoids bloom out not unlike the red paeoney itself; the pains are often intolerable, the patient constantly walks or rolls on the floor in agony, especially worse after a stool, fissures that bite and itch and burn; very painful sensitive ulcers exuding serum and blood. Sudden pasty diarrhea with faintness in abdomen and burning in anus after stool, returning after six hours, then internal chilliness, generally a few hours afterwards he felt the worst. Stools thin frequent.

FEMALE SEXUAL ORGANS: The external genitalia of the female becomes painful, congested and swollen.

URINARY ORGANS: In the urinary organs there is constriction in the neck of the bladder so that urine passed only in drops. Frequent copious micturation burning and scanty urine.

CHEST: In the chest there is much sticking pain worse on motion and during respiration. Pain beneath the heart as from anxiety. Pain under the sternum is a persistant symptom. Rush of blood, congestion and heat in chest, pulse contracted.

NECK, BACK, LIMBS: They have sticking jerking shooting tearing pains neuralgic in character. The fingers and toes have much suffering. Cramp in the ulna at the wrist, tense feeling in muscles at elbow on flexing the arm. Shooting and tingling in the fingers. Finger felt cold dead after an injury, shriveled, yellow and without sensation. Lower limbs have many symptoms of pain and weakness such as cramps and shooting pains hindering walking by day and rest at night. Chronic ulcer of the leg serpiginous spreading at edges with severe shooting pains. Ulcer on left great toe and on dorsum of foot from tight boots. Painful corns. Swelling of toes with contraction, intermittent jerking pains through them. Generally worse from motion and exertion, evening, warm room, and rainy weather. Many complaints are worse after sleep, or come on during sleep.

SLEEP: Sleepiness all afternoon, starting on falling asleep, even during the day; sleep restless and unremembered dreams; restless disturbed sleep the first night of the proving by burning at epigastrium, afterward by voluptuous dreams with emissions or by anxious and vivid dreams of death. Sleep unrefreshing, disturbed by frightful dreams: of death or quarreling, anxious, vivid, wonderful and amorous with emissions. Dreams of a ghost sitting upon his chest, and oppressing his breath so that he often woke groaning.

A close study and knowledge of this unique remedy will reward the precriber with many cures, especially in severe rectal complaints that cannot be obtained by any other agency.

Strychninum and its Preparations[1]

Strychninum sulphuricum

Facial neuralgia and neuralgic headache will often refuse to be benefited by the ordinary doses of Nux-v. in use by our school, but will promptly disappear under the use of the 3x of Stry-s. In one very obstinate case Stry-val. cured after other perparations failed.

Of the various preparations of Stry-s. is generally used. It is probably the most certain of all.

I often use the Stry-p. when the cerebral functions are involved, or when the symptoms seem to call for Ph-ac. or Phos.

The Citrate of iron and Strychnia is a favorite preparation with many of our school. It is perhaps the best in all cases where anemia is a predominant symptom. The use of this double salt obviates the alternation of Strychnia with Ferr. I usually prescribe it in the 1x trituration.

In many cases of exhaustion of brain power, or in women in whom a high state of nervous erethism exists, I have seen brilliant curative results attend the use of the Stry-val., in the 21 trituration or dilution.

Strychninum arsenate[2]

Introduced into Homeopathic Literature by Dr. E. M. Hale
Triturations.

Chronic diarrhea in a child with paralytic conditons of bladder, rectum and lower extremities.

Certain forms of paralysis where Ars. and Strychnia both appear to be indicated.

Strychnia phosphorica or Strychninum phosphoricum[3]

Eleven students of the Iowa State University Homeopathic School, under supervision of Dr. George Royal, have made a good proving of Stry-p., under the general rules adopted by the O. O. and L. Society, which may be summarized as follows:

---

1. From the handwritten manuscript of Dr. Grimmer, exact date unknown. Most of the contents was taken from: Hale, Edwin M.; Materia Medica and Special Therepeutics of the New Remedies. Vol. II, F.E. Boericke, Hahnemann Publishing House, Philadelphia. 1886. - Editor.
2. Douglass M.E: Characteristics of the Homeopathic Materia Medica, Boericke & Runyon Co., New York, 1901, page 839.
3. Hansen Oscar M.D.: Text Book of Materia Medica and Therapeutics of Rare Homeopathic Remdies: The Homeopathic Publishing Company, London, 1899.

STRYCHNIA PHOSPHORICA OR STRYCHNINUM PHOSPHORICUM ...

The drug seems to act through the cerebro-spinal nervous system.

Twitching, trembling of muscles, lack of co-ordination, still, weak, or complete loss of power, vertigo and fainting.

Mentally, much silly laughter.

Very irregular pulse, from 50 to 132, face flushed, skin at times cold and clammy.

Sub-normal temperature, as low as 97.

Markedly worse from motion; better from rest and open air.

The proving points to chorea, locomotor ataxis, paralysis, tetanus and hysteria. Potencies proved: 30th, 6th, 3rd and 1st; all acted. From the Homeopathic Recorder.

CHARACTERISTIC SYMPTOMS AND THERAPEUTICS: Neurasthenia spinalis from anemia of the spinal cord with paralysis. Is an excellent remedy. Spinal irritation with burning, aching, and weakness in the spine, the pain extending to the front of the chest. Tenderness on pressure in the mid-dorsal region. Sleeplessness, cold feet. Feet, hands, and axillae covered with clammy perspiration.

STRYCHNINUM OR STRYCHNINUM SULPHURICUM[1]

Much of our knowledge of this drug comes to us by observations made from the abuses of its empirical adminstration in the treatment of heart and nervous diseases. It is indeed homeopathic to many patients suffering from such complaints. But even in these cases, the drug must not be given over too long a period and in the crude form if serious symptoms would be avoided. It acts profoundly on the brain and spinal cord, producing mental disturbances and symptoms of illusions, hallucinations, and mental excitement merging into weakness and paralysis. The nerves everywhere are markedly affected such as optic nerve paralysis and sclerosis. Induration of the posterior columns and nerve roots of the spinal cord are frequent centers of attack by the drug. From all this we can recommend it to the neurologist for study and use.

Inumerable cases of poisonings with strychnine have been recorded, and these cases furnish us with a rich array of symptoms, which with the provings even though fragmentary and incomplete give us a good image of sickness for the homeopathic use of this medicine.

Perhaps the most characteristic and certain action of the drug is its power to produce convulsions and spasms of a tetanic nature; and these spasms are all made worse by light, noise, or the least jar, showing how completely all the special senses are involved. A case of poisoning presents one of the most gruesome and terrorizing pictures of sickness to be met with; lying on the back, which is the only tolerable position with body rigid, jaws set, hands flexed and the whole muscular system convulsed with short jerky spasms, which continue for a short time and then remit, the muscles remaining contracted and hard as wood during the intervals between the paroxysms. As the disease advances a set expression, the risus sardonicus, is assumed together with a condition of opisthotonos and cries of terror, hippocratic countenance, frothing of the mouth complete this picture generally ending in death by asphyxia.

To quote Clarke, the clinical application of the remedy comprises a large and varied group of complaints and conditions. Amaurosis. Aorta, pain in. Aphonia. Asthama. Athetosis. Bladder, paralysis of, and pains in. Breasts, pains in. Cough, explosive. Cramps. Diaphragm, spasms of.

---

1. From the handwritten manuscript of Dr. Grimmer, exact date unknown. A large part of this article was taken from the recorded provings in Clarke's DICTIONARY OF PRACTICAL MATERIA MEDICA. - Editor.

Emphysema. Enuresis. Exophthalmos. Eyes; optic nerve, sclerosis of. Headache. Hemiplegia. Influenza. Joints, stiffness of. Laryngeal, crises of. Locomotor ataxia. Malar bones, pains in. Neurasthenia. Night blindness. Paraplegia. Proctalgia. Rheumatism. Scrotum, abcess of. Spinal irritation. Tetanus.

Of course many of the symptoms are very similar to those of Nux-v. We will try to give you the more characteristic and uncommon symptoms omitting the common ones. Another condition that is somewhat unusual is a chorea persisting during sleep the opposite of AGAR.[1] Electric like shocks occuring whenever the prover was touched or when any one lightly shook the bed. A touch on any part of body produced a voluptuous sensation. Hale recommends the salts of strychnine in the tetanic convulsions of cerebro-spinal meningitis. Neuralgic pains around the eyes and face coming suddenly at intervals.

Spasms of the esophagus in hysterical women.

Brain exhaustion of women in whom high nervous erethism exists.

Cooper suggest its use in the spasmodic coughs that often follow influenza.

Under peculiar sensations are: Feeling as if the head and face were enlarged. As if an iron cap were on the head. Paralyzed feeling in left half of head and face. Scalp sore as if hair had been pulled. As if nerves were suddenly pulled out of teeth. As of a lump in the throat. As if water dripped off right elbow at intervals, and off right shoulder. As if chopped in half at the waist at night. The pains and sensations come suddenly and return at *intervals*. Sudden palpitation. Darting, pinching, lancinating fulgurating electric pains. Gurgling noise in rectum with electric darts was noted in one prover. Many pains center around the lips and eyes. Pains and chills occur in the occiput and nape and run down the whole lengh of the spine. Itching of whole body, and violent itching of the roof of the mouth. Jerking, twitchings, and shocks in all parts run through the pathogenesis.

Stiffness is a leading feature and Cooper gives "rheumatism with stiff joints" as an indication. Symptoms are < morning, by touch, noise, motion, exertion, walking, draft of air, after meals; > lying on the back.

ANTIDOTES: Hale suggests PASSI. as being antidotal. HYOS. for the drowsiness, respiratory affections (Clarke). TAB., CHLF., CAMPH. and ACON. have been advised. OXYGEN inhalations have been effective anti-

---

1.   Kent, Repertory p. 1348. - Editor.

dotes in animals. The rectal symptoms are best relieved by SULPH. CHAM. 1M has cured the convulsions in one case of poisoning.

RELATIONS: NUX-V. and IGN. are the closest anologues. ARS., BELL., BRUC., CHAM., HYOS., LYC., STRAM., SULPH. may be compared symptomatologically.

MIND: The mental symptoms are striking and valuable. Delirium like that of hydrophobia, like delirium tremens. Frightened. Shrinks from persons, from currents of air. Shouted out: "They are coming for me". Extreme nervous excitability; painful nervousness. Immoderate fits of laughing, with light, swimming sensation and giddiness. Moaning, sobbing, screaming. Exceedingly despondent. Irritable. Confusion of ideas. Loss of memory. Consciousness perfect till death; though there may also be loss of consciousness.

HEAD: There is much vertigo with roaring of the ears while lying with nausea. Jerking of the head forward and backward. Veins of the head, neck and face turgid; red, protruding eyes. Violent headache with bursting pains in the forehead, especially the left side. Or there may be stupid headache with extreme drowsiness. Sensation of iron cap on head. Violent thumping pains in head especially the right half and over the left eye. Shattered sensation with drowsiness. Sharp darting pains in left temple and around back of left ear. Sudden pain and pressure in vertex and left eye. Peculiar paralyzed feeling in left half of face and head. Constant pains in back of head and nape of neck. Sore pains in scalp as if the hair had been pulled. Intense itching of scalp and nape.

EYES: This is a valuable remedy for the eye specialist to study and use homeopathically. Eyes highly congested and in constant motion, as in great affright. Eyes red; injected and protruding. Eyes sunken; rolling, distorted, turned to one side, turned to the right and fixed, with dilated insensible pupils and red conjuntiva. Aching, smarting, dull pain in eyes with misty vision. Burning in eyes, worse from light. Feeling as if eyes were suddenly stiffened and drawn back. Intense, sudden, burning pain in eyes and lids. Cold feeling in eyes. Rolling of eyes as if they were two cold bullets. Tender bruised feeling over left eye. Rapid pulsation over left eye; in left upper lid, with weakness, swelling discharge. Increased lachrymation. Needle like pains in balls of eyes. Pupils dilated eyes staring or pupils contracted. Vision dim, confused misty; persistant amaurosis. Sparks before eyes, balckish, white or red. Increased peripheric sensibility for blue. Enlargement of the field of vision. Everything seemed to turn green and he fell to the floor.

EARS: In the external ears there is a creeping tingling sensation. Sudden burning, itching in the ears, nose lips and eyes. Intense aching behind ears and down spine. Sharp darting pains behind right ear, behind ears and back of head and spine. Digging pain deep in left ear. Intense fullness in ears. Hearing extremely sensitive, hears the slightest sounds. Roaring; burning; noise like wind.

FACE: Nose and face swollen and burning hot; eyes half closed as if stung by bees. Face pale distorted. Muscles stiff. Risus sardonicus. Expression of extreme terror. Face livid, flushed and bathed with cold clammy sweat. Short needle like pains in cheek bones, pains shooting into the teeth, especially the left side. Lips, blue livid, swollen, retracted. Trismus. Stiffening of jaws affecting speech. Dull pains in jaws generally shooting into the temples.

TEETH: Teeth clenched. Toothache at midnight in left upper teeth, shooting into cheek bone, as if nerves were suddenly pulled out, at night, Drawing, shooting pains.

MOUTH: Tongue dry and papillae erect; dry with white moisture on edges; gums, lips, and roof of mouth violet, hot, sore. Taste bad, feverish, hot and bitter. Frothing at the mouth. Violent itching in roof of mouth. Mouth filled with frothy saliva. Articulation difficult. Speech indistinct or lost.

THROAT: Choking sensation in throat as if something were held tightly around it. Dry spasmodic contracted feeling; intense difficulty in swallowing. Feeling as of a lump in throat, < evening. Soreness and scraping left side. Every attempt to swallow caused violent spasms of muscles of pharynx. Severe dull pains in muscles and glands of neck and at back of ears.

STOMACH: Unusually good appetite, enjoys her food amazingly. Thirst intense, feverish. Eructations: of bitter wind before vomiting, bitter, greasy, with bad taste. Nausea, almost constant retching. Violent vomiting. Vomiting thin colorless liquid. Heavy feeling in stomach. Intense pain in pit of stomach. Intense twitching, violent jerks, spasms. Spasm of pit of stomach suddenly while at dinner lasting an hour with severe pain and feeling of suffocation compelling to loosen clothes. Burning along esophagus and stomach. Immediately felt a burning sensation in stomach for about a minute, then felt as if the blood ran cold.

ABDOMEN: Aching with sick feeling in abdomen. Sharp needle like pain in left hypochondruim. Abdominal muscles rigid in tetanic spasms. Sore contracted buised feeling. Rumbling. Griping, cutting gnawing pain in the bowels. Sharp, cutting pain in right lower and left upper half of abdomen. Uneasiness in bowels and constipation. Sharp needle like pains in left groin.

RECTUM: Gurgling sounds in rectum with spasms of darting pain compelling to sit on the ground as if shot. Two dart like shocks from a strong galvanic battery before going to bed. Spasmodic jumping in anus. Diarrhea, copious and watery. Feces discharged involuntarily during the spasms. Stool lumpy and dry, flatus smelling like fresh putty. Stools lumpy with mucus. Very obstinate constipation with griping.

URINARY ORGANS: Contraction of bladder; it expelled urine apparently as fast as it was secreted. Bladder paralyzed. Painful pressure extending down thighs from back of bladder down rectum; from front wall of bladder along urethrea, pains finally leaving bladder and settling in glans penis. Scalding in urethra. Constant urging. Urine either copious or scanty, variable. Dark like beer, thick red sediment albuminous-looking masses floating in it.

MALE SEXUAL ORGANS: In the male the left spermatic cord is painful and the left testicle swelled, painful only on standing or walking; hard and swollen, later burning pain on left side of scrotum where the skin was tense on the testicle and a large abcess formed in the dartos and cellular tissue; this was opened by a small incision and yielded a very large quantity of semi-transparent fluid partly mixed with blood, after the discharge of which the size of the testicle became somewhat less.

FEMALE SEXUAL ORGANS: In the female while falling asleep quite suddenly several hysterical jerks as from the womb with burning irritating heat and violent pulsation in the passages. Also feeling of great pressure and bearing down. Darting pain and thrilling sensation in vagina with momentary pulsation coming on at intervals. Violent tearing pains in womb at intervals. Menses at proper times, lasted only two days and scanty flow. Any touch on the body, it mattered not where, excited a voluptuous sensation.

RESPIRATORY ORGANS: The respiratory organs persents some marked symptoms. Spasms of muscles about larynx and anus; she felt and looks as if strangled; the muscles on each side of larynx became tense like cords. Spasms of respiratory muscles, breathing irregular, intermittent, difficult. Voice weak, low, hoarse. Aphonia. Occasionally spasmodic explosive cough. Breathing hurried, difficult, choking, tight with great pain in precordia. Sobbing, moaning. Asphyxia.

CHEST: Walls of chest fixed. Oppression, chest moves en masse, is hyper-resonant. Tightness. Pain: severe, sharp, contractive, spasmodic darting on chest, neck and back. Severe stabbing pains in right breat passing through to back at intervals. Also in left breast.

HEART: The heart comes in for a number of symptoms. There is tightness about the precordia. During the day dull pain, shifting along line of aortic arch. Fluttering sensation about heart with faintness. Sudden palpitation. Tumultous action of heart. Feeling as of heart coming into throat. Heart fluttering like a wounded bird. Pulse irregular, accelerated, corded, tense, strong, full, rapid, nearly extinct in the paroxysms.

NECK AND BACK: Neck swollen. Jugular vein distended. Neck stiff, muscles like rigid cords. Painful stiffness extending down the back. Darting knife like pains in muscles of neck and top of shoulders, chest and abdomen with sick feeling. Back stiff. Convulsive jerks in back and spinal column. Intense icy coldness in entire back. Agonizing gnawing pain in back, neck and muscles of the legs. Suddenly violent cutting in back at waist line as though she was chopped in half, extending right and left to stomach at night.

EXTREMITIES: Fingers and toes violet colored, fingers spasmodically drawn in, toes drawn back. Limbs out-stretched and rigid at times jerking movements. Cramps. Darting pains in muscles. Rheumatic pains in arms and legs. Crawling in limbs after spasms. In the upper and lower limbs are found the same convulsive, sharp, drawing pains, with stiffness and contraction. Cramping, agonizing gnawing pains in the muscles especially of the thighs. twitching and tingling.

GENERALS: Spasmodic convulsive twitching. Every muscle in the body in a state of convulsive twitching. Violent, electric like starting and shuddering; followed by opisthotonos. Shocks so violent in the muscles that the right thigh was dislocated. Convulsions recurring regularly. Every attempt to move threatened a convulsion. Convulsive jerks on falling asleep. In convulsion, skin hot, bathed in perspiration and steaming. Can lie in no position but on back, any other positions brings on convulsions. An attempt to take liquids produced violent spasmodic fit preventing swallowing it, here we see the likeness of a typical advanced case of *rabies*. General aggravation at night and from 8 - 10 p.m.

SKIN: Skin pale at first, then livid and bluish. Formication. Burning tingling with intense itching of skin over the whole body especially severe over scalp, face, arms and legs.

SLEEP: Yawning with extreme drowsiness. Sleepless from internal anxiety and uneasiness or from dread of rectal spasms; with visions of dead persons. Extreme restlessness and talking in sleep with peculiar working in back of brain. Restless nights with profuse perspiration. Dreams disagreeable. Strange wanderings of the imagination.

FEVER: Extreme chilliness and drowsiness. Peculiar creeping chilliness all over with a tremulous sensation in the jaws. Extreme chilliness even in a warm room. Icy coldness. A single cold chill down entire length of spine. Extremities cold and perspiration flowing in a stream from head and chest. Fever of adynamic type, or intermittent type. Intolerable sense of heat over whole body, though some parts cold to the feel. Burning heat with hot sweat in the early effects of the proving; in later stages cold sweats obtain. Cold sweat with convulsive shocks and increased shaking and stiffening.

From the foregoing array of terrible symptoms and sufferings we may readily trace the certain path of its use and power to cure in some of the more severe and advanced cases of *tetanus* and *rabies* where terror and spasm preceed death. In chronic disease of the spine and nervous system STRY. is destined to be a valuable remedy in the hands of the discerning. In an old case of locomotor ataxy, this remedy in the 1M potency enabled the patient to leave his wheel chair and walk again.

Another interesting clinical feature is that it has cured several cases of *tapeworm*. One in a little girl seven years of age where the usual vermicides and specifics for tape worm had failed to cure. After the administration of this remedy in the 200 and 1 M potencies doses given at intervals of from a month to six weeks apart this little patient, (after a lapse of two years) has had no more segments or mucus expelled, and the child is in better health than in years before.

THUJA[1]

THUJ. is one of the most useful and far-reaching remedies of the Materia Medica whose therapeutic worth was discovered and developed by Hahnemann. He placed it at the head of the anti-sycotic group.

Boenninghausen found it curative and prophylactic in an epidemic of small-pox[2], and Burnett because of the fact of that curative action applied it successfully as the best antidote against the ravages of vaccinosis, the disease resulting from the poison of small-pox vaccine introduced directly into the blood. From Burnett's time to the present, THUJ. has been a benediction and at times a life saver, especially for the evil effects following small-pox vaccination.

Truly the beautiful "tree of life" is endowed, by the Creator's faith, with the twin properties: the force of destruction and degeneration on the one hand and the benign power of regeneration and healthfulness on the other, the manner in which this inherent force is applied determining the end that is obtained. By the intelligent use of the Law of Similars together with the employment of the homeopathic technique of preparing and prescribing the similar remedy, can the force of destruction and disintegration be changed and transmuted as if by magic, into healing streams of energy, to dissipate disease and restore the bloom of health.

When the medical world learns these simple facts, humanity can then be freed from innumerable sufferings attendant upon the abuse and misuse of drastic experimental drugs, of crude vaccines and serums introduced directly into the bloom stream acting as foreign materials and proteins to fester and poison the fountain of life and pile up added evil in the human economy.

As we look around throughout the realm of nature, we behold everywhere the double aspects of action and reaction, of negative and positive forces, of good and evil at work to promote the progress of growth and evolution toward the goal of better things. Hence all objects, minerals, plants and animals contain within themselves these same dual qualities. Every human being has the possibility of disease or health, of evil or good inherent in his life process operation in retaliation to envi-

---

1. THE HOMEOPATHIC RECORDER, Vol. LXIII, No. 12, June 1948, p. 262. See also "Thuja" by Elizabeth W. Hubbard, THE HOMEOPATHIC RECORDER, Vol. LXIII, No. 10, April, 1948, pgs 224 ff.

2. Von Boenninghausen, C.M.F. The Lesser Writings, translated from the original German by Prof. L.H. Tafel. Boericke and Tafel, Philadelphia, 1908, pgs 3,4.

ronment. Every plant and mineral has the dual power of producing good or evil in its nature when applied to the economy of man. Divine Providence has vouchsafed to man the power to choose and endowed him with intelligence and discrimination to mold his life in accordance with the laws and order of the universe. Thus, man may use the destructive powers in drugs to dissipate the destructive processes inherent in his organism by employing the Law of Similars and the unique technique of its application. From these observations we learn that crude drugs bring out the inherent evils of disease in man as evidenced by provings, and potentized drugs dissipate those evils and restore the harmony and power of life processes in their relation to environment.

Now to proceed with the story of THUJ.: We are told that this tree loves to abide in wet swampy places, and its habitat extends from Pennsylvania northward to Canada, and it is not by accident that the symptoms and conditions produced by this drug are brought on or made worse by exposure to wet and dampness. Grauvogl listed THUJ. in his hydrogeniod graph which contains such remedies as CALC., DULC., NAT-S. and RHUS-T. - all having aggravations from cold wet weather and from exposure to the same.

Thuja is not just an anti-sycotic, that is, a constitutional gonorrheal remedy, manifesting excrecences warts (especially fig warts) dark-colored spots, cauliflower-like growth which are soft fetid and emitting an ordor like herring brine (sometimes a sweetish odor is noted), growth tending to bleed easily; also marked and extensive catarrhal states, both chronic and acute, are produced and cured with this medicine. Besides these manifestations of sycosis, many symptoms and states relating to syphilis are found. Also in the pathogenesis may be noted many chronic skin eruptions that are psoric in nature. Thus we behold in this unique remedy a blending of all the miasms described by Hahnemann in his chronic diseases together with the added evils resulting from the universal poisoning of humanity by vaccination.

From this general outline it is likely that many prescribers have failed to get the most in the way of cure by neglecting a full and complete study of this remedy's proving, together with its chemical confirmations in the field of cure at the hands of the old masters, Hahnemann, Boeninghausen, Burnett and Clarke whose observation and use of the curative action of THUJ. present a volume of brilliant cures of a great number of disease conditions embracing both acute and chronic manifestations. In fact, the wide extent of the proving and cured confirmations is too vast to present in a brief medical paper; so only the highlights of the therapeutics will be given with the hope that sufficient interest may be awakened to stimulate a more detailed study by physicians everywhere.

A remedy well-proven and clinically developed presents a great array of mental, emotional an nervous symptoms and states. THUJ. is rich in many strange, rare and peculiar symptoms. Such symptoms are the joy of the homeopathic prescriber.[1]

MIND: Those having *fixed ideas*, especially of an unusual nature such as: as if the *soul were seperated from the body*, or that the *limbs were brittle like glass and would break easily*. Or the sensation of a *living animal in the abdomen*. Sensation as if the whole *body is very thin and delicate and could not resist the least violence. As if the body would be dissolved.* The *insane will not be touched or approached.* Imbecility after vaccination, mental depression and anxious apprehensions regarding the future; everything appears troublesome and repugnant.

The merest trifle occasions pensiveness: *music causes him to weep*, with trembling of the feet. Hurried with ill humor, talks hastily. Averse to any kind of mental labor. Mental depression after child birth.

Very depressed, sad and irritable. *Scrupulous about small things.* Feels she can not exist any longer; shunning everybody. Aversion to life. Moroseness and peevishness, perversions of the will, the love of life is gone. Over-excited quarrelsome; easily angered about trifles.

The child is *excessively obstinate. In reading and writing the patient uses wrong expressions.* Talks hastily and *swallows words.* Thoughtlessness, forgetfulness, slowness of speech and reflection for words when in conversation. Incapacity for reflection. Cretinism, an indication of profound effects on the endocrine chain.

HEAD: Sense of intoxication and much vertigo, especially on closing the eyes. Head: suffering of many kinds. Pains are congestive compressive, as if a hoop or band encircled the head, or sharp pains as if nail were driven into the vertex. Head pain > from looking upwards or sideways or turning head backwards. Headaches brought on or < from sexual excesses, or from heating or overlifting. Headaches > exercising in the open air, < stooping, > bending backward. Dull stupefying headaches. Pressive headaches with shocks in the forehead and temples. Headache < afternoon and at 3:00 a.m., < at rest, > after perspiartion. Neuralgic types of headache; nervous, sycotic or syphilitic headaches.

---

1. Much what follows is taken from Clarke: DICTIONARY OF PRACTICAL MATERIA MEDICA. - Editor.

Meningitis of sycotic children may require Thuj. Headaches with sun stroke, especially with the sycotic constitution.

Hair becomes hard, dry and lusterless and falls; extremely sensitive scalp even the hair at night when lying in bed is painful in the neuralgia of the head. Wants the head and face wrapped up warm. Scalp itching and very tender to even the pressure of the hat. Dry, herpetic eruptions of scalp with dandruff extending to the eyebrows. Perspiration smelling like honey on uncovered parts of the head, face and hands with dryness of the covered parts. Pityriasis affecting forhead, face and ears and neck.

EYES: Thuj. has paralytic weakness of the eyelids and lower limbs. Many eye symptoms are cured with this remedy. Stitches through left eye to brain, malignant balanorrhea; wart-like excrescence on iris. Inflammation of cornea; vascular tumor of the cornea. Episcleritis, sclerochoroiditis, staphyloma, ophthalmia, neonatorum, phlyctenular conjunctivitis. Conjunctivitis of left eye with violent pain across forehead and outer side of eyeball constantly recurring from childhood and following the supression of a skin eruption. Fungus tumor in the orbit. Granular lids with wart-like granulations. Epithelioma of left lower lid. Ptosis, lids fall down several times a day. Eyelids feel heavy as lead. Styes, tarsal tumors, chalazae; red painful nodosities on margins of the lids.

Purulent and itching pimples between the eyebrows, condylomata in eye-brows. Nocturnal agglutination of the lids; weakness of the eyes, obscure sight, dim sight, as if through a cloud or veil. Diplopia, myopia, black dancing specks before eyes; floating stripes; sees green stripes which frighten her. Flames of light, mostly yellow and many other perversions of sight.

EARS: The ears are the source of much troubles and pain. Catarrhal and other discharges purulent, offensive oozing from ears. Polyps and other growths. The same severe catarrhal states and conditions are found in the nose.

NOSE: Nose red and hot or swollen; tumid, red eruption on nose. Painful pressure at root of nose. Dry or fluent coryza with cough and hoarseness. Fetid green discharges, green mucous mixed with pus and blood, or thick green mucous. Chronic catarrh after measles, scarlatina, or variola. Ozena, warts on nose.

FACE: Heat of face or burning redness. Redness of face with fine nets of veins as if marbled; this condition is also found over the limbs. Greasy skin of face (GRAPH. and TUB.). Pains in bones if face. Neuralgia of trigeminus after suppressed gonorrhea. Facial pains spreading to neck and head. Scabious, itching eruption on face. Red, painful nodosities on temples. Tumors and warts on the lips. Flat ulcers on inside of lips and corners of the mouth. Fungus on left lower jaw, more angry in damp weather; swelling of submaxillary glands. Toothache after drinking tea; many complaints are worse from the excess of tea and THUJ. is the best antidote.

MOUTH: Carious teeth and very sensitive inflamed swollen gums with losseness of the teeth. Aphthae and ulcers in the mouth which feels as if burned. Salvation with swollen salivary glands. Swelling of the tongue, painful ulcers on tongue; condylomata under tongue, varicose veins under the tongue. Sweet taste with gonorrhea; slowness of speech.

THROAT: Painful sore throat with dryness and necessity to swallow. Swelling of tonsils and throat with ulcers like chancres. Large accumulation of mucous in the throat that is tenacious and hawked up with difficulty. Exophthalmic goiter.

STOMACH: The appetite is impaired and taste perverted, either sweet or like rotten eggs. Craves salt. Food never seems salty enough. Desires cold drings and food. Unable to eat breakfast, a keynote of Burnett's. Aversion to fresh meat and potatoes, speedy satiety when eating (LYC.), aggravated by onions (also LYC.). Many distresses after eating.

Bitter or putrid risings and greasy substances. Nausea and vomiting of acid serum and of food. Indurations of stomach and abdomen.

ABDOMEN: Soreness in hepatic region, pressing and constrictive pains through the whole abdomen. Sensation as if something was alive in the abdomen. Intussusception of the intestines; obstinate constipation; tenesmus with rigidity of the penis. Diarrhea, pale yellow, watery, forcibly expelled with much noisy wind and colic; worse after eating; very exhausting with short and difficult breathing; anxiety, intermitting pulse, acute pressive pain in the back.

RECTUM: Rapid disappearance of fat; periodic diarrhea at the same hour; stools oily or greasy, with the passing stool sensation as if burning lead were passing through. Burning soreness in rectum lasting all day. Painful contraction of anus during evacuation. Condylomata at anus. Hemorrhoidal tumor, swollen and painful, worse while sitting. Fistula in ano; fissure of anus.

URINARY ORGANS: Kidneys inflamed, feet swollen, diabetes. Violent burning in fundus of bladder. Frequent urging to urinate with interrupted stream. Bladder and rectum feel paralyzed, lacking power to expel; involuntary emission of urine.

MALE GENITALIA: The genitalia of both sexes are the site of much suffering, the characteristic stigmata of the venereal poisons are prominent. Warts, chancres, ulceration, polypi, cauliflower excrescences, and offensive catarrhal discharges that are painful and burning with swellings, and morbid growths abound.

FEMALE GENITALIA: In the female, varicosities that are painful and burning. With the menses the breasts are painful and swollen; violent motion of the child in the womb during gestation. Abortion at the end of the third month is a feature of THUJ. Labor pains weak or ceasing, contractibility hindered by sycotic complications.

RESPIRATORY ORGANS: The respiratory tract presents many distressing symptoms and conditions. The voice is weak or low. Sensation of a skin in the larynx; polypus of the vocal cord, shortness of breath from mucous in the trachea. Asthma, worse at night, with red face, coughing spells with sensation of adhesion of the lungs. Asthma with gonorrhea without having been exposed to contagion. Asthma with little cough. Asthma of sycotic children. Respiration short and quick, worse from deep inspiration and talking, relieved lying on affected side. Convulsive asthma. Cough in the morning excited by a choking sensation. Sputa green, tasting like old cheese. Spasms of lungs from drinking cold water.

Oppression and dyspnoea; pain in chest as from internal adhesion; hemorrhage from lungs copious and terribly offensive. Cramp in heart with violent and audible palpitation of heart, especially climbing stairs. Anxious palpitation or visible palpitation without anxiety.

BACK AND LIMBS: The neck, back and limbs are recipient of much suffering and weakness too numerous to mention here. THUJ. is a paralytic remedy. However among afflictions of these parts is gonorrheal rheumatism and left-sided sciatica with the affected leg atrophied. Emaciation and deadness of affected parts.

SLEEP: Sleep and dream symptoms are important and often guiding. Sleep retarded because of agitation and dry heat. Nocturnal sleeplessness with agitation and coldness of the body. Unrefreshing nocturnal sleep. Distressing, anxious dreams, of danger, of death and the dead, of falling from a height soon after falling asleep. Starting and crying out in sleep. Sleeplessness with apparitions as soon as he closes his eyes, which vanish when he opens them; lascivious dreams without emission of semen, but with painful erections on waking.

FEVER, CHILL AND SWEAT: Perspiration at commencement of sleep. Perspiration on parts uncovered with dry heat of covered parts; perspiration after the chill without intervening heat; persiration at times oily, staining th clothes yellow, or fetid, or smelling sweet like honey. Perspiration only during sleep.

GENERALITIES: Typically a left-sided remedy, < by touch, > by pressure; rubbing >. Closing eyes < the vertigo. Overlifting < the head pains. Lying on affected side > the asthma. Motion >. < extension and letting limbs hang down. < at 3.00 a.m., early morning (the sycotic hour). < at night, < cold water, damp weather, change, draught, overheating, sun's rays, bright light, warmth of bed. Warmth < except the rheumatism which is > by cold. < after eating, especially breakfast, tea, coffee, fat food and onions. < after coitus. < blowing nose. < during increasing moon; from sun and bright light.

Causation of complaint: Vaccination; gonorrhea badly treated or suppressed; sunstroke; sexual excess; tea; coffee; beer; sweets; tobacco; fat meats; onions; SULPH. and MERC.

New Remedies and New Aspects of Old Remedies[1]

Euphorbium, Malaria officinalis, Paeonia, Kali thiocyanatum

The Homeopathic Materia Medica is so rich in therapeutic worth that one wonders what need is there for new remedies. But as we use the Materia Medica and study its vast storehouse of knowledge we discover new and valuable aspects to our well proven polycrests and many of our partial and fragmentarily proven remedies need further study and development as such study often brings most happy results in difficult and baffling cases of illness.

Regarding new remedies it is patent that we need many more of the type corresponding to the chronic diseases that are constantly increasing and which, because of the complexities of living conditions now prevailing, becoming more resistant to treatment - such as cancer and the various blood diseases and many others of the degenerative type, to say nothing of the great increase in mental and nervous breakdowns. Insanity and psychopathic abnormalities are increasing so fast that it is becoming difficult to house and care for them properly. Hence the bad effects of overcrowding and inadequate personnel to treat and care for them and all this tends to aggravate rather than help these unfortunates.

A few examples are set forth here to illustrate the possibility of curative power residing in the remedy best adapted to the individual patient for whom it is selected.

Euphorbium

Euph. is one of our fairly well proven remedies and it has been found useful in a goodly number of chronic and difficult diseases, including cancer and bone diseases. Especially has it been efficacious in the relief of the severe burning pains of cancer. Clarke describes a desperate case of sarcoma of the pelvic bones that found relief in repeated doses of this remedy, 6th potency.

---

1. The Homeopathic Recorder, Vol. LXVIII, No. 6, December, 1952, p. 15. The original article also covered the two Cadm-o. and Oci., which were published earlier. Therefore we deleted the paragraph on Cadm-o. which is printed it in the article "Differentiating Symptoms of Some of the Cadmium Salts" p. 13. The text of Oci. has been incorporated in the article "Neglected and Little Used Remedies" p. 117 to keep the materia medica of Oci. in one place. - Editor.

EUPHORBIUM ...

In its pathogenesis can be found the prostration and weakness with the burning pains and restlessness that belong to ARS. The pains are worse during rest and at night like ARS.; the patient is chilly and shudders with the cold. The anxiety in EUPH. is not as marked as the dreadful fear of death found in the ARS. provings. It is easy to differentiate between these two very similar remedies by their polarity.[1] EUPH. being negative magnetically and ARS. being bi-polar. Diseases that are magnetically positive such as cancer require a remedy from the magnetically negative group, the totality of symptoms finally decides.

A case of an aged lady in her seventies had been under careful homeopathic prescribing for several years with only a moderate degree of help. A sudden acute condition came on which caused her family to be alarmed. Her physician was not available at the time so a local physician (allopathic) was called in to attend her. She was rushed to the hospital and given all the tests and soon her family was told that she had cancer of the liver in late stages and nothing could be done but palliation until the end.

The old lady full of faith and assurance that her homeopathic doctor could help her insisted on going back to this treatment. The family feeling there was nothing to loose consented and sent for a remedy as the patient was unable to come to the office. A small sample of blood on blotting paper was submitted and EUPH. came through, symptomatically and magnetically. It was given in the 10M with astounding results. The jaundice and weakness cleared rapidly, the emaciation was changed to plumpness and all pain and discomfort ceased enabling the patient to sleep and enjoy all her usual routine even to the resumption of household duties. Two years have gone by and the patient remains well and happy; this may not be a cure but at least there has been several years of comfortable living.

EUPH. should be studied more, as I believe it to be one of our so-called forgotten remedies. Gangrene, with burning pain, of old persons who are weak and cold; erysipelatous bullosa; persistant stomach ulcers that fail to respond to the more usual remedies like PHOS. and ARS. will heal under EUPH. Indolent ulcers that burn like coals of fire and resist the usually well selected remedies will heal under this remedy.

---

1. See "Recent Concepts and New Formulas in Medicine" p. 679 and "Importance of Electronic Reactions to Future Medicine" p. 683. - Editor.

EUPHORBIUM ...

A chronic cough that comes on as soon as the patient touches the bed, coming in two violent attacks and continued as long as she remained lying down; cough was accompanied by pain in right temple; cold feet and a pain in the heel. After failure of many remedies EUPH. drop doses of tincture in a glass of water, to be sipped occasionally gave instant relief, but the patient had to continue the remedy or the cough returned.[1]

Sudden starting up in bed as from an electric shock is an unusual symptom that belongs to this remedy. Periodic cramps and convulsions with loss of consciousness is a feature. Most symptoms are worse at night and in the morning. Rest aggravates, motion ameliorate RHUS-T., ARS. and KALI-I.). Heat aggravates, cool applications ameliorate, a differentiating symptom from ARS.

We have presented only a very brief synopsis of this wonderful remedy. It will repay the physician magnificently for his study of it.

MALARIA OFFICINALIS

MALAR.: This remedy has been called the vegetable Pyrogen and it seems appropriate, as it is produced from decaying vegetation, while Pyrogen is the product of decaying flesh. This remedy is magnetically neutral and fits in with neutral diseases such as flu, T. B. and malaria.

There are instances where malaria has cured tubercular disease. As great an authority as Hering relates an experience of his own in a converse sense. He was exposed to the swampy Isthmus of Panama for nine days, on the ship's return several of the sailors who were like him exposed to the swampy influence, were prostrated with Panama fever, while Hering who had formerly suffered from tubercular disease of the lungs was unaffected by the experience.

Dr. Bowen of Indiana[2], the producer and prover of this remarkable remedy gave to a lady apparently in the last stages of consumption, herself the last survivor of five, the rest of her family having died of consumption as well as several of the preceding generation, a dose of a watery solution of the remedy. On the fifth day she had a fairly perceptible chill and a harder one on the sixth and seventh day. Antidotes were required but when cured of her malaria, her tuberculosis infection was also cured.

---

1. Clarke's Dictionary of Practical Materia Medica, p. 738, Münninghoff case report. - Editor
2. See Clarke: Dictionary of Practical Materia Medica, Vol. II, p. 392 ff.

MALARIA OFFICINALIS ...

Another case of Bowen's was Mrs. R. 45 years old, weight 245 lbs. She could scarcely walk from rheumatism in her back and limbs. This was of two years standing. MALAR. 1x was given, ten pills three or four times a day; in a week all rheumatism and lameness were gone.

Mr. S., foreman in a large saw mill where his work involved frequent wettings, had rheumatism of malarial nature worse by Quinine and external applications. He was given MALAR. 1x, in three days he was better and soon had relief from pain and was greatly improved in general health.

Mr. I. S. age fifty-five. Veteran and pensioner, bronzed in color. Unable to walk for years. He had heart, chest and hemorrhoidal troubles which were remedied but still he could not walk or get out of a chair. His back had been injured while in the army. RUTA and RHUS-T. enabled him to get up and take one or two steps. Bowen concluded that the complaint was really rheumatism of malarial origin and gave MALAR. 1x, ten pills three or four times a day. In a week the patient went to Bowen's home and walked up and down a flight of steps alone. In five more days he walked three miles in one morning. He put on flesh and seemed ten years younger.

Dr. Yingling was equally successful with the use of this remedy in potencies ranging to the 1M.

The clinical application of this remarkable remedy demonstrates its value and effectfulness in serious states of illness after the failure of other remedies. It needs further provings and study. It has proven effective in very resistant, relapsing types of fever, especially those based on tubercular or malarial causation.

PAEONIA

PAEON.: This is another little remedy too often over-looked by the profession in the treatment of hemorrhoids, fissure and ulcerating conditions of the rectum.

The female sexual organs are markedly disturbed with this remedy. The external genitals are swollen and painful.

Sleep is greatly disturbed with dreams, many unremembered but others voluptuous with emissions or anxious vivid dreams of death or frightful death of relatives which make sleep unrefreshing.

Paeonia ...

Rat., Nit-ac. and Sil. need be compared with this remedy in the special conditions mentioned those refering to rectal and hemorrhoidal complaints.

Kali thiocyanatum

Another new remedy that needs proving and developing to place it where it belongs in the realm of cure is Kali-thio-cyanide (KCNS). It is magnetically negative and corresponds to a wide range of chronic conditions such as severe types of nerve and blood disorders. In crude laboratory experiments on rats a highly interesting result was obtained, proving its intricate tie up with the vital processes of life. Those members of a litter that were given regulated doses of this drug obtained a life span one-third greater than those of the same litter not receiving the drug. We have no proven indications for its homeopathic use, but clinically when prescribed by the blood selection it has cured inveterate cases of arthritis and severe types of heart and kidney disease after the failure of other carefully selected homeopathic remedies.

Conclusion

The object of this paper is to call attention to these remedies for further study and trial by as many doctors as possible thereby gaining more knowledge quickly for future use.

Neglected and Little Used Remedies[1]

Eryngium aquaticum, Erythrinus, Erythroxylon coca, Ocimum canum

The Homeopathic Materia Medica is a treasury of medical knowledge for the cure of the sick and is of inestimable value. For years much of its contents has remained dormant and undeveloped for the benefit of human needs. A short review of some of these neglected jewels in the homeopathic treasury might stimulate study and provings for more perfect and extended use of these agents of cure.

Some of our good homeopaths have contended that our Materia Medica is too big and cumbersome to handle because of limited time in the lives of every busy prescriber. But more proficient use of repertories and the application of the new technique and approach of the electro-magnetic classification of remedies save much time and labor and make for greater accuracy in prescribing.

All remedies, in fact all substances in nature, fall into four definite classes relative to polarity, viz positive, negative, bi-polar and neutral. The blood of each patient falls into one of these polarity groups. When the patient's polarity is known, three fourths of the remedies in the Materia Medica are removed from study in the case; only the required polarity group that the polarity of the patient's blood requires is needed for further study repertorial, symptomatic, etc. By this method we can use many little proved remedies in a specific case with wonderful effect, with increased accuracy, and with much time saved.

Eryngium aquaticum

Ery-a. is electro-magnetically negative, of wide range of action and very little used. It acts extensively on the mucous membranes everywhere, producing thick yellow discharges from eyes, ears, nose, mouth, bowels, urethra and vagina. Hemorrhages from stomach and bowels.

It antidotes the effects of blows like Arn.

It has cured renal colic with calculli on left side. Seminal and prostatic weakness.

Clarke lists among cured symptoms and conditions conjunctivitis, constipation, cough, diarrhea, dropsy, gleet, gonorrhea, hemorrhoids,

---

1. From the handwritten manuscript of Dr. Grimmer, dated October 1952. - Editor.

ERYNGIUM AQUATICUM ...

influenza, laryngitis, leucorrhea, renal colic, sclerotitis, sexual weakness, strabismus, spermatorrhea, incontinence of the urine and wounds.

MIND: The mind is dull and confused without the ability to concentrate, and if the effort is persisted in, a heavy full pain is brought on.

HEAD: In the head there is vertigo with expanding sensation in the frontal region above the eyes. Stooping causes dimness of sight; sharp shooting pain over left eye; when sitting in a stooped position, pain leaves eye, passes into neck and along muscles of shoulder and beneath scapula. Shooting in coronary region and in right side of face from eyes to teeth in the morning. Dull dragging pain in occiput, neck and shoulders; when less severe in head is worse in shoulder. Scalp sore, combing hair is painful.

EYES: Eyes burning and sensitive to light. Bad effects from exposure to strong light, squinting; sclero-iritis, watery or purulent discharge.

Purulent inflammation of left eye; purulent sticking discharges causing gumming of the lids; conjunctiva, granular and rough. Muscles of eyes feel stiff, pain on moving them quickly.

EARS: bruised; tearing pain; as if ears were being torn off. Inflammation of eustachian tube; left ear swollen inside and outside; tender to pressure; constant aching and bleeding readily; thick white, bloody, foul smelling pus. Continued singing and ringing with creaking sound in left ear.

NOSE: Profuse thich yellow discharge from the nose.

MOUTH: Thick, tenacious, disagreeable mucous in mouth.

THROAT: Smarting raw pain along left side of throat with dry tongue. Intense redness or slight swelling without pain, profuse secretion of thick white mucous.

STOMACH: Anorexia, nausea followed by acrid eructations. Hollow empty feeling in stomach with heavy dragging pain. Spitting up bright arterial blood mixed with black clots, with burning in epigastrium after a blow on stomach. Burning in stomach or esophagus after taking the drug.

ABDOMEN: Severe colicky or cramping pains in small intestines. Severe pain in left groin and testicle.

RECTUM: Mucous diarrhea of children; constipation; stools dark leaden color, dry and very hard; tenesmus at stool with a sensation of cutting as they pass through anus. Hemorrhoids and prolapsus ani.

Eryngium aquaticum ...

Urinary Organs: Frequent desire to urinate; stinging burning pain in urethra, behind glans, during urination. Must urinate every five minutes. Urine dropping away all the time and burning like fire. Renal colic.

Male Genitalia: In the male, desire suppressed then excited with lewd dreams and pollutions; discharge of prostatic fluid from slightest causes. Spermatorrhea from onanism and excessive indulgence. Emissions at night with erections followed by great lassitude and depression. Partial impotence, emissions without erections day and night followed by great lassitude after injury to testicles. Gonorrhea with painful erections, gleet.

Female Genitalia: Leucorrhea.

Respiratory organs: Chronic laryngitis, short hacking cough; cough with sensation of constriction in throat; oppression of chest; feeling of fullness, inability to take a long breath.

Erythrinus

Eryth. is electro-magnetically negative. It is a kind of red mullet of South America and a tincture of the fish. Dr. Burnett is the authority for the action of this remedy. He based its use from the effects on sailors who ate the fish. They came out with a peculiar red rash which became chronic and which the doctors took for a form of syphilis. Dr. Burnett cured, with it, a case of pityriasis rubra appearing in a large patch on the chest and benefitted other cases. He believes this form of skin affection to be a manifestation of syphilis in the second generation, the father of the patient he cured having had syphilis. Aur-m. is the complementary remedy. Eryth. needs further proving as it well might be a remedy highly valuable in forms of chronic skin disease.

Erythroxylon coca

Coca is another magnetically negative remedy that is not used as much as it should be. It could be used to great advantage in certain types of sickness. It should be a wonderful remedy in states of nervous exhaustion due to both mental and physical strain.

Peculiar sensations and hallucinations are present. Sensation under the skin as if small foreign bodies were present, something like grains of sand; or crawling on skin as if bugs were crawling or a feeling of a worm or worms under the skin. Imagines that in the skin are worms moving

Erythroxylon coca ...

along; these worms are only seen on the prover's own linen or in his skin or crawling along his pen holder. He does not see these things on other people's clothes, nor on clean linen, only associated with things pertaining to his own person.

MIND: The chronic mentals are those of deep depression, melancholy, hypochondriasis, mental depression with drowsiness. Prefers solitude and darkness. Muddled feeling in the brain, loss of energy, great mental excitement in the acute states.

VERTIGO: Vertigo and fainting with tension across forehead like a rubber band.

HEAD: Headache just over the eyebrows not constant, worse raising head or turning eyes up. Shocks in head; dull feeling in occiput with vertigo, worse lying down; the only possible position is on his face. Occiput painful and tender to touch, aggravated by coughing. Headache with chilliness, with dryness of throat relieved after eating and at sunset.

EYES: Intolerance of light with dilated pupils; dark cloud before eyes eyes deeply reddened until bloody tears gushed out. White, dark and fiery spots before the eyes, flickering or flashing in the field of vision. Indistinct vision soon followed by headache with nausea. Aching pain behind the eyes causing feeling as if squinting inwardly.

EARS: In the ears sounds of buzzing or humming with fever.

NOSE: Epistaxis passing from right to left nostril; sense of smell greatly diminished.

MOUTH AND THROAT: Dry mouth on awakening. Uvula feels swollen, swallowing difficult.

STOMACH: This drug retards hunger and thirst and enabled the Indians to perform long periods of exertion, running, climbing mountains, etc. without the sense of fatigue. Loss of appetite for solid foods; craves spirits and tobacco. Ailments from salt food. Flatus rises with such force it seems the esophagus would be rent by it. Emptyness or fullness felt in stomach. Confirmed dyspepsia especially in hypochondriacs.

ABDOMEN: Pressure and tension in the abdomen after meals. Flatulence, violent bellyache with tympanitic distension.

STOOL AND ANUS: Flatus from bowels smell like burnt gunpowder. Dysentery. Constipation from inactivity of rectum, stools dry like walnuts; piles painful on walking or sitting. Sphincters relaxed.

Erythroxylon coca ...

Urinary Organs: Fine stitches in female urethra before urinating. Frequent desire with increased flow, frequency at night. Nocturnal enuresis; film on urine; urine smells like sweat; yellowish red flocculent deposits; oily scum on surface of urine.

Male Genitalia: In the male, sensation as if the penis was absent. Coldness; gone sensation; relaxation of external parts; emissions; nervous prostration from sexual excesses. Spermatorrhea; partial impotence; satyriasis.

Female Genitalia: Menstrual flow of the female comes in gushes waking her from sound sleep; nymphomania during menses and after parturition.

Respiratory Organs: In the respiratory organs there is weakness of voice. Phthisis of the larynx when from irritability of the pharynx, the stomach will retain no food. Rapid breathing. Painful shortness of the breath at night. Short breath in athletes or those using alcohol or tobacco in excess. Hemoptysis. On coughing there is pain in occiput. Cough from cold air or fast walking. Expectoration of small lumps like boiled starch, immediately after rising in the morning.

Chest: Sudden attacks of cramps in the chest; becomes cold and unable to continue the ascent (mountain climbing). Intense oppression in chest. Rush of blood to chest with slight headache. Emphysema.

Heart: Palpitation of heart with flushing, violent and audible palpitation;angina pectoris from climbing or over exertion; pulse greatly accelerated and intermittent, looses one beat in four.

Limbs: Feeling of internal coldness with numbness of hands and feet, weakness of the extremities.

Skin: Scarlatina like rash over body, especially the neck.

Sleep: Inclination to sleep but can find no rest. Great drowsiness.

Fever, Chill and Perspiration: Sense of flushing especially up back with palpitation. Chilliness and headache in the afternoon. At night heat and sleeplessness with throbbing in the arteries. Flushes of heat on the back and burning in abdomen. Extreme weariness accompanies the fever. Night sweats.

Ocimum canum[1]

Oci. Magnetically bi-polar. A most valuable remedy for afflictions of the kidneys and bladder and especially for the relief and cure of renal calculus and gravel. Renal colic of the most severe type where stones
lodged in the urinary passages and blocked the urinary flow.

We owe this remedy to Mure, who tells us that it is used in Brazil as a specific for diseases of the kidneys, bladder and urethra. Renal colic with violent vomiting every fifteen minutes. Red urine with brick-dust sediment after the attack. The urine may be saffron color, or thick purulent with an intolerable smell of musk. In renal colic this remedy has been curative after many of our better proven remedies have failed.

Our proving is very fragmentary. A few clinical observations may serve as indications; swelling of the inguinal glands; (even bubo has been cured). Diarrhea, several attacks daily. The urine is turbid depositing a white and albuminous sediment after renal attacks. Burning during micturition; urine saffron or red (bloody) with brick dust sediment. Cramping pains in kidneys; renal colic right or left with violent vomiting causing the patient to twist and turn about, wrings her hands, screams and groans during an attack.

In the male sexual organs there is heat, swelling and excessive sensitivity of the left testicle.

In the female sexual organs lancinations in the labia majora. Swelling of the whole vulva; falling of the vagina so as to issue even from the vulva. Itching of the breasts; engorgement of the mammary glands. The tips of the breasts are very painful, and the least contact extorts a cry. Compressive pain in the breast as in the case of wet nurses.

Numbness of the right thigh for two days. It is employed in baths for rheumatism.

Acts on skin as an irritant.

Dreams about being poisoned, dreams about her parents, friends, children.

Is a sudorific, it is used in bilious remittent fevers.

The scope of usefulness for this remedy would be much enhanced with further provings. Physicians do not use this remedy as much as they should. It is one of our best remedies for very serious and painful complaints.

---

1. See footnote p. 112. - Editor.

CLINICAL NOVELTIES[1]

OXYDENDRON ARBOREUM; SCROPHULARIA NODOSA; PARTHENIUM; SOLANUM INTEGRI

Some random notes on a few little used and little known remedies will be of interest if not of use. However, if homeopathic provings could be made of them a valuable asset to the Homeopathic Materia Medica would be obtained, with new and powerful agents of cure.

OXYDENDRON ARBOREUM

The little known remedy OXYD., or Sorrell or Elk tree - growing in the rich woods of the Alleghanies, Natural order: Ericaceae (tribe Andreomedia). Made into a tincture of the leaves. Clinical use in Dropsy - ascites and anasarca.

Clarke says OXYD. is the only species of its genus.

There are no provings: and only one reported cure by M. E. Douglass in a woman of a general dropsy - ascites and anasarca which dated from an attack of measles treated with ice drinks and ice applications seven months before; the urine was nearly suppressed but contained little albumen; menses suppressed; great difficulty of breathing even when sitting, lying down impossible; the skin of the legs burst in several places. After APOC. and several carefully chosen remedies failed to help, Oxydendron tincture - three drams in a tumbler of water - three teaspoonfuls of the mixture every three hours was given with relief of the respiration in forty-eight hours. After ten days the patient was able to lie down in bed; in the interval, RHUS-T. was given to combat an erysipelas of left leg. In two months the patient was free of dropsy and felt perfectly well though much emaciated.

William Boericke mentions prostatic enlargement. Vesical calculi and irritation of neck of bladder as being amenable to its action.

My experience with this remedy was in the case of a young married man, 23 years of age who came to my office November 19, 1942 suffering with acute diffuse nephritis which followed the extraction of a large number of infected teeth; extremities were badly swollen with considerable ascites. The only thing complained of was many dizzy headaches; blood pressure 160/90; heart sounds weak and fast but regular; urine albuminous and loaded with granular and hyaline casts. The general

---

1. THE HOMEOPATHIC RECORDER, Vol. LXIV, No. 5, November 1948, p. 126.

Oxydendron arboreum ...

health had always been good. The patient had been treated several months before I saw him by regular physicians of the old school. There were no therauptic symptoms only common and diagnostic symptoms were present for the selection of the remedy. AUR-I. 10M, MERC-S. 10M, and KALI-AR. 10M were given within an interval of about ten days apart. After each remedy the patient grew worse, becoming more bloated with fluid and gradually finding it harder to get his breath. After a month he was a pitiable sight, distended to abnormal proportions and unable to lie down, and found it almost impossible to move.

Apparently this was an incurable case, but in desperation the patient consented to a test of his blood for remedy selection. OXYD. was the only remedy in several hundred of the polarity group to which his blood belonged to come through. It was given in the two hundredth potency with most amazing and rapid improvement in the patient's symptoms and well being. The potency was repeated in 3 weeks and later several doses of the 10M were given at month intervals, followed by the 50M and CM potencies to complete the cure in about 6 months when the patient returned to his work as a truck driver, and has remained on the job until the present time. Some three years have elapsed with the patient remaining strong and well but still considerably under weight, (135 lbs.) for his height (6 feet).

From this brief review of the little known drug we could expect much greater things from its use by a complete homeopathic proving.

Scrrophularia nodosa

SCROPH-N. is another remedy needing a complete proving to bring out tremendous powers of cure. It has specific affinity for the breast, dissipating tumors after CON. fails. The glands are markedly affected; also its action on the skin is strong. Eczema in and around the ears. Pruritus vaginae, lupoid ulceration, scrofulous swelling (CIST.), painful hemorrhoids, tubercular testis, ephithelioma, nodosities in the breasts (SCIR.) are some of the clinical conditions this remedy has proved curative in. Clarke's Dictionary gives the fullest account of its uses and symptoms but a full proving is really needed to obtain the best values inherent in this wonderful remedy.

PARTHENIUM

PARTH. or Escoba amaraga (Bitter-broom) is another fragment of a proving. We should have a wider and more specific knowledge of, to be had only by a Hahnemannian proving.

Dr. W. Boericke summerizes what is known of this remedy briefly, to wit: A Cuban remedy for fevers, especially malarial fevers. Increased flow of milk, Amenorrhea and general debility. Cheyne-Stokes breathing, after Quinine. Headaches extending to nose (feels swelled, pain in frontal eminence). Eyes heavy, eye balls ache. Ringing in ears. Pain at root of nose. Aching in teeth, teeth feel on edge, or too long. Disordered vision. Tinnitus and pain in ears. Pain in left hypochondrium. Spleen affections.

Modalities: Worse after sleep, sudden motion. Better, after rising and walking about. Compare: CHIN., CEAN., HELIA.

SOLANUM INTEGRI

In the Solanaceae group are found some of our most wonderful remedies for the cure of a wide variety of human ills. But perhaps the greatest one of this group which our literature has no mention of is the SOLANIUM INTEGRI, the love apple or wild tomato, growing wild in the waste lands of Florida.

Several years ago, while visiting there, I procured one of the plants with their fruit and sent it to our able pharmacist and good friend Mr. Ehrhart of Chicago for identification and preparation of tincture and potencies of this plant, having first tested the whole plant and fruit for its polarity and vibratory rates of disease contained therein.

It belongs to the positive group and corresponds to rates of malignant disease of various types such as tuberculosis and degenerative types of disease. In the past this remedy in potency only, 30th and higher by means of testing it over the patients blood to ascertain its homeopathic relation to each specific case tested. The results in a great number of seriously ill cases have been uniformly good.

The most outstanding cases were those of chronic bronchial asthma. One very unusual case of a doctor, who has suffered for almost a lifetime and had tried all forms of medication for relief including good Homeopathic prescribing with only occassional slight relief. One month after one dose of the 30th potency of SOLANIUM INTEGRI the patient reported being almost entirely free of asthma and felt better

SOLANUM INTEGRI ...

than ever before in his life. The patient is still improving after 6 months and is now on the ten thousandth potency of the remedy.

Surely here is another remedy that, when proved homeopathically, will be a mighty weapon in the hands of the physician to relieve and cure one of the most intractable and terrible diseases: asthma.

CONCLUSION

We trust these rambling notes may not be too tiresome for your attention and that we may form a proving class to really bring out the great possibilities of cure all these remedies possess.

The Spider Poisons[1]

The ARACHNIDA species provides healing qualities of wide range and unique conditions, with terrible states of mind and body not found in the same degree in other medical agents. A close study of these medicines produced from the spider family will enable the prescriber to cure where other agents have failed.

The object of this paper is to call attention to the importance and value of these remedies rather than recount a detailed statement of the numerous symptoms which can easily be obtained from the Materia Medica. Carke's Dictionary records the fullest and best treatise to be had.

Aranea diadema

ARAN. (the Cross Spider) is one of our neglected and forgotten remedies not mentioned by Anschutz in his volume of NEW, OLD AND FORGOTTEN REMEDIES.

This remedy is of wide-range and profoundly deep in action, curing conditions which are of long standing, chronic and of an obstinate resisting nature to the ordinary remedies; in other words, it cures after other seemingly indicated remedies fail.

It deeply affects the nervous system, the blood and circulatory system, the bones and the glands, especially the liver and spleen. It depresses the mental sphere profoundly, causing deep despondency and longing for death like AUR.

It belongs to GRAUVOGL'S HYDROGENOID group of remedies in its extreme sensitiveness to wet, cold, rainy weather and even bad effects from bathing. Remedies like CALC., DULC., RHUS-T. and NAT-S. are in this group. It is a hemorrhagic remedy producing long-lasting, copious and too frequent menses. Metrorrhagia, bright colored blood. Dysmenia, spasms commencing in stomach. Viscous leucorrhea.

From the respiratory organs violent hemoptysis in anemic debilitated subjects. Hemorrhage from wounds. Punctured wounds. General weakness even to a state of exhaustion is noted.

---

1. From the handwritten manuscript of Dr. Grimmer, exact date unknown. The major part of this article is taken from: Clarke, John H., A DICTIONARY OF PRACTICAL MATERIA MEDICA; The London Homeopathic Publishing Co., London 1900. - Editor.

ARANEA DIADEMA ...

Pain is an outstanding feature of this remedy, the pains are periodic at clock-like regular intervals like CEDR., but CEDR. is worse in hot climates and ARAN. is aggravated in cold, wet or rainy weather.

The pains are severe and often violent, making rest impossible and driving the patient out of bed like ARS., RHUS-T., SYPH. and TARENT.

Severe frontal headache relieved by smoking tobacco and going out into the open air. Headache with confusion, vertigo and flickering before the eyes, worse sitting up, must lie down; confusion when studying; pressure as if in the bones of the right temple with pressure of the hand relieving. Headache with burning eyes and heat of face. Glimmering and glittering before the eyes preceding headache. Burning, stinging and shooting pain in the eyes.

In the teeth and mouth there is much suffering. Painfulness of the teeth as soon as he goes to bed in the evening. Sharp, sensitive sensation as of cold in the teeth (incisors) every day at the same hour. Sudden violent pains in teeth of whole upper and lower jaws at night immediately after lying down.

Instantly a painful sensation as though arising from several points darted along the tongue painfully affecting the tongue, jaws and head, like an instantaneous electric shock. Tongue seemed almost paralyzed, utterance thick and heavy and the pains at root of tongue and in lower jaw, especially at the joint are most excruciating. Bitter taste with coated tongue relieved by smoking. Thirst during fever and during the greater part of the other sufferings. Dejection and lassitude with thirst, coryza with thirst.

Eating causes headache and spasms, vomiting with fever; epigastrium painful to pressure. Swelling of the spleen after intermittant fever suppressed by QUININE. Enlarged spleen with chilliness. Fullness and heaviness in the abdomen as from a stone with a sinking sensation in the epigastrium. Borborygmus in the abdomen and heaviness in the thighs every day at the same time.

This is a powerful remedy for the malaria cachexia where the acute attacks are brought on or aggravated by cold wet, rainy weather. Or when the attacks appear annually in the spring or autumn with the change from warmth to damp stormy weather.

The symptomatology of this remedy can be summed up into a few general features, viz. mental despondency, physical exhaustion, perio-

ARANEA DIADEMA ...

dicity, hemorrhagic tendencies, anemia, coldness and lack of vital heat, chronic deep-seated complaints.

ARANEARIUM TELA (TELA)

TELA (Cobweb of the Black Spider) furnishes us with an unusual but fragmentary remedy for sleeplessness. It rapidly lowers the frequency of the pulse rate and further tests and use make it a valuable remedy to reduce high blood pressure.

In some people it has produced a calm and delightful state of feeling followed by a disposition to sleep. The most delicious tranquillity resembling the action of OP. and followed by no bad effects. Twenty grains given to an old, infirm asthmatic produced slight but pleasant delirium. Muscular energy is increased, could not be kept in bed but danced and jumped about the room all night.

ARANEA SCINENCIA

ARAN-SC. (a Grey Spider) found in Kentucky on old walls does not spin a web. The most noted symptoms of this spider is a constant twitching of the under eyelids which brings it in relation to the choreic nature of MYGAL. The eyes are inflamed, weak, watery with swollen lids; rather profuse flow of saliva, sweet taste. Much dull stupid headache of considerable intensity, especially in the posterior part of head; unable to rest for it; could not collect thoughts with it. Felt as if he had been drinking. (This could suggest a helpful agent to relieve the effects of a hang-over.) Sleepiness, all symptoms worse in a warm room. Compare other spider remedies, AGAR., CARB-V., PULS., APIS, SULPH., KALI-S., all worse in a warm room.

LATRODECTUS KATIPO

LAT-K. is a native of New Zealand and some parts of California. Symptoms recorded are from the effects of the bites. The seat of the bite becomes immediately painful and swelling usually occurs. In some cases the swelling does not come on until some days after the bite.

In one case five days after the bite a scarlet papulous rash appeared on both extremities burning like fire. Lassitude, faintness, twitching and in one case trismus were noted. The symptoms were somewhat slow in evolution and in one, that of a girl bitten on the abdomen, death did not occur until six weeks after the bite.

Latrodectus katipo ...

MIND: Delirium half smothered by imperfect intoxication; nervous depression.

FACE: Anxious expression of the face, extreme pallor changing to blue tint of face and body. Jaws became stiff very soon, could not open mouth to eat and could scarcely articulate; *note the similarity to tetanus.*

STOMACH: Lost all desire for food after a fortnight, lingered six weeks and died.

ABDOMEN: Very severe drawing or cramping sensation in the abdomen.

RESPIRATION: Respirations almost ceased.

HEART: Almost pulseless, pulse scarcely more than twelve or fourteen beats per minute.

LOWER LIMBS: Severe shaking, burning pains extended from bite on foot up the limbs and seemed to center about the heel. Feet felt as if rudely lacerated by a dull instrument, waking him from sleep immediately.

GENERALITIES: Suffered long, wasting and losing all energy, having the appearance of one going into a decline. It was three months before he rallied and six before he recovered. Nervous twitching all over body, suddenly became faint and pallid. Large amounts of whiskey produced little impression except a feeling as though the affected side was drunk.

SKIN: A small red spot like a flea bite appeared on the skin. Bitten surface raised was large and round as a tea cup, the raised part white with red halo with pain, swelling and pain relieved by spirits of ammonia. The ammonia relieved the pain but not the swelling which was the size and shape of a hen's egg.

The bite remained a small purple point for nine days, on the tenth it began to swell and turn white like a bee sting. Pain and swelling rapidly increases, dorsum of foot and ankle like a puff ball. Red streak running up leg typical of a streptococcus infection from infected wounds. A bright, scarlet papular eruption on both lower limbs, stinging and burning like fire.

FEVER: Extremities cold and flaccid. A cold, clammy sweat covered the left lower extremity and in the morning sweat covered both limbs.

The respiratory centers in the brain are markedly affected under the action of this remedy as well as the cardio-vascular centers and ganglia which control and regulate the heart function. In fact this is true of all

Latrodectus katipo ...

the spider poisons in varying degrees, greatest under the black widow, Lat-m. and least under Ther.

Latrodectus mactans

Lat-m. (the Black Widow) virus produces a typical replica of a severe attack of angina pectoris.

MIND: Extreme anxiety, screams fearfully exclaiming she will soon loose her breath and die.

STOMACH: The face and the vomiting of black vomit and a sinking sensation at the epigastrium.

STOOL: Two copious stools were similar to the black vomit.

RESPIRATORY ORGANS: Extreme apnea. Respiration only occasional, gasping.

HEART: Violent precordial pains extending to axilla and down left arm to fingers with numbness, later arm is almost paralysed. The pulse is 130 and so frequent it could not be counted and so feeble it could scarcely be felt. Screams with the pain and fears death.

GENERALITIES: When cupped the blood flowed like water and would not coagulate not even when tamin was added the next day. In thirty-six hours from the time the was bitten, he took three and one-half quart bottles of the best rectified whiskey without the least sign of intoxication. Itching and redness of the part bitten, at first without pain but violent pain soon followed at site of bite on back of left hand and extended in short time up forearm and arm to shoulder and thence to precordial region. Lay apparently moribund.

SKIN: Skin cold as marble.

Mygale

MYGAL. (a large black Cuban spider) has been clinically proved useful in chordee and gonorrhea as well as in aggravated cases of chorea. It has been of great use in carbuncles. This is not listed in Clarke. It affects the nerves, blood and lymphatics in marked degree. Clarke states "The pathogenetic data of MYGAL. consists of a proving by a young lady and the effect of a bite on a man."

In the latter case, inflammation ensued which spread along the lympathics; violet and afterwards green discoloration; chill followed by fever, dry mouth and great thirst; trembling, dyspnoea, despondency and fear of death.

Mygale ...

The prover developed sadness, dry mouth, nausea with great palpitation, dim sight and great general weakness, increased flow of urine, scalding and stinging in the urethea. This last symptom has led to the successful use of Mygal. in gonorrhea, chordee, and syphilis.

The trembling observed in the man suggests its use in nervous cases; but the sphere of Mygal. in chorea has been developed from the clinical side. In the cases cured with it, twitching and contractions of facial muscles have been very prominent. Convulsive movements of the head to right side, twitching of one side of the body; mostly right. (Ther. is mainly left sided). The twitching may be so violent as to prevent walking. Limbs are quiet during sleep (Agar.). Movements are < in the morning. Nausea and strong palpitation should be an indication. Symptoms are < by eating, < sitting. (Legs may be in constant motion.)

Delirious, talks about his business. Sad, despondent with sad expression, fear of death, nausea with dim sight; palpatation strong; acute ear pain. Constant twitching of muscles of face. Difficult breathing. Restless sleep all night with ridiculous dreams. Severe chill lasting thirty minutes, then fever and trembling of limbs.

Scorpio[1]

Scor. (the scorpion), a member of the spider family. Its poison is painful and even dangerous especially to children. Clinically it has proven useful in salivation, strabismus, tetanus.

The symptoms of the schema are from the effects of the stings; there are no provings[2]. Pain and swelling of the injured part are first experienced and constitutional symptoms follow. These include sleepiness, prostration and possible tetanus. Strabismus has been observed in some cases and the pupils are dilated. Among the symptoms noted are frequent sneezing, trismus, copious saliva and meteorism.

Scolopendra

Scol. (the centipede) though not of the spider family, it secrets a virus more similar to the spider toxins than any other insect produces. It has been used clinically in angina pectoris, convulsions and malig-

---

1. The symptoms in this schema are from various species and are found in Allen's Encyclopedia.
2. Recently an extensive proving of Androctonus amurreuxi hebraeus (another scorpion) was done by Jeremy Sherr. The Society of Homeopaths, Northhampton, England, 1990

Scolopendra ...

nant pustule. The writer has employed it successfully in a case of a vicious looking ulcer the size of a dime affecting the hard palate. It was of six months duration and very painful, making eating difficult. It had been diagnosed epithelioma by the patient's dentist after biopsy. In less than two months the ulcer was healed and the patient was much improved in health. Several doses of Scol. 10M wrought the cure.

The effects of the centipede bite have been observed on several patients. Swelling, pain, inflammation and gangrene of the bitten part, with appearance like malignant pustule in one case, were constant symptoms. Vomiting and precordial anxiety occurred and in one fatal case the paroxysms of vomiting increased in intensity till the child in a convulsive struggle ceased to breathe. A noted symptom; no perspiration of the right (bitten) arm for three months.

Among the symptoms listed vertigo, headache, vomiting of a pale yellow matter continued at frequent intervals with increasing violence until death. Arm greatly swollen, erysipelatous blush extending over half the arm, black-dotted impression in two rows, three-quarters of an inch apart raised in dark lines extending from dot to dot, five and one-half inches long showing the entrance of every foot, pain deep and dull. No perspiration on the bitten arm for three months. Instant complaint which grew rapidly worse which was described by the child as being "all-over". The child, a girl of four died in eight hours. On the skin a large red spot becoming black in the middle of which an eschar formed as large as a five franc piece. The whole affection resembled a malignant pustule and was associated with swelling of the lymphatic glands. Violent itching followed by violent pain in the bitten part.

Tarentula hispanica

Tarent.: The best known and most widely used of the spider poisons. It cures many chronic and intractable difficult conditions of disease.

The clinical use of the remedy listed by Clarke is proof of its wide range and deep action. Angina pectoris. Callosities. Chorea. Coccygodynia. Corneal opacities. Cystitis. Depressed Spirits. Diphteria. Dysmenorrhoea. Epistaxis. Erotomaina. Fibroma. Headache. Hiccough. Hysteria. Intermittents. Kleptomania. Levitation. Locomotor ataxia. Mamia. Meniere's disease. Migraine. Onanism. Ovarian enlargement. Paralysis agitans. Physometra. Proctalgia. Pruritis pudenda. Quinsy.

TARENTULA HISPANICA ...

Septic diseases. Spinal irritation. Spinal sclerosis. Tumors. Uterine cancer. Uterine neuralgia. Vertebrae tumors.

The mental and emotional symptoms are striking, unique and highly characteristic. The intense restlessness of the patient and especially of his lower extremities constitutes a certain and strong indication for its use. It affects the sexual sphere of both sexes profoundly causing uncontrollable desire and even mania. Yet intercourse intensifies the suffering of both sexes.

Music ameliorates the mental and physical sufferings in a remarkable degree. Also profuse perspiration seems to relieve at least the convulsive paroxysms and restless mania ended in profuse perspiration after the playing of music. Friction or rubbing the head and various parts comfort and relieve. Many of the mental symptoms are associated with sexual disorders. The sexual desire was so excited in a woman that when playing or dancing with men she hugged them before everybody and was angry when reproved, but did it again. Hysterical, alternating moods, laughing, crying, joking and profound melancholy. Though friction relieves many symptoms the spinal nerves are extremely sensitive to the least touch which cause spasmodic pain in the head and heart regions. This patient suffers paroxysms of insanity, presses her head, pulls her hair, repeated after intermissions, threatening manners and speech, restlessness of the legs, mocking laughter and joy expressed in her face; comes out of the attack with severe headache, eyes staring and wide open, sees small figures hovering before her eyes and moves her hands. Great excitement caused by music, one hour after it has general and copious sweat. Hysteria with bitter belching, < by moaning, > by sighing with repeated yawning. Ludicrous and lascivious visions of monsters, animals, faces, insects, ghosts. The colors red, yellow and green and particularly black produce heavy mist before the eyes. Sees strangers in the room. Great taciturnity and irritability. Desire to strike himself and others. Excessive gaiety, laughs at the slightest cause. Maniacally happy mood, joy and strong emotion when seeing beloved persons. Sings until hoarse and exhausted, fits of nervous laughter followed by screams. Profound grief and anxiety. Desires to take things which do not belong to her. Indifference, disgust and sadness from morning until 3 p.m. were marked, from 3 p.m. to evening the gay disposition returned. Wants to be without light, and without being spoken to. Irri-

TARENTULA HISPANICA ...

tability, rage, fury, mischievous, destructive, ennui, fear of impending calamity. Little intelligence and poor memory.

Many strange sensations afflict this patient. The neuralgia in the head are intense, as if thousands of needles were pricking to the brain, worse by touch, noise and strong light. Relieved by rubbing head against the pillow. Sensations as if hammered in the head and many parts. Sensations as if a hair in the eye; as if singing like a tea kettle in the ear; as if the lower teeth would fall out; as if a living body in the stomach were rising to the throat; as if there were not sufficient space in the hypogastrium; painful uneasiness in the coccyx; motion in uterus as of a foetus; as if heart turned and twisted around; heart as if squeezed and compressed; as if insects creeping and crawling.

TARENT. is suited to persons of hysterical and choreic tendencies who are foxy, mischieveous and destructive. Tickling, burning, numbness are prominent sensations. There is a great lack of vital heat and debilitating sweats that are cold. Aggravated by touch and rest yet must walk around even though made worse by it. Can run better than walk, worse at night. Worse washing head or wetting hands in cold water. Coitus aggravates. Light and sleep aggravate. Ameliorated by rubbing; motion > the headache but < uterine and coccyx pains. Fresh air and warm water relieve, riding in a carriage relieves the pain in spermatic cords. Epistaxis relieved throbbing in carotids. Falls, unrequited love, bad news, scolding, punishment and sepsis are contributing causes of complaints.

TARENTULA CUBENSIS

TARENT-C. (The Cuban Tarentula). This poison effects first the blood and cellular tissues profoundly and later the nervous system from the toxemia supervening. Its clinical use has been applied to carbuncle, chorea and intermittents.

Carbuncle even to sloughing with great prostration and diarrhea. Intermittent fever with evening exacerbation. A keynote symptom is atrocious pains.

A case of chorea in a girl of twelve; choreic movements confined to the left side and worse at night cured with the 6th centesimal potency. Anxiety, delirium, headache, diarrhea, retention of the urine and general toxemia are present. The bite is painless, the person is not sensible of it until the next day, when an inflamed pimple is found surrounded

Tarentula cubensis ...

by a scarlet areola; from the pimple to some other part of the body a red erysipelatous line is seen marking the line followed by the spider over the skin after biting. The pimple swells, the inflamed areola spreads, chills and fever set in with copious sweat and retention of the urine. The pimple becomes a hard, large and exceedingly painful abscess ending by mortification of the integuments over it and having several small openings discharging a thick sanious matter containing pieces of mortified cellular tissue fasciae and tendons; the openings by growing run into one another forming a large cavity.

At this period the fever takes the intermittent type with evening exacerbations. In two cases involving delicate children the bite proved fatal, but the majority recover in from three to six weeks. Chills followed by intense burning fever supervene on the second or third day with great thirst, anxiety, restlessness, headache, delirium, copious perspiration and retention of urine. Later the fever takes the intermittent type, with evening paroxysms accompanied by diarrhea and great prostration.

Theridion

Ther. (The Orange Spider). This remedy was introduced and proved by Hering. While similar in nature and scope to the other spiders it has many distinctive symptoms belonging to itself.

It effects the bones in a marked degree producing necrosis and caries and curing the same. It has cured Meniere's disease and ozena. Its effect on the nervous system is more intense than that of the other spiders and perhaps no other of our numerous remedies now known can equal the extreme sensibility to sensory impressions unless it be Mosch. in some respects and Bell. in others.

The extreme sensitiveness to noise, even slight noises are felt in the teeth. Jar and vibration of all kinds effect this subject more than that found in any other medicine. It is even greater than that found in Bell.

The vertigo of this remedy is unique in that it is worse from closing the eyes, even though there is great sensitiveness to light. The eyes are one of the centers strongly affected with much suffering occurring here. Riding in a carriage or a boat aggravates. With this highly sensitive, nervous individual there is weakness, trembling, coldness, anxiety, faintness and cold sweat.

THERIDION ...

H. C. Allen states that in scrofulosis when the seemingly best remedies fail to relieve this remedy may help.

There are hallucinations of sight and hearing. Luminious vibrations and rushing sounds. Aggravations from closing the eyes are associated with symptoms affecting the head and stomach being the leading indication for its use in seasickness and the sickness of pregnancy. Time passing too slowly is a symptoms of value for the selection of the remedy, although the text states: "Time appears to pass rapidly, although he does little." This remedy strongly affects the lungs and has cured phthisis florida in a number of cases.

Peculiar sensations of the remedy are: As if her head was another strange head; as if vertex did not belong to her; as if a veil before her eyes; as if too much air passed into nose and mouth; mouth as if furred, benumbed; as if someone tapped her on the groin when raising the leg; as if a lump were lying in perineal region; like labor pains in lower abdomen; as if a child were bounding in the body; as if something in the oesophagus were slipping towards epigastrium; as if bones were broken and would fall asunder; as if dying. Burning pains and itching are common. A stitch high up in apex of left chest has proved a guiding symptom in the cure of cases of phthisis. Burning in the liver region has lead to the cure of abscess and even cancer of that organ. The symptoms are < by touch, pressure, on ship board, riding in a carriage, closing eyes, jar, least noise; lying causes pain deep in brain. > by flickering before eyes. < by stooping, rising, motion, exertion, going up or down stairs, walking < the complaints of this patient. After washing clothes, nausea and fainting. < every night. Warm water > the nausea and retching. Warmth >. Cold <. Cold water feels too cold. Groin pains are worse from coition. Headache < after stool. Left side is most affected.

CONCLUSION

After a study of these fearful poisons and noting the tremendous upheavals produced by them, endangering life itself, disorganizing the bloodstream and disturbing the nervous system for months and even years after a single bite (one dose) as it were, of an infinitely small amount of the toxin one need no longer doubt the power of the small dose to heal whenever it is applicable (i.e. homeopathic) to the given case. It is indeed an overwhelming proof of the truth and worth of the homeopathic principle.

Unusual Remedies[1]

Toxicophis; Teucrium scorodina; Tilia; Congo Red

This paper should have been entitled unproven remedies. Such remedies may be used in cases that present no guiding symptoms for the selection of any known proven remedy. The knowledge of these drugs was chiefly obtained by their selection over the blood of the sick patients; and the symptoms given are those that were cured by the given drug. Some of the symptoms were the results of poisoning (as in snake bite).

Toxicophis

One of which is recorded under Toxicophis, the virus of the moccasin snake, in Clarke's Dictionary, page 1448.

CHARACTERISTICS: After the bite of this serpent, if the victim lives, symptoms of pain and fever recur annually at exactly the same period for many years with decreasing intensity each year. In one case the pain spread to other parts after some years.

LOWER LIMBS: Right leg became painful and swelled rapidly; for several years the pain was confined to the knee of the bitten limb. In a few years it left the knee and seized the hip and finally attacked the shoulder.

Note the chronic nature extending over years and the direction of the symptoms from below upwards and the exact periodicity of complaints. All these present a definite key in the treatment of related complaints. For eighteen years after the bite, one case continued to have an annual recurrence of symptoms of severe pain, but without swelling occurring at the same time of year.

Clinical Cases

CASE I. One case of sarcoma of the rectum in a five year old boy cured with this remedy. The tumor was painless but growing rapidly before the intervention of this remedy in the *30th potency*. The child presented few symptoms, the most marked being a persistant noctural enuresis which also was cured with the remedy. The general symptoms

---

1. From the handwritten manuscript of Dr. Grimmer, exact date unknown. A short discussion of Merc-k-i. in this paper was combined with the main article "Merc-iod. cum Kali-Iod." p. 143. - Editor.

TOXICOPHIS ...

of toxemia and apathy were present, complexion dark with a peculiar cachectic aspect. The child remains well after nearly three years.

CASE 2.[1] Another case of sarcoma of the tibia and fibula where this remedy was one of a series of four to restore the patient to health. A boy age nine. Father had had a severe syphlitic infection prior to marriage, treated homeopathically for an insufficient period. This boy, the oldest of a family of four, was the only unhealthy member. He first started with an iritis which was treated at the North Western medical clinic until the child was almost totally blind. KALI-BI. in several potencies cleared up the iritis and dissolved the scars over the pupils and gave back perfect vision as well as improving the general health for awhile. About a year later the boy was brought back to me with enlarged and ulcerated, cervical glands of the neck one of which had been surgically treated; but other glands becoming involed, I was asked to treat the case again. NAT-SIL-F. M and 10M were given at long intervals apart and the glands of the neck were entirely cured for a while; but returned again with open discharging glands of the neck in about three months. NAT-SIL-F. 50M given with very little benefit and a new condition evolved involving both bones of the right leg, with extreme pain and swelling over a localized area in center of shin bone; X-ray revealed a sarcoma involving both bones. Over the blood the remedy TOXI. came through. This was given 30th potency with immediate relief of both the adenitis and the pain and swelling of the leg; later TOXI. 200 was given with complete secedence of all the then present symptoms, but swelling and pain soon began in the other leg, which did not subside under a higher potency of TOXI., This demanded a new remedy, which was MERC-K-I., a double salt of mercury and potassium with only a fragmentary proving. This remedy given in the 10M three doses at intervals of from six to eight weeks has entirely restored this boy for the past five months. The last dose was given March 10 of this year. (MERC-K-I. has followed TOXI. in several cases).

CASE 3. A case of continuous progressive destructive osteo-neuritis of many years standing that had resisted many treatments and methods in a fifty year old man was cured by a few doses of TOXI. 30 and 200.

When I first applied to Mr. Erhart for TOXI., I was surprised to learn that he did not have it, but he promised to get it for me. This he was

---

1. Cf. "Homeopathy Versus the Specialist" p. 398. - Editor.

Toxicophis ...

unable to do after trying to get it from both our American and European pharmacies. I decided if necessary I would take a trip to Florida where these snakes abound to procure some of this virus, but was saved the trip through a relative who then lived in Florida. He procured a fine specimen and sent the head in alcohol to Mr. Erhart, who extraced the virus with a close call to himself, as in doing it he pricked his finger on one of the fangs above the poison sac; his prompt action in cutting the wound and applying an antidote doubtless saved him serious trouble.

Teucrium scorodonia

Teucr-s. is not proven. But to quote Clarke's Dictionary which cites the testimony of some reliable authorities who laud it as an anti-tubercular remedy of unusual merit. Dr. Criquelion of Mons[1] tells how Dr. Marting one day in the Ardennes[1] had occasion to examine a man of thirty who was apparently in the last stage of consumption and had a cavity in one apex; Marting gave his opinion that the man had not long to live. A year later being in the same district he called at the house and inquired of a man whom he saw there apparently in perfect health what had become of the invalid. "I am he" was the reply. It was the fact, though it took some time to convince Marting of it. An old woman had recommened him to make a tisane of the wood Germander (Teucr-s.) which grew abundantly about there. He had taken it daily and got well.

A similar case says Cooper was told me by a distinguished scientist. Teucr-s. is allied to Marrubium vulgare (common or white horehound) a well known cough remedy and to Nepeta glechoma (Grand Ivy) which was formerly much used with snail jelly for chest affecyons. Martiny introduced Teucr-s. into his practice and used a tisane [2]of it with much success in bronchorrhea and consumptive affections with tuberculous elements and muco-purulent expectoration. Clarke verifies the last observation of its use having used it in five to ten drops of the tincture two or three times each day. Criquelion points out that Teucr-s. has been used as a subcutaneous injection in tuberculine cases as a substitute of Tub-k. Criquelion had a patient, a farmer of scrofulous habit, high color, thick neck who had had for ten years an enlarged testicle the size of a quince which he diagnosed to be tuberculous. Teucr-s. 6 was given, one drop in four teaspoonfuls of water a teaspoonful

---

1. In Belgium
2. i.e. a tea. - Editor.

TEUCRIUM SCORODONIA ...

three quarters of an hour before each meal. After three months the testicle was softer; in six months it had almost returned to its proper size.

Clarke compares BAC., TEUCR., HELX.

In the potencies I have cured a case of very chronic frequently recurring headaches in a young woman. Worse at the periods, which were very painful with protracted flow; all these symptoms passed leaving the patient in robust health. I have also cured a number of chronic coughs in children of tuberculous parentage who had enlarged cervical glands and presented many other tubercular features.

TILIA

A neglected remedy with quite a proving is a valuable asset in the treatment of pelvic disorders of women. TIL. is a tincture made from the fresh blossoms of the lime tree and was proved by the Austrian Society.

Clarke summarizes the proving in a graphic and epigrammatic way as follows :

CHARACTERISTICS: The most striking characteristic is an intense sore feeling about the abdomen and profuse warm sweat which gives no relief. This has led to its successful use in cases of peritonitis. In addition to this are marked bearing down symptoms in the whole genito-urinary and rectal regions; especially in the uterus and these combined with others have indicated TIL. in puerperal metritis and other disorders of the female generative sphere. An intense facial neuralgia was developed in the proving and also a very aggravated condition of skin irritation with pimples of the lichen order.

SOME PECULIAR SYMPTOMS ARE: As if a piece of cold iron pierced through right eye, causing burning; burning as if a piece of ice were drawn over ear and face; as if something living were under the skin of face; tearing in anterior muscles of thigh as if they were too short. There are a number of pains above the root of the nose; epistaxis of thin pale blood which coagulated quickly. The left side was most affected; great sensitiveness to draft of air was induced; the symptoms were < afternoon and evening, talking, walking, sneezing, stooping. Cold water >. > in a cool room, walking about in open air, closing eyes, by coffee.

Pain in the head was > by application of cold water, pain in jaw was <. Heat of bed < skin symptoms.

TILIA ...

The mental symptoms: Melancholy, disposed to weep; love sick; dread of society; irritable, disinclined to work, together with the relief from walking in the open air and cold applications reminds one of PULS.

Sweat without relief of symptoms is like MERC. The severe bearing down symptoms of the pelvis suggest LIL-T. and SEP. as comparisons. Symptoms left sided predominating speaks of LACH. The great sensitiveness to jar and touch looks like BELL. The creeping as if something were alive under the skin strongly suggest COCA. The sensitiveness to a draft of air brings to our mind HEP. and SIL. This likeness to the proving of so many other well proven and frequently used drugs stamps TIL. with the possibility of great use when we can understand and apply it properly.

CASE: I have cured a case of severe menstrual headache in a woman with a small fibroid of the uterus with TIL. 45M doses given at long intervals. The tumor disappeared and the patient rarely has any but light headaches.

CONGO RED

CONGO RED an aniline dye, has no homeopathic proving; its only therapuetic use was by Abrams, applied locally over cancerous growths to inhibit their growth.

Clinically in high potencies this drug has cured several cases of breast cancer involving the whole breast which took on a stoney hardness. The affected breast became much smaller than normal under the action of the drug. It acts best in warm blooded patients and resembles iodine in the above mentioned effects. CON., CARB-AN., CALC-F. and SIL. would be compared in stony hardness of the mammary glands.

MERC-IOD. CUM KALI-IOD.[1]

MERC-K-I., double iodide of mercury and potassium chemical formula HgK_2I_4 is a far more valuable and powerful and broader remedy than Hale ever dreamed of, or that one might glean from the fragmentary proving recorded in Clarke's Dictionary, Volume II, page 459. We are indebted to Hale for the introduction of this remedy into our Materia Medica. Hale recommended it as effective in combating the prostrating sequelae of flu and kindred diseases, all of which is true, but the range and depth of action of this wonderful medicine in its curative power, surpasses anything Hale ever dreamed of.

Its first and acute manifestations are on the catarrhal membranes of the nose, throat, eyes, and respiratory tract. Hale recommends it for the treatment of inveterate colds and Clarke confirms that experience.

Clarke says it may be used where indications for the three elements of this salt are present, viz. mercury, iodine and potassium.[2]

Cooper commends it in acute facial paralysis from cold. J.R. Haynes praises its curative effects in many cases of catarrhal flu, and he further says if it does not quickly relieve and permanently cure it is of no use to repeat it.

Among some of the acute diseases that often need this remedy are malignant forms of flu, diptheria, and low types of fever in patients having a tubercular or syphilitic background, upon which are engrafted the aforementioned acute diseases.

This remedy has recently proved curative in two cases of undulant fever. Recovery took place in a few weeks after the administration of the remedy and leaving the blood free of flutins, which are said to persist for years after recovery, under other than homeopathic means of cure, or in those cases when recovery takes place under the natural limitations of the disease.[3]

The tissues upon which this drug manifests its strongest action are the blood, glands, bones, nerves, skin, and mucus membranes.

Like MERC. and KALI-I., its symptoms and conditions of disease are markedly < at night; this is especially true of the bone and nerve pains. It has the nightly aggravations common to MERC. and SYPH.. Arthritis,

---

1. From the handwritten manuscript of Dr. Grimmer, exact date unknown. A short discussion of MERC-K-I. in the previous article "Unusual Remedies" p. 138 was combined with the discussion here. - Editor.
2. Mostly in the form of MERC. and KALI-I. - Editor.
3. See "Undulant Fever" p. 481 in the chapter "Special Diseases". - Editor.

neuritis, and all painful complaints worse at night and resisting other remedies, should make you study this remedy.

It has cured catarrhal complaints of a very chronic nature; also nasal polyps. It should be a wonderful sinus remedy as well as a valuable remedy in certain chronic rheumatic states.

There is marked irritability of mind and extreme restlessness. The patient is sensitive to both extremes of temperature (like MERC.).

Eruptions of a most chronic nature such as psoriasis will yield to this remedy when it is homeopathically indicated.

Weakness, anemia, and emaciation are prominent features.

Chronic forms of headache, violent in character, based on a syphilitic or tubercular groundwork, have yielded to the power of this remedy.

It must be compared and studied with the AURUM SALTS, other MERCURY combinations, KALI-I., and the nosodes SYPH. and TUB-K. in order to appreciate its nature and depth of action.

Sarcoma of the bones, adenitis of tubercular and malignant types, Hodgkin's disease, late stages and manifestations of tertiary syphilis are a few of the chronic forms of sickness that have yielded to the magic of this medicine.

This wonderful remedy has many times complimented and finished cases after the favorable action of TOXI. (Osteo-sarcoma).[1]

It is among our most powerful antisyphilitics and strongly related to T.B. and Sarcoma. In the awful continuous, crushing pains that sometimes accompany deep sarcomatous growths or those involving the boney structures, this is my most reliable help, often completely relieving for long periods.

Enough has been shown here in its empirical use to justify a full homeopathic proving of this drug. With the consummation of such a proving, we can add another valuable weapon to our already potent armamentarium against disease. The indications given in our literature are far too meager to be followed or successfully used from a homeopathic standpoint; yet in spite of this fact some unbelieveable cures of so called incurable conditions have been accomplished with this medicine given along crude empirical lines. The homeopathic scientist should do finer and more specific work in his wonderfully selective field of therapeutics.

---

1. Cf. "Toxicophis" p. 138 in article "Unusual Remedies". - Editor.

Homeopathic War Remedies[1]

Medical scientists are much concerned about the *fearsome* effects of atomic explosions on the population of the large industrial and residential centers. What remedies, if any, can be employed to palliate or neutralize such forces and their chain reactions? The homeopathic materia medica has in its scope remedies to meet and at least modify in part some of the evils produced by atomic explosions. Any survivor not too close to the center of the explosion would be helped and comforted by the remedy Arn. given in any potency as soon as possible after the explosion. Arn. for concussions and contusions has been the first and best remedy in homeopathic hands for the past one hundred and fifty years.

After the concussion is met, the effect from radiation must be dealt with, and the remedy Phos. is by far the first and best as an antidote to all forms of radiation, be it radium, x-ray, or atomic radiation. Phos. meets the destructive effects produced on the capillary circulation and later on the blood elements as well. Phos. is a remedy for deep burns as well as for ulcerations of a serious nature; even gangrene has often been cured with this remedy.

If every individual who possibly might be exposed to the horrors of such forces would provide himself with, and carry on his person, a small vial of homeopathic Arn. to be taken as soon as possible after an explosion and another vial of homeopathic Phos. to be taken one-half hour after the Arn. was taken, he would have with him a first-aid help of the greatest value. These two simple homeopathic remedies universally taken would save many lives and prevent much suffering and prolonged illness.

We will mention a few other well known and widely proven homeopathic remedies for specific conditions: Arn. for bruises of the soft tissues; Hyper. for injury to nerve centers and tissues; Canth. for burns; Calen. for lacerated wounds; Led. for punctured wounds; Staph. for incised wounds; Symph. for broken bones and also promotes rapid healing even in the sickly and the aged; Pyrog. for septic woulds that rapidly involve the heart and other vital centers of the body. Sil. will remove small particles of glass and other substances from the tissues where surgery is often difficult to apply successfully without lacerating too much tissue.

---

1. "Editorial" in The Homeopathic Recorder, Vol. LXVI, No. 9, March, 1951, p. 262.

For the evil effects that often come after the giving of the various shots demanded by the armed forces, homeopathy has effective and satisfying antidotes. Shock followed by severe pain in head and nape with fever often follows the tetanus shots. MAG-P. will bring comfort in a surprisingly short time to these victims. ARS. antidotes the evil effects and distressing symptoms that follow the yellow fever shots. BRY. takes care of the bad effects following the typhoid and paratyphoid shots. BAPT. antidotes the typhus shots. MALAND. is the best antidote for the violent acute inflammations and swellings with alarming fever that often follow smallpox vaccination.

ACON., ARN., BELL., CARB-V. (hemorrhages with shock), MILL., PHOS. and the snake poisons; (LACH., ELAPS, CROT-H.) all are a group of hemorrhage remedies that would save many lives if given on their specific indication.

Nervous soldiers who are full of fear of death or other horrors and anxieties would soon be helped to face their ordeals with strength and resolution if given a dose of ACON.

The above-mentioned remedies constitute only a fraction of the homeopathic materia medica that could be employed for the good of the defenders of the republic. In these times of high costs and ever-mounting prices, homeopathy presents the most economic type of medicine as well as the most effective in curing power that has ever been discovered.

Prophylaxis

HOMEOPATHIC PROPHYLAXIS[1]

Preventive medicines occupies a prominent place today and it is logical that it should because prevention makes cure unnecessary. As the Law of Similars excells in the power to cure it excells more forcibly and certainly in the art of disease prevention.

Especially in the realm of children's diseases have the prophylaxis attempts been chiefly directed and with some degree of apparent success. I say apparent because there is need for refinements in the technique of administration and in the preparations of the theraputic agents employed as there is still much to be desired in results obtained by present methods. It is true that the agents employed bear a crude similarity to the homeopathic principle and because of this crudity of preparation and administration we meet with much disappointment and considerable consequential evil effects that follow their use.

Homeopathic prophylaxis never causes anaphylaxis or shock, never results in secondary infection, never leaves in its wake serum or vaccine disease or any other severe reaction; it simply protects surely and gently. While the homeopathic law provides specific remedies for specific disease conditions such as BELL. for scarlet fever, DIPH. and MERC-CY. for diphtheria, CARB-V. and CUPR. for whooping cough, LATH. and GELS. for poliomyelitis, VARIO. for small pox, etc., it reaches a much higher degree of efficiency when the remedy for the GENUS EPIDEMICUS is given for protection than is obtained by the disease specific.

To illustrate: an epidemic of scarlet fever may have more cases with a rough or a purplish rash than those having the typical smooth shining red rash that BELL. is specific in. Where the typical rough darker rash prevails remedies like AIL. and PHYT. and SULPH. will give more certain protection, but after the single epidemic remedy is found that brings the highest protection over all others.

In diphtheria protection DIPH. is the number one prophylaxis remedy but in some severe epidemics of the past MERC-CY. has proven to be very effective as well as curative in the disease.

In whooping cough CARB-V. has been a reliable protection in hundreds of cases of young children and infants. But some epidemics require remedies like DROS. and CUPR. and then they afford the most certain protection.

---

1. THE HOMEOPATHIC RECORDER, Vol. LXV, No. 6, December 1949, p. 154.

The remedy LATH. has given the most certain protection in thousands of exposed cases to polio through many epidemics over the last forty years. It easily heads the list of homeopathic remedies for protection against the dreaded polio. This remedy has the same affinity to the same centers in the spinal cord and brain that the polio virus and acts as the most perfect antidote both for protection and cure. This single instrument in Homeopathy's citadel of power should command world wide recognition both from the medical profession and the laity at large.

Against small pox VARIO. is an effective weapon, but we have others that proved curative and effective prophylaxis agents in many epidemics of the past such as SARR., ANT-T., VAC. and MALAND. ANT-T. in the third trituration rubbed on an abrasion of the skin produces a typical vaccination scar. MALAND. is the most potent antidote to the dangerous septicemia sometimes following vaccination and THUJ. is the best antidote against the chronic effects after vaccination.

It is strange so little has been said by homeopathic doctors familiar with the wide spread possibilities of homeopathic prophylaxis. Especially in the face of so many harmful and even deadly accidents that have followed the application of the prevailing methods of protection against acute epidemic diseases. As true healers and educators of progressive medicine it is our duty to give to the world this knowledge for its protection and well being. It is also our duty to invite physicians of all schools of healing to test fully the homeopathic art of protection against epidemic diseases if nothing else. If such tests were honestly made by sincere men of all schools of healing, homeopathy would reach its place in the sun.

Prophylactic Medicine Allopathic and Homeopathic[1]

To the sanitary engineer, and not the allopathic doctor, belongs credit for whatever real success has been accomplished in disease prevention. Centuries of blundering and groping by the rule of "trial and error" (mostly error) by so-called medical scientists has only brought multiplied miseries, increased sickness and shortened lives to millions of unsuspecting victims. The marked lessening of epidemic diseases such as smallpox, diphtheria, scarlet fever, etc., has been entirely due to better sanitation, hygiene and isolation. Before the Dick test or the scarlet fever inocculations were applied, the disease scarlet fever was declining greatly in prevalence and virulency; the same is true of diphtheria; nevertheless, the death rate from that disease still runs about 12% in spite of the highly praised curative powers of anti-toxine, which now is almost universally given because of pressure from health authorities everywhere.

Alexis Carrel in his book "Man the Unknown" states that medical science has succeeded in saving more infants and protecting the youth from the ravages of acute self-limiting disease, but that more people are dying in early middle life of chronic degenerative diseases, cancer, kidney and heart diseases, than ever before. And in the light of physiologic law, it is logical to conclude that the everlasting bombardment of the blood stream from infancy, and early youth, to maturity, with the numerous vaccines and serums, all products of disease, together with the noxious and deadly coal tar and sulpha drugs, known by dozens of trade names that make up the armamentarium of Allopathic medicine, might well be the causative factor in the alarming increase of the so-called degenerative diseases. To those diseases might be added the constant increase of mental and nervous disorders now afflicting the human race, brought on and aggravated by coal-tar sedatives and bromides. In recent years there has been a marked increase in so-called rare and unusual blood diseases almost all fatal. It is a recognized fact even by the old school vendors and prescribers of these coal tar drugs, that they produce marked changes in the blood elements of those who partake of them.

Probably the most vital and important medical problem to confront the race now and in the future is that of malaria. And here again outside of sanitation, medical science has no medicine to cure this alarming

---

1. The Homeopathic Recorder, Vol. LIX, No. 9, March 1944, p. 396.

and rapidly spreading disease. The drastic treatment used to control the chills only suppresses the disease by driving it into the vital centers of the organisms. Every soldier or individual infected with malaria is a certain potential chronic invalid for the rest of his life unless he is fortunate enough to receive the homeopathic remedy needed to cure his individual case.

The best prophylactic treatment against all disease, both acute and chronic, is building up vital resistance, by producing a harmonious physiologic process in the body organism. And the homeopathic remedy does just that thing, with no trace of consequential drug or serum miasm involved. Children and young adults treated homeopathically develop immunity against all acute disorder or throw them off, leaving better health behind. And older people live longer and in greater comfort to perform their accustomed uses easier and more satisfactorily.

Homeopathy has developed a number of prophylactic remedies against infectious and contagious diseases, such as smallpox, scarlet fever, diphtheria, infantile paralysis, as well as wonderful emergency remedies against trauma, lacerations, cuts and broken bones, burns, brain and spinal concussions, all of which would be invaluable for use in the army and navy, did not a fanatical and prejudiced medical oligarchy prevent such use.

And the defenders of the nation who prefer such treatment and refuse to accept the orthodox treatment of empirical medicine are jailed and disgraced for no other crime than daring to think and reason for themselves, the supposed right of every American. What hypocrites Americans are, shouting to the world in brazen tones about the glories of the "four freedoms," while piling insults, humiliation and physical torture on the brave men who offer their lives on the world's battlefields against the enemies of the nation.

Never before has the world needed the benign touch of homeopathic healing as it does now and will need in the near future, and our most passionate wish is to see this system given the chance to prove again and again its claims of superior success in both prophylaxis and cure.

Homeopathic Prophylaxis No. 1[1]

In the field of preventative medicine Homeopathy stands supreme, because it is the only system of medicine that deals with constitutional causes. Hygiene, sanitation and dietary science are valuable assets in promoting and maintaining health both for the individual and for society as a whole. The sanitary engineer has been the greatest factor in the control and eradication of epidemic disease notably, typhoid, malaria and yellow fever. Undoubtedly the decrease in epidemics of small pox, scarlet fever and diphtheria are more largely due to better sanitation, control of sewerage and the protection of the drinking water along with dairy and food inspection than to the so called protective vaccines and serums that have been so loudly proclaimed and so extensively used. Infact, these so called protective agents are far from being an unmixed good, as they produce many severe reactions deleterious to health.

From the time of Hahnemann BELL. has been a constant successful preventative of scarlet fever of the smooth type. The coarse type has found its best prophylactic remedies in AIL., RHUS-T., PHYT. and SULPH., each varying with the prevailing epidemic.

Diphtheria has been successfully controlled by MERC-CY. and DIPH., and marvelous results were obtained with these drugs in the days when no sanitation or hygiene was practiced to any extent if at all.

Protection against **whooping cough** is best obtained by the epidemic remedy but much routine protection may be accomplished by remedies like CARB-V., CUPR., DROS., and PERT.

Poliomyelitis also finds its best protection from the prevailing epedemic remedy such as GELS., COCC., CUR. and LATH. Of these the most constant specific is LATH. and clinically it has been almost one hundred percent effective in the prevention of polio in the past fifty years at the hands of many homeopathic physicians.

Hahnemann's prophylactic remedies against **cholera** were CAMPH., CUPR. and VERAT. and they are equally effective today.

Severe types of **yellow fever** found the curative and protective remedies in ARS., CROT-H. For the bad effects of the yellow fever shots given by the army ARS. proved highly efficient.

Every Homeopath knows the power of Boenninghausen's big three for **croup**: ACON., HEP. and SPONG., and they are still highly efficient

---

1. From the handwritten manuscript of Dr. Grimmer, dated 1953. This article probably appeared in THE JOURNAL OF A.I.H. about 1953; but I cannot find the journal. - Editor

and certain in action. Along with this group it would be well to remember that Samb. nigra and Lach. with their specific indications are often needed remedies in the more serious cases of croup.

In those places where **small-pox** still exists, namely the Philippine's, Japan and many of the Asiatic countries remedies like Thuj., Ant-t., Sil., Sarr. and Vario. are mighty forces for both cure and protection aggainst this dread disease.

It is always a safe rule in any epidemic of disease to select for protective purposes those remedies most frequently indicated and and curative in the prevailing epidemic. Some of the worst epidemics of **flu** notably those of 1917 and 18 found a narrow group of remedies needed or indicated. Ars., Bry., Carb-v., Gels., Eup-per., Lach., Rhus-t., Phos., Sep. and Sulph. constituted a common group that proved highly efficacious. Late in that epidemic around the Chicago area Ars., Bry., Carb-v., and Sulph. were the most needed remedies.

After working awhile in an epidemic the physician is able to save much time and labor in the selection of the best remedies needed because he will find a few remedies, sometime only two or three, running through his cases and these are the remedies that will prove protective against the disease to those who are exposed to it and have not yet come down with it. So much for acute disease prophylaxis which is highly efficacious without any detrimental side effects so frequently found under vaccine and serum protection.

In the realm of chronic constitutional and inheritable diseases Homeopathy stands alone in its power to prevent degenerative changes in the body organism. Children given careful Homeopathic treatment, especially at an early age, will develop splendid bodies and sound minds and escape early heart and kidney disease, cancer, leukemia and anemia. They will develop a nervous system capable of standing the stress and strain of the complexities of our present time.

Of course with the Homeopathic medicine they must be taught the need of temperate living, proper diet with good physical and mental hygiene. Especially must they avoid excesses in alcohol and tobacco as well as the intake of pain killing and depressing coal tar and phenobarbital drugs. They must be protected against the numerous serums and vaccines prevailing today if they would avoid having cancer or other blood-destroying and degenerative diseases. Many times if these things have been forced on them by law or taken through ignorance they will have to be antidoted with proper Homeopathic antidotes before health can be restored.

A source of much severe chronic suffering such as asthma, chronic skin and intestinal diseases are aggravated and made incurable by **aluminium toxines** produced by cooking utensils made with aluminium and its alloys, or from the intake of water softened by aluminium chloride. These patients will not get well of their chronic troubles even with seemingly well selected Homeopathic remedies until after the aluminium toxines are antidoted and irradicated with potencies of CADM-O.

If the medical profession in general would heed the significance of the above mentioned facts and avail themselves of Homeopathic help and knowledge the public health would be much better conserved and a world of suffering would cease with better health and happiness prevailing.

President's Message Homoeopathic Prophylaxis No. 2[1]

In the past two decades there has been a constantly growing interest in the application of preventive medicine. The degree of success attained by these methods, aside from the beneficial effect of better sanitation and sewage disposal, is a debatable question. Most of the good accomplished in the control of epidemic disease, especially typhoid, can be ascribed to sanitary measures protecting food and water supply from sewage contamination, and that has been an outstanding success. Typhoid has been almost entirely eliminated from our midst and most of the other epidemic deseases such as diphtheria, scarlet fever, etc. are all much milder in their ravages.

Polio presents the only exception. It seems to defy the efforts of the sanitary engineer and the medical specialist alike as it rages on unchecked and in some aspects is even stronger. Formerly children were almost exclusively the victims whereas recently many adults have fallen prey to its crippling power.

Experimental vaccines to date have proven disappointing in spite of exaggerated claims for their efficiency in the protection and cure of the disease. The antibiotics or so-called "wonder drugs" have been disappointing and even harmful in many instances and they soon loose their power to cure permanently. They are said to be inadequate to cope with the so-called virus diseases. In contrast to the uncertainties of allopathic prophylaxis, Homoeopathy has developed a protective array of remedies against many forms of both acute and chronic disease.

Homoeopathic prophylaxis began with Hahnemann who states in the Organon that BELL. affords a splendid protection against the smooth rash of **scarlet fever** and, from his time to the present, homoeopathic doctors have prevented thousands of children from falling victims to scarlet fever. There is a coarse variety of scarlet fever that may require PHYT. and still another, a very malignant type, where the eruption is scant and purplish and where the glands and mucous membranes are mostly involved with extensive ulceration and the patient is greatly devitalized; the curative and prophylactic remedy here is AIL. From these observations we learn that the epidemic remedies are always the best for preventive measures. Boenninghausen, Hahnemann's most apt and ardent student, discovered the powers of THUJ. as one of the great protectors against smallpox and also for the pernicious effects of

---

1. From the handwritten manuscript of Dr. Grimmer, dated 1953. - Editor

smallpox vaccination and to this day THUJ. is one of the top drugs against these evils.

Diphtheria had and has its best protection in MERC-CY. and DIPH., the diphtheria nosode. DIPH. has been very efficacious in ridding so-called carriers of their infective germs.

BAPT. has performed the same service for **typhoid** carriers.

Before the so-called discoveries of Pasteur with his anti-rabies vaccine, the homoeopathic physician, *Constantine Hering,* had potentized the saliva of the mad dog and gave the world a successful prophylactic and cure for **rabies:** LYSS. (HYDROPHOBINUM). Homoeopathy has successfully cured numerous cases down through the years simply and with certainty and with little expense or suffering for the patients.

Burnett cured many cases of tuberculosis in children and young adults as well as protected many more against the disease with the remedy BAC.. Homoeopathy has developed many more tubercular nosodes all valuable for certain special forms of the disease, especially in its chronic aspects which constitute the groundwork for many of the intractible, chronic diseases of today.

MAG-P. is a specific against tetanus and has cured many severe and advanced cases in the convulsive stage and this remedy also antidotes the frequently severe effects that follow the injection of the anti-tetanus serum.

For the adverse effects of the yellow fever shots ARS. affords splendid relief and BRY. is sufficiently potent against the injections of typhoid to restore order.

All homoeopaths know the value of THUJ. against the ill results following smallpox vaccination. For the bad effects of diphtheria prophylaxis, MERC-CY. is adequate. BELL. meets the evils of the Dick vaccine. A great many young service men have been comforted and helped through the ordeal of serum "shooting" by homoeopathic protection against this evil.

Homoeopathy affords the best first aid treatment against burns, bruises, strains and broken bones: CANTH. for burns, ARN. for bruises, HYPER. for nerve injuries, RHUS-T. for strains and SYMPH. to aid in the rapid knitting of broken bones (this remedy is also useful for the effects of blows and injuries to the eye ball). For the sting of bees, wasps and other insects CARB-AC. in potency affords certain and rapid relief. Medical experts of traditional medicine tell us that atropine, the alkaloid of BELL., is the best antidote against the radiation from atom bombs, but homoeopathic science has demonstrated that potentized PHOS. is the most effective agent against the radiations of x-ray and radium which are identical with the radiation effects of the atom bomb.

Perhaps the protective agent that the world most ardently waits for is the one against polio and, strange as it may seem, that agent has been with us and successfully operating for the past fifty years. The remedy, LAT-S., obtained from the wild pea, according to Dr. W. Boericke, presents the most perfect likeness of the polio disease, not only symptomatically and clinically but pathologically as well, and affects the identical centers and areas of the spinal cord the polio virus does. In the hands of many homoeopathic physicians this remedy has successfully protected thousands. The essayist has used it for the past forty years in many epidemics and given it to many hundreds as a protective measure and not one case ever came down with polio. Other homoeopathic doctors of my acquaintance have had the same results.

The simplicity and effectiveness of the homoeopathic potency stands out like the most resplendent jewel in the diadem of the healing art. In every epidemic disease there are some few atypical cases that will call for a specific remedy to effect the cure. Many years ago, Dr. Wolf of Chicago brought to me the blood specimen of a twelve-year-old boy who was paralyzed in all his limbs and was unconscious from polio, a bulbar case. There were few, if any, guiding therapeutic symptoms to prescribe on but from the polarity of the blood a single unusual remedy was selected. NAT-AR. in the ten thousandth potency was given. This produced an amazing reaction of cure in the space of a few days. In a few hours after the remedy was given, consciousness returned and the paralysis was gone in forty-eight hours. This rapid recovery left not the slightest atrophy or disfunction of the muscular tissues anywhere in the body and the child was around and fully recovered in two weeks.

When the remedy that is truly homoeopathic is given, curative action stops disease processes so quickly that no damage is done to the nerve tissues because the disease is checked before it has had time to impair or destroy the delicate nerve cells and tissues attacked by polio.

Amazing as the curative results obtained in acute and accidental conditions of sickness are, when we are privileged to observe the miracles of cure found in chronic disease we are filled with wonder almost beyond belief. Chronic disease is never self-limiting to end in spontaneous cure as most acute diseases do. These chronic chronic cases do not get well by themselves under unassisted natural processes, they only yield to the most scientific homoeopathic treatment.

To cope successfully with chronic disease, the homoeopathic prescriber requires years of experience and training in his chosen art and science. Not only must he be a master of the vast Materia Medica, but he must be highly trained and versed in the principles of homoeopathic philosophy; he must be a keen observer and logical thinker, able to translate the language of the proven remedies to fit the pathogenesis of each given case of illness coming to him. He must know the natural scope and pace of action of sickness and he must be able to select remedies of like attributes and symptoms to fit the needs of each patient he treats. Lastly, he must be able to know the significance and importance of suppressions. When he is endowed with these needed essentials, he is a master prescriber able to meet and overcome chronic and inheritable weakness and maladjustments and perform miracles of cure under natural law.

Here in this field of chronic disease we can exploit the advantages of prevention over the necessity of cure. Many chronic conditions such as cancer, arthritis, kidney, heart and lung disease can be prevented and aborted in the early stages of these afflictions by expert homoeopathic treatment. This fact is the most valuable asset that Homoeopathy brings to the needs of suffering humanity today and to all the future.

Children born and reared under correct and inspired homoeopathic care and guidance soon become free of all sickness and develop normal mental and physical processes that ultimate in healthy bodies and happy personalities.

With these known facts before us it is not hard to envision a superior type of humanity grown under the auspices of three generations of homeopathic treatment. As homoeopathic philosophy and care is more universally accepted, the progress of the race will come faster to build a better world.

As we note the importance of good health and vital power to all the affairs of life, it behooves us all, for the sake of our children and their children, to make every effort to preserve the God-given principles of homoeopathic healing for all the future.

Prevention and Cure of Heart Disease by Homeopathy[1]

While Homeopathy has no one specific remedy for heart disease, it is rich in many remedies whose provings indicate their use and applicability to all the various types of cardiac disease classified. We will take up some of the more important phases of prophylaxis first, which after all is a superior form of cure.

After nearly fifty years of observation and work with the sick in the broad field of general medicine the writer is convinced that the injudicious and almost universal use and addiction of the numerous coal-tar drugs, the barbitals, aspirin, anacin, midols and numerous others that have come down through the years, the more drastic types being those following World War II. One such as Acetanilid, Pyramidox, Phenacetin, etc., constitute one of the important factors in the wide spread increase of heart disease as well as cancer and other degenerative diseases such as leukemia and anemia. These drugs literally wiped out thousands during the great flu epidemic of that war period. The greatest harm comes from the ease and cheapness with which these agents of destruction can be obtained. Without guidance or advice of a physician any layman can go to the nearest drug store or supermarket and get a supply. In fact, he need not do that if he has a lady friend along, for most of the women nowadays carry a supply of aspirin or anacin with them to use for any slight distress or pain. Many are addicts and need no excuse to take the drug, often putting it in coke or beer or other alcoholic beverages. It is true that many of these addicts live many years and carry on with the help of the drugs before the ravages of disease show up in the form of a drastic blood change or a gastric ulcer, a damaged kidney or heart to say nothing of impaired mentality and memory. These drugs are known by all medical men to be depressants and suppressants as well as destroyers of certain blood elements producing the conditions of destroyed blood platelets. They also prevent and weaken nerve function of the organism by inhibiting the sensibility to pain as well as affecting adversely the thermal centers in the brain, suppressing fevers and preventing the natural advantage high temperature brings to the organism in its fight against toxemias and infections; in fewer words: they interfere in the natural reactions and processes of body function against disease.

---

1. The Homeopathic Recorder, Vol. LXVII, No. 7, January 1952, p. 191.

If the organization for the study and prevention of heart disease financed by the American public would but stress this one evil of coal-tar drugs, its easy distribution and ready use by the gullable multitudes guided by radio announcers and advertizing agents of the manufacturing chemists, whose only interest is profit regardless of the harm produced, they would accomplish more results in the prevention of heart and other degenerative diseases than a century of present day research and laboratory procedure could. Perhaps the fear of offending the tremendously large and powerful commercial interest of these manufacturers and vendors of universal ill health may be the reason the public is deprived of so much valuable knowledge.

In the early and functional stage of disease such as the numerous types of headache, neuralgia, beginning arthritic pain as well as febrile and infective diseases, if instead of taking any of these numerous suppressive coal-tar drugs a simple Homeopathic remedy could be taken, the conditions of sickness would be more permanently eradicated with no sequence remaining. It is common knowledge that many heart lesions follow acute infections especially of a rheumatic nature. It is common practice outside of Homeopathic procedure to use some one of these numerous coal-tar derivatives for the relief of pain and fever. The sufferers of insomnia and frayed-out nerves often become addicts of the above mentioned drugs and wind up mental and nervous wrecks if not victims of heart, cancer or blood disease. If enough physicians of all schools of medicine would impress on their patients the inherent danger the use of these subtle yet drastic drugs engender it would not be long before an organized educational program would bring to the public the necessity for the control and use of these agents only with a physicians advice. Such a program would prevent much heart and other degenerative diseases and prove to be a prophylactic factor of great value.

Needless to add that correct habits of living, pertaining to diet, ventilation, hygiene, both mental and physical, the avoidance of excesses with sufficient rest and recreation all of which is endorsed by all schools of medical thought may well be included as a prophylactic factor.

The third and most important prophylactic factor in the prevention of heart and all other degenerative forms of disease is the application of the constitutional Homeopathic remedy. The sooner in the life of the individual this application is made the better the results obtained. The Homeopathic remedy is the only force capable of neutralizing in the organism inherited toxines of disease and normalizing the physiologic processes of spirit, mind and body to produce harmony, which is health and vital resistance. All this enables the individual to exist in comfort and adjust to his changing environment without friction, and to live out his full life span. The Homeopathic treatment of functional heart conditions is comparatively easy for the physician and highly satisfactory for the patient because results are one hundred per cent good.

In the organic forms of heart disease the treatment is more difficult and complex and the results in cure from a pathological standpoint are practically nil. But from the point of palliation, comfort and prolongation of life often with a splendid ability to carry on in life's affairs, the results are most gratifying. No system of treatment removes serious heart pathology but the Homeopathic remedy brings more comfort and longer life than any other treatment known to man.

To enumerate the numerous remedies and their specific symptoms for the treatment of various forms of heart disease would require a book of large volume. For that reason we will submit to you for study some of the valuable remedies that many years of practice of many Homeopathic physicians have given the world for the relief and even cure of patients suffering with this increasing malady.

In this day of drug slugging and drastic medication with an ever-increasing array of new experimental chemical specifics, the conditions of many patients are made worse by these means. With the added burden of a vitiated blood stream the victim of a heart disease has greatly lessened chances for help or recovery as his ability to react to curative remedies is much impaired. For this class of patient with few or no therapeutic symptoms for the selection of a remedy, and where natural manifestations of sickness have been suppressed and an overwhelmed vital force is barely struggling to exist a potency of CARB-V. will bring outstanding results.

CARBO VEGETABLIS

CARB-V. is the best single antidote to coal-tar drugs and all fumes and gases which reduce the power of the blood cells to perform their function in the exchange of oxygen and carbon dioxide. The CARB-V. patient suffers from great air hunger and his general body weakness is accentuated in the weakness of his lungs and their respiratory function. It has cured dilation of the heart. It effects muscle tone through the blood stream, bringing improved nourishment to the weakened cells. CARB-V. is one of the remedies to revive the flagging vital force which fails to react to remedies that are seemingly indicated but fail to arouse

CARBO VEGETABLIS ...

curative reaction. Lack of vital reaction is a keynote and fits the general picture of the provings. Clarke in his Dictionary of Practical Materia Medica lists this remedy high in its clinical application in the cure of heart disease. Volumes could be written about the power and symptoms of this wonderful remedy, but the object of this paper is to call attention of physicians to it for study which can be profitably persued in our rich Homeopathic literature.

CRATAEGUS OXYACANTHIA

CRAT. is a remedy with a very fragmentary Homeopathic proving, but it has been extensively used by Homeopathic physicians with marked success in many forms of heart disease such as *angina pectoris, failing heart muscles with hypertrophy*, etc. The mental state is one of irritability, crossness and melancholy. "Weak, rapid pulse, dyspnea, dropsy dependent on failure of heart whether from valvular affection or from anemia." (Clarke)

The slightest exertion aggravates or brings on the symptoms. The drug may cause nausea when given in the tincture unless given during or immediately after a meal; thus nausea with weakness may well be a leading indication. Clarke says: "CRAT. is the nearest approach to a positive heart tonic that I know of.

This remedy has mostly been used in five to ten-drop doses of the tincture. But Dr. Wilbur Bond of Greenfork, Indiana, some years ago reported a number of nice cures with this remedy in high potency and the writer has had cases cured with it in potencies thus confirming its power in potency when applicable. This valuable drug should have a complete Hahnemannian proving. This remedy seems to accomplish all that digitalis does in material doses without the consequential heart poison that the accumulated effects of digitalis produces.

DIGITALIS

DIG., however, is one of our most effective remedies in certain forms of serious heart disease characterized by a *slow intermittent pulse or a violent palpitation with extreme anguish and anxiety*. Cyanosis is also a marked symptom. DIG. is a broad remedy covering many other complaints either associated with or outside the heart affections. It has been clinically applied to amaurosis angina pectoris, asthma, Bright's disease, cyanosis, delirium tremens, dropsy, fever, gonorrhea, headache, heart

DIGITALIS ...

affections, hydrocele, hydrocephalus, impotence, jaundice, lung congestions, lost memory, meningitis, noises in head, paraphimosis, prostate enlargement, ptyalism, spermatorrhea, toothache, urinary disorders and vision disorders.

The remedy picture is summed up into three main features by Clarke as follows: Slow intermittent pulse, enlarged, sore, painful liver; white pasty stools. Along with these is prostration from slight exertion. The mental condition is anxious, low spirited, tearful, wants to be alone. Jaundiced appearance is often found in complaints needing this remedy and it is frequently a source of comfort to those suffering from enlarged prostates with painful and difficult urinary complaints. There are a number of characteristic keynote symptoms that when present in any given case will serve as a reliable indication for its selection. Sudden sensation as if the heart stood still or would stop if the patient moves; (GELS. has the opposite feeling, as if the heart would stop beating if she did not keep moving about). The mere sight or smell of food excites violent nausea with clean tongue, thirst for water with absence of fever. Deathly sinking at epigastrium. Complaints from emotional disturbances that are referred to the heart and epigastrium.

CACTUS GRANDIFLORUS

CACT. is one of our most effective remedies in the treatment of painful and serious conditions of the heart. Its symptoms are characterized by squeezing, constricting pains especially referred to the heart and chest regions. But these constrictions may be found in many other conditions and parts of the body, such as painful constriction of the esophagus preventing swallowing or exciting a constant desire to swallow. Suffocative constriction of throat with full throbbing carotid, constriction or pulsation in scrobiculus, copius hematemesis; constriction of rectum with sense of great weight and urging to evacuate a great quantity but nothing passes; copious hemorrhages from anus. Constriction of neck of bladder with constant urge to void urine; urine passes by drops with great burning. Constriction of vagina preventing coition. Constriction, burning pains and a sense of weight or pressure in all the parts affected. Difficult oppressed breathing with the constricting chest pains associated with dreadful fear and anxiety present some of the important aspects of this remedy.

SNAKE POISONS

All the serpent poisons present indications for the many types of heart disease. Perhaps the ones more frequently used are LACH. and NAJA. To go into the interesting origin and history of LACH. together with its vast symtomology is beyond the scope of this paper. I will only touch upon some of its clinical high lights and symptoms and leave the fuller study to those who are interested enough to give the time and make the effort required to obtain a rich amount of useful knowledge for the cure of the sick.

LACHESIS

LACH. is especially useful in women around the climateric period who suffer with cardiac difficulties associated with flushing of heat sometimes alternating with chills down the back. Weakness and faintness are common with marked aggravation during and after sleep. Also irregular profuse and painful menstrual periods generally too frequent and copious.

This remedy is predominately a left sided medicine with some few exceptions. Some of the headaches are worse on the right side and relieved by closing the eyes and from sleep. The pains are pulsating, constricting and burning. There is a rich array of mental symptoms. Great anguish and unbearable anxiety which is relieved in the open air. Fear and presentiment of death.

Distrust, suspicion and jealousy. Mental depression and melancholy, concerned about his illness, sense of persecution, thinks he is hated and despised. Fear of being poisoned. Thinks he is someone else. In the hands of a stronger power. That he is dead and preparations are being made for his funeral. Averse to people. Restless and uneasy. Does not wish to attend to business but wants to be off somewhere all the time. Indolence with dislike and unfitness for any labor either mental or physical. A state of ecstacy and exaltation inducing tears. Desires to meditate and to compose intellectual works. Frantic loquacity with elevated language. Extreme sensitiveness to impressions and great irritability. Mistakes in speaking and writing. Weakness of memory, extreme forgetfulness. Timidity of character with variableness and indecision. Confusion as to time. Imbecility and loss of every mental faculty. Nocturnal delirium with much talking or with murmuring. Dementia and loss of consciousness.

LACHESIS ...

Heart symptoms are palpitation with fainting and anxiety, sometimes excited by cramp-like pains, with cough and suffocation. Feels as if heart hung by a thread and every heart beat would tear it off; irregularity of beats, constriction in region of the heart. Spasm in the heart (with aneurism of right carotid and disagreeable pulsation in the ears).

As if the heart were too large for its containing cavity. Stitches in region of heart with shortness of breath. Fainting fits and cold sweats. Faint feeling about the heart, with heats up spine and flushing of the face. Faintings, giddiness and palpitation constantly recurring. Lying on left side aggravates the heart pain.

NAJA

NAJA, the cobra venom presents many of the general features of the other snake poisons but it has some distinct differences in modality and action belonging to its own pathogenesis.

This remedy affects profoundly the medulla oblongata and cerebellum and the whole nervous system.

Its cardiac symptoms are those of depression and uneasiness about the heart. Fluttering and palpitation of heart. Audible palpitation of heart. Pulse slow and irregular in rhythm and force; weak and thready, scarcely perceptible or rapid and full one hundred and twenty. Some beats tolerably full and strong, afterwards thirty two, irregular in rhythm and force, some of the beats full and bounding. One striking modality: great relief of pain and breathing lying on the right side.

General modalities are extreme sensitiveness to cold. Languor, fatigue and torpor. Organs feel as if drawn together, especially the ovary and heart. Depression of both mental and physical powers. Symptoms worse from stimulants, relieved walking in open air. Swelling of body, local inflamations. Appearance as if intoxicated. Convulsive movement of mouth and limbs, rolling about as if weak and faint. Moaned, grasped his throat, tossed his head from side to side and moved his arms and legs uneasily. Unnatural quiet, with groans and complaints of slight pain in the bitten arm. Sensation of wasting away. Swooning fits. Loss of sense of feeling.

Suicidal insanity, irresolute, melancholia. Insanity, suddenly to cut his own head in two with an axe. Loss of consciousness, speechless, comatose. Clinically this remedy has been used for angina pectoris, asthma, dyspnea, hay fever, headache, heart affections, spasmodic

NAJA ...

stricture of the oesophagus, ovarian affections, plague, spinal irritation, sore throat. This remedy cured a well developed case of breast cancer, diagnosis confirmed by biopsy.[1]

CENCHERIS CONTORTRIX

CENCH. This remedy has been somewhat overlooked and neglected by Homeopaths, perhaps because of its incomplete proving. But it competes in value in heart complaints with Lachesis, its nearest analogue. Clarke gives us some nice points of distinction between these two remedies. LACH. affects the left ovary more than the right. CENCH. the right more.CENCH. has difficult empty swallowing, with easy swallowing of solids and liquids. LACH. can swallow solids, not liquids. Both remedies have extreme sensitiveness to tight clothing around neck and waist.

With lost memory there is lethargy. Anxiety; feels she will die suddenly. Alternating moods. Dreamy, absent minded. Took the wrong car without realizing where she was going. Suspicious, thinks her husband is going to put her in an insane asylum every day from three to eight p.m. for ten days, yet she knew it was a delusion.

The dreams of CENCH. are vivid and horrible, cannot be shaken off during waking hours. Often they are lascivious.

There is a feeling as if the whole body was enlarged, especially the heart feels as if it were distended to fill the whole chest. At 3 p.m. sensation of fluttering followed by feeling that the heart fell down into abdomen then pulse became feeble, with heat lasting until after midnight.

The sexual desire of both sexes is much increased under the influence of this remedy.

This remedy produces bag-like swelling above the eyes and below the brow like KALI-C.

LATRODECTUS MACTANS

The spider poisons give us some effective heart remedies, the most often indicated is LAT-M., the Black Widow, whose symptomatology and clinical application places it among the valuable remedies for angina pectoris. It causes extreme anxiety, screams fearfully exclaiming that she would loose her breath and die. Violent precordial pain extending to axilla and down left arm and forearm to fingers with numbness of the extremity and apnea. The left arm is almost paralyzed with the

---

1. Case by Dr. Grimmer - see see Case 7 Mrs. A. M. age 30 pgs 425 ff.

LATRODECTUS MACTANS ...

pain. Pulse so fast it could not be counted and so feeble it could scarcely be felt. Expression of deep anxiety on face. Nausea followed by severe abdominal pain. Vomited black vomit copiously. With the nausea and severe pain there was a sinking sensation at the epigastrium. The profound effect on the blood was shown. When cupped the blood flowed like water and would not coagulate, not even with the addition of tannin. In thirty-six hours from the time he was bitten, he drank three and a half quart bottles of the best rectified whiskey without the least sign of intoxication. A moribund state set in with the skin cold as marble.

ACONITE

It would be remiss not to mention ACON. among our valuable remedies in the treatment of patients suffering from disturbances of the heart, and not all of these troubles are acute and functional. Many chronic conditions of the glands, the blood, and the nerves as well as the heart will yield to the magic power of this medicine. The restlessness, anxiety and awful fear of death, with the sudden violent onset of the disease with severe unbearable pain often associated with tingling or numbness of the painful parts occurring in full blooded plethoric individuals furnish a picture needing ACON. Extreme sensitiveness to noise, touch, light or jar. A condition of clairvoyance sometimes occurs predicting the day and hour of death. The heart palpitates with great anxiety and heat of body chiefly in the face and great weariness of limbs. Sensation of compression and blows in region of the heart. Inflammation of the heart, chronic diseases of the heart with continued pressure in the left side of chest. Oppressed breathing when moving fast and ascending stairs. Stitches in the region of the heart, attacks of fainting and tingling in the fingers, pulse full, strong, hard or slow, feeble, threadlike with anxiety. This is the banner remedy for the bad effects of fright.

We have only scratched the surface of the Materia Medica of the remedies used in the Homeopathic treatment of heart ailments. If we were asked to compile a repertory of heart remedies we would have to include every remedy in the whole Materia Medica to avoid leaving something of use out of the list. Any remedy fitting the constitutional history and symptoms of the patient would be the needed one to bring about curative conditions.

MALARIA PROPHYLAXIS[1]

From the most remote times, malaria has altered the course of empires, and shaped the destiny of nations[2]. Even types of civilization have survived or fallen because of the devastating power of this universal and seemingly unconquered force. The Greeks in the siege of Troy, it is claimed, found the ravages of malaria more dangerous and deadly than their Trojan enemies. Hannibal's defeat and retreat before the gates of Rome was entirely due to this ubiquitous and enervating disease. And at this time America's victory or defeat in the Pacific may well depend upon the successful control of this subtle but mighty influence that smites friend and foe alike, for it is and has been from earliest history man's most destructive enemy and the greatest obstacle in his march on the road of progress and civilization.

Scientific medicine admits its weakness and its inability to cure the countless victims of the malarial poison. Quinine, most often relied on, is rarely if ever curative but it is a powerful suppressant, that is, the drug disease masks the malarial disease, and renders it more or less quietus in its manifestations. The usual high fever, chill and sweat may be replaced by anemia and weakness complicated with chronic forms of spleen and liver disease when large and continuous doses of quinine are given, thus producing a complication and fusion of natural and drug disease, (suppressed malaria).

Every homeopathic prescriber knows the certain curative power of the indicated remedy. While any one of our proven polycrests may be indicated in a given case of malaria by the totality of its symptoms thus indicating a wide range of remedies for study, the fact is that at least ninety percent of malarial cases will find the curative remedy in a list of less than a dozen remedies which are as follows:

ARS., CHIN., CAUST., EUP-PER., GELS., NAT-M., NUX-V., RHUS-T., SEP., SULPH., TUB. And from these eleven remedies, three may be taken that will cure about seventy five percent of all malarial infections.

ARS., CHIN., and NAT-M. given in proper form and sequence would not only prove curative in the majority of cases but would be effective prophylactics as a general protection against the disease. The most

---

1.   From the handwritten manuscript of Dr. Grimmer, exact date unknown. - Editor.
2.   The Fouth Horseman by Nikifaroukh, A; MacMillan 1992. This book will clarify much of the epidemiology of the worst of the scourges (epidemics) that have befallen man and provides important information for the whole medical profession and even more particularly to homeopaths. - Editor.

effective single remedy (almost specific) for all malarial disease complicated with Quinine poisoning, is the remedy NAT-M.; CAUST. is more specific in cases where paralysis of single parts of the whole body has resulted from the combined effects of malaria and quinine.

To protect one against the ravages of this dread destroyer one should have a dose of NAT-M. 30 or higher once a week for a month or six weeks before entering the malarial districts.

On getting into the infected territory a dose of ARS. 30th potency to be taken once a week for a month, but if malarial symptoms appear while on the ARS. treatment then a dose of CHIN. 30th or higher for three days. If malaria symptoms persist a higher potency of NAT-M. once a week will eradicate the disease in most cases.

This method of applying homeopathic remedies in malaria is not entirely homeopathic, but for army routine made up of indifferent prescribers it will bring a hundred fold more success and comfort to the afflicted than the present routine army methods now bring. We have treated both acute and chronic forms of the malaria disease from India, Africa as well as cases from Southern Illinois, Missouri and Mississippi valley with a hundred percent of cures and no failures. And the homeopathic literature abounds with thousands of verifications in lasting cures. It is regretable that a hidebound orthodoxy in medicine and fanatical red tape of army medical directors, prevents the brave defenders of American liberty from receiving the certain benign effects and cure of the only real scientific medicine ever known, Homeopathy.

HOMEOPATHY'S PROPHYLAXIS AGAINST POLIO[1]

Much has been done to save life and rehabilitate the crippled victims of this ruthless affliction. The iron lung has brought many hopeless cases through from certain death to life only to leave them in a fearfully maimed and helpless state. The famous Snite case is an example of living many years by means of the artificial respiration offered by the iron lung. Not all, however, have the means at hand to make life as bearable under such trying conditions as this man had. Physio-therapy, massage, spinal manipulations, hot packs, hydro therapy, etc., together with surgical techniques of muscle building and conservation have done much to mitigate the crippling and weakness that follow a severe attack of polio.

Perhaps as much if not more than any other factor in the treatment of Polio is the psychological aid given to instill courage and persistency in the seemingly unending battle to get well with the application of an intelligent system of exercise which often obtains startling and unexpected results in cure and restoration. But there are cases like that of the late President Franklin D. Roosevelt where no therapy, either mental or physical, can in any way restore withered muscles or paralyzed parts and the weakness persists until the end of life.

The medical treatment of polio has been disappointing and strikingly inefficient with two exceptions; viz: The psychosomatic aspect of medicine has aided greatly in instilling courage and hope to give force to the other adjuvants of treatment mentioned before, such as physio-therapy, etc. Serums and vaccines have proven useless and even harmful in some cases. The "wonder drugs"[2] have only added weakness. Barbituates and other sedatives and depressants have inhibited the vital processes of the body and prevented it from reacting to the curative stimuli of hydro-therapy, massage and other physical agents.

The notable exception in medical treatment which has been highly successful in the treatment of polio for the past forty years, the results of which have been entirely ignored by the medical profession is the Homeopathic system of medication. It is exceptional when a polio case results in death under Homeopathic care. Even the worst cases pulled through in the days before the iron lung was known, and severe crippling was and is the exception as a sequela of the infection. So quickly

---

1. THE LAYMAN SPEAKS, Vol. 5, No. 3, March 1952.
2. Wonder drugs (= antibiotics) have no effect on viral disease such as polio. - Editor.

does the Homeopathic remedy neutralize the infective virus in the blood stream that there is not time for the deadly force to affect the nerves of the patients.

But Homeopathy has much more than a large percentage of cures to give the world in its warfare against this dread destroyer. It has a highly successful prophylactic against the spread and contagion of polio in the remedy LATH. This remedy in its provings on healthy human beings produced identical states and symptoms that the polio virus causes. It likewise affects the same nerve roots in the spinal cord (lateral and anterior coloumns - Boericke) to cause the same pathology found in the victims of polio.

Clinically in the past forty years, Homeopathic physicians[1] have successfully protected thousands of children with this simple Homeopathic remedy. These facts have been brought to the attention of the medical world many times in the past decade but without arousing enough interest to test them out for the good of humanity. Research medicine has vainly tried to produce a serum of vaccine against this ever increasing menace to life and limb.

In the past this disease was found almost exclusively among children and young adults but in recent epidemics more and more adults and especially young pregnant women[2] have been attacked.

In the past five years the writer has developed a technique for the administration of the Homeopathic prophylactic against polio that has, up-to-date registered one hundred per cent efficient.[3] This remedy is readily obtainable from any or all of the leading Homeopathic pharmacies of the country. These are Ehrhart and Karl in Chicago; Boericke and Tafel in Philadelphia and Chicago; Luyties in St. Louis and Homeopathic pharmacies in San Francisco and Los Angeles, California and to each of these pharmacies will be mailed a copy of the Homeopathic technique for prophylactics against polio.

The reason for this action is the lack of interest and indifference manifested by the organized medical profession in the past to the vital claims based on numerous clinical experiences and offered to the world

---

1. Dr Grimmer was a major pioneer in the use of Lat-s. as a polio prophylactic and in his own practice over 30,000 children and adults were successfully immunized in fifty years without any side effects. In the days where there was no allopathic polio vaccine this was a major scientific advance. - Editor.
2. Pregnancy increases the risk of contracting paralytic polio myelitis. Cecil Textbook of Medicine. 1982, page 2094, Saunders & Co, Philadelphia. - Editor.
3. See "Repertory Rubrics for Kent's Repertory from Grimmer" p. 859, prepared by the editor.

of medicine to verify or disprove. If this knowledge is as valuable to the needs of the world as the writer is absolutely certain it is, the world should and will have it freely because untold suffering and heart-rending terror will be averted for thousands with the application of a sure, safe protection against this awesome malady.

TECHNIQUE FOR HOMEOPATHIC PROPHYLAXIS AGAINST POLIO

All seeking protection by the Homeopathic method must observe strictly several rules of procedure during the time of treatment and immunization.

1) First, they must abstain from all other medication both topical and internal by injection, olfaction or rubbing in or on the skin. All camphorated or mentholated concoctions or deodorants and perspiration suppressants must be avoided in order to permit the Homeopathic remedy to do its work quickly and effectively. If these rules are not observed the results cannot be certain and complete as they should be.

2) Secondly: A careful nutritious diet of fruit, vegetables and dairy products with a minimum of starches and sweets (except the natural sweets such as honey and fruit sweets) should be given. Especially harmful are the white cane sugar and chocolate preparations. These should be definitely interdicted.

3) For the protective medication a proper spacing of the doses administered together with a graduation of potencies are required for the best results.

4) **For Children from One to Three Years of Age** a single dose of the 30th potency of LATHYRUS-SATIVA once a month for a period of three months during the epidemic. **Two months** after the third dose of the 30th potency is given the 200th potency may be given and repeated again in another two months. **Two months after** the second 200th potency is given than a single dose of the one thousandth potency should be given. Thereafter, only a **single dose of the ten thousandth** potency **twice a year** will be needed for the following **five years** to insure protection for life.

5) **For older children and adults** the spacing of the doses in the same potencies are the same for the first three months after which longer

Technique for Homeopathic Prophylaxis Against Polio ...

intervals between doses can intervene; such as doses of the one thousandth every six months for several years.

If this simple procedure could be universally carried out for a few years it is my firm belief that polio at most would consist only of isolated cases, and those of a mild self-limiting type, with no sequela of deformity or weakness resulting.

Of course proper sanitation and sewerage disposal which prevent the contamination of drinking water and milk supply will aid greatly in the prevention of epidemics of the disease.

The Homeopathic remedy plus diet and sanitation are the forces that will render polio extinct and only a frightful memory in the annals of medicine.

HOMEOPATHIC REMEDIES FOR THE CURE AND PREVENTION OF POLIO[1]

While this is a discussion of the remedies, related to the disease it might be well to remind you of a few cardinal facts recently developed by researchers concerning our subject.

The theory sponsored by the Rockefeller Institute, that flies are the carriers, is no longer accepted by laboratory experts. It is now generally believed by them, that the discharges from the mouth and nose of infected persons are the most likely sources of infection. This, like the time old story of the chicken and the egg, presents to the inquiring philosopher an unsatisfactory and make-shift answer as to which came first the affected individual or the germ or virus. At any rate they are still looking for the specific organism among the filtrateable lists of diseases; it has not yet been discovered or isolated[2]. This is the fact that baffles the treatment methods of our brothers of the Old School. They tell me they are fighting an enemy in the dark and their methods of procedure are purely experimental and more or less uncertain and negative in results. They have found out by experimenting on monkeys that the blood of healthy adults contains neutralizing substances (anti-bodies) to the toxines of the disease, capable of producing a degree of immunity when injected into susceptible organisms; but as a curative agent (using serums) this process is very limited in extent, unless the blood serum is used early in the sickness; this fact stresses the need for an early and accurate diagnosis, not always as easy as some writers imply.

However, there are certain important factors in the study of this sickness that every physician should bear in mind.

SIGNS AND SYMPTOMS OF POLIO

1) To quote from the July-September issue of the Illinois Health Quarterly: Observation has shown a large number of cases to be of a mild type likely due to the better resistance of some individuals, which run a short course of fever, with disturbed digestion, headaches, lassitude etc., leaving the patient free of paralytic symptoms after recovery. This class of cases present symptoms common to many acute infectious diseases in their incipiency, hence, it is nec-

---

1. From the handwritten manuscript of Dr. Grimmer, exact date unknown. - Editor.
2. This article was written many years before the viral nature of polio was known. Of course the nature of the polio virus (a small enteric picorna virus) is now fairly well understood. - Editor.

Signs and Symptoms of Polio ...

essary to know some of the physical signs that accompany this specific illness.

2) As a rule there is greater prostration or weakness than the amount of fever present would justify, this is usually under 102⁰ F (39⁰ C). The flushed face is anxious and frequently there is pallor about the nose and mouth.[1]

3) The throat is mildly infected, but not enough so, to account for the patient's condition. The pulse is usually rapid and out of proportion to the temperature. The rest of the physical examination is negative apart from the nervous system.

4) There is frequently a rather coarse tremor when the child moves, which may be very striking. There is a distinct rigidity of the neck; this is not as marked as that usually seen in meningitis. The patient tilts the head on the neck but does not bend the neck on the shoulders. As a result the head can be brought about half way forward, when resistance is encountered and the patient complains of pain. More constant and more characteristic than the stiffness of the neck is a stiffness of the spine. This is best brought out by having the patient sit up in bed and try to bend the head down onto the knees. The average child ill with other infections is very flexible and has no difficulty in doing this. If these patients bend forward at all, it is from the hips, with the spine held rigidly.[2]

5) Many of them cannot assume a comfortable sitting position without propping themselves up on their arms. Anterior flexion of the spine often causes a drawing pain in the lumbar region, Kernig's sign is not usually marked at this stage, but the deep reflexes are frequently increased rather than diminished as they are later.

6) A cerebral tache is almost always present, not infrequently becoming a purplish, irregular blotching line of half an inch or more in width. It is the presence of these signs and symptoms which justifies a probable diagnosis of anterior poliomyelitis and calls for the final step in diagnosis. This step is the examination of the spinal fluid.

---

1. KR p. 360R, 361L - Editor.
2. KR p. 474R, 946R, 947L - Editor.

SIGNS AND SYMPTOMS OF POLIO ...

7) The fluid is usually under moderately increased pressure (from 150 to 200 mm of water). Microscopically the fluid appears to be clear, but when viewed by transmitted light, it presents a faint haziness which has been described by Zingher as a ground glass appearance. There is an increase of cells, usually between 50 and 250 but occasionally as high as 700 to 800 or as low as 20. These cells may be largely polymorphonuclear early, but later are lymphocytes. There is an increase in globulin.

8) Other acute infections accompanied by meningitis may stimulate the clinical picture of early infantile paralysis, but usually the cause of meningeal irritation becomes evident on physical examination. However in the event of doubt the lumbar puncture as a rule, gives a normal spinal fluid. Tuberculosis and syphilitic meningitis or encephalitis may give a spinal fluid which may be confusing; however the clinical picture is usually sufficiently different that one may avoid mistakes. To the homeopathist the signs and symptoms just detailed, are most valuable, not only from a diagnostic point, but for the search of the curative remedy as well. The painful, uncertain and more or less dangerous spinal puncture procedure will never be needed by the competent homeopath; because the mild non-paralytic cases yield so quickly to the curative remedy that a diagnosis cannot be made before the cure is complete, and in those cases that have developed paralysis the diagnosis is already made and the indicated remedy is the only concern and need left.

ISOLATION

The recommendations for a strict isolation and quarantine of these patients cannot be too closely observed and followed for the protection of others, and for the prevention of a spread of the disease to epidemic proportions. Personally however, I believe the disease is spread by morbific agents in the atmosphere and that quarantine is more a matter of precaution rather than of real use. And our best guarantee for protection individually and collectively, will be found in a homeopathic prophylactic, chosen from the prevailing epidemic remedies of the time and place where the disease is found.

ISOLATION ...

I have had twenty five years of experience with the homeopathic remedies, wherein, many hundreds of cases were seen and treated with no deaths and only one case of crippling, resulting. (That case had been under old school care with the constant use of morphine to control the pain and nervous symptoms for over a week and the child was paralysed and unconscious with death impending, when I was called in on the case. He did not die but was badly maimed in both extremeties). Such results as these should convince one of the superiority of homeopathic treatment.

For prophylactic purposes, I have always given the epidemic remedy - i.e. the remedy of the genus epidemicus - after I had found it, but where no epidemic remedy is known, we have in LATH., a powerful and certain protection against the ravages of this frightful malady. Over 5000 children have been easily and positively protected by this remedy in my hands; given once a week in the 30th potency, during the period of the epidemic. Later years, I have given the 10M. potency at intervals of 30 days with complete protection ("Homeopathy's Prophylaxis Against Polio" p. 171). Many of these children had been directly exposed to the disease, yet evinced no symptoms of sickness while under the remedy. Contrast all this with the more or less uncertain and dangerous method of blood serum treatment and one wonders why homeopathy is not universally employed.

Dr. Henry Bascom Thomas, is authority for the statement, that a positive diagnosis of infantile paralysis, is frequently very difficult to make, before the paralysis appears. He further states, there is no evidence that medicines or serums have any effect of lessening paralysis after the onset of the second stage. What a pity that such men, who have attained so high a place cannot bring themselves to investigate, the curative results of homeopathic methods.

HOMEOPATHIC TREATMENT

We will now proceed with homeopathic remedies and their indications. In the early stages of sickness anyone of our polycrests may be indicated and given and recovery will be certain and rapid. For convenience in remedy study, we may divide the remedies into two groups corresponding to the two first stages of the disease. The first group is the larger one comprising seventy five of our best proven polycrests, they are related to the acute symptoms that come on early, also they include

HOMEOPATHIC TREATMENT ...

the mild non-paralytic types that are met with in a large number of acute manifestations of illness.

I will merely name this group because you all know their indications.

Acon., agar., abrot., aeth., alum., ant-t., apis, arn., ars., arum-t., asaf., bell., brom., bry., cham., canth., carb-v., caust., chlor., cimic., cina., coff., coloc., dulc., eup-per., ferr-p., fagu., gels., hell., hep., hyos., ip., jab., kali-br., kali-i., kali-p., kalm., lac-c., lach., lath., led., lob., lyc., lyss., merc., merc-i-f., merc-i-r., merc-cy., nat-ar., nat-m., nux-m., nux-v., olnd., op., phos., plb., phys., phyt., podo., psor., puls., pyrog., rhus-t., sang., sil., spig., stram., sulph., tab., tarent., thuj., valer., verat., verat-v., zinc.

A good working knowledge of these remedies will enable the clinician to cope with ninety five percent of all acute ailments met with in general practice and all the leading remedies for infantile paralysis are here included.

A keen homeopathic prescriber will abort nearly every case he sees in the first twenty four hours of sickness. It is in those cases where the paralytic symptoms are already present when the physician is first called that the exact similimum is so necessary, if life is to be secured and crippling is to be avoided. And these are the remedies that are more precious than material riches, for they are the keys to life and health, but each must be selected by the Master prescriber for the individual patient if perfect results are to be obtained. For life is not only in the balance, but a life of healthful strength instead of a maimed weakling that may linger on the correct remedy chosen out of this valuable group of seventy five remedies.

WHY HAVE POLIO?[1]

So called regular medicine has failed disastrously to answer the question: Why have Polio? Millions of dollars have been collected from a sympathetic public and spent for so-called research, the chief results of which have been the destruction and suffering of millions of defenseless monkeys; several hundred thousand are required annually to make the vaccine.

Surely no one can logically or truthfully claim any degree of immunity for the Salk vaccine in the light of the present experiment with its many dire and fatal side effects, together with the fact that epidemics of the disease are raging as never before in Boston, and everywhere this so-called protective agent was widely used there has been no appreciable diminuation of the scourge. In spite of the painstaking care to make the Salk vaccine theoretically safe many contacts of vaccinated cases have been stricken down with the bulbar type of the disease and died, thus proving the imminent danger from its use.

This is not the first time that a vaccine has proven ineffective and dangerous. Some twenty or thirty years ago the Michael Reese Hospital of Chicago produced and experimented with a vaccine for protection against polio with much the same unhappy results.

Regardless of these incontestable facts the organized propaganda for the March of Dimes has the brazen, unscrupulous audacity to place placards in public places, food stores, etc., announcing that the Salk vaccine is safe and effective. Indeed it has proven safe and good for the vendors of toxines and effective in spreading epidemic disease.

We hope the criticism herein offered against the use of the Salk vaccine will prove constructive, as it is based on the results produced which must stand as proven fact. The work for a highly effective and at the same time one hundred percent safe prophylactic against polio, free from all side effects, will continue until it is found and proven to the world.

We know that the homeopathic law of similars has the answer to polio prevention, safely, surely, economically and with no consequential side effects. In the past fifty years measuring my experience in the medical field, homeopathic physicians have immunized many hundreds of thousands of patients against this dread disease with very few, if any, failures. In my individual practice I succeeded in immunizing

---

1.   THE LAYMAN SPEAKS, excact date unknown. - Editor.

not less than fifty thousand cases without a single failure. Such a record based on an established law of cure, viz., the Law of Similiars, promulgated by Samuel Hahnnemann one hundred and sixty years ago is sufficient reason for our faith.

To elucidate the Law of Similiars for a clearer understanding of the same and especially for those unacquainted with the subject, I will give a brief summary of its action. To start with, remedial agents are first given to humans in approximate health and all subsequent reactions are noted: symptoms produced, mental, emotional and physical, changes observed in the blood and other body secretions and excretions. In fact all deviations from the normal state of health are noted and recorded. This constitutes a proving and is incorporated into the Homeopathic Materia Medica. Each single remedy is proven separately on humans (not on dumb animals). Some provings on animals have been made to note the pathologic changes wrought in the tissue cells of the animal body.

Among the numerous homeopathic provings the drug LATH. has been well proven. Some of its most drastic action is found in the poisonous effects of humans who ate it in their food and became paralyzed in their lower limbs, simulating the worst cases of paralytic polio and the same nerve roots in the spinal cord (anterior horn cells) of the victims were involved that takes place under the action of the polio virus. Clinically this remedy when used in homeopathic form or attenuated doses, has cured many cases of the disease as well as immunized thousands against it.

Immunologists tell us that the puncture from even a sterile needle may trigger into activity an incubating latent polio into an active and virulent form of the disease. This fact alone makes all hypodermic injections of serums or vaccines a dangerous and unscientific proceedure. Already there is a suggestion to prepare the vaccine so it can be administered by mouth much after the methods employed by homeopathy in the administration of their nosodes (remedies prepared in potentized form from disease producing secretions and tissues). The administration of remedies by mouth avoids another added danger which exists when a foreign protein is injected into the blood stream; death has occassionally followed this proceedure and no one can measure the infinite harm done to thousands of these victims of pseudo science who survived the first impact of the shock to their systems.

It is apparent that the hazards involved in the protection against disease is as great or even greater than the ravages of the disease itself under the present standard of techniques in preparing and administering their protective vaccines.

In striking contrast the homeopathic approach and technique is truely scientific, safe, highly efficient, and economical in its application. Homeopathy teaches us no one remedy can be curative in all cases in any specific disease condition and that the individual's characteristic symptoms are always the true guide for the selection of the curative remedy.

However in epidemic disease a relatively few remedies and sometimes onlyone remedy) may be needed. In the polio disease there are only a few of the well proven remedies that correspond to the symptomatic and pathological nature of the disease in their pathogenesis and clinical confirmations.

Heading the list of such remedies is Lath. (the wild pea) which through the past half century has proven to be a most efficient prophylactic[1] against this dreadful malady. This remedy can be easily procured by physicians in the desired potencies at any of our homeopathic pharmacies in the country: Ehrhart and Karl and Boericke and Tafel in Chicago, Luyties in Saint Louis, Boericke and Tafel in New York and Philadelphia, Boericke and Runyon in San Francisco and Los Angeles.

DIET: An investigation in the south some years ago established the fact that excessive amounts of cane sugar in the diet predisposes subjects to a susceptibility to the disease. It then behoves us to regulate the diet, especially of children, curtailing all articles rich in cane sugar such as pastries, candy, soft drinks, etc. and substitute fruits and vegetables and their juices in abundance, thereby enriching the natural vitamin intake which aids body resistance to disease.

It must always be remembered that the **deep constitutional remedy** is the **most effective protection** against all acute infectious disease conditions and **it alone is sufficient**.

Polio is no longer a scourge and threat to children alone as more and more adults are stricken with each epidemic. Pregnant women are more susceptible than the non-pregnant. How much excess of alcoholic drinks may have to do with the increase of the infection in male adults has not been determined but it may be a factor. Excessive fatigue and strain and exposure to temperature extremes are other exciting agents by reducing body resistance to all disease influences.[2]

---

1. The technique for immunization against polio is laid out in the article "Homeopathy's Prophylaxis Against Polio" p. 171 ff. - Editor.

Homeopathic research is now studying another remedy: Coyotillo, native of Mexico, which was introduced by Dr. Garcia-Trevino of Mexico to his homeopathic colleagues. From its highly poisonous effects on animals and humans who have eaten the fruit and seeds of the plant which produces complete paralysis of the lower extremities and death in a short time, twenty four to forty eight hours after its intake. A strange and significant factor concerning the properties of the plant is that animals poisoned with the seeds have recovered after they are given a decoction of the root of the plant. We need and will soon have a full proving of this potentially valuable remedy to add power and hope to our already extensive Materia Medica. In its toxic manifestations it simulates the worst cases of bulbar polio.

Because the steady increase in the spread and virulence of the disease is sufficient reason for the healers in every branch and type of the healing art to be interested in the prophylaxis and cure of this scourge, because many lives may be saved to perform their destined uses in the world are why I have the great privilege of presenting this paper before this fine scientific group.

---

2. Tonsilectomy predisposes to infection with the polio virus. See CECIL TEXTBOOK OF MEDCINE, page 2094, Saunders & Co., Philadelphia, 1982 - Editor.

HOMEOPATHIC PROTECTION FROM POLIO[1]

The constant alarming increase of polio epidemics in the last decade renders any certain protective agent against the ravages of this disease a most welcome boom to the public. Homeopathy provides that beneficial measure in the remedy LATH. This remedy has been well proven on healthy humans and its clinical application in many epidemics in the past fifty years places it at the top, both as a curative and prophylactic drug against polio and other spinal diseases of a serious type.

Pathologically and symptomatically LATH. presents a striking likeness of the polio sickness. It attacks the nerve roots in the anterior column of the spine in identically the same way the polio virus does and its paralytic action and muscular atrophy presents similar states and symptoms found in polio victims. Hence, it is the logical and scientific answer to the prevention and cure of polio.

In the **bulbar type** of the disease OP. in homeopathic form is the remedy needed as a complimentary to cure. It is said if the bulbar type case recovers there is not the consequent crippling that follows recovery from severe spinal cases. Before the days of the iron lung homeopaths saved the severest cases with remedies like **OP.** and ANT-T..; this in no way depreciates the value and use of the iron lung.

Also the **spinal cases that were badly crippled after recovery** were greatly benefited by remedies like CALC-P. and CALC-S. before the advent of the Kenny cure which has proven very helpful and well worthwhile, involving massage manipulation and hot packs (mechanical therapy).

As true healers we should avail ourselves of every useful means at hand to help the patient. True physicians accept without prejudice every proven advance in medicine for the good of the race.

However, much of modern medicine dominated as it is today by powerful commercial interests is propaganda put out for selfish purposes and not for the public good; in fact much of the so-called scientific advancement such as the wonder drugs have produced great harm and have been repudiated even by the venders and advocates who dispensed them.

But to get back to polio. It has been observed that in recent epidemics more and more adults and especially young pregnant women have been attacked with the disease. This is only another reason that a safe,

---

1. From the handwritten manuscript of Dr. Grimmer, exact date unknown. - Editor.

sure antidote with no adverse side effects or consequential results from its use constitutes a most desirable and valuable asset for the irradication of polio, as well as an advance in true scientific medicine.

To apply the homeopathic method of protection against polio is very simple and easy. During the epidemic months when polio prevails a small dose of the 30th potency of LATH. given every two weeks (and no other medication permitted) will immunize any human subject against polio for the first season.

For protection against the disease the second or following season will require a higher potency of the remedy, the 200 given a month apart. The third season will require the one thousand potency of the remedy given a month apart. Thereafter, only a single dose of the ten thousand potency at the beginning of the season will immunize for life.

If every physician in the land will apply the simple homeopathic formula by prescribing LATH. as directed in this brief paper the land in a few years will be freed of the dread terror of poliomyelitis.

Not only is LATH. symptomatically and pathologically similar in nature to the polio virus but it is electro magnetically similar as both the virus and the remedy are neutral in action. Thus the chain of similarity is complete making the remedy a perfect neutralizer of the disease.

In closing it might be well to state for those not informed that this drug can be obtained in the desired potencies from any homeopathic pharmacy. Ehrhart and Karl and Boericke and Tafel both of Chicago are two pharmacies willing and able to furnish this remedy properly and reliably prepared.

Philosophy

Pillars of Homeopathic Philosophy[1]

This book is written for my children and their children, and for many friends and my former patients who are unable to obtain homeopathic treatment because of the lack of homeopathic physicians in many places in our country today.

It must be known that in order to make a successful prescription it is necessary to apply the Materia Medica in conjunction with the homeopathic philosophy in order to guide the future actions of the prescriber. The re-actions that follow the administration of the remedy are highly informative to those able to interpret their meaning accurately. After a good prescription the symptoms leave from above downward, from within outward, from center to circumference, from more vital to less vital parts of the body. When symptoms leave in this way the prescriber can feel certain of a good prescription that should bring curative results. If symptoms depart in an opposite direction the prescription was faulty and inaccurate.

As a rule self medication cannot be endorsed except in cases of emergency, and where a competent homeopathic physician cannot be had. The prescriber must know that all symptoms are not of equal value; the mental, emotional symptoms are the most valuable for prescribing. Symptoms affecting the patient as a whole, such as the effects of heat and cold, storms, etc. are next in value. These symptoms are known as generals. Symptoms affecting special parts and organs of the body are known as particulars; they are less valuable for use in prescribing.

We know that the homeopathic remedy cannot cure every case of disease because other means along with the remedy must be used, such as proper diet of vital food containing the organic minerals and vitamins; in fact much of human sickness stems from processed food lacking the essential vital elements.

The homeopathic remedy does what nothing else can do; it antidotes the deep seated constitutional inherited toxins that affects every human being in the world. Proper regular exercise is another aid to good health. But the most important thing to know and remember for both doctor and patient is the fact that no healing is obtained without the Will and Blessing of our Heavenly Father.

---

1. These three pages were meant to be the beginnings of a preface to a book on Materia Medica which Dr. Grimmer started a few days before his death in 1967 and of which only 6 pages were written. - Editor.

With these facts in mind we are ready with faith and reverence to take up the study of Materia Medica in our search for the Similimum in each individual case of sickness it is our privilage to help.

For those desiring to become more proficient in prescribing the Homeopathic Materia, the following books will prove very helpful; Hahnemann's Organon, Kent's Philosophy, Boericke's Materia Medica, H.C. Allen's Keynotes of Homeopathic Remedies. A careful and persistent study of these books will aid greatly in successful prescribing of the Homeopathic Materia Medica.

In the domain of sickness there are five diseases that may be called killers and when they are advanced to the chronic state they rarely, if ever, are cured although they may be palliated, and the sufferings lessened by proper treatment. These killing diseases are: Cancer, which may affect any tissue or organ of the body; cardio-vascular disease, which may end in heart failure; cerebro-spinal disease, which may end in apoplectic stroke and paralysis; kidney disease often ends in coma and death, and chronic respiratory diseases ending in death. Any remedy in the Materia Medica may be needed in any given case, but the one that is needed can only be determined by the totality of the general characteristic symptoms of the case. From four to six general characteristic symptoms of any case will reflect the spirit of the totality and its removal by the best remedy.

We will now proceed with our remedy study. From the early beginnings of homeopathy its ranks have been divided and torn by the question of potency to be used, its whether the high or the low potencies was more efficient to cure the sick. It is now known that all the potencies are needed to do the best work in curing sick people. In a general way, the lower potencies do better work in the acute forms of sickness. Most cases of chronic disease require a succession of potencies to cure cases of disease.

THE BLESSED "GIFT OF GOD"[1]

Remedies prepared from living things fresh from the Creator's hands; proved remedies that must be given according to the Law of Similars. If the symptoms of these remedies are studied and applied faithfully, healing results will surely follow. The physician fortunate enough to know and apply them in love and faith in the Heavenly Father is twice blest, first by the Lord of heaven and earth and second by grateful, happy, healed patients.

Because of the lack of enough homeopathic physicians in the United States to meet the needs of many people wanting homeopathic treatment, this knowledge is given to the laity for their healing needs. These remedies can all be obtained at Ehrhart and Karl's Homeopathic Pharmacy, 17 North Wabash Avenue, Chicago, Illinois.

Many cure producing remedies are obtained from the so-called non-living minerals and metals; their curative powers are released by the process of potentization developed by Dr. Samuel Hahnemann over one hundred fifty years ago. Every substance throughout the whole domain of nature contains occult cure-producing powers.

Experienced prescribers know that all symptoms are not of equal value in finding the best remedy for each individual case of sickness.

The mental and emotional symptoms and disturbances of the sick individual such as the fears, the hates, perverted loves, the frustrations, disappointments, grief, etc. are most important in the search for the best remedy.

Symptoms and states of mind that affect the patient as a whole are known as generals. Those symptoms that affect special parts and organs of the body are known as particulars, and are less valuable for prescribing purposes.

Symptoms peculiar to the individual known as characteristics are of high grade value in the selection of the remedy.

The modalities: time and circumstances of the aggravations and ameliorations of the patient's symptoms is another essential feature in every case.

Those prescribing homeopathic medicines will note certain specific results occurring in the symptomatology of the patient after each prescription. After a good prescription, the symptoms of the patient will depart in the inverse order of their coming; the last to come will be the

---

1.   From the handwritten manuscript of Dr. Grimmer, exact date unknown. - Editor.

first to go, and they depart from above downward, from within out, from center to circumference, from the vital centers to the external tissues, such as the skin and mucous membranes. A case from practice will illustrate:

A six year old child suffering almost constantly with severe asthmatic attack that came soon after the suppression of an eczema of the scalp, which developed soon after the child's birth. A single dose of SULPH. 10M brought back the eruption on the scalp and permanently cured the asthma, and soon after this the eczema as well was cured.

It is just as necessary for the prescriber to know the homeopathic philosophy as it is to know the symptomatology of the Homeopathic Materia Medica. Both must be used together to obtain the best results in the domain of cure. The homeopathic literature contains many fine books, written by outstanding homeopathic physicians, but they were written for the use of the doctors. This book is written for the instruction, and use of lay people in need of homeopathic treatment where no homeopathic doctor is available. Only the essential symptoms for successful prescribing are given in this work to conserve space and time: hence this is but a synopsis of the Materia Medica of remedies described that follow.

Perhaps the most important factor in the search for the best remedy will be found to be the causative element of the patient's sickness, such as the effects of shock, of fright, of injuries, of grief, of disappointed love and all forms of frustration together with the baneful effects of hate, envy and greed.

There are two books that treat of the art and science of homeopathic prescribing, viz, the "Organon" by Hahnemann and Kent's "Philosophy". These books are indispensible for those who seek perfection in prescribing homeopathically. These books can be obtained at Ehrhart and Karl.

When seeking to restore and maintain health we must know the value of food that is vital and nourishing and that contains the organic minerals and vitamins found only in the natural plants and grains grown in and on soils enriched by scientific preparation and treatment. Today we are subjected to too much processed and devitalized foods. Hence the difficulty in maintaining good health.

Another important asset in the enjoyment of good health is deep rhythmic breathing which oxidizes and purifies the blood to give it prophylactic power against disease. Regular systematic exercise is also a contributing asset to good health. But more important than anything else is living in the blessing of the first and second commandments which are epitomized in the last words of our Savior Jesus Christ before the crucifixion, to love one another as he loved us.

It is apparent that good health depends on a number of things working together for the healing and happiness of the embodied man spiritually, mentally and physically all blended as one and dedicated to the heavenly Father and all His children everywhere in the world. From what we have seen, we know that remedies alone cannot completely cure all the sickness afflicting mankind, neither can proper food alone nor deep breathing and exercise alone. What potentized remedies do (and I nothing else can do) is to antidote the inherited toxins coming down through succeeding generations to keep mankind sick. These toxins can be irradicated by the right remedy.

REASONS FOR THE NEED OF HOMEOPATHIC PHILOSOPHY[1]

The fact that homeopathic physicians have stated that the study of homeopathic philosophy is not of sufficient value to justify the labor and effort involved in such study is the reason for the title of this paper.

It might be well to have some standard definition of philosophy in order to clarify the work we wish to present. Webster defines philosophy as follows: "First: the love of wisdom; second: the knowledge of phenomena as explained by and resolved into causes and reasons, powers and laws; third: a systematic body of general conceptions and principles, ordinarily with implication of their practical application as a practical philosophy of life; fourth: practical wisdom, calmness of temper and judgment, equanimity."

Will Durant in his book entitled *The Story of Philosophy*[2] clearly and charmingly shows how the status and progress of individuals, states, races, and eras have corresponded to the type of philosophic concepts they imbibed. Furthermore, he reveals that only with the aid and light of philosophic truth has there been any advance in the conduct and accomplishments of the race. To quote a brief excerpt from the introduction to his book: "Every science begins as philosophy and ends as art; it arises in hypothesis and flows into achievement. Philosophy is a hypothetical interpretation of the unknown (as in metaphysics) or of the inexactly known, as in ethics or political philosophy; it is the front trench in the siege of truth. Science is the captured territory, and behind it are those secure regions in which knowledge and art build our imperfect and marvelous world. Philosophy seems to stand still, perplexed; but only because she leaves the fruits of victory to her daughters, the sciences, and herself passes on divinely discontent, to the uncertain and unexplained."

I will present a few of its practical and commonplace phases for your consideration.

First and paramount above all other reasons for the existance and use of homeopathic philosophy is the distinctive concept it holds of the nature of health and disease. This concept is essential in homeopathic practice as is the "Law of Similars"; in fact, it is indispensable for the

---

1. This article was presented in a regional meeting and never published. From the handwritten manuscript of Dr. Grimmer, exact date unknown - Editor.
2. DURANT, WILL; The Story of Philosophy; New revised edition, Garden City Publishing, 1933, 592 p.

successful application of the law, involving in its scope the evolution and prognosis in all sick states before, during, and after the administration of the similar remedy.

Without the Hahnemannian perception of the vital force and its relation to health and sickness[1], the application and use of the law are restricted and confined to very narrow limitations. To know that health is harmony in the play of vital processes[2] and that disease has its beginnings in the disturbance of this harmony is the fundamental tenet of our philosophy. In more modern terms, ill health begins in some unbalance of the electro-magnetic processes which precipitate a changed body chemistry; this change if not soon reversed results in tissue changes, morbid anatomy or pathology, the end results of disease.

However, traditional medicine regards pathology as the disease itself and seeks to extirpate it, thinking thereby to cure the patient. Here we see the opposing philosophies of the two schools of medical thought. One the homeopathic, recognizing and operating on the functional or causative plane of life; the other school, the mechanical operates on the material plane, which corresponds to the effects of disease only.

The homeopathic concept of life processes alone can explain the reason for the similar remedy in the minimum dose and the phenomena of health and sickness in all of its ramifications.

The observations of many able prescribers over a long period have given us a number of aphorisms that are invaluable to the homeopathist in the successful application of the true art of healing. Hahnemann's observation that symptoms get well in the inverse order of their coming under the action of the similium has been confirmed by thousands of prescribers. Hering's observation of symptoms departing from above downward, from within outward, from center to circumference is another often confirmed observation. Kent in his philosophy of homeopathics has given us twelve observations following the administration of the homeopathic remedy, which every homeopathic doctor should know and remember.[3]

1) Prolonged aggravation and final decline of the patient. This is an indication of incurable disease or that tissue changes in vital organs

---

1. Organon §8 - 16. - Editor.
2. Organon §9. - Editor.
3. Cf: Kent, J.T., Lectures on Homeopathic Philosophy. Lecture XXXV. Prognosis after Observing the Action of the Remedy. Ehrhart and Karl Chicago. - Editor.

have progressed too far to be arrested or restored. The anti-psoric was too deep; it has established destruction.

2) Long aggravation; but final and slow improvement. Usually this indicates the beginning of some marked tissue changes in some organ.

3) The sharp aggravation followed by a rapid improvement of the patient. Long relief of symptoms with a general improvement in the state of the patient's health is probably the most frequently noted and is a sure indication of the selection of the best remedy.

4) A prolonged amelioration with no aggravation indicates the correct remedy given in the perfectly attuned potency.

5) The amelioration coming first followed by the aggravation afterwards indicates either an incurable disease or a remedy only superficial in action to the case. Such remedies frequently repeated may easily act as suppressants producing irreparable harm to the patient.

6) Too short relief of symptoms. In acute cases this may mean a desperate condition (high grade inflammation; organs threatened by rapid processes); in chronic cases this means there are structural changes and organs are destroyed or being destroyed or in a very precarious condition.

7) Full time amelioration of symptoms; yet no special relief of the patient. This indicates latent conditions, or latent existing organic conditions. Or patients have an organ missing or diseased and cannot rise above their own pitch. This is a suitable homeopathic palliation.

8) Cases where symptoms of every remedy given appear without benefit to the patient's symptoms or general health denotes one of great susceptibility to all miasmatic or morbid influences and will prove a very difficult one to cure of his chronic states. Such patients are natural provers and remedies should not be given above the 30th potency or below the 6th.[1]

---

1. Dr. Kent observed that you may often cure their acute troubles by a 30th or 200th and relieve their chronic troubles by a 30th, 200th or 500th potency.

9) Action of the medicines upon provers. Healthy provers are always benefited by provings.[1]

10) New symptoms appearing after the remedy: If a great number of new symptoms appear after the administration of a remedy, the prescription will generally prove an unfavorable one - it did not sustain a true homeopathic relation.

11) Old symptoms reappear: Good prescription, disease curable - Hering's Law.

12) Symptoms take wrong direction (from circumference to center). The remedy must be antidoted at once as it is a suppressant.

From all this we see another use and perhaps the greatest one for the existence of Homeopathic Philosophy: It teaches one to observe facts and their sequence and to reason distinctively and logically, thereby perfecting our science and growing in wisdom.

---

1. §141 Organon - see especially the footnote 103 to §141 - Editor.

WHY PHILOSOPHY?[1]

This is a question often asked both in and out of conventions. Reviewing the ascent of man from primitive times, and noting the milestones that mark his progress along the path of civilization, we are struck with the part that philosophy plays in all his achievements spiritually, intellectually and socially.

It is a recognized fact, that without a logical system of thinking and planning, no accomplishment in science, art or sociology is possible. And how much more applicable must this be in the domain of therapeutics.

Philosophy treats of law and orderly thinking from cause to effect, correlating observed facts and reducing them to formulae for use and expansion. Homeopathy based on the known therapeutic "*Law of Similars*" cannot evolve to its highest use without a philosophy to correlate the thousands of observed facts related to drug provings, and subsequent cures resulting from the application of the law to the sick.

So much has been written about this very important subject by the masters who have gone before: Hahnemann, Hering, Dunham, Kent, Boger, are but a few that I need to mention to show how futile my efforts must be to bring anything new or original to you about the philosophy of Homeopathy. And so well have they perfected this necessary characteristic of our therapeutics that the best I can offer is a brief review of some of the important essentials of our philosophy culled from the writing and teachings of these immortals.

Perhaps the first essential is to perceive with Hahnemann the nature of sickness and its relationship to health. Unless one knows the order and sequence involved in the creation of the human organism he cannot be a master healer. It is fitting to recognize that the vital force or energy is prior to the physical body and is its builder and sustainer through life[2]. This animating principle or vital force when flowing in order and unhampered, spells harmony or health in mind and body, and produces normal physiologic, biochemical action that results in normal histology and normal anatomical structure. Any inharmony of the vital force activating the physiologic processes ends in pathology or morbid anatomy. Hence to remove the pathologic end results of

---

1. This article appeared in THE HOMEOPATHIC RECORDER, Vol. LVII, No. 2, August, 1941, page 60. Article by same title but different text see pgs 201 ff.
2. §9 Organon.

morbific vital action is only dealing with effects and not causes of disease. It is only necessary to change and direct the disturbed vital force to its normal healthy state in order to free the body of disease and promote health.[1]

A second essential is to know what is curable in sickness together with what is curative in medicines, and to recognize when they are properly prepared and scientifically selected for each given case of sickness.[2]

A third essential is the taking of a comprehensive and complete case history of the patient, recording his individual symptoms of sickness past and present, with their times of exacerbation and amelioration. An image of his mental and emotional states must be environment such as heat, cold, weather changes, etc. Added to all this must be as complete a family history as can be obtained.[3]

In obtaining such a history the physician must not ask any direct questions or suggest any line of thought to his patient. Remember any question answered by "yes or no" is incorrectly put and is of doubtful value. Every symptom properly obtained becomes a fact that, linked with the completed chain of facts (symptoms), presents an image of disease that may be duplicated by the likeness of one of our proven drugs. When one can transcribe such a case record into the language of drug provings, he will learn what is curable in disease as well as the curative powers of remedies. He will know how to observe the pace and directions of symptoms of disease and of drug provings as well.

Another essential that must be followed faithfully to assure the complete working of a successful prescription is a knowledge of the order and direction of cure. That is symptoms get well in the reverse order of their coming, they depart from center to circumference, from above downward, from more to less vital parts of the body. Old symptoms, long forgotten, frequently return and pass under the action of the curative remedy. Suppressed symptoms, especially catarrhal and skin diseases of a chronic nature, reappear with a relief of internal symptoms and states after the administration of the indicated remedy.[4]

---

1. §10 - 16 Organon - Editor.
2. §3 Organon - Editor.
3. §82 - 99 Organon - Editor.
4. And these suppressions in turn finally disappear under the indicated remedy to leave behind perfect health. -- Editor.

Every homeopathic physician should be thoroughly familiar with the nature of each of the chronic miasms and their importance in the causation and maintenance of disease, both acute and chronic.

Lastly, it is essential that the homeopathist, more than any other physician, should be alert to the changing theories and so-called scientific discoveries in medicines. This is especially true concerning the numerous new drugs, serums, and chemical poisons, that are flooding the public at this time. From the earliest time in medical history, humanity has suffered more from experimental attempts of cure than it has from the ravages of the diseases at which the cures were directed. At the present time, many of these drugs are especially pernicious, leaving an insidious train of chronic blood and nerve degenerations after the abusive experimental use on thousands of human guinea pigs who are the hapless victims of empirical medicine which readily lends itself to an unscrupulous racket rightly labeled commercialized medicine.

A few don'ts might be thrown in here as profitable reminders for the physician to heed. Kent warned to never leave a remedy that benefited a case until after a higher potency of it has failed to act. A few cases are on record where a lower potency has acted after the higher had failed but these later observations occurred in the course of acute disease; typhoid, etc. In the course of chronic disease when new symptoms appear even though when quite numerous, do not change or interfere with the remedy while the patient is better. In the selection of remedies from a case record, choose the generalities, those symptoms characteristic of the patient, the emotional symptoms, the general body reactions to environment, the desires and aversions, the sex symptoms as being important for repertory or other study. In this society it should be and is, superfluous to admonish against the prescribing for diagnostic names of disease instead of for the sick patient. With diagnoses admittedly 50 per cent erroneous, such a basis is absurd and useless to the homeopath for prescribing purposes. There are many more dont's that may be found in the writings and teachings of the host of mighty men and women who have gone before us, leaving behind them for the future of the race a priceless heritage, that we in gratitude and humility should make every sacrifice to preserve and expand, by adding out little mites to the common fund of their God sent knowledge for the healing of the nations. Under the benign ministrations of Homeopathy will come a better race where peace, understanding and good will shall prevail over the earth, and all men shall live united as one family under the Fatherhood of God.

WHY PHILOSOPHY?[1]

No idea, project or science, can advance or expand without a philosophic background or foundation to promote its growth and permanency in the activities of our expanding world.

Our literature is so rich in many fine papers on homeopathic philosophy from the pens of our greatest physicians and thinkers, to say nothing of Hahnemann's *Organon* and Kent's *Homeopathic Philosophy,* that it seems puerile and egotistical or presumptious on my part, to present a paper on this subject that can add anything new or original or even of value to the volumes of keen observations and logical conclusions from which laws and rules have been deducted and expounded for the use of all present and future homeopathic physicians everywhere. The best I can offer is a cursory review of some of the important highlights that have been presented time to time in the past.

Taking the Case: A case properly taken makes the correct prescription easier to find, and insures greater accuracy with consequent better success in terms of cure.

Only indirect questioning of the patient must be employed; any question that is answered by yes or no has been wrongly put and the answer is of little, if any, value to prescribe on.

Direct questions tend to invoke answers without sufficient thought on the part of the patient and in certain impressionable types of patients, a direct question may suggest symptoms or conditions not really present.

The patient should be permitted to relate the account of his sick history and symptoms without interruption exept when he strays from the subject. When he has finished his story, then the indirect questions may be put to him.

In case taking the physician must bring to bear to the fullest, his powers of observation and he must employ the use of sight, hearing, smell, even taste and touch in order to obtain an accurate picture of the sick patient that will enable him to match his symptoms with the one specific remedy in the materia medica that can effect a cure by the law of similars.

---

1. JOURNAL OF THE AMERICAN INSTITUTE OF HOMEOPATHY, Vol. 53; Nos. 9-10; Sept., Oct., 1960, p. 133 and also in THE LAYMAN SPEAKS, Vol. XVII, Jan. 1964, p. 15. Article by same title but different text see pgs 198 ff.

In the search for the indicated remedy, the characteristic mental and emotional symptoms are of highest rank. The loves and hates (perverted loves) are very valuable in remedy selection. Included are the symptoms of fear, anger and frustration, and the effects these emotions leave on the economy of the patient, these all blend into the realm of causation behind the patient's illness.

The physical general symptoms which express the patient's reaction to environmental forces, such as heat, cold, storm, noise, etc. together with the food desires and aversions, are next in importance; perhaps somewhat more valuable are the symptoms of the sexual spheres because the loves and emotional side of life are involved. The hemorrhages and discharges are important in general symptoms because the whole economy of the patient is involved in their elaboration. The most valuable of all symptoms are the strange, rare and peculiar[1].

All these aforementioned symptoms relate closely to the patient as a whole and are of much greater value in the realm of prescribing than are the particular symptoms relating to the parts or organs of the body.

After the Case is Taken: After the correct prescription is made, certain states and changes in the symptomatology of the patient may be noted.

First an improvement in the general state of the patient and his symptoms are seen; often the first reaction of the remedy is an aggravation of symptoms followed by marked and continued improvement. The return of old symptoms such as skin eruptions, discharges from some of the body orifices, the return of malarial states that had been suppressed by quinine, rheumatic or neuralgic pains, chronic headaches and many other conditions that had been palliated by powerful pain killing drugs are favorable signs.

Such return of old symptoms and conditions can always be hailed as an indication that the correct prescription was made and that the vital centers are relieved with the appearance of surface manifestations. Symptoms under the homeopathic remedy proceed from within outward, from above downward, from center to circumference, from internal vital organs to mucous membranes and the outer skin, and in the reverse order of their appearance. (Hering's Law)

When such manifestations occur they must not be interfered with by other medication until the time comes for a repetition of the curative remedy. The repetition of the curative remedy and the time lapse between doses is vitally important and fraught with uncertainty,

---

1. §153 Organon - Editor.

because in recent times there are so many interfering elements that cut short the action of our remedies[1] so that repetition or complementary remedies are often needed at much shorter periods than what occurred in the earlier times of homeopathic prescribing.

In times when such interferences are absent, the action of the curative dose will continue from a month to six weeks, in some instances much longer with a continued improvement in the symptoms and general state of the patient.

Some of the frequent interfering forces to homeopathic remedies outside of camphor and menthol, are alumina and flourides which come by way of aluminum cooking utensils, the alumina flourides put into the public water supply and the flouride used in dental work and in tooth pastes. These are drastic poisons that not only stop the action of curative medicines, but pollute the blood stream of thousands of innocent, helpless victims with a subtle destructive sick-making power, very difficult to antidote or eradicate from the body once it has accumulated to a point of saturation. Destructive processes that ultimate in many forms of malignant disease, crippling forms of arthritis, ulcerative conditions, gangrenous states, severe forms of lung, cardiac and renal diseases - may be induced and aggravated by this universal poison.

Another universal poison becoming more and more recognized by scientists is that of radiation. Already the high strates of the earth's atmosphere, with the rainfall and all the oceans are more or less charged with radio-active strontium. This poison also cuts short and inhibits the action of curative medicines.

Adulterated foods, drastic drugging, often self-administered, are other factors in the cause of impaired health and inhibited action of curative medicines.

Hahnemannian Homeopathy as practiced by its best trained prescribers can better cope with these wide spread subtle sick-producing forces, that may well constitute a most serious threat to the existance of all the Earth's inhabitants. At least universal health is menaced with a chain of untoward suffering in its wake.

Homeopathy recognizes laws and principles in all its procedures in its quest of cure. There is no science known to man that is not employed in the processes of homeopathic techniques; the most advanced type of physics is required in the manufacture of our medicines. We were the first in the field of psychosomatic medicine and we

---

1. See article "Things that Interfere with the Homeopathic Prescription" p. 293 ff. - Editor.

stand unrivaled in our recognition and practice of the higher spiritual laws fresh from the goodness of Divine Providence.

Friends and advocates of homeopathic healing, ours is a rare privilege to practice this effective form of healing. To be principled and gifted in its knowledge is a blessing to both patient and physician. We must perfect our uses that we may become keener prescribers. To accomplish these ends best, we need unremitting study of our vast materia medica and the philosophy of Hahnemann and Kent with a sublime trust in the Heavenly Father.

ESSENTIALS OF HOMEOPATHIC PHILOSOPHY[1]

After all the profound and clearly stated papers and treatises emanating from the great leaders in our school on this vital subject of the philosophy, that distinguishes us and sets us apart from all other schools of healing, it seems almost a waste of time on my part to attempt to bring you anything of value not heretofore given. But inspired by those immortals, I will try in a humble way to impart to you what has appealed to me as the essential features of our philosophy. These enable us to excell in the noble art of healing because these essentials bring us a more logical concept of life in its relation to health and to disease, together with its cause and cure.

If we can raise our consciousness to the mental plane of Hahnemann and his faithful disciples, Boeninghausen, Hering, Dunham, Kent, Lippe and many others, we will more easily perceive the true nature of sickness, and at the same time be better armed to cope with it.

There are at least four important factors in the study and application of the indicated remedy to the sick that must be understood, if one would become a successful homeopathic prescriber; and these may well constitute the essentials of homeopathic philosophy.

The first essential is the homeopathic concept of life itself, manifested in health and in disease, involving in its scope both cause and cure.

The second is the successful and complete taking of the case, according to proper scientific modes of procedure, the gathering together and classification of symptoms in their relative order and power to build up a symptom picture, whose likeness can be found only in one of the drug provings hidden away in the vast storehouse of the homeopathic Materia Medica.

Third, a knowledge of the relative value of all symptoms obtained both subjectively and objectively. Fourth, the ability to observe keenly and accurately the order in which symptoms come under the progress of disease, and conversely, the order of their departure under the influence of the *homeopathic* remedy.

The Hahnemannian perception of life, even today, is not grasped by many of the acknowledged leaders of scientific thought, who are unable to lift their noses from among the worms of the earth. In spite of the discoveries made by the great physicists of the day, medical thought, in

---

1. THE HOMEOPATHIC RECORDER, Vol. LIII, No. 4, 1938, pgs. 26 ff.

the main, vegetates in the material dogmas of the earth-bound, instead of vibrating in unison with the throb of creation. Unless we, with Hahnemann, perceive that which builds and is prior to the material body, that which animates and vivifies it, that which is a spark of the Great First Cause, the mysterious wonderful life force, laughed at by the ignorant and scoffed at by the egotistical because it escapes the lens of the miscroscope and eludes the findings of the test tube, unless we catch the subtle meaning of this mystic force, we will fail to meet the needs of homeopathic wisdom and consequently fail to cure many types of sickness; nor will we reach the heights of knowledge, where the beacon light of truth beckons and shines to guide our unwary steps from the pitfalls of sophistry and error.

Unless we know that the type of body growing and developing through infancy and childhood to mature life is the result of a certain rhythmic flow of life force, we must fail in the realm of causation.

When the rhythm of this vital stream, in its constant round through the organism, is checked or changed by some morbific agent, there soon supervenes a change in the chemistry and growth of body cells. In place of the normally developed histology that results from the normal flow of vital force, there comes disfunction or disease action, which soon ultimates in pathologic processes and morbid anatomy. Thus, in the language of Dr. Kent disease is first a "change of state" ultimating in disfunction of vital processes to be soon followed by morbid cell growth or tissue changes.[1]

We must know from the provings of our drugs on healthy human beings (not on rats and guinea pigs, whose emotions and mental reactions even the great scientists and laboratory experts have failed to note or record) that drugs have the power of altering first a change of mental and moral processes, together with changes in the function of the body organism; and later, if their use is persisted in, tissue changes will ensue. And because drugs have the power to alter vital processes from health to disease, conversely they can, if prepared and given in accordance with the homeopathic law, bring health and harmony back to the afflicted and the suffering ones, but harmonizing the flow of life force.

Normal life force equals electro-magnetic balance throughout the organism, which insures perfect chemistry, ultimating in normal cell growth and repair. Abnormal or deranged life force equals electro-mag-

---

1. Kent LHP Lecture XIX paragraph 5 ff. - Editor.

Grimmer's Work

netic imbalance which brings destructive chemical changes in the organism that ultimate in pathologic processes and morbid anatomy.

When these subtleties of life, in health and in disease, are understood and accepted, Homeopathy opens up before our vision like a flood of light, and we are willing and ready to carry the heavy burden of labor involved, in the patient and painstaking care necessary in taking case histories, and in the long, tedious study of comparative similars for the selection of the one remedy needed for each individual case of sickness. But in this laborious and exacting work, the Masters, who have gone before, have left us a kindly heritage in methods and forms of procedure, which insure accuracy and save much time and toil.

The second proposition relating to the taking of the case, and proceeding after the manner in which evidence is amassed in a court of law, but without asking direct questions to the patient or his relatives and friends, is one of the vital parts in the development of correct homeopathic practice[1]. H. C. Allen is reported to have said that a case well taken equals nine-tenths of the work involved in the search for the indicated remedy. Any symptom elicited by a question that can be answered by yes or no is of doubtful value, because such questions enable the patient to answer without due reflection, or they may suggest to his sick mind symptoms and states he does not suffer from; hence, his answers may be misleading. All questions must be put in such a way that will require answers only after due reflection and consideration has been given by the patient.

For example: In order to ascertain the group of remedies, hot or cold, to which the patient belongs, we may be compelled to ask a number of questions in an indirect way as follows: How sensitive to cold are you? How sensitive to extreme heat are you? How does a hot closed room affect you? How much clothing do you need in cold weather? If symptoms are obtained throughout in this manner, they are far more reliable; and they assume the status of proven facts, which provides a solid foundation to build our symptom picture on, whose nearest likeness must then be sought in the Materia Medica, for the indicated remedy.

When the case has been carefully and fully taken in the proper way, we are ready to utilize our knowledge of the relative value of symptoms, which is the third essential. Hahnemann speaks of the characteristic symptoms of a case or of a drug proving as being the most valuable in

---

1. §87 Organon - Editor.

the search for the curative remedy[1]. And among these characteristics, he listed as strongest and best these symptoms relating to the mind, such as the fears, the delusions, deliriums and aberrations of the mental processes. (How wonderfully correct these observations are, every homeopathic prescriber knows).[2]

Then follow the physical characteristics, preferably those symptoms that cannot be explained from the presence of any pathologic or anatomic derangement, because the latter falls in a large common group. It is well to know symptoms belonging to this common group, that by contract we may better recognize the much smaller but infinitely more valuable group containing the strong, rare and peculiar symptoms, because these are the key symptoms around which cluster the symptoms of the whole case and by which the homeopath may with greater certainty find the curative remedy. Symptoms found in the provings of many remedies, symptoms diagnostic of great common group of symptoms and are relatively inferior in value for prescribing purposes.

Kent, in his Homeopathic Philosophy, classified the Hahnemannian symptoms in a very logical and orderly way as follows:[3] First, two grand symptom groups called Generals and Particulars, the former relating to the patient as a whole, including both mental and physical, common and uncommon; and the latter group relating solely to the organs and parts of the body and given lesser value in the selection of the indicated remedy.

Kent divided the high grade mental symptoms into three groups: The first and strongest in value are those pertaining to the will, which involves all perversions of the loves, including fears, hatreds, desires and aversions of the mind. The second group registers abnormal processes of the understanding, such as delirium, delusions, irrational thought, weakness and inability of concentration. And the third group relates to the disturbances of the memory, which he called the outer cortex of the mind.

Next in importance after the mental symptoms are the physical generals, consisting of the patient's responses to environment, heat, cold, weather changes, electric and wind, storms, the desires and aversions of the stomach, the sex perversions and disturbances. Pathological condi-

---

1. §153 Organon - Editor.
2. §210, 211 Organon - Editor.
3. "Repertory Study" p. 246

tions that are the ultimates of long-perverted life force belong in this group.

The group listed as particulars involves the symptoms relating to various parts and organs of the body. And ramifying all through these groups from first to last, there are the two grand divisions of symptoms, the rare, strange and more or less unusual, and the great group of common symptoms. A working knowledge of these various groups and their relative value of power and importance in the case enables the prescriber to select the valuable therapeutic symptoms for **prescribing purposes,** as well as to distinguish symptoms mostly valuable for **diagnostic purposes.**

The last essential is one of observing the order in which disease symptoms appear and in which they go after the remedy has acted. Hahnemann states that under the action of the homeopathic remedy symptoms disappear in the inverse order of their coming, that is, the last to come are the first to go. And Hering added to the above another observation concerning the order in which symptoms leave the patient when under the influence of the homeopathic remedy. It is as follows: Symptoms, pains and disease processes leave the patient from above downward and from within outward or from center to circumference.

The recognition of the above observations will serve as indicators for the accuracy of the homeopathic prescription. To illustrate: A case of diptheria where the disease travels from right to left will recover under natural processes in the same order that it comes; that is, the right tonsil will clear up first and the left one last. Under the power of the homeopathic remedy, the last tonsil to become involved will be the first to clear up, symptoms going in reverse order to their coming. An inflamed eye will get well under the action of the indicated remedy in the same way, symptoms going in the reverse order of their appearance, thus avoiding the need for the dangerous use of material doses of atropin for the purpose of dilating the pupils to prevent adhesions. Under the indicated remedy, inflamatory processes heal, leaving no adhesions behind.

Many forms of suppression will be lifted from the sick economy by the homeopathic remedy; such as: the reappearance of skin eruptions that were suppressed by metallic salves; catarrhal complaints and gonorrheal discharges suppressed by injections, followed by rheumatic troubles; leucorrheal flow checked by local treatments succeeded by ovarian and uterine growths; the so-called cure of malaria by massive amounts of quinine leaving chronic liver, spleen or blood disease as a sequel; the treatment of insomnia and chronic forms of headache, a multiplicity of neuralgic and rheumatic pains, by some of the numerous coal-tar derivatives - the chief cause for the great increase in heart and kidney disease of the last two decades.

Every properly taken case history will mark the time and order of these signs and symptoms and their reappearance under treatment, indicating that the proper remedy was selected and that the case is curable.

It is surprising how often we are asked by homeopathic doctors, especially among our younger graduates, of what practical use is the philosophic tenets of our school. Why waste time and energy defending certain doctrines and theories evolved by men of earlier generations when modern science is moving forward so rapidly with new discoveries and new concepts relating to the form and nature of matter and the universe? The answer is obvious - for the same reason that we spend time studying the works of Newton, Copernicus, Galileo and many others of vision, contemporaries with the founders of Homeopathy.

A law once discovered remains the same throughout all time, regardless of passing changes, and basic principle like mathematics does not alter their nature and action to suit the changing opinions of men. If we know these fundamentals with their orderly processes based on law, we are better armed to discover and remove causes. These things serve as indications of the correctness of our prescriptions and show when the remedy action ceases and a repetition of the same or a complimentary remedy is needed.

Because the universal language of symptoms brings all knowledge needed for treatment of the sick, we need but learn and know their mystic message to grow wise and helpful to the helpless and afflicted. And because Homeopathy is a basic law concerning life processes, is proof to the intelligent and independent observer and thinker that it is true and co-existant and cooperative with all other laws of the cosmos; it is also a part of the universal whole. It cannot be annihilated; it cannot be altered, but remains the same yesterday, today and forever.

Our Expanding Homeopathic Philosophy[1]

As new truths are discovered and new concepts of disease causation are evolved from a new array of proven facts, we turn to the cardinal principles of Homeopathics to note what consistency exists between the new found claims and the often proved doctrine, for all facets of the truth are consistant and complimentary.

Homeopathics deals with man and his parts in sickness and in health, his nature, his attributes and his reactions to the stiumulants of environment. It seeks to know the causes of his ailments and the remedies that can prevent or cure them. Homeopathy teaches that man has an internal force or vehicle that activates his external body and that he lives on flames expressed by his emotional, rational and spiritual drives, coincidental with his physical existence.

We have learned that man is born into the world with weaknesses and a predisposition to certain types of constitutional sickness transmitted from his progenitors who transgressed the laws of creation and left a heritage of imperfection and weakness to be expressed in sin and suffering in the children. Holy writ tells us that the sins of the fathers are visited on the children until the third generation. Thus one of the cardinal features of homeopathic philosophy is verified by the word itself.

Late advances in the science of physics explains why and how the homeopathic potencies (small doses) can produce the astounding results in cure noted by so many able prescribers. We are told by the savants of physics that matter and energy are interchangeable under varying conditions and that both are characterized by their specific rates of vibration[2]; in fine all matter from its crudest to its finest form and expression, is vibratory in nature. Energy or force of all kinds is matter transformed to higher rates of vibration.

Homeopathic potencies consist of matter raised to extremely high rates of vibration simulating the quality and vibratory rate of the life force that animates the human body. These forces are not only vibratory, but they have directional flow or polarity also. Polarity is the determining factor or cause of all the affinities and repulsions in the

---

1. Journal of the American Institute of Homeopathy, Vol. 48, No.9., Sept., 1955, pp. 274 ff..
2. Albert Einstein characterized this in his famous equation $E=mc^2$ where E is the energy liberated by matter of mass and c is the velocity of light (about 300.000 km/sec). Thus one sees clearly the tremendous energy that is liberated when even a very tiny mass is converted into energy. - Editor.

whole realm of nature; the cohesive properties of matter, chemical affinities and gravitational pull between the heavenly bodies, are all expressions of polarity.

Thus we see that the finest grain of sand made up primarily of tiny electrons and the mightest sun whirling in space are both governed by the same mysterious but mighty inexorable force, that force emanating from God whose guiding omnipotent intelligence holds and binds the fabric of the Cosmos in perfect unity and order.

This universal law of electro magnetic polarity performs an important role in homeopathics. The remedies of our Materia Medica are classified into four groups according to their polarity, viz negative, positive, neutral and bi-polar and the blood of all patient will come in one of these four groups.

An individual whose blood test is negative with an intensity measuring 12 hundredths of an ohm in electrical resistance will be found at least in approximately good health, or one under the influence of the similimum will give the normal negative polarity reading as long as the remedy continues to act. The similimum will restore all abnormal polarities to the normal with an abatement of all adverse symptoms and improved health in the whole clinical picture as long as the remedy holds and acts. The selection of remedies for the sick with the aid of the polarimeter has been verified by a number of good prescribers.

When the polarity of the patient is known the search for the similimum is then reduced to one-fourth of the remedies of the Materia Medica because the similimum can only be found in that polarity group demanded by the polarity of the patients blood.

The observation herein stated have been confirmed in many thousands of cases over a period of more than thirty years and substantiated by a number of homeopathic physicians.

When the patient has been on the indicated remedy for some time and symptoms are changing, old ones returning and new states and symptoms coming up, with perhaps some sharp aggravations annoying both to the patient and doctor, it is most assuring to the doctor and his patient to ascertain by a quick simple test of the patients polarity to know whether or not the remedy is still working curatively.

If the polarity registers 12 hundreds of an ohm, negative, the remedy is holding and working and must not be interfered with. If the polarity has gone back to what it was when the last remedy was given then the same remedy or one of its analogues will come in over the patient's blood. The remedy that restores the polarity again to normal reading, negative 12 hundredths of an ohm of electrical resistance is the similimum. If the polarity has changed, then a remedy belonging to the changed polarity group must be selected and given. In this way the best complimentary remedy can be found in any given case.

In these times of constant drug abuses and of food, air and water contaminations with chemical poisoning and processing, remedies are frequently antidoted and the curative rhythm in the patient's vital processes broken and changed requiring a suitable remedy to meet the changed polarity and changed body chemistry. The ever changing blood chemistry of the patient is directly under the influence of the patients polarity state. As long as the blood registers 12 hundredths ohms of electrical resistance, negative, the blood chemistry will perform its many important functions normally and efficently.

This new aspect of the blood synchronizing so perfectly with our special philosophy of homeopathics lends an added bit of power and certainity to the great realm of healing. From the statements made concerning the importance of the polarity of the blood I trust it will not be construed that I advocate the substitution of this relative new method of remedy finding for the tried and true concepts and principles established by Hahnemann and so richly expanded by the many master prescribers and teachers of our glorious science and art that followed him so staunchly and well. Because I wish to stress the fact, that unless one is deeply and completely versed and indoctrinated in the homeopathic philosophy and assiduously and unremittingly studies the great constantly expanding Materia Medica he will attain but little satisfaction in terms of cure. To make a success in prescribing with this new adjunct one must be completely trained in homeopathic philosophy that he may never loose sight of the patient as the one all important objective in every case of illness.

First and foremost the careful painstaking work of taking the case history is the most essential factor in successful prescribing. Dr. H. C. Allen once remarked that a case well taken constitutes one half to three-fourths of the work in finding the indicated remedy. In the eyes of the master homeopath it is a constant and reliable index of the patient's progress toward health in the unfoldment and evolution of the symptoms as they appear and leave the complete story of a successful homeopathic prescription recorded.

As the title of this paper implies, Homeopathic Philosophy is an expanding philosophy, capable of receiving new additions of truth as long as they are compatible with and complimentary to the basic principles of the doctrines. Because the law of magnetic polarity is consistent with the law of cure and its workings confirms so much of known homeopathic philosophy, is the reason for bringing to the attention of the homeopathic profession this treatise of facts for their consideration and constructive criticism. Whatever your decision, singly or as a group may be, this important subject is with us to accept or reject as our reason may direct.

Personally I feel it is a great asset for the success of our cause because vast experience has proved it to be of inestimable value in finding the needed remedy especially in difficult cases presenting a paucity of therapeutic symptoms or those cases burdened with pathologic tissue changes and with only common and diagnostic symptoms to prescribe on. The late and illustrious Dr. Guy Stearns was an enthusiastic advocate of this concept of prescribing, which he described in a masterly scientific paper entitled "The Approach to Reality."[1]

No matter how much of worth we possess in our wonderous homeopathic methods and principles of cure, we still should be receptive to all additional aids for the purpose of cure as long as these new adjuncts do not conflict with our proven laws and procedures and as long as they prove valuable with the test of time and by the results in cure that are achieved.

The question often occurs to many, how can the homeopathic remedy eradicate the inherited toxins of disease? The answer is simple when we consider the mode by which all traits and characteristics are transmitted from generation to generation.

The microscopic group of molecules known as genes are one of the marvels of creation, for in those tiny bundles are packed the individualizing characteristics and traits and the physical appearance of the species race and individual that are transmitted through time and eternity unchanged and incapable of being changed except by powerful radiant energy forces affecting the genes bringing about a state of mutation as it is called, which breaks the fixed chain and pattern of inheritance and produces individuals differing from their species and progenitors. The homeopathic potency is the only force adaptable enough to the nature and smallness of these microscopic bodies to influence their action by eradicating the inherited toxins that tend to inhibit their harmonious activity. In other words the homeopathic potency produces a mild form of mutation which dissipates the toxins of inherited disease and results

---

1.   THE HOMEOPATHIC RECORDER, Vol. LV, No. 11, November 1940, p. 3. - Editor.

in the production of a more perfected individual. Because the homeopathic potency can harmonize all vital processes including the activity and function of the genes is reason enough to conclude that this same subtle but potent force does eradicate inherited constitutional diseases from the individual and the race when intelligently applied[1].

From the days of Hahnemann to the present time master prescribers have stressed the importance of mental and emotional symptoms as being most valuable for the selection of the needed remedy to effect the cure. Today the new aspect of medicine called psychosomatic tells us how frustrations and fears, anger and hatred form the etiologic background for most of the chronic diseases such as cancer and crippling arthritis now affecting the race.

When an individual becomes normalized by the homeopathic cure, the deeper side of his being, the will and the understanding or the rational mind are balanced. Then the man begins to control his desires and emotions and becomes more the master of his destiny and his environment. With the change in the mental and moral sphere, his physical health improves with a high degree of resistance to acute maladies of all kinds. He regulates his life habits and appetites, avoids deleterious foods and drink, becomes temperate in all things, takes adequate exercise and sufficient rest, supplies his blood stream with abundance of fresh air. Finally he cultivates an atmosphere of cheerfulness and a sense of humor all of which enables him to meet every challenge besetting life's highway wherever he turns in these fate packed times. Such is the transition from constitutional weakness and suffering to homeopathic health and comfort.

Much concern is expressed in the world today about the atomic explosions now going on for experimental purposes by the United States and Russia and great fears are engendered by the possible prospect of an atomic war. The wide spread devastating destruction such a war would bring might well be surpassed by a universal annihilating radiation completely destroying all animal life on the planet.

No remedy of proven value has been given the world for radiation sickness by our old school colleagues. It is well to remind our homeopathic doctors that our potencies of Phos. provides the best antidote for

---

1. Our master prescribers Kent, Grimmer, Hering, Lippe, Hahnemann, Boger dreamed of purifying the human race and lifting our species to a race living in spiritual harmony and peace under spiritual and natural laws in a world free of chronic diseases. But alas their vision was marred by lower instincts of the present allopathic medical establishment and the pharmaceutical industry. - Editor.

radiation sickness yet discovered. We are told that though Geiger counters all through the midwest, even around the neighborhood of Chicage continue to register increasing amounts of radiation dust, we need have no fears as the amounts are far too light to affect one anymore than a radium dial watch could. Some of us saw some very sick patients whose illness was caused from wearing radium dial watches when they were more popular than they are now. By discarding the watches and taking a potency of Phos. their heath was restored.

Here is a situation where homeopathic science could easily prove its superior worth. Perhaps the most outstanding feature of homeopathic therapeutics is its efficacy in the realm of disease prevention. Not only are acute epidemic diseases prevented but all types of chronic sicknesses are inhibited and prevented by careful and really scientific homeopathic prescribing.

The application of the homeopathic remedy to the ills and needs of the growing child has most far reaching and beneficial results in the child's growth and development, enabling it to attain a normal, healthy and happy maturity with an unusual power of resistance to all sick making forces in its environment[1]. More wonderful still, the magic impact of the similimum will dissipate the inherited toxins of disharmony that affect all mankind everywhere, even as the sunshine dissipates the frozen waste of snow and leaves a verdant garden growing in its place.

A life force freed of the toxins engendered from inherited ills can and does build into the human economy only normal blood chemistry and normal tissue cells. Into such a constitution and body there is no room for the pathologic changes and end results of cancer, athritis, diabetes, organic kidney and heart disease to develop. Morbid fears, frustration, complexes and emotional instability all can be greatly modified if not entirely irradicated by this potent gift of Divine Power, the similimum. We need but the faith, the energy and intelligence to find and properly apply it. Then all this is curable under God.

---

1. These lines remind one of the similar lines in Kent's great lecture on Carb-v. cf. Kent, James Tylor: Lectures on Homeopathic Materia Medica, Fourth Edition, Boericke and Tafel, Philadelphia, 1956. - Editor.

Logic and Philosophy[1]

It is self evident that logic and philosophy must be intimately related and complimentary in scope. **Philosophy** has been defined by Webster as "the knowledge of the causes of all phenomena both of mind and matter" also as "a particular philosophic system". Other definitions are "the love of wisdom as leading to the search for it; hence knowledge of general principles as explaining facts and existences." "The general laws that furnish the rational explanation of anything; practical wisdom, reasoned science and metaphysics, a mental philosophy". All these definitions convey some idea of the importance and value of philosophic standards when applied to any science or system of procedure. And this should apply more forcefully in the practice of medicine than in any other human endeavor or enterprise. **Logic** is defined as "the science of correct and accurate thinking or reasoning, especially by inference". From the preceeding observations we see how essential it is that a rational system or method of procedure obtains in the practice of the art and science of medicine.

Homeopathy stands alone as a medical system involving and recognizing a philosophy of life in its relation to inherited causes and its reactions to environmental influences and to all sorts of stimuli. Life and the forces operating upon it produce certain observed changes and conditions in the physical, mental and emotional spheres of man. The observed facts, involving the laws and sequences of causes and effects, require logical deductions to explain the phenomena of health or disease co-existant with life. Homeopathy also teaches us to discover the means and measures of preventing disease and insuring health for the happiness and progress of the race.

Homeopathy is distinctive in its study of man in his completeness and in its recognition of mechanisms more subtle and more complex than anything the physical body of man presents to the five senses. These subtle mechanisms are prior to, and dominate, build and repair the physical body, and enable it to live and function on the physical plane of existence in matter. Homeopathy in the all important study of man does not exclude the use of the knowledge of anatomy, physiology, chemistry, biology and many other accepted and proven scientific procedures relating to the study of health and disease. Together with these things, it employs forces and mechanisms that can only be per-

---

1. The Homeopathic Recorder, Vol. LVIII, No. 1, July, 1942, Editorial, p. 49.

ceived and used through the media of, and upon plains of the super physical. Failure to comprehend and interpret the reactions (of that animating spark or force called life) to heredity and environment excludes us from the realm of causes and leaves us uncertain and confused in the whirlpool of effects.

The realm of causes exists beyond the ken of the five senses, and only their effects are with us on the plane of matter. The materialistic scientist views the physical body as a complex automatic mechanism, activated by electro-magnetic forces through the processes of oxidation. Consciousness with its mental and emotional manifestations are regarded as but bio-chemical end results elaborated by this same automatic organism. The dynamistic philosopher sees the material body as the result of life forces, influencing growth and development and dominated by the conscious mind as the highest manifestation of the ego, which has envolved from the great eternal first cause, the Creator.

Traditional medicine regards disease as a material entity, or a toxemia or a pathologic change in the tissues of the body, and in their treatment employ mechanical or surgical measures or crude chemicals in an attempt to cure or correct the trouble.

Homeopathy perceives disease as but a change in the harmonious flow of life forces, the dynamis of the body, thereby producing a series of changes first in the subtle nerve centers whose vibrant energies produce all the astounding complex chemical changes of the fluids and tissues ultimating in disease or pathology. When the mysterious messenger of life flows harmoniously and uninterruptedly, health is blooming; when it is checked or disturbed, disease prevails and death is at hand. This dynamis or life force, flowing from the source of creative energy, vivifies and animates all nature, through mineral, plant and animal kingdoms, thus making all of us kin and more or less inter-dependant and related. Given a relatively perfect mechanism activated by a dynamis flowing in harmony and attunement with its environment we may be assured of a state of health resulting. Such relatively perfect mechanisms are those bodies blessed by good inheritance for then the dynamises have been orderly and strong from the time of conception; hence growth and development have proceeded in a normal way to ultimate in the birth of healthy beings able to meet changing forces of environment successfully and thus escape sickness or retardation of growth and development.

The homeopathic concept of illness involves equally subtle instruments and forces to restore harmony in the play of life energy when it has been disturbed by any morbific agent or cause. Homeopathic remedies, by reason of the process of potentization and because of the fact that each remedy has been proven or tested on relatively healthy human beings, are each a specialized charge of polarized energy - electrolytes of a specific nature, selected to meet the needs of each individual case of disease, whose activities are first manifested in the deep centers of the nervous system where the mystic currents of life forces concentrate at these power stations of the body to be distributed in an orderly even stream in accordance with the body's needs along the course of the efferent system of nerves to the remotest parts of the organism.

Some illustrations and comparisons of methods will better describe two different concepts of the modus operandi of cure:

In the treatment of malaria the old school give massive doses of quinine to kill the plasmodia of malaria in the blood stream and they actually succeed in doing it, but at a great cost in health and suffering which results from the combined effect of the disease and the drug together creating a new combination of symptoms and body changes; true there may be no more chills or fever, but in their place many forms of neuralgic pains of a chronic nature are frequently produced, or chronic liver, spleen and blood changes all of a chronic baffling and resistant nature results. These states are recognized by homeopaths as suppressions and not cures. The homeopath administers his remedies in accordance with a proven law called the Law of Similars: every case of sickness is studied as an individual case regardless of its diagnostic name and though a large number of cases may be suffering from a malarial infection each one presents a symptom picture calling for its own specific remedy because each individual with symptoms, idiosyncrasies and reactions peculiar to himself reacts differently to the malarial poison and for that reason requires his own specific antidote or remedy.

Another illustration is in the treatment of syphilis. So called regular medicine attacks lues by administering powerful drugs such as arsenicals, mercurials, bismuth preparations and iodides all in drastic dosages injected directly into the blood stream[1] with the object of destroying the spirocheta claimed to be the specific cause of the disease, even though often certain nerve, brain and spinal conditions of a most serious nature may fail to show the presence of the spirocheta in the blood or spinal fluid, with negative Wasserman and Kahn tests. Such cases are

---

1. Today the allopathic treatment of syphilis involves large doses of antibiotics. - Editor.

especially apt to appear after a course of drastic old school anti-syphilitic treatment. Again we see suppression instead of cure; these are victims of the combined effects of syphilis and artificial drug disease: Paresis, locomotor ataxia and numerous other nerve and blood diseases continue to present a hideous train of evil subtilities for "scientific" medicine to ponder over as a result of its handiwork. As a result of all this, we witness periodical changes in treatment and the introduction of new experimental drugs without the guidance of law or philosophy, only a blind, blundering, haphazard empirical series of unending trials and errors to pile up suffering and disappointment and accumulated evils and weakness in the race, piling up constantly, increasing suffering and impaired health to be transmitted down through the generations.

Old school medicine is making a great noise about the control of syphilis, but aside from the educational phase of their program calling attention to the dangers and seriousness of the infection they are doing infinitely greater harm than they are good in the false assumption of the Wasserman blood test as the criterion of treatment for lues. Without a chemical history of the infection and the following sequence of symptoms and body changes such as the chancre, sore throat and typical eruptions, loss of hair and a host of symptoms and signs, the diagnosis of syphilis is not justified on a Wasserman reaction alone. And the drastic nature of the treatment must produce great harm in many cases. Were it not for the selfish blight of commercialism, this monstrous practice would not flourish as it now does. But manufacturing chemists and political and industrial doctors permit their insatiable greed to blind them to wholesale suffering and impoverishment among their hapless victims.

Homeopathy observes the order and pace, direction and development in the symptoms and changes of disease whether it be an artificial drug disease (proving) or a natural one. Some of the observations are highly interesting and of great value to both patient and physician. One of the outstanding observations is that chronic diseases first attack the centers of the organism and then proceed to manifest at the periphery (the externals). Thus both acute and chronic diseases have periods of so called incubation (central action) and later show forth in their characteristic symptoms. The manifestations of chronic disease at the periphery is the body's way of protecting the internal organs of man from damage by ultimating disease in the least important part of man. Thus many chronic intestinal complaints and asthmatic difficulties are often the result of suppressing skin eruption with powerful salves, because by such treatment the chronic disease is, so to say, driven into the internal skin or mucous membranes of the lungs, intestines, or some other mucous lining.

Another important observation is that symptoms get well in the reverse order of their coming, that is, the last to appear are the first to go, under the action of the homeopathic remedy. The reverse of this takes place when nature unassisted brings about recovery, the last symptoms to come being the last to get well.

THE POWER OF INFINITESIMALS[1]

When we view the material universe in concrete forms we fail to perceive the urge of action and reaction residing in infinitesimal units throughout the whole realm of nature. As we follow the physicist from solid forms of matter to matter in a liquid state and then into gaseous forms and finally into its electro-magnetic and radio-active forms we are cognizant of the increased energy and power of matter in these successive steps above mentioned (viz. from solid to radioactive processes). To illustrate, we need only compare the relative power residing in an ounce of coal as compared to an equal amount of radium. The heat and light energy in the small quantity of coal is soon expended leaving a residue of potash and carbon. While an ounce of Radium will produce light and heat for a million years without appreciable diminution in weight or form. We cannot separate the so called imponderable forms of energy, light, electricity, magnetism, etc., from the infinitesimals because such forms of energy are composed of infinitesimal units, electrons[2] which are recognized as the ultimate units of all atoms in the material world.

Not so long ago we were taught that atoms were the ultimate division of matter, we are now told that the electron holds that place and there are some who even dispute this statement.

Professor See, a great astronomer and mathematician speaks of the etheon, a thousand times smaller than the electron - these small units filling interstellar space within whose vastness float the numerous solar systems and their retinue of planets making up the universe. The most wonderful vivifying and potently catalysing force in the universe is light in its many gradations of polarity ranging from infra-red on out beyond the ultra violet into the realm of high frequency rays, X-rays, and finally the mysterious and only recently discovered cosmic ray coming from somewhere outside our solar system. Little as yet is known about this strange force beyond the fact that its penetrating power carries it through six feet of solid lead, (the X-ray being able to penetrate only a few inches of lead foil), and its vibratory frequency exceeds that of the X-ray a hundred fold.

---

1. The handwritten manuscript has no date, but was probably written in 1947 and it seems it was never published. - Editor.
2. At the time of writing (about 1947) some of the newer concepts of physics were unknown. - Editor.

Without light all organic forms of matter would perish and most inorganic chemical combinations would cease. With the presence of light come higher forms of life and intelligence. The various polarities of light affect various forms of life. For instance in the spheres of the infra-red area called the heat and chemical areas exist all planes of inorganic chemistry; in the spheres or spectrum of the white rays including the ultra violet, are found the planes of organic chemistry and higher life forms that best flourish in these strata; beyond the ultraviolet are the destructive rays where mere evolution as it were, is reversed and matter undergoes changes from highly active to denser forms as is shown in the gradual and almost imperceptible process of radium disintegration into lead. One form of polarized light, moonlight[1] or reflected light, affects certain enzymes of starch causing it to change into sugar. Also certain pathogenic bacteria thrive in polarized light, these same forms of bacteria perish in the white rays of sunlight and most rapidly in the ultraviolet rays. The various color rays are only the result of a change in the rate of vibrations or frequency of the light waves.

The speed of light is only surpassed by one other force in the universe, namely human thought. When we shall know more about the therapeutic powers of light in all its gradation and polarities and perfect a technique of application we will have no more sickness, ignorance nor unhappiness in our midst.

Next to light in power to change and build new combinations of material forms are the chemical catalysts. These catalysts do not enter into the chemical changes and compounds: their mere presence produces the chemical phenomenon and without their presence these chemical unions would not take place. We are indebted to Mr Fred Lodge, chemist for Armour for most of the chemical catalysts mentioned here tonight. To quote Mr. Lodge.

HARDENING OF FATS: Such oily fats as cottonseed oil may be materially hardened by causing additional hydrogen to combine with the carbon of the oil so that in fact a stearine is formed. Such a product is "Crisco", extensively used in our kitchens. If a stream of hydrogen gas is passed through the hot oil alone, no change takes place. However, if a little finely divided, metallic nickel is present, a chemical action is at once set up, the carbon in the compound takes on more hydrogen and becomes a stearine, instead of an oil. Only two tenths of one percent of

---

1. The remedy LUNA has had quite an extensive proving and clinical use in modern Homeopathy - Editor.

nickel is necessary to insure the reaction and this nickel does not enter into the reaction except as a catalyst. The hot stearine is run through filter presses and the nickel entirely recovered, less than four parts per million being left in the final product. (One part in a million is equivalent to the 6X potency.)

OXIDATION OF AMMONIA: When ammonia gas and hydrogen are mixed with air and passed through a fine gauze of platinum, previously heated, the oxygen of the air combines with the nitrogen and hydrogen to form nitric acid, a compound directly opposite in character to the alkaline ammonia. That the platinum does not appear as a component part of the final product is shown by the fact that the process may be carried on continuously for months without any renewal of platinum.

OXIDATION OF SULPHUR DIOXIDE TO SULPHUR TRIOXIDE: When the hot sulphur dioxide gases resulting from the burning of the sulphur and containing, of course, excess air are brought in contact with metallic platinum in the form of platinum black, or in contact with oxides of iron or aluminum or vanadium, the oxygen of the air combines with the sulphur dioxide to form sulphur trioxide the gases are reasonably pure, the catalyst functions indefinitely especially so in the case of platinum, as plants have been in operation continuously for more than ten years without any change of the platinum catalyst.

PRODUCTION OF PETROLEUM FROM COAL: A process is in operation in Europe producing different grades of petroleum from coal by means of a catalyst. The coal is finely ground and mixed into a paste with oil, and a small amount of some catalyst, such as iron oxide. This is introduced into a steel cylinder, externally heated. Hydrogen under a considerable pressure is admitted to the cylinder, whereupon because of the catalytic action, the hydrogen and carbon of the coal combine to form various hydrocarbons including several grades of oils. In this process, the iron oxide catalyst is not recovered because of its low value, but is allowed to go with the ash. Note that the mere presence of the true catalyst is alone sufficient to bring about certain chemical unions impossible of forming without catalytic aid.

Examples of minute quantities affecting the properties of substance are: Soft malleable iron plus 2% carbon equal carbon steel. Steel plus a few percent of chromium and nickel equal stainless steel.

Enzymes are powerful agents acting as catalysts that perform tasks of the greatest importance in the affairs of life and its multitudinous processes. When any one of the numerous digestive and blood ferments are lacking, physical life soon ebbs. The various endocrine glands secrete, in infinitesimal quantities, special ferments or enzymes to perform special functions in the body organism. But for the existence of one of these enzymes the Volstead act with its long train of evils would never been inflicted upon an already over burdened humanity.

The occult subtle and infinitely fine substances called vitamins that have such a bearing on nutrition, growth, and development are so infinitesimal that they are hardly recognized other than by their stupendous effects when present or absent.

The smallness and power of bacteria need not be elaborated here but some interesting things may be said about bacteriophage. This virus found first in polluted water of rivers or lakes where typhoid and other intestinal disease bacteria abound, is observed thus by the electron microscope; in nature it is capable of killing pathogenic micro-organisms in a test tube and antidoting their effects in the human body. Today in Europe and in South America the bacteriophages active against typhoid and dysentery are being used in research related to these diseases.

A few facts concerning the power of the tiny things dwelling in the realm of the electron microscope will help to elucidate the title of my paper.

From the December number of jottings published by Boericke and Tafel, we are told that potentized SIL. is necessary to sustain life. Diatoms are organisms that are found through out the world in all fresh and salt water. Diatoms are the basic food for the organisms next higher in the scale of life and therefore are the foundations on which all marine life is built. In the open oceans diatoms occur in greatest abundance where there is an admixture of muddy water from some river and where the salinity is relatively low. Their abundance appears to be related to the pressure of colloidal silica in these areas rather than to temperature for they are found abundantly in the tropics as well as toward the poles.

A few quotations from the Journal of the American Medical Association printed in the November issue of the Homeopathic Recorder will prove interesting, instructive and sustaining to some of our weak kneed homeopaths. A milligram of thyroxin produces a 2% rise in basal metabolism in a man weighing 154 lbs. Speaking of botulinum the fatal dose is diminished to $3x10^{-21}$ grams, some dilution for this journal to admit. A therapeutic dose of $2x10^{-5}$ mg of tuberculin is recomended, future treatment being based on reaction (not bad Homeopathy). Dr. Brans in his article on exophthalmic goiter says that one milligram of thyroxin will produce symptoms. Lieb stimulated the uterine contractions of a guinea pig with 10^{-3} mg of quinine solution. Dr. Ringer speaking of amyl-nitrite, began treatment with a minim dose but found it too strong and was obliged to reduce it to one third of a minim. He continues, the 10th nay, even the 30th of a minim will in some cases counteract flushing. Claude Bernard said every substance which in large doses abolished the property of an organic element stimulates it when given in small doses. Christiansen of Harvard writes, the effective therapeutic dose should be far below the toxic dose. The extraordinary distinct radiographs taken of the 60th trituration of RAD-BR. by Boericke and Tafel some years ago knocked into a cocked hat the old threadbare claim that there was no medicine in the 30th potency.

A few quotations from Crile in his Bipolar Theory of Living Processes will illustrate the infinitely small units of which the animal organism is composed. It is estimated that there are twenty-eight trillion bipolar electric cells in the human body independent units, yet intrinisically wired and bound together and under the dominance and control of the organism as a whole to form the most wonderful automatic self repairing and sustaining mechanism, a veritable epitome of the universe. This wonderous body is admirably constructed for the work it has to perform in all the multitudinous processes of life (for its perpetuation and reproduction) and functions as an electro-chemical machine. These tiny units, some of them ultramicroscopic in size and made up of electronic and colloidal elements, are so constitued to perform their specific labors in the body economy by means of the elaboration and discharge of electric energy through oxidation processes. Each bipolar unit or cell is representative of the organism as a whole in its structure and inherent qualities of automatic repair and reproduction by means of electro-chemical laws. This unit is made up of the nucleus the acid element, and cytoplasm the alkaline element, and separated by a semi permeable film of very low conductivity. These characteristics of the cell indicate a difference in electric potential between the nucleus and the cytoplasm. This is the bipolar mechanism: the nucleus being the positive element, the cytoplasm the negative element. The oxidation in the nucleus appears to be on a higher scale than the oxidation occuring in the cytoplasm and therefore as the electric tension increases in the nucleus the current breaks through, the potential in the nucleus falls consequently the current is interrupted. Since the potential is immediately restored by oxidation we perceive that an interrupted current passes continually from the positive nucleus to the negative cytoplasm and as a result a charge is accumulated on the surface films. These films of ininite thinness and of high dielectric constant are pecularily adapted to the storage and adaptive discharge of electric energy. The extreme thinness of these films is needed because the work of the cell depends on its capacity for oxidation; oxidation in turn depends on the electric energy seated between the nucleus and the cytoplasm, this energy depends on the voltage of the cell and on the electric charge the lipid films will hold. The electric charge the lipid film will hold is dependent on the thinness of the film, the thinner the film, the greater the charge. Dr. Fricke has found that the film which surrounds the cells is on the order of 10^{-7} of a centimeter thick, and that the lipid film has electric capacity of a high order; viz., 0.8 microfarads per square centimeter. We may consider, then that electricity keeps the "flame of life" burning in the cell and that the flame oxidation supplies the electricity which is the "vital force" of the animal. In accordance with this conception, therefore, the cell is an automatic mechanism. Life as we view it is the expression of the activity of this automatic mechanism.

It is of infinite advantage to have the organism made up of trillions of units called cells instead of an equal mass in a single unit. The advantage of the greater surface area of the lipid films surrounding the microscopic cells (as compared with that of a single cell of equal mass) is the corresponding increase in working capacity and a corresponding increase in the amount of oxidation. Sir Arthur Thompson has estimated the total surface area of the 28 trillion cells to be equivalent to nine acres. Meynert estimated that there are 10^9 cells in the cerebral cortex, the total surface area of the cortical cells would be about 3 square meters, the total area would have a capacity equivelent to that of a Leyden glass jar 0.3 millimeters in thickness with a surface area of 114,000 square meters, (the area of a city block.)

Further consideration of the cell as a bipolar electrochemical unit indicates the dividing line between the living and non living. In accordance with this conception, the term of electric energy on the membranes with a resultant polarization together with a mechanism for the release of that energy to perform work. There is no more energy per mass in the living than in the non-living. In the living, energy is captured and same amount of energy exists, but is balanced; equalized, inert, non-living.

In the light of all these astonishing facts and the plausible theories based upon them we homeopaths hold the golden key of theraupeutic worth to unlock the storehouses of healing for the race. Every onward step of science forward sheds more light on the claims and tenants of Homeopathy and confirms every detail. Mathematics in positive terms proves our claims for the power of potencies. Physics and chemistry proclaim in ever increasing volume that the wonderous effects of our attenuated medicines are but catalysts of stupendous efficiency. Formerly our claims of cure were a cause for laughter and ridicule from the unthinking who were unable mentally to grasp such delicate and intricate phenomema, but now every advance in real science and the unfolding of new laws and forces, climaxed by 150 years of glorious achievements all indicate our claims and entitle us to a place in the sun among the servants and benefactors of the race.

FINER FORCES IN MEDICINE[1]

Since the discovery and application of homeopathic remedies for the treatment of the sick, especially the use of those remedies in their highly potentized state one hundred fifty years ago, little else but ridicule has been given us by the world of medical science for our claims of the subtle powers residing in the unseen side of nature.

Recently, however, a number of startling things have been revealed and given the public concerning the application of finer forces in the diagnosis and cure of disease. According to recent newspaper accounts, at the Mayo Clinic they have succeeded in making rapid and accurate diagnoses and differentiations of the common cold, flu and poliomyelitis by noting the behavior of the streptococcus germs placed in a magnetic field under a dark lense.

Experiments reported by the *Yale Journal of Biology and Medicine*, December, 1936, by employing a vacuum tube microvolt meter for the measurement of bioelectric phenomena, "have brought out many interesting facts relating to the state of health in cells, tissues, organs and organisms. The experimenter claims that, every excess of action, every change in physical state of the protoplasm of any organ or of any area in the embryo, or in egg, produces - it is believed - an electrical disturbance. These currents probably play a larger part in the determination of rates of growth, in the orientation or polarization of the cells and the differentiation of the organism, in its polarity, in other words than has been supposed." Discovery of the fact that ultra-microscopic organisms carry electric charges of definite polarities thereby enabling the investigator to identify toxemias of infinitesimal quanties together with the recognition of the bioelectric phenomena involved in the processes of all living things may easily explain part of the *modus operandi* of highly potentized homeopathic remedies.

Dr. Guy Stearns and others have demonstrated that homeopathic potencies are electro-magnetic forces consisting of oscillatory frequencies equal to those of magnetism which is said to average as high as 18,000,000,000,000,000,000 (18×10^{18}) oscillations per second.

Potencies are likewise of definite polarities identified in accordance with the drug substance employed. They, the potencies, can impart their properties to an unbelievably larger amount of fluid, water or alcohol by diffusion, rendering those substances equally active in magnetic

---

1. THE HOMEOPATHIC RECORDER, Vol. LIII, No. 3, March, 1938, p. 46.

power to themselves. Thus a very small amount of the infinitesimal substance introduced into the living body rapidly spreads throughout its whole fluid contents from the deepest centers to the outermost parts harmonizing disturbed vibratory rates in the organism by producing a state of resonance in the body circuits. When the electro magnetic circuits or currents of the body are established in order, a balanced orderly chemical activity prevails; and while said orderly chemical processes are maintained, the processes of growth and repair ultimate in normal cell development histology. When these processes are reversed from center to circumference, first a change in the electromagnetic currents of the organism takes place immediately followed by change of body chemistry soon followed by tissue or end changes to ultimate in pathology.

More and more clinical evidence is increasing from various sources of the power of highly potentized remedies in the eradication of disease and the establishment and maintenance of health.

We need cite only the experiments and claims of Beir of Germany and his irritational theory of disease and its cure by attenuated drugs. Also the more recent experiments of McDonald of England and his hydration theory of disease and its cure where potencies ranging up to the 30th are used to effect definite and satisfactory cures. Both these scientists have acknowledged the truth and efficacy of homeopathic fundamentals. All of which brings vividly to our minds those soul-stirring words of the poet:

Truth crushed to earth, will rise again,

The eternal years of God are hers

Error, stung writhes in pain,

And dies amidst her worshippers.

THE OCCULT SIDE OF HOMEOPATHIC PHILOSOPHY[1]

The aspect of our philosophy that deals of the life side of existence in its relation to the form side might be termed occult because it operates within the scope of the imponderable forces of nature.

All energies of the cosmos are vibratory in character and are prior to and causative of all forms and ultimates in matter. Hence the "Life Force" (Vital Force or Dynamis or Vital Principle of Hahnemann) constitutes one of the distinctive features of homeopathy, because it exists and operates in the sphere of the imponderables. Unless the physician can perceive and grasp the significance and importance of life processes, in the realm of health and disease his knowledge of the Law of Similars will avail him little in the realm of cure.

Involved with this "Life Force" of Hahnemann are a number of bodies or vehicles intermingling and ramifying throughout and in conjunction with the physical body of man and corresponding to the physical aspects of nature. These several bodies are classified by occult students and scientists as, first: the physical or chemical body which is subdivided into a made up of several subdivisions and variations of matter.

We all know that the material world including the body of man is composed roughly of solids, water, gases and ethers. These solids, water and gases, make up the chemical band of nature, and from this division all the forms of mineral, plant, animal, including man, are derived. This is the physical body which corresponds to the crust of the earth.

Intermingling with the physical body of nature and man, is the etheric body, comprising four aspects or divisions, each with its specific function to perform in the rhythmic march of nature. The etheric region of nature and man, while still physical, is invisible and intangible where our ordinary senses fail us, hence material science has no cognizance of this aspect of nature because no instrument has yet been devised to register the vibrations or energies flowing from this sphere. Likely some of the so-called electronic reactions of Abrams are vibrations from this plane. Only the trained clairvoyant can see the energies operating on this and other higher planes of life to be mentioned later on; he can see all the processes of life operating on all these plans of nature separately and in unison throughout all the vast intangible causative realms of nature.

---

1. THE HOMEOPATHIC RECORDER, Vol. LXII, No. 7, Jan. 1947, p. 195.

THE ETHERIC REGION IS MADE UP OF <u>FOUR SUBDIVISIONS</u> WITH SPECIFIC FUNCTIONS OF EACH: 1) <u>CHEMICAL</u>; 2) <u>LIFE</u>; 3) <u>LIGHT</u> AND 4) <u>REFLECTING</u>.

1) The *chemical ether* is both positive and negative in its manifestations. The forces which cause *assimilation* and *excretion* work through it; assimilation is carried on along the positive pole of the chemical ether attracting the needed elements in their proper proportions to build and repair the physical body. Elimination of waste material is carried on by the action of the negative pole of the chemical ether.

2) The *life ether* promotes the forces of the *propagation* of the species. Like the chemical ether it works along positive and negative poles, the forces which work along the positive pole of this ether are those which work in the female during gestation; they enable her to do the positive work of bringing forth a new being. On the other hand, the forces working along the negative pole enable the *male* to produce semen. In the work on the impregnated ovum of the animal and man, or upon the seed of the plant, the forces working along the positive pole of the life ether produce male plants, animals and men; while the forces which express themselves through the negative pole generate *females*.

3) Next is the *light ether* having positive and negative manifestations as have the other ethers. The forces which play along its positive pole are the forces which generate the *blood heat* in the higher species of animal and in man, which make them individual sources of heat. The forces which work along the negative pole of the light ether are those operating through *the senses*, manifesting as the passive functionsof sight, hearing, feeling, tasting and smelling. They also build and nourish the eye. In the cold blooded animals the positive pole of the light ether is the avenue of the forces which circulate the blood, and the negative forces have the same functions in regard to the eye as in the case of the higher animals and man. Where eyes are lacking, the forces working in the negative pole of the light ether are perhaps building or nourishing other sense organs.

In plants the forces which work along the *positive pole* of the light ether cause the *circulation* of the juices of the plant. Thus in winter, when the light ether is not charged with sunlight as in summer, the

232

sap ceases to flow until the summer sun again invests the light ether with its force. The forces which work along the *negative pole* of the light ether deposit the chlorophyll, the green substance of the plant and also colors the flowers. In fact, all *color* in all the kingdoms of nature is deposited by means of the negative pole of the light ether. Therefore, animal have the deepest color on the back and flowers are deepest colored on the side turned toward the light. In the polar regions of the earth, where the rays of the sun are weak, all color is lighter and in some cases is so sparingly deposited that in winter it is withdrawn altogether and the animals become white.

4) The *reflecting ether* is the fourth of the ethers. Everything that has ever happened has left behind it an ineffaceable picture in this reflecting ether. These pictures impressed in the reflecting ether constitute what is known as the *memory* of nature. This ether is also the medium through which thought makes an impression upon the human brain. It is most intimately connected with the fourth subdivision of the world of thought.This is the highest of the four subdivisions contained in the region of concrete thought and is the home world of the human mind. Here a much clearer version of the memory of nature is found than in the reflecting ether.

The *desire world* in nature corresponds to the desire body in man and like all other realms in nature is made up of seven divisions or regions. Desire stuff in the desire world persists through its seven subdivisions or regions as material for the embodiment of desire. As the chemical region is the realm of form and as the etheric region is the home of the forces carrying on life activities in those forms, enabling them to live, move and propagate, so the forces in the desire world working in the quickened desire body, impel it to move in this or that direction.

If there were only the activities of the chemical and etheric regions of the physical world, there would be forms having life, able to move, but with no incentive for so doing. This *incentive* is supplied by the cosmic forces active in the desire world and without this activity playing through every fibre of the vitalized body, urging action in this direction or that, there would be no experience and no *moral growth*. The functions of the different ethers would take care of the growth of the form, but moral growth would be entirely lacking. *Evolution* would be an impossibility, both as to form and life for it is only in response to the requirements of *spiritual growth* that forms evolve to higher states. Thus we see the great importance of this realm of nature.

Desires, wishes, passions and feelings express themselves in the matter of the different regions of the desire world as form and feature express themselves in the chemical region of the physical world. They take forms which last for a longer or shorter time, according to the intensity of the desire, wish or feeling embodied in them. In the desire world the distinction between the forces and the matter is not so definite and apparent as in the physical world. There force and matter are almost identical and interchangeable. To a certain extent the desire world consists of force matter. As desires and emotions are the driving and activating forces of life, it is easy to see the importance (for a homeopathic physician) of an intimate knowledge of this subject, especially in applying remedies having similar emotions involved in any special case he may be treating.

But in nature and in man, there are deeper and stronger forces yet to probe and observe: The *world of thought*, consisting of seven regions of varying qualities and densities, and like the physical world, it is divided into two main divisions, viz., the region of concrete thought comprising the four most dense regions, and the region of abstract thought comprising the three regions of finest substance.

This world of thought is the central one of the five worlds from which man obtains his vehicles. Here spirit and body meet. It is also the highest of the three worlds in which man's evolution is being carried forward at the present time, the two higher worlds being practically in abeyance as yet, so far as man is concerned. Here in this world of thought reside imagination and will which enable the man to control the emotional impulses of the desire world and to invent and improve along original lines in the things affecting his life. Here is the seat of philosophy, abstract reason, mathematics, etc.; here also exits the innumerable vibrations of tone and color that generate the sublime tones of harmonious music. Here poetry has its birthplace; and life in all its brightest and richest manifestations exist.

The *vital force from the sun* which surrounds us as a colorless fluid, is absorbed by the vital body through the etheric counterpart of the spleen, wherein it undergoes a curious transformation of color. It becomes pale rose hued and spreads along the nerves all over the dense body. It is to the nervous system what the force of electricity is to a telegraph system. Though there be wires, instruments and telegraph operators all in order, if electricity is lacking no message can be sent. The ego, the brain, and the nervous system may be seemingly in perfect order, but if the vital force be lacking to carry the massage of the ego through the nerves to the muscles, the dense body will remain inert. This is exactly what happens when part of the dense body becomes paralyzed. The vital or etheric body has become diseased and the vital force can no longer flow to those parts. In most cases of sickness, the trouble is with the finer invisible vehicles. That is why homeopathic potencies corresponding in fineness and similar in nature to these vehicles can better reach these invisible centers and establish states of harmony, therein enabling the flow of the vital force to restore with its vivifying power weakened calls and tissues throughout the whole economy of the body, from center to circumference, from within outward, from the realms of thought and emotions to the chemistry of the crude body.

I want to speak of another manifestation in the life of man associated with his various vehicles including his physical body and that is the aura or human atmosphere, as it is called by Walter J. Kilner. This scientist has devised chemical screens whereby the human aura may be visible to the naked eye; and more, the eye may be trained, after the aura has been seen by the aid of screens, so that it can be seen without chemical or other assistance. The color, size and texture of the aura give good indications of the character of the subject and his states of health of disease as well. Occultists tell us that all that belongs to man, including his inheritance, his character and his evolutionary progress, summed up in health states, desire nature, thought power, and spiritual advancement, are found and known by those gifted with a state of consciousness to perceive and read the aura. Thus the achievement of Mr. Kilner may well be a great boon to the suffering and the sick as well as the advancing physician who welcomes every vestige of new knowledge that helps him understand the mystery of life and its uses and goals.

No discussions of occult man would be complete without some statement concerning the blood, the man in solution. The blood not only carries all nutrition and the purifying oxygen to the remotest cells of the body but it distributes the regenerating vital force of the sun as well and thereby constantly perpetuates the life cycle. It is closely associated with the aura connecting man's present with his past generations and his future advance in evolution.

Dr. Rudolph Steiner wrote "The grand work for the formation of the blood, with all its attendant system of blood vessels, appears very late in the development of the embryo," and from this natural science has rightly concluded that the formation of blood occurred late in the evolution of the universe. Not until the human embryo has repeated in itself all the earlier stages of human growth thus attaining to the condition in which the world was before the formation of blood, is it ready to perform this crowning act of evolution, the transmitting and uplifting of all that has gone before into the very special fluid which we call blood.

Manly Hall says,

The consciousness of man was released through the blood, that is, the action of the blood resulted in certain modifications of the bodily fabric. These modifications were of the nature of refinements, affording greater opportunity for the expression of the subtle impulses from the soul.

Consciousness moved from the simple to the complex, as demonstrated by Herbert Spencer. Man moved the focus of his awareness from heredity to environment, from inward to outward perception. His first blood consciousness was entirely subjective, that is, the blood lived in him. Gradually this has changed and now man lives in his blood.

The composite blood of the present man, containing within it the strains from many ancient sources, has relulted in the cosmopolitan quality of the modern mind.

Released from bondage to these phantoms of the blood stream, the thought is turned to the assimilation of knowledge derived from the phenomenal universe. It does not necessarily follow, however, that the blood has ceased to exert an influence for in its present state, that is emancipation from ancestral influence, it has formed into a new chemistry and is a suitable carrier for the impulses of the ego.

The blood has become the instrument of self expression and as such carries within its subtle body the dictums of the intellectual genius. As the blood once revealed the past, so now it foretells the future; for within it are set up the vibrations and patterns by which the future estate of man is to be determined. The blood is now a medium by which external phenomenal circumstances are carried inward to be incorporated into consciousness, and by which the consciousness in its turn, flows outward to determine and direct the activity of the personality.

We have only skimmed the surface of a very small part of this fascinating subject; it would require volumes to describe in full occult relations of the blood, the organs and the endocrines of the human body to the structure and soul of unbounded nature all animated and governed by that Great First Cause, Deity, with his countless hierarchies and appointed helpers throughout his universal realm.

We are indebted to Max Hendel, the author of the *Rosicrucian Cosmo Conception,* a volume treating of the evolution and involution of man physically and spiritually and his relation and place in Nature's economy, for much of the above information; also to Manly Hall, author of *Man, The Grand Symbol of the Mysteries and Healing, The Divine Art* for the statements and thoughts concerning the blood and its occult significance; also to Walter J. Kilney for the statement concerning the aura described in his book entitled *The Human Atmosphere.*

If the writer of this brief sketch treating of the occult forces in man can stimulate investigation along these lines in the ranks of medicine, especially the homeopathic branch, he will feel well paid for the efford of bringing this subject to the attention of his colleagues.

Occult Causes and Material Effects[1]

Throughout the whole realm of nature every manifestation and change presented to the five senses operating on the material plane of existence is but the effect of some subtle unseen force of causation functioning on the super plane of the Cosmos. It matters little what name we may call this super animated realm of cause: the mental, astral and spiritual planes of existence are all terms used to express unseen states of being wherein all manifestations in the physical world are germinated and produced.

If two grains of wheat, one synthetic, the exact replica of the natural grain, are planted in the earth and subjected to the sun's vivifying rays and the earth's magnetic and chemical forces, two vastly different results ensue. The same subtle forces are at work on two bodies chemically and anatomically alike, but one responds by a manifestation of life growth, expansion and development; the other's reaction is death, decomposition and oblivion. This difference in effects obtain because the synthetic grain of the chemist lacks the animated spark of the mysterious life force residing in the natural grain. And this unseen life force or spark can only be known on the material plane by its manifestation, expressed in a favorable environment with the proper stimuli: it defies all synthetic definition and analysis. Behind all natural phenomena - seasonal, metereological, tidal and terrestrial - are definite but unseen causes.

Every particle of matter in the universe even to the smallest electron is subject and obedient to the same laws operating beyond the ken of the five senses. The greatest sun whirling in remotest space has no more free will than the tiniest electron vibrating in a single cell of the human body. Both are confined to the definite limits of their influential spheres.

Time, space, intelligence or consciousness, substance, vibration, polarity, rhythym, tune or harmony are the cardinal features and requisites of an expanding universe. All these terms, except consciousness, may be reduced to mathematical formulation. A study of the infinitesmals in nature presents a perfect likeness of the vast suns of interstellar space.

Man has been aptly called an epitome of the universe. An organization made up of many systems (organs) and individual cells (units)

---

1. From the handwritten manuscript of Dr. Grimmer, exact date unknown. - Editor.

independent yet fused together for cooperative work for the common good of the organism as a whole.

The convulsions of nature that periodically afflict us in the form of tornadoes, earthquakes and storms are only a change of state or potential in the electrical and magnetic forces behind all physical phenomena in nature. As long as there is equilibrium and harmony in the flow of these forces, all is peace and serenity or health and comfort. And when the flow of these forces is again disturbed, violence and unharmony or disease obtains until equilibrium again recurs.

In the world of science today there is much confusion and disagreement concerning a determinate answer to the phenomena of the physical universe. Compton and others are inclined to admit that something of the metaphysical must enter into their theories to obtain the answer, while Einstein and Planck persist in the belief that an absolute answer may be had in physical processes alone, and that may be expressed in mathematical terms. In the world of medicine we observe a still greater state of chaos and confusion. The scientific medical man believes only what is cognizant through his five senses; and as we have shown, nothing of cause exists on that plane; it follows that definite knowledge concerning man and the universe around him cannot be known to him.

The testimony of the five senses is subject to illusions and error. Our eyes tell us that the sun rises and sets, but absolute knowledge of astronomy teaches us that the Earth's motion on its axis is the cause of day and night and that the rising and setting sun is only apparent.

Until we measure man and the universe in this same scale of absolute knowledge, we will be confused both scientifically and medically. Until we are able to perceive the finer forces operating in nature back of all concrete form, we cannot contact cause. The realm of the five senses is the realm of effects, and any effect directed there is lost as far as modifying or preventing inevitable results.

Changes in the physical world or in the physical body of man can only be modified or influenced by changing the causative forces, unseen and unknown save by the conscious intelligence of the cosmos or man. Consciousness in varying degree of lucidity is an attribute of every entity in nature throughout the animal, vegetable and mineral kingdoms. Internally consciousness is inextricably bound up with the life force or essence of things and beings; externally it is associated with the aura. Scientists have proven by delicate electric tests and stimuli that plants have sensation and even suffer pain and experience pleasure and that they have circulatiory and nervous systems. The chemical reactions, affinities, and revulsions of the mineral elements with their spectroscopic responses may well be ascribed to a modified degree of consciousness. The auras of humans, animals, plants and minerals have long been demonstrable facts; thus we are dealing with actualities and not mere metaphysical theories.

Even science, which always lags behind advanced thought, (since it accepts only that which is proven) is now beginning to recognize that we live in a conscious universe. And while mathematics may designate and describe or reduce to a formula the units of the physical worlds, it is inadequate to so circumscribe consciousness.

The so-called medical scientist, however, is innocently oblivious to the part and place of consciousness in nature; and if he does give a passing glance at the consciousness of man, it is to relegate it to a remote and unimportant place in his studies.

Homeopathy since its inception has recognized consciousness[1] in all its manifestations and especially with its internal associate the vital force as the dominating factor of life, health and disease. We see consciousness departing with the ebbing of the vital force from this physical plane. We see the perversions of affections, and their deep emotional disturbance, the illusions of the sense, the delusions and deliriums, and aberations of the emotional mind that come with manifestations of disease when the vital force flows in disorder. All these things are shown and recorded in the pathogenesis of each of our proven remedies.

Also accompanying these things are vast changes in the physical body, pathological conditions which have been cured many times by many different prescribers in the past one hundred and fifty years with the application of the homeopathically indicated remedy, given in highly attenuated unseen form, to change the disturbed flow of vital force to a state of harmony and tune.

Not only does the indicated remedy bring harmony and tune to the individual body of the sick man, but it brings him in tune and accord with the Cosmos, the environment he lives in. When in his sickness certain foods disturb him and certain pollens and emanations aggravate him, after the administration of the needed remedy these things no longer affect him adversely. He is in tune with himself within, and with the universe without. Thus, the life force may be so modified that one may seem to live in a changed world, but it is the man, not the world,

---

1. Organon § 9 ff. - Editor.

that has changed. He has been brought into harmony with all nature. And these changes may be noted in all planes of his being (or as the occultists express it: "In all his bodies or vehicles") so that the moral and mental processes, together with an uplift throughout the physical body can be observed and felt by the patient.

These facts teach us that man, when sick, is sick through all his planes and that healing must proceed from within and toward the surface. Hence the observation (Hering's Law): "From within out, from center to cirumference, from above down, from more vital to less vital parts".

When we shall know more about the internal forces residing in external things and more about the internal vital force of man, then we shall accomplish greater things in the realm of healing. Inherited weaknesses and predispositions will fade away like winter's snow beneath the summer sun. When enough of humanity shall know and recognize the importance of Homeopathic Philosophy and its application to the sick, especially to the sick weakly child, then shall we behold the new race. Then will come the conquest over all mental and physical defects. Insanity, epilepsy, cancer and tuberculosis will be but nightmares of the past, and out of this will grow a race of super men and women living in harmony among themselves and in tune with the infinite.

HEREDITY, ENVIRONMENT, HOMEOPATHY[1]

All individuals are born with a certain inherited racial or family weakness, a tendency to disease. Hahnemann expressed this fact in terms of Psora, Syphilis, Sycosis, to which modern physicians may add Serum disease and Drug Miasms. These inherited agents and acquired toxins prevent the normal harmonious rhythmic flow of the life forces to an abnormal weakened interrupted stream, depriving the blood and body cells of proper nutrition (composed of hormones, enzymes, and endocrine secretions) for growth, repair and protective power against acute or environmental disease viz: infections, poisons, etc.

When Psora is eliminated from the individual, his life force flows in such harmony through his body that complete health of mind and body is obtained, thus endowing him with power to resist unhealthy conditions of environment successfully and enabling him to build up immunity against toxins and infections of various kinds. Without the presence of Psora, acute or environmental disease can make no headway or abide long in the human organism.

A child born of parents whose bodies have been cleansed of Psora by homeopathic treatment will possess superior mental, emotional and physical qualities over those less fortunately born.

The potentized homeopathic remedy is the only force so far discovered by man that is capable of modifying or eliminating the inherited toxins resulting from Psora and its chain of secondary toxins viz: disease acquired in the environment and added to the ravages of Psora.

Both the psoric and homeopathic forces are vibratory in nature and act along parallel lines on a similar magnetic polarity, hence the mutual destruction and obliteration of both forces when they melt in the deep centers of the organism where all vital life processes emerge.

These vibratory forces each with its own specific rate of vibration and its distinctive polarity produce all the affinities, the attractions and repulsions prevading throughout all nature to cause the multitudinous phenomena of growth and decay, of health and disease, of stress and storm, of sunshine and calm, ramifying the animated cosmos.

---

1. "Editorial" in THE HOMEOPATHIC RECORDER, Vol. LXIII, No. 9, March, 1948, p. 214.

The Sphere of the Repertory in the Practice of Medicine[1]

The sphere of the repertory is as broad as the Homeopathic Materia Medica itself. Repertory study is especially valuable in the treatment of chronic diseases, because absolute accuracy in prescribing is necessary to success in these chronic forms of sickness.

Osler is quoted as saying that ninety-five per cent of acute sickness is self-limiting and will recover even though no physician be present. The above statement, however, does not coincide with the statistics of Allopathic losses in pneumonia, which in some epidemics reached a death rate of forty percent. Perhaps, had no physician been present, these losses would have been much less appalling. If the claims of several non-medical cults are taken as a check, we are justified in believing that flu and pneumonia cases at least are a much safer insurance risk when they are deprived of the "privilege" of allopathic or so-called regular treatment.

The fact is that chronic disease, as Hahnemann pointed out a hundred years ago, is not self-limiting and does not tend to recover,[2] although better diet and sanitary surroundings will modify temporarily most forms of chronic illness. Their direction is toward death and only the mighty power of the homeopathic similimum can turn the tides of life ebbing deathward back toward the flood of glowing health.

Admitting that only the exact remedy can cure in chronic diseases,to do our full duty by the sick, it behooves us to use every means and method that makes for accuracy in prescribing. The reason chronic diseases present so many difficulties in the finding of the right remedy is because the symptom pictures or images of such sufferers present so many features that are common to the provings of all our deep acting medicines: the minerals, the metals, the snake and animal poisons, the nosodes and the basic vegetable substances (like Lyc.). All these medicines affect man very slowly and deeply, changing his internals before external manifestations appear.

Acute diseases on the other hand, present much more distinct and characteristic pictures comparatively easily recognized in the provings of the acute remedies as for example: Acon. with its violent anxiety, heat and restlessness, sudden onset, etc., or Bell. with its peculiarly disturbed mental sphere. Arn., Bry., Gels., Ip. and Rhus-t. all present

---

1. From the handwritten manuscript of Dr. Grimmer, exact date unknown. - Editor.
2. Organon §78. - Editor.

symptom pictures, so specific that the merest tyro in homeopathic prescribing finds no difficulty in recognizing them. And the more these beautiful instruments are used by the conscientious prescriber the easier the work becomes and the grander and more satisfying the results obtained.

However, one need not limit repertory work and study to chronic or special diseases by any means. By special disease is meant diseases of organs, as eye, ear, nose and throat. Furthermore, the use of the repertory in milder forms of illness is much easier than in chronic diseases and leads one even more swiftly to the similimum, the action of which (in mild illness) is far more spectacular (because mild illnesses have a natural tendency to get well and the similimum catalyzes the process). In finding guiding symptoms of the special parts of the body the repertory is especially useful. Such a study will enrich ones knowledge of the materia medica, and enlarge ones vision of the possibilities of internal medication. If our homeopathic specialists could only be induced to devote a little of their time to the study of the effects of our proven remedies on the organs of special sense, they would stop chasing the will-o'-the-wisps of empirical traditional medicine which is mouldy with the chill, death and damp of the dark ages. And they would be rewarded with much better results in their work.

To be successful in repertory work as well as in any other form of homeopathic prescribing, one must be well versed in the homeopathic philosophy as promulgated by Hahnemann, and enriched by Kent. The primary essential is case taking, and unless the case is properly taken, your knowledge of the repertory and the materia medica is of little avail. The reason why homeopathy is dying out among the present generation is because these fundamental principals have not been taught by the teachers of the past twenty-five years. They have been traitors to the sacred cause of truth, either unknowingly or from a bigotted and prejudiced training. They, like the political trimmers of the day, prefer to sail along the path of passive resistance, the path of false teachings that attracts and delights the multitude which is represented by the self styled scientific medicine of the day.

With this group who make up the majority whose tenents are constantly changing and uncertain, the science of today is the disappointment and fraud of tomorrow. Yet like leaves in a whirlpool, they are constantly buffeted and eddyed around, without guide or compass, and they have not the will to change the course leading them to the destroying vortex. Every allopathic prescription made by a homeopathic graduate is a falsity and a crime against a beneficient cause. However, there is a brighter side to the future of homeopathy. In spite of the machinations and the delinquencies of her so-called votaries and instructors and in spite of the many, many crimes committed in her name, in spite of all of these things, homeopathy shall live and be dominant.

The repertory of today is a mighty monument of truth and of great use to sick humanity. Its compilers (especially Dr. James Tyler Kent) deserve our ever-lasting gratitude and esteem for the love and labor they extended in its construction. How much more complete may the future repertory be if we work honestly and sincerely, in accordance with our laws in its construction.

The dawn of a new day is breaking whose light shall penetrate and illuminate all the dark, dismal precincts of medicine, and destroy the incubus of superstition and error so long oppressing. The wonderous, vital force of Hahnemann, so long the mark of ridicule by materialistic minds, can now be measured in all its changes and perturbations in health and in diseases by Abrams' electronic reactions of the blood.[1] And more: Every drug in all its numerous potencies, from the crudest to the highest and finest, will be measured as to its electronic energy and its uses, perfectly and completely adjusted to the needs of the sick, with devices so simple and accurate that a child can be taught to apply them.

---

1. See artcle "Recent Concepts and New Formulas in Medicine" p. 679 ff. - Editor.

Repertory Study[1]

A great many excellent papers have been written on this important subject and everything has been said that there is to say about it. I hope repetition will not be too triesome for those familiar with this work. In order that it may not be boring, and for those less acquainted with this valuable asset to homeopathic prescribing I will deal only with the essentials of repertory technique.

First and foremost, in this phase of homeopathic prescribing, as in all other approaches of methods of arriving at the needed remedy, the similimum, the case must be fully and properly taken. Symptoms must be obtained by indirect approach; any symptom answered by "yes" or "no" is of doubtful value.[2] Secondly, a knowledge of the relative value of symptoms is imperative to arrive at the successful prescription by analytical study and logic. In fact the correct classification and grouping of symptoms in a given case constitutes the greatest essential in arriving at the homeopathic remedy for that case.

Symptoms of all cases fall into two primary groups:

General

Particular

The GENERAL symptoms are those pertaining to the patient as a whole; such as his mental and emotional states, his fears, hates loves, and desires, symptoms of the will and the understanding emanating from the deep centers of life - the innermost - and hence the most valuable.

The physical generals, somewhat less in importance and value, are those of the body organism reacting to environment such as the temperature and weather changes. The time of aggravation or amelioration both diurnal and seasonable, periodicity, etc. are included in the physical generals. The appetite for food and drink, food desires and aversions, susceptibilities and allergies may be included here. The symptoms of the sexual sphere fall in with this group. The discharges and hemorrhages from the orifices of the body are grouped here also as the whole economy is elaborated to produce them.

The second and less important group of symptoms are known as PARTICULARS, because they pertain to the organs and parts of the body.

---

1. JOURNAL OF THE AMERICAN INSTITUTE OF HOMEOPATHY, vol. 46, No. 6, June 1953, p. 169.
2. §87 Organon - Editor.

The aforementioned two groups are in turn divided into two groups of symptoms viz COMMON and UNCOMMON. Thus:

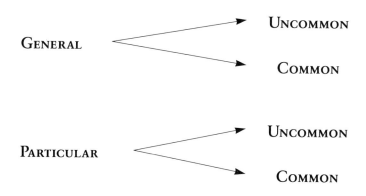

The COMMON symptoms are those common to the provings of many remedies or those common to disease states (pathologic and diagnostic such as fever, pain etc.) with no modifying concomitants. For the purpose of prescribing the common symptoms are valueless as guides for the selection of the correct remedy.

The UNCOMMON are those that are unusual, rare and peculiar, or those that are highly characteristic of the provings of a certain drug and when found in a case are valuable guides for the selection of the homeopathic remedy.[1]

The right remedy will only be found in the totality of the high grade general symptoms together with the characteristic and unusual or rare particular symptoms of the case. That is, the remedy needed to cure must run trough all the mental and physical generals as well as in the high grade uncommon particulars.[2]

To illustrate: A cold patient lacking vital heat that is restless, with marked fear of death will need the remedy that runs highest through the three rubrics: 1) Lacking vital heat, 2) Restlessness, and 3) Fear of death. The remedies found in high grade in the rubric "Lack of vital heat" are as follows and total 100.

---

1.   Organon §153 - Editor.
2.   Organon §154 - Editor.

Lack of Vital Heat[1] (Kent Repertory, page 1366) *Aesc., agar., alum., alumn., am-c., am-m., ant-c.,* **Aran.,** *arg-met., arg-n.,* **Ars.,** *ars-i., asar., aur.,* **Bar-c.,** *bar-m., bor., brom., bufo., cadm-s.,* **Calc., Calc-ar.,** *calc-f.,* **Calc-p.,** *calc-s.,* **Camph.,** *carb-an., carb-v., caul.,* **Caust.,** *chel., chin., cimic., cinnb.,* **Cist.,** *cocc., con., cupr.,* **Crot-c.,** *dig.,* **Dulc.,** *elaps,* **Ferr.,** *ferr-ar.,* **Graph.,** *guaj.,* **Hell., Hep.,** *ip.,* **Kali-ar., Kali-bi., Kali-c., Kali-p.,** *kalm., kreos., lach., lac-d.,* **Led.,** *lyc., mag-c.,* **Mag-p.,** *mang., med., merc., mez., mosch., naja, nat-ar., nat-m., nat-p.,* **Nit-ac.,** *nux-m.,* **Nux-v.,** *ol-j., petr.,* **Ph-ac., Phos.,** *plb.,* **Psor., Pyrog.,** *ran-b., rhod.,* **Rhus-t.,** *rumx., sabad., senec., sep.,* **Sil.,** *spig., stann., staph., stront., sulph., sul-ac., sumb., tarent., ther., thuj., tub.*

The remedies in the first rubric "lack of vital heat", must run through the second rubric, "restlessness", as follows, in the high grade type. Some one remedy in this rubric is the one needed to cure. All remedies not running through both rubrics are dropped.

Restlessness (Kent, page 72): *Arg-m.,* **Arg-n., Ars., Ars-i., Calc.,** *carb-v., caust.,* **Ferr., Ferr-ar.,** *graph., guaj.,* **Kali-ars., Kreos., Lyc.,** *med.,* **Merc.,** *nat-a., phos.,* **Pyrog., Rhus-t., Sep., Sil., Staph., Sulph., Zinc.**

In the second rubric "restlessness", only twenty five remedies run through both rubrics. The third rubric "fear of death", now leaves but seven remedies running through the rubrics. Thus we have reduced the number of remedies in the case from one hundred to seven!

Fear of Death (Kent, page 44): *Arg-n.,* **Ars., Calc.,** *caust., lyc.,* **Phos.,** *rhus-t.*

If we take a fourth rubric: "Fear of the dark", our number is reduced to three.

Fear of the Dark (Kent, page 43): *Calc., lyc., phos.*

A fifth rubric: "Fear of solitude or of being alone" brings in only two remedies.

Fear of Being Alone (Kent, page 43): **Lyc., Phos.**

From here we go to the materia medica to make our choice between these two remedies not a difficult problem when the case is worked down to two or three remedies. In this way we can see how the needed remedy runs all through the case.

---

1. Some remedies in Kent's rubric were upgraded to second or third degree by Dr. Grimmer from his experience - ex: Cadm-s.

A simple little diagram of four circles[1] with branches given of will enable one to visualize the groupings and relative value of symptoms for the selection of the homeopathic remedy.

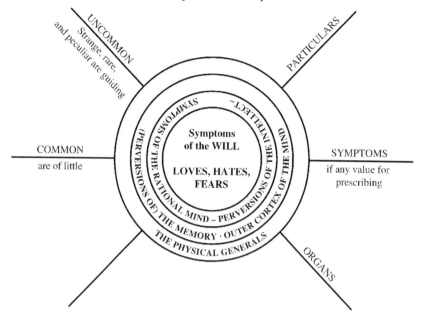

Repertory prescribing makes for greater accuracy and in the long run is a time saver; and with its use one grows in the knowledge of the materia medica, all of which brings abundance in the realm of cure by perfecting the physician in his chosen sevice.

1. Grimmer, A.H: The Essentials of Homeopathic Philosophy, THE HOMEOPATHIC RECORDER, Vol. XXXII, No. 9, September 15, 1917, pgs. 392-397, cf. especially pgs. 394 - 395. The printed article in JAIH, June 1953, did not include this diagram which is in the hand written manuscript and was also found in the 1917 article of the HOMEOPATHIC RECORDER cited above.

Object and Need for a Repertory Compendium[I]

The object and need for a repertory compend is to simplify the use of the great repertory of Kent. One of the apt criticisms concerning homeopathic medicine is the vastness of the homeopathic materia medicia with its great array of symptoms, many of them confusing and apparently contradictory. For instance in the pathogenesis of certain remedies may be found both constipation and diarrhea, aggravations from both heat and cold, from motion and rest. There are many other such instances, but these will suffice to show our meaning to the homeopathic investigator and stress the need for clarity and brevity in the procedure for the search of the similimum in every given case presented. The great repertory (of Kent) was conceived and built along the lines to conform to the homeopathic concept of the Hahnemannian philosophy as protrayed in the Organon and futher elucidated in Kent's Homeopathic Philosophy.

The first and most important step in the art of prescribing is the taking of the case. Each and every symptom obtained relating to the family and personal history must be absolutely accurate beyond all doubt. In that way every symptom obtained becomes an established fact and when the symptom picture is complete there is an array of facts to compare with the proven facts of the materia medica. It is obvious that unless such care and accuracy is pursued in the gathering of symptoms for study and comparison with the materia medica, curative results must be uncertain and even nil.

The method of questioning the patient when obtaining the case history is of vital importance. Any question answered by yes or no has been wrongly put and the answer is uncertain and of little or no value[2]. Questions must be asked in such a way as not to suggest possible ailments; sick folks are often very suggestible and impressionable, and when they answer yes or no without thought the answer may be inaccurate and misleading. Hence, the indirect method of questioning must be employed. Often four or five indirect questions must be asked to ascertain one important fact relating to the patient. For instance to obtain the patient's reaction to temperature changes we may ask indirectly as follows: How are you affected by the extreme cold of winter? How much clothing do you require in cold weather? How does cold,

---

1.   From the handwritten manuscript of Dr. Grimmer, exact date unknown. - Editor.
2.   §87 Organon - Editor.

rainy weather affect you? How easily do you catch cold?[1] The same procedure can be taken in questioning the patient's reaction to the extreme heat of summer, of a hot room, warm wraps, etc. Answers to symptoms and conditions obtained in this way are accurate and reliable because the patient has had to think about the question before giving his answer and no suggestive influence has clouded his answers.

When the symptoms of the case, properly obtained are gathered together to complete a picture of the case we are ready to evaluate the relative value of the symptoms for the selection of the curative remedy. Both Hahnemann and Kent stress the importance of characteristic symptoms. They are those symptoms peculiar to the nature of the patient's sickness.

Likewise they stressed the value of mental and emotional symptoms, the desires, the hates and fears, the appetites, the food cravings and aversions and the symptoms relating to the sexual sphere. The body's reaction and response to the impacts of environment such as heat, cold and temperature changes. All these are classified as general symptoms because they are related to those things affecting the patient as a whole. Those symptoms that are related to the body parts and organs are known as particulars. It is obvious that the general symptoms must be more important and valuable for remedy selection than particulars because the former represents the body organism as a unit while particulars only relate to parts or organs of the body.

It must be noted that all symptoms of every case are made up in two distinct groups, namely, common and uncommon, the latter group comprise those symptoms that are *unusual, rare, strange* and *peculiar* and distinctive of the patient.[2] They are his symptoms and they are found in fewer of the proven remedies. They are among the most valuable for the search of the homeopathic remedy. The common symptoms are those that are common to many diseases and complaints, diagnostic and pathologic symptoms, symptoms common in the provings of many remedies, none distinctive nor characteristic of any one remedy or of the case under study.

The symptoms that pertain to the mind and the emotions rank first in importance because the mind and the will is the center of the whole being during his earth life. Next in line are the physical generals. They

---

1. It is also well not to ask these questions in consecutive order but to space them apart so that the patient has to rethink each question. - Editor.
2. See Hahnemann: Organon § 153. - Editor.

are expressed in the patient's reaction to environment such as the effects of weather and temperature changes, heat, cold, storms, dampness, light, noise, odors, taste, etc., times of aggravations and ameliorations, causations (such as injuries, shock, emotional and physical, anger, fear, grief, etc.)[1]. The symptoms of the sexual sphere belong in this group as they are closely related to the autonomic nervous system and the endocrine chain. Hemorrhages and the discharges from the various orifices of the body are physical generals because the body organism is involved in their elaboration. Pulse and temperature readings and their characteristics are generals because they result from the organisms reaction to the impacts of environment such as infections, shock and the stresses of life. As stated before the particular symptoms are those related to the body parts and are of inferior rank for the search of the homeopathic remedy.

The remedy provings, conducted by Hahnemann and his students, which make up the Homeopathic materia medica and the construction of the repertory are all conceived and built in harmony with the principles of the homeopathic philosophy. Hence, in prescribing the physician must proceed along the same lines to achieve success with the homeopathic remedies.

The repertory compend will follow the general scheme of the great repertory but in a somewhat abbreviated manner and the combining of various important groups of repertory rubrics will give the busy practitioner valuable rubrics of remedies that may well contain the remedies covering a large proportion of their cases worked out to a small group of remedies for individual study.

The following repertory index should be made:

First the mind and emotional symptoms, then the physical generals made up of the patient's reaction to the impacts of environment, the appetites, desires and aversions, the sexual symptoms and desires and aversions, hemorrhages and body discharges, lastly eruptions and skin manifestations, then causations including injuries, bruises, cuts, strains, burns, etc. Pathological groupings will be given only in remedies of the first and second rank. The same is true of all particular symptoms

---

1. Actually "psychosomatic" causes such as emotional excitement, anger, fear, grief, etc., should be considered of first rank together with the mental symptoms. Physical causes such as injury, trauma, etc., should also be accorded a high rank, though not as high as "psychosomatic" causes. - Editor.

because the curative remedy must be in the high grade groups when the case is worked through the high grade generals.

At the end of the printed matter in the book is added a good number of blank pages to enable the physician to add additional symptoms and rubrics containing small groups of appropriate remedies to meet cases in practice needing such remedies. This will enable the repertory compend to expand in value and use.

ASTRO-PHYSICS AND HOMEOPATHY[1]

Astro-physics is a recent extension of physics and chemistry embracing radio, science and more remotely biology in its scope. All of them, however, emphasize the complete unity of the Cosmos operating under law. These sciences also teach us of the close interplay and relationship of the vastly great with the infinitely small throughout all nature. The mightiest sun swinging through the depth of space and the tiniest atom spinning around the central nucleus alike are brought into being and governed with the same force of intellegence and power coming from the Creator.

The interchange of energy and matter and the harmony and activities behind the constant flux and change involved in the evolution of all growth and development, great or small, taking place in time and space throughout the universal order excites our wonder and admiration. The march of the planets around the solar orb and the earth rotating on its axis provide us with the measured units of time, of seasons and cycles, bringing light out of darkness, maturing the germinating seed of plants, trees, fruits, flowers and grain to give substance and beauty to our environment for our every need.

The phenomena of cycles are associated with many of the mysteries of life, including the cycle of life itself, the cycles of regularly recurring natural phenomena such as the yearly meteor showers when the earth passes through certain signs of the zodiac, Leo in August, Scorpio in November and the regular advent of the seventeen year reappearance of the locusts in destructive numbers. Even in the destructive side of nature there are cycles such as earthquake cycles, tornado cycles, epidemic cycles of disease, war cycles, cycles of economic depressions, maximum sun spot cycles every twelve years corresponding to the revolution of the planet Jupiter. All these cycles are known to coincide with certain positions and mutual relationships of the sun and the planets in the Zodiac together with their mundane position in relation to the earth. Even cyclonic events in history may be foretold by those versed in the science of mundane astrology.

But the physician is more concerned with the phenomena of planetary and solar action affecting the life, growth and health of plants, animals and human lives collectively and individually. Hippocrates, the father of medicine, observed that many types of fever and acute disease ran their course, progressed and declined with the lunar phases. The

---

1. THE HOMEOPATHIC RECORDER, Vol. LXIX No. 7, January, 1954, p. 170.

period of gestation of the human animal corresponds closely to nine lunar months duration from the time of conception to birth time. A great deal of sea life corresponds with the lunar revolution as well as the tides of the oceans and seas everywhere over the earth. Certain plants grow and thrive better with an increasingly bright moon; for example, those that grow above the earth like maize and other grains and shrubs, while the so-called root crop such as potatoes, carrots, turnips, etc. are more productive when germinated and grown under a decreasing, darkening moon. The so-called mass psychology is influenced and even governed by planetary law. Crimes of violence and cruelty will coincide with an adverse aspect of position of the planet Mars. Airplane accidents where fire and falling are involved and sudden failure of mechanical parts are causative factors will find those days and those times heavily marked by the planets Uranus and Saturn. The time (i.e. *moment*) when one falls sick will surely indicate the nature, progress and termination of that illness to one trained in the lore of the stars. In fact, all the critical years and events of an individual's life may be known as they are blue-printed by the changing play of the planets in his birth chart or horoscope throughout his life.

All this sounds like blind fate swinging without resistance on its way, but this is true only for the animal and the lower order of man who obeys the animal impulses and urges of his nature. For the evolved man, who directs his will with intelligence and in accordance with the higher laws of divine order, adverse stellar forces may be much modified or entirely avoided. The evolved man has learned to protect himself from the violence of the elements as well as from the ravages of pestilence and famine, and he can avoid most of the threatened evils in his birth chart by building up his health and stamina, avoiding accidents, and nullifying the destructive forces around him with corrective thinking and living, together with the application of the homeopathic remedy.

Man becomes sick when his life force is flowing against the harmonious tide of the Cosmos. Be it either strain, infection, of faulty living as the exciting cause, the most effective means of restoring the harmonious flow of the life force in the individual is the homeopathic remedy. It is the most potent and certain force yet discovered to replace order and harmony where chaos and disorder hold sway. The transition from health to sickness and vice-versa is a very simple and imperceptible process; a reversal in the direction or an impediment in the steady flow of life energy is the change that precedes any chemical or physical change in the cells or tissues of the body organism. Instantly after the administration of the *homeopathic*[1] remedy a normalized polarity obtains; that is, the direction of the life force flows in harmony with cosmic order, and health results. Hence, in sicknesses being cured under the Homeopathic remedy, we behold the often observed action: the symptoms going away in the reverse order of their coming and from center to cirumference, from above down etc. (Hering's Law).

Some of our very able prescribers and scholars have endeavored to explain the subtle forces that Homeopathy deals with through the mediums of advanced physics, organic chemistry and biology, hoping in that way to awaken interest in the minds of men belonging to the dominate group of healers. It is a fact that these sciences have made some steps that could enable them to envision the Homeopathic concepts of life and sickness and its cure.

The physicist in speaking of the smallness of the atom (which may be measured by about 1/3000 of the wave length of yellow light) further states the comparison is significant, because the wave length roughly indicated the dimensions of the smallest grain still recognizable in the microscope. Thus it will be seen such a grain still contains thousands of millions of atoms. Lord Kelvin said "that if you could take the molecules in a glass of water, then pour contents of the glass into the ocean and stir the latter thoroughly (just who would do the stirring he did not say) so as to distribute the marked molecules uniformly throughout the seven seas, if then you took a glass of water anywhere out of the ocean, you would find in it about a hundred of your marked molecules." With these facts before them, why all the ridicule about the smallness of Homeopathic potency and dose? Thus far the physicist has taken a step in proving that in the minute things of the universe reside powers of undreamed proportion and expansion, as shown by the fission of the atom.

The biologist likewise has uncovered some very illuminating yet still unexplainable facts in investigating some of the minute things close to the nucleolus of life and life expression and in discussing the gene, that microscopic group of specialized atoms which carries in its tiny compass the mysterious but potent property of transmitting for centuries without cange the inherited traits and likeness of the species and the individual. Only under the force of powerful radiation can these tiny potent reservoirs of power be made to alter their nature or deviate from the fixed pattern of their existence and function; and when influenced by powerful x-ray or radium radiation, a state known as mutation takes

---

1. i.e. homeopathic to the patient. - Editor.

place breaking the fixed pattern of their nature to produce atypical and other forms and traits in the inherited line.

The more familiar we become with the related science the more sure we feel that homeopathic truth will sooner or later be recognized and accepted as an unvarying law of cure. But it is well to remember that these sciences are still expanding and gaining fresh knowledge. Thirty years before the discovery of the x-ray, a different view was held concerning the property and construction of matter both organic and inorganic. With the development of the quantum theory, originally proposed by Max Planck in 1900 and consumated in 1926 by Heitler and London, many obscure things concerning matter and energy have been cleared away.

But there are many things treated by Homeopathy that exist and operate outside and beyond the dominion of physics and chemistry, while biology touches only some of the fringes of the subject. I refer to the will and the consciousness of man as well as the dominating life force fresh from the Creator without which the body organism would be but a mass of decaying matter settling down to inanimate substance. The one thing common to all is their conformity to law and order, which in itself is a coordinating influence toward unity of purpose for the common good. As our vision broadens, we are lifted up to higher vistas with wider horizons to give us an awareness of the mighty unseen forces operating without friction or hinderance throughout the material universe. Everything created is for mutual purpose and use. The plant grows on and devours and refines the mineral for the use of the more highly developed and endowed animal including man, and the animal is sacrificed for the purpose of man's needs and growth. Lastly, man under God must give up his instinctive desires, that he may obtain spiritual growth and worth, thereby enabling him to serve others of his kind less fortunately endowed. Thus moves the great cycle of universal order through time and space omnipotent and eternal to bring about the lesser cycles of perturbation and change, evolution and growth of species and races of plants, animals and men. This is a passing view of material nature, the realm of effects. In the unseen realm of cause dwell the real and abiding values where intellectual growth and artistic perfections and spiritual attainments all have their origin and inception.

Homeopathy operates on both the material plane where all physical changes and effects are noted and, it also digs deep into the unseen realm of causation where only philosophic concepts can make us aware of its potent and mysterious workings.

Observations Relative to the Curative Action of Remedies[1]

Our knowledge of remedy action primarily comes from the results produced and obtained by provings. This is especially true of the Hahnemannian method of ascertaining the curative possibilities residing in each single drug substance. Within the compass of these provings are included the results observed from poisoning.

Modern science has added its might by noting the pathological end results obtained through animal experimentation. But the value of the last named is somewhat doubtful, at least in some cases, because of the different effects produced on some animals and on humans especially by certain drugs. For instance, the rabbit and the sheep can eat deadly night-shade with apparent nutritional benefit and no bad effects while man and the horse suffer serious or fatal reactions to the drug belladonna or its alkaloid atropin.

The reason homeopathic proving methods are more valuable than others is because the moral and mental changes noted in provers, while under a drug's influence, are the most essential factors of sickness as well as the most valuable for the selection of the curative medicine, and because such changes are also noted in many states of disease. Even cases of mental disease ending fatally where no brain pathology was noted by post mortem had evinced marked disturbance in the moral and mental spheres during life. In fact, all chronic diseases, if studied carefully, will show decided and characteristic mental symptoms long before physical changes can be discovered in the body by any laboratory test now known.

However, recently by an electrical contrivance called the encephalograph[2], which measures and classifies the brain waves or electrical impulses both in health and disease, changes in mental health can be accurately known. And, stranger still, it is claimed that this instrument registers an individual rate that is as differentiating as are finger prints; however, the brain waves do change in the same individual with age, health and even emotional states. It is further stated that this appliance notes changes taking place under the action of drugs and chemicals, certain chemicals being capable of restoring normal brain impulses in abnormal cases and vice-versa. Certain drugs will change healthy rates

1. The Homeopathic Recorder, Vol. LIII, No. 12, December 1938, p. 3.
2. EEG - Editor.

to abnormal ones. This instrument is now being used extensively by psychiatrists diagnostically as well as for the selection of curative agents for individual cases. All this is confirmatiory of the great "Law of Similars".

The proverbial hopefulness and cheerfulness of those suffering from tubercular disease, the profound gloom and despondency of those with liver trouble, and the anxious fear evinced by certain cardiac complaints are but illustrative instances of the relationship of mental symptoms to specific disease. From this brief survey we can see how necessary it is to have full and complete provings of all our drugs and to study and restudy these provings until they become living pictures and entities of human sufferers stamped indelibly upon our consciousness, so that when these images are met at the sick bed we may recognize them and give the needed remedy with swiftness and precision.

When we have acquired a large full knowledge of drug provings and have added to that knowledge the ability to elicit a good history of the symptoms of sickness in each individual case, including all phisical findings and laboratory reports of blood or other tissue changes, we are then able to give an intelligent and really scientific prescription based upon a fully proven natural law. Only when the above mentioned conditions are met are we able to make certain observations following the administration of the homeopathic remedy indicated at that time.

In the study of provings as well as in the study of the symptoms and progress of diseases we may note a certain pace of action and progression. Some remedies like ACON. and BELL. correspond to the sudden rapid and more or less violent activities and manifestations of acute disease. While others like the minerals and metals produce a syndrome similar to the progress of chronic disease starts. And others like the snake and animal poisons simulate diseases where blood and tissue changes are distinctive features of the illness.

When the physician is able to fit the suitable remedy to any given case of sickness, he will be able to note certain reactions in his patient after the administration of the homeopathic remedy. First, he may note a more or less definite initial aggravation of the symptoms; yet often even during this period of aggravation, the patient himself is stronger and more fit[1]. Another common observation noted is that the last

---

1. For example, if it be a fever, the temperature may actually increase initially (aggravation of symptoms) and yet the patient feels better (as is obvious by his increased cheerfulness and well being). - Editor.

symptoms that appeared will be the first to improve or leave. An inflamed or ulcerating eye will react favorably first after the correct remedy. A sore throat where the progress has been from right to left will under the correct remedy get well from left to right, the inverse order of appearance. If such progress does not take place in that direction of symptoms, the reverse order of their coming, the case is one of recovery by nature's unaided powers; and the physician can claim no credit for his remedy.

Often after the homeopathic remedy is given, old symptoms and conditions recur, for example, an eruption that had been suppressed ("cured?") by topical applications even years before. If such eruptions recur in those suffering from bronchial asthma or chronic intestinal disease, the later states are immediately relieved, and the eruption will go more slowly under the same remedy if it be allowed to act undisturbed by other medication. Another common observation noted is that conditions and symptoms proceed from the centers to the cirumference or toward the extremities, from more vital to less vital centers, from within outward. Such are eruptions of various types, catarrhal and other discharges (especially gonorrheal), which have been stopped, not cured, by suppressive methods or local treatments. These reappear like grim ghosts of the past unhappy period.

Generally the remedy that restores these manifestations will eradicate them with more time and application, but in severe cases where there has been a blending of the miasms, complicated with drug suppressions, other complimentary remedies will be indicated by the evolution of the symptoms and needed to complete the cure. Cases suffering a prolonged aggravation with no relief following are likely to be incurable. However, remedy interference (by the application of camphor, use of cathartics and other drugs such as aspirin and the barbitol preperations for palliative purposes) may produce such results.

Some sensitive patients will prove every remedy given in a high potency and will fail to have their sickness cured. Such patients must be given the indicated drug very low (say the 3rd to the 30th potency or even drop doses of the tincture) a single dose at a time with long intervals elapsing between doses in order to bring about curative action.

Incurables will avoid severe aggravations and get palliation of their symptoms and prolonging of life if their physician prescribes remedies of a more superficial nature in potencies not above the 30th. To illustrate, a badly diseased heart will almost invariably do better under drop doses of the tincture than under high potencies. The latter stir up such violent reactions in incurable cases that great and unnecessary suffering may be produced.

Occasionally following the administration of the homeopathic remedy, the patient will show only a steady gentle inprovement of all symptoms and states with no aggravation or reaction whatever. Such cases have received a proper remedy in the exact potency needed to produce so happy a result.

There are many more observations the masters have made that might be cited, but sufficient evidence has been presented to prove the value of careful observation after the administration of the homeopathic remedy. By such observations we may know the accuracy of prescriptions; also the curability of our patients as well as the time to repeat or change our remedies. We may predict many things to a certainty by a watchful check on the evolution of symptom pictures after the indicated remedy is given. Homeopathic processes express nature's orderly and benign forces in the body organism working toward harmony and health.

It only remains for the physician to study and know the mystic language of signs and symptoms along with the other proven methods of medical procedure to enable him to excel as a healer of the sick and a true benefactor of the race. And no greater privilege can be given to a man than that of the power of healing, that can comfort the suffering and afflicted who appeal to us for help on this earth journey over life's troublesome storm-tossed seas.[1]

---

1. We recommend to read the article from James Tyler Kent: Lectures on Homeopathic Philosophy, Lecture XXXV: Prognosis after Observating the Action of the Remedy. - Editor.

REVIEW OF HOMEOPATHIC PHILOSOPHY.[1]

The beginning of Homeopathic Philosophy began with Hahnemann, the rediscoverer of the Law of Similars. Others before him, most notably Hippocrates, the "Father of Medicine", envisioned this law, but never developed its expansive possibilities and unlimited use in the realm of cure.

But Hahnemann did more than rediscover and extend a therapeutic law, and by proving and recording the symptoms of over a hundred remedies, he built the foundation of the extensive Materia Medica of today.

He also sought for causes and investigated natural pnenomena concerning the etiology of disease. After much labor and study he perceived that the fundamental causes of all chronic sickness stemmed from what he called the three miasms: Psora, Syphilis and Sycosis. These are racial in scope and prevail wherever human beings are found but in a more limited degree in the remote islands of the South Seas before the white and yellow races contacted them.

Acute diseases come on primarily as an outburst or acute exacerbation of one or more of the chronic miasms which so weakened the life or vital force of the subject that environmental influences, infections, chilling, over-heating, lack of sanitation, spoiled food and water, vitiated air, etc. contributes to the sickness individually and epidemically.

One of Hahnemann's basic tenets is the recognition and acceptance of the "Vital Force", that indestructible and eternal energy which stems directly from Deity and animates all life, growth, development and motion in the Cosmos. In the absence of the vital force there is decay and death of the body organism[2] All repair and growth is dependent on the harmonious uninterrupted flow of this vital energy and all disease results from interruptions and disturbance of this same vital energy.[3]

Hahnemann recognized forms of illness which he termed indispositions brought on by faulty living conditions such as defective ventilation, lack of sanitation, impure and insufficient food, bad water, etc.[4]

Hahnemann was the first to evaluate the relative importance of symptoms for the selection of the indicated remedy. His technique of

1. Journal of the American Institute of Homeopathy, Vol. 45, No. 6, p. 119, June, 1952.
2. §10 Organon - Editor.
3. §11 Organon - Editor.
4. §77 Organon - Editor.

taking the case history of the patient is practiced and followed today in medical hospitals and institutions everywhere.

Hahnemann was one of the first men of medicine to advocate a more rational and humane treatment of the insane; he recognized the close link between mental aberations and incompentency with physical disease and with the necessity of treating the being as a whole.[1] He envisioned the individual organism both in health and disease as a unit of many complex parts and functions animated and sustained by an imponderable force[2].

Hahnemann was the first to note the prevalency and danger of suppression of disease manifestations, especially when related to the suppression of skin eruptions by powerful astringents and metallic ointments.[3] From these phenomena he established the relation of external manifestations of disease and internal health. Hence the observation of symptoms of disease disappearing under the action of the homeopathic remedy from center to cirumference and from above down, and in the reverse order of their coming, the last to come being the first to go.

Hahnemannian concepts are fundamental tenents of psychosomatic medicine which is the latest advance in Old School medical thought and practice in as much as Hahnemann perceived the mental and emotional reactions of life to be the more important factors in health and disease as well as being most valuable for the selection of the indicated remedy in the realm of cure.

Many excellent papers on Homeopathic Philosophy have been contributed by a number of Hahnemann's eminent followers: Boeninghausen, Hering, Dunham, Roberts, Close, Kent and many others who were writers and teachers of homeopathic teaching and practice. Dr. James Tyler Kent in his book on Homeopathic Philosophy added a number (twelve to be exact) of observations concerning the reactions in the patient after the administration of the indicated remedy.[4] These are highly enlightening and valuable to those who practice strict homeopathic prescribing. Kent's book elaborated and explained the Hahnemannian doctrine much in detail and will take its place beside the

---

1. §214 - 230 ORGANON - Editor.
2. §9 ff. - Editor.
3. §202 ff. - Editor.
4. Lecture XXXV. - Editor.

Organon as a strong contributing force influencing the trend of medical thought toward logic and progress.

From the times of Hahnemann to Kent there was little thought or effort to bring Homeopathy into the focus and scope of the general sciences especially those of physics and chemistry. But beginning with Fincke the first mention was made of the relation of the homeopathic potencies to the force of vibration, x-ray, radiant energy, radium, etc. The discovery of these elements and energies opened up new vistas in the great realm of physics changing scientific concepts from rank materialism to something of a more tolerant attitude toward the finer forces in nature and their effects operating on the occult plain of causation.

Coming down to our time, we have two outstanding men who recognized the fact that Homeopathy could not advance or be accepted by scientific minds unless its place in the field of physics can be established. These men, Dr. Charles Bryant and the late Dr. Fred Morgan, have done much to elucidate the relative place and force of homepathic theraputics in the realm of physics.

New knowledge and simpler techniques in the application of the vibratory forces of the remedy will soon bring more accuracy in prescribing and a markedly greater increase of cures. It has now been established that the magnetic polarities and vibratory rates of remedies correspond to the polarities and vibrations of disease. Thus when the proper remedy corresponding to the magnetic and vibratory nature of the disease is given a sick patient, equilibrium is instantly brought about, with a harmonious play of the vital processes and the restoration of body chemistry thus eradicating disease with health remaining.

This new technique in no way lessens the need for the study of the homeopathic similimum or the proving of remedies on healty human beings. Now more than ever do we need a knowledge of Homeopathic Philosophy to guide us in our work and to render it all the more successful and efficient. But acceptance of this new advance in Homeopathic prescribing based on known laws of physics will be easier understood and accepted by those imbued with scientific knowledge. With a scientific basis for our work Homeopathy will spread its gentle benign power over the world to bring forth a healthier, better, more efficient race of men and women to rule the world of the future in peace and justice.

Case Taking[1]

Mr. Chairman, friends and colleagues of the Southern Homeopathic Convention, through the helpful kindness of our gracious and charming colleague, Dr. Ruth Rogers, I am privileged to address you vocally by way of the tape recorder which she has so generously provided.

Case taking is the most important element in a successful Homeopathic prescription. It is the ability of the prescriber to obtain a complete and accurate history of the sick patient including both his personal and family history, together with all the symptoms present in the case. Dr. H. C. Allen remarked that a case well taken, insured accuracy and efficiency in the selection of the similimum. When the symptom picture with the case history is completed, it is ready for analytical study.

It is common knowledge that all symptoms are not of equal value for the selection of the curative remedy. Hahnemann and all the master prescribers and teachers that followed him have stressed the value and importance of the mental and emotional symptoms as being of highest rank in any given case in the search for the curative remedy. Dr. Kent, a strict follower of Hahnemann's concepts, formulated a system of symptom analysis logical and consistent with the Homeopathic philosophy which has been established by clinical observation for over one hundred years by the best Homeopathic scholars and prescribers of the Homeopathic science and art.

In every case of sickness and in all provings of remedies, there are two distinct groups of symptoms classified as generals and particulars. The general symptoms are those that pertain to the patient as a whole, such as the type of hemorrhages, discharges and excretions from the patient. These are generals because the economy as a whole is involved in their elaboration. Mental and emotional states, the body's reaction to envionment, such as, heat and cold, the food desires and aversions, the sex functions, desires and aversions, anything or any condition affecting the patient's entire economy is included in the list of generals. Particular symptoms are those affecting organs or parts of the body organism primarily.

As stated before the high grade general symptoms are those pertaining to the mind and emotions, such as the fears and mental aberrations,

---

1. Address to the Southern Homeopathic Convention, exact date unknown. Reproduced from the handwritten manuscript of Dr. Grimmer. - Editor.

illusions etc., impaired mind function, impaired memory and difficult concentration.[1]

The physical generals are next in order of value: the effects on the patient from the extremes of temperature, heat and cold, storms, rains, snows, electric and wind stroms, and the extent of their sick producing effects on the patient. All these things affect the patient as a whole. Where the personal pronoun "I" is used to describe the symptom, it makes it a general. Where the possessive pronoun "my" is used to describe the particular part or place of the body affected, it is a particular symptom.

Throughout the whole symptom picture of both generals and particulars there are two distinct groups known as common symptoms and characteristic symptoms, the latter which contain the unusual and rare symptoms. These are highly valuable for prescribing purposes.[2] The common are of little value in prescribing as they are those common in the provings of many drugs and common to the symptoms of many diseases (diagnostic). The characteristic are those symptoms peculiar to each individual remedy or to the individual patient under study. A symptom found only in the provings of few drugs is rare and, if a mental or high grade physical general, may be very valuable for the selection of the similimum. A symptom unrelated to any anatomical or physiological condition is unusual and may be listed under the rare and peculiar, hence valuable for remedy selection.

A simplified means of charting symptoms may aid one to perceive the relative importance of symptoms for the selection of the curative remedy in any given case.[3]

The mental symptoms may be classed into several groups relative to their value as follows: symptoms pertaining to the will which include the loves and hates (perverted loves) with resentments, frustrations, jealousies and inhibitions. These constitute the deepest and most central symptoms of the being. Here is included the love of life and when that is disturbed to the point of suicide we see a most profound inharmony in the center of being, presenting a symptom of first value typified by the remedy AUR. which takes away all desire to exist and be. The other group pertains to the rational mind and to the perversions of the intellectual and reasoning processes. Here we get symptoms expressing irra-

---

1. and those symptoms that are strong, rare, peculiar - Editor.
2. Hahnemann, Samuel: Organon §153. - Editor.
3. See article "Repertory Study" p. 246. - Editor.

tional concepts of living, with faulty reasoning that may end in harmful results. Insane statements and actions, irresponsible conclusions and acts belong to this second group. ARG-MET. is typical of this group. In Clarke, silver is listed as a remedy for brain fag and he states that it affects the mental processes mere than the affections. Kent also mentions its effects on the rational mind especially.

The method of questioning the patient while taking the case is an important procedure in order to avoid error and to obtain the true facts in every case of sickness. Remember that every question answered by the patient with "yes" or "no", has been wrongly put by the physician and is of little, if any value for prescribing purposes. Every symptom obtained from the patient to be a verified fact must come in an answer to indirect questioning. A direct question permits the patient to answer without adequate thought, it also may suggest to an impressionable person conditions that do not exist. For instance, the physician wishing to know the patient's temperature reactions may need to ask several indirect questions, such as how does the heat of summer affect you and your symptoms? What effect does cold of winter have on you? How much covering or clothing do you require in cold weather? How does rain or snow effect you? Thus a number of indirect questions may be needed to establish one important general fact or symptom which can place the patient beyond all doubt either into the hot or cold group of patients or into that smaller group who are sensitive to both extremes of temperature.[1] When the sum total of symptoms of the case are procurred in this way the prescriber has an array of established facts to compare with the established facts of the Materia Medica for study and comparison. By this procedure the chance for error is reduced, with greater certainty for an accurate and successful prescription.

The successful Homeopathic prescriber must take on the role of an astute detective in his search for symptoms and facts that are accurate and true. Again he must be an impartial judge of these facts and harmonize them with the facts of the Materia Medica; he must be free of prejudice and develop the art of logical thinking.[2] His task is far from easy, but his reward is great in satisfaction, for every successful prescription in fraught with good to the patient and delight to the doctor. The doctor who treats his patient with the art and science of Homeopathy is a

---

1. The appropriate rubric for this may be found in Kent's Repertory III or later editions, p. 1349, "Cold, heat and cold" - Editor.
2. §83. - Editor.

medical idealist recognizing the deeper and more subtle aspects of human sickness and its cure. He accepts the fact that the patient is sick mentally and emotionally as well as physically. He also sees his patient as an individual unit requiring special individual study for the one individual remedy needed for his special case of sickness no matter what the diagnostic name of his illness may be. The Homeopathic physician avoids supressing local manifestations of disease especially those of mucous membranes and skin, knowing that great harm and suffering can come to the patient from such suppression.[1]

The Homeopathist is a philosopher, noting the ill effects of disturbed emotions and faulty thinking on the physiologic processes of the body organism, first producing functional disorder that in time will ultimate in pathologic changes in the tissues and organs of the body.[2] Competent medical authorities now claim that the deadly, crippling ravages of arthritic disease are caused and aggravated by all sorts of wrong, harmful and unholy thinking and this is not so strange, when we realize that no conscious action takes place that is not preceeded by a thought process or impulse. "As a man thinketh in his heart so he is." Hahnemann's recognition of the importance and relationship of the mental and emotional states and symptoms to disease, has in more recent times been verified and substantiated by the observations and claims of the psycho-somatic branch of medical thought that tells us, all constitutional disease, mental and physical, has its origin in maladjusted and perverted modes of thinking. Clinical evidence in all schools of medical and healing thought have verified these claims.

The Homeopathic physician, because of the subtle power of his healing instruments (potentized remedies), has acquired an element of faith not found in the general run of the healing profession. Christ tells us if we have the faith comparable to the size of a mustard seed we can remove mountains. From our study of man we know he has a mind and a body as well as an immortal soul. This immortal soul binds him with Deity through time and eternity. This unity with Deity is the distinguishing quality that seperates man from the purely animal world, or rather the animal in him has evolved into the realms of the spiritual world. Because of his composite nature, man exists in various realms of nature which may be summarized into physical and spiritual, and because of these facts, he has need of both physical (natural) and spirit-

---

1.   §202 - Editor.
2.   §210, 211 - Editor.

ual nourishment and medication to promote his growth and well being on all the planes of his existence. The similimum, in potentized form, can bring harmony into all of life's processes by normalizing the vital force of the sick individual, and thus open the way for the spiritual influxes emanating from the Lord to insure permanent cure in the deepest centers of being." In the healthy condition of man, the spiritual vital force, the dynamis that animates the material body, rules with unbounded sway, and retains all parts of the organism in admirable, harmonious, vital operation, as regards both sensations and functions, so that our indwelling, reason-gifted mind can freely employ this living healthy instrument[1] for the higher purposes of our existence".[2] Every true healer knows that the efficacy of faith in the power and goodness of GOD that may reside in both patient and doctor, is the all potent factor in cure regardless of the therapy that may be employed. Homeopathic philosophy recognizes the value of both the scientific and spiritual aspects of healing. Hence its wide application and use in the sphere of sickness.

We beg your indulgance and pardon for this divergence into the domain of philosophy, but we believe that it will help us all, by provoking comment and friendly criticism concerning its use and application in the vital field of healing. Also a true concept of the relative value of symptoms in the domain of sickness is revealed. These philosophic concepts of the etiology and cure of human illness are valuable. If we would attain the highest use in Homeopathic prescribing we must perfect ourselves in a knowledge of the language of symptoms which expresses the sufferings and needs of our patients in the many forms of human sickness. Homeopathy more completely meets the needs of sick humanity than the cruder forms of healing. To the new born infant and growing child as well as the matured adult down to the sunset golden time of advancing age, the Homeopathic remedy is a GOD sent boon of healing and comfort.

In closing, I wish to proclaim from the house tops of the world my praise and Thanksgiving to our heavenly Father for this precious gift of healing and to invoke His blessings for those who live by and practice this benign art as well as for those who abide in its sublime tenents.[3]

---

1. i.e. the body - Editor.
2. Hahnemann: Organon, § 9. - Editor.
3. We recommend to study the following works: 1. Hahnemann, Samuel: Organon. 2. Kent, J. T.: Lectures in Homeopathic Philosophy. 3. Kent, J. T.: Repertory of Homeopathic Materia Medic and Grimmer's article "Repertory Study" p. 246. Editor.

THE ESSENTIALS FOR A HOMEOPATHIC PRESCRIPTION[1]

Every homeopathic doctor knows that if he can select the true similimum in any given case he can obtain maximum results in terms of cure. But many difficulties must be overcome in the search for the best homeopathic remedy. The most important factor in homeopathic procedure is the successful taking of the case and there is no better technique than the one devised by Hahnemann for such work. Let the patient tell the story of his case without interruption and when he has finished, the questions by the physician (for details and clarification of the history and symptoms) come next in order.[2]

No direct or leading questions should be asked. Any question answered by "yes" or "no" has been wrongly put, and the answers are of doubtful value for remedy selection. Every symptom of the pathogenesis must stand out as an indubitable fact. At times a number of indirect questions must be put to the patient in order to obtain the correct status of a single symptom. This is especially true when the symptom is either a strong mental or a high grade general symptom qualifying strongly the nature of the patient and his illness.

A case fully and properly taken will yield not less than six or eight strong characterizing symptoms and from this group the curative remedy will be found.

After the case is taken comes the task of grading the symptoms according to their relative value and importance for remedy selection. The method of classifying and grading symptoms for remedy finding as outlined by the late Dr. J. T. Kent is logical and has produced outstanding results in accuracy in obtaining the similmum.

The symptoms are divided into general and particular groups of symptoms:

The generals are those symptoms describing the ailments of the patient as a whole, symptoms relating to the mind, the emotions, desires and mental processes, such as reason, memory etc. Also the physical generals which relate to the body's response to the forces of environment as the effects of heat, cold, weather changes, open air, or lack of the same, closed rooms, etc. Included in the physical generals are the food desires and aversions that proceed from the stomach, but

---

1. Exact date unknown, but written Nov. 1953 for HOMEOPATIA MAGAZINE, H.L. Roux director; Rio Baniba 118; Buenos Aires; Argentine. - Editor.
2. §82 - 99 - Editor.

nevertheless they are general because the body as a whole is involved in this process. The discharges, including hemorrhages from the orifice of the body are all general symptoms because the organization as a whole is the contracting factor in their elaboration. The sexual symptoms are likewise generals because they are desires or aversions of the patient. The sleep and dream symptoms belong to the general group for the same reasons outlined in the aforementioned groups. Symptoms known as particulars are those relating exclusively to the organs and parts of the body, and are less valuable for prescribing purposes.

Another grand division of symptoms running throughout both general and particular groups are two more groups known as common on the one hand and as characteristics or distinguishing on the other.

The common symptoms are those common to the provings of many remedies and those common to the symptoms of many diseases. Diagnostic symptoms are common and all these symptoms are of little value in the selection of the homeopathic remedy.

The characterizing symptoms are those that are rare, strange, unusual and peculiar. When they occur in a case of sickness the curative remedy needed for that case must contain these symptoms in its proving. At times one of these outstanding characteristic symptoms in conjunction with the rest of the totality of the symptoms may well point the way to the homeopathic specific.

There exists a class of symptoms known as keynotes over which much heated controversy has occurred in the past concerning their value in remedy selection. Much depends on whether the keynote is a general or a particular. If a general it might well be a useful guide in conjunction with the totality of the case for the finding of the curative remedy. If a particular, it would be of doubtful use. In the main the study of the keynotes may be useful as leaders to study the case and if the keynote is a general and is consistent with the rest of the totality of the symptoms a successful prescription would result[1].

The similimum is only found in the totality of the symptoms presented but its detection is much simplified by the high grade of characteristic symptoms embraced in that totality. When the similimum is found and prescribed the homeopathic physicians justified in expecting rapid, gentle and satisfactory results in curative action.

---

1. Actually Guernsey's original paper was never carefully studied and grossly misunderstood. Guernsey followed Hahnemann's method and his "Keynpte system" involved a careful case taking and assembling the "characteristic symptoms" of the case (§153). Her referred to these characteristic symptoms as Keynotes. - Editor.

But in these days of food and water adulterations and chemical processes, humanity is afflicted with an unceasing stream of health destroying agents many of them antidotal to the action of curative remedies which renders the homeopathic work difficult and often futile. Aluminum toxin is one of the most common of the inhibiting agents to homeopathic remedies. Patients poisoned with this substance can obtain but little good from the best homeopathic remedy until the homeopathic antidote has been given. That antidote is CADM-O. in any potency above or equal to the 30.

The toxin of aluminum is frequently found in the blood of many cancer patients hence it is one of the predisposing factors of irritation occurring in a majority of the unfortunate victims of cancer, hence CADM-O. is one of our most frequent and effective remedies for this condition. Other exciting factors in cancer causation are the indiscriminate and excessive application of the so called wonder drugs (antibiotics) and coal tar derivatives together with the universal and often forceful use of serums and vaccines, products of disease shot directly into the blood stream of the victims. How can the crude products of disease promote anything but sickness and suffering? When will the medical men, the guardians of health repudiate this universal outrage against nature and get back to a program of sanity and trust in Divine Providence? More faith in the power of the life force, that God given principle of life, and less reliance on experimental chemicals will produce more health and reduce suffering and hurtful expense among the multitude.

A few words of commendation for our homeopathic pharmacists are in order here. Their faithful painstaking care in the preparation of our remedies and potencies is without doubt the most certain element for our successful fight against disease. Without the guarantee of the purity and verity of our numerous drugs, of what use all our tedious labors in case taking and remedy selection by way of repertory and unending materia medica study. Too little thought has been given this important phase of our profession and not enough recognition has been granted for the grand work our pharmacists have performed for the whole homeopathic profession as well as for the good of the homeopathic lay world who depend so much an accurate homeopathic prescribing for their well being and happiness.

I am well aware this subject has been dwelt on many times before, but it is of such vast importance to the continued growth and success of homeopathy everywhere that repetition can do only good.

THE RELATIVE VALUE OF SYMPTOMS[1]

When a case has been fully and properly taken, it is time to evaluate the symptoms in the order of their importance.

Prior to such an appraisal the taking of the case and the manner and method employed to obtain the symptoms of the case is most vital in importance. Symptoms obtained without the Hahnemannian technique are of doubtful value and may be false and misleading. Any and all given symptoms must represent a statement of facts, and these facts must be brought forth after the manner of judicial procedure.

The patient tells his story without interruption unless he is loquacious and wandering, when he must be carefully guided to his task with an indirect line of questioning by the physician.[2]

Direct questions tend to suggest, and the patient may answer without sufficient thought. Any question answered by yes or no to the Homeopath is of doubtful value.[3]

Sometimes the physician may be compelled to ask three or four indirect questions to ascertain the verity or sureness of one symptom. To illustrate: In order to know that temperature group the patient belongs to, the physician will ask how sensitive to cold are you. How are you affected by a hot room? How does the sun's heat affect you? How much clothing do you require to keep warm? How are you affected by changes of weather? What can you say about the temperature of your hands and feet? In this way the physician can with certainty ascertain to which group his patient belongs. Is he a cold patient with deficient vital heat,[4] or is he warm blooded and made worse by over heating, or is he one who is sensitive to the both extremes of temperature?[5] The mental and emotional symptoms may be obtained in a similar way. How easily moved to tears are you? How does music affect you? How does noise or light affect you? How does darkness affect you? How restless are you? What can you say of your memory? Thus when symptoms are obtained in this way, they are genuine and reliable and constitute facts which can be fitted to the facts of the Materia Medica.

When the symptoms of a case history are obtained properly, then the physician may begin to appraise and weigh the relative value of the

---

1. THE HOMEOPATHIC RECORDER, Vol. LXVII, No. 6, Dec. 1951, p. 159.
2. §84 - Editor.
3. §87 - Editor.
4. Kent's Repertory = KR p. 1366. - Editor.
5. KR p. 1399. Editor.

symptoms for the selection of the homeopathic remedy. The writer has followed the general outline for the grading and evaluating of symptoms devised by Dr. James Tyler Kent and found that method logical and concise and most helpful in the selection of the needed remedy.[1]

In that plan there are three classes of symptoms as follows: General, which relate to the patient as a whole, such as his bodily reaction to environment, his mental and emotional states, his aversions and desires, his body secretions and discharges. Particulars, which relate to organs and parts. Common, which are common to the provings of many remedies or to disease conditions (diagnostic).

These three groups of symptoms are each made up of three grades[2]: First, Second and Third.[3] Thus the first grade generals are those that are rare and peculiar or those that are characteristic of the remedy. The symptoms that relate to the will, the loves, the hates, the fears, the desires and aversions belong to the high or first grade. The second grade are those pertaining to the rational mind or intellect, the body reactions to environment, the physical appetites, the sexual symptoms, the body secretions and discharge, because such are elaborated by the organism as a whole, the modalities as to time and condition of aggravation and amelioration. The third grade are the common symptoms found in disease such as headache, malaise, fever, chill, sweat, etc., or those symptoms common to the provings of many remedies. Common symptoms may be expressed in general symptoms of the patient as a whole, or they may be found in the particular parts of the body.[4]

The high grade particulars are those that are rare and unusual, such as inflammation with little or no pain, thirst without fever itching skin with no eruption. The modalities constitute the second grade and the common symptoms the third grade.

This is but a brief outline of classifying symptoms for remedy selection.

But all the teachers and master prescribers from Hahnemann down have stressed the unusual and rare symptoms as the ones of impor-

---

1. KLHP: Lectures XXX - XXXIII - Editor.
2. See also Currim, Ahmed N: Guide to Kent's Repertory, Hahnemann Institute, 1996.
3. KLHP: Lectures XXXII and XXXIII - Editor.
4. Actually Kent defined grades 1,2,3 in Lecture XXXIII in a certain way as regards provings and cures made - Here the word "grade" as used by Dr. Grimmer really should be replaced by the word "importance" to avoid confusion with the technical word "grade" defined be Kent. - Editor.

tance, because they are characteristic of the sick patient as well as of the remedy he needs for his cure.

This subject has been presented many times more by much more proficient teachers and prescribers than I am, but I bring to you my humble efforts and trust we have some discussion on this very vital subject that all together we may bring forth better and simpler means to reach the desired goal - a surer and quicker way to find the similimum.

After the First Prescription[I]

If the case has been fully taken, the administration of the homeo-pathic remedy will produce certain and definite reactions and changes in the symptom picture within a period of time, varying from a few hours to several days or even weeks depending upon the nature of the sickness and the reactive powers of the individual patient. If the case be acute, a few hours will bring beginning changes; if chronic, days or week may pass before changes come.

The most common observation noted is the aggravation of the symptoms (from slight to intense in different individuals); this aggrava-tion is followed by steady and progressive improvement of the patient and his symptoms[2], often for weeks or even months. When a prescrip-tion is followed by such a happy combination of circumstances, we may be sure it was strictly homeopathic, and these cases with rare exception will need no other remedy to effect a cure or no second pre-scription.

However, after the first prescription when sufficient time has elapsed to bring about a return of the symptoms likely in a much milder and often somewhat changed degree, the remedy will need to be repeated in the same potency. And later again, after a considerable time, a repeti-tion of the remedy is required by the return of symptoms, and then experience has taught that better and more lasting results are obtained if the potency of the same remedy be raised to a much higher plane. This method of remedy and increase of potency may be repeated a large number of times until the patient has been carried through the range of potencies from the 1M to the MM, when most cases will be dismissed cured.

Occasionally a case persists to manifest the symptom picture in a much modified degree after being through the range of potencies. Then the prescriber may go back down the scale of potencies to the 30th or 200th potency and repeat the progressive march of the potencies of the same remedy selected at the first study, because a remedy that will per-sist to act favorably through the range of potencies is the remedy homeopathic to that case, and rarely will any other remedy be needed for that particular patient.

---

1. From the handwritten manuscript of Dr. Grimmer, exact date unknown. - Editor.
2. Kent: Lectures on Homeopathic Philosophy - Lecture XXXV. Editor.

The exceptions are those cases where there is a blending of the miasms complicated with drug disease. If a drug disease complicates, it may be necessary to give a homeopathic antidote, even in a series of potencies or until such time as the patient is free of drug symptoms, when a return to the homeopathic constitutional remedy will be needed. More often the drug disease must be disposed of before the natural disease can be successfully treated[1].

In the case of a complication of miasms, the first prescription must correspond to the initial [2]symptoms of the patient. After he is free from these initial symptoms, and a new picture presents itself, a remedy con-plimentary to the first remedy and homeopathic to the new picture must be administered.

Before a new remedy is given, a re-study of the case must be made and as great or even greater discrimination is needed for the selection of the second remedy of a chronic case that is beginning to flow in order. A safe rule to follow is the injunction once expressed by Dr. Kent "never leave a remedy that has acted curatively until it fails to act in a higher potency". This is not the exact quotation, but it expresses the idea he wished to convey. Sometimes a change in the symptoms may come, and still the first remedy prescribed may continue to be homeo-pathic to the case. If the patient as a whole has improved and the changed symptoms are old ones returning, or if they proceed from within out from more to less vital parts or if old skin eruptions or dis-charges re-appear, the remedy should not be changed but allowed to act until improvement ceases; and then it may be repeated in a higher potency if several repetitions have already been made. The physician must definitely know that the first remedy has ceased to function before he hazards a second remedy in a case started to flow in order if he does not want to bring confusion into his case and perhaps spoil it.[3]

Cases have been observed where no aggravation follows the adminis-tration of the remedy, only a steady and long amelioration of the symp-toms with a sense of well being in the patient. Such cases have received the similium in the exact potency suited to that patient, and needless to say no other remedy will be necessary for that case.[4]

---

1. Kent: ibid Lecture XXVI. - Editor.
2. i.e. most recent - Editor.
3. Kent ibid Lecture XXXVI - paragraph 11. - Editor.
4. Kent Lecture XXXV. - Editor.

Other cases will show a protraced aggravation of symptoms with no improvement following. Such cases are either incurable and have received too deep a remedy, or they are sensitives who prove every remedy given them.

If pathologic and other factors indicate the possibility of incurability, a superficial remedy must be selected for palliation.

If a state of hypersusceptibility be present, the remedies must be given in a very low potency but still in the single dose and only repeated at sufficient long intervals to obtain curative results; after a time the potency may be increased if the action has been homeopathic.

Another observation has been noted where following the remedy, a short period of relief was followed by an aggravation of symptoms or a return to the original state. If such a prescription has not been interfered with by other drugs taken intentionally or accidentally (as in form of camphor of other chemical fumes), or if cathartics or analgesic drugs (either coal tar derivatives or narcotics) have not been taken, the prescription was wrong and unfortunate for both patient and doctor.[1]

It is presumed the doctor had corrected all faulty living habits and conditions before he made the prescription, for if he failed to do so, his remedy might well have been rendered nil or its action cut short by unhygienic conditions and bad dietary habits.

A wrong prescription in a deeply chronic case or a seriously sick acute case may well be fatal or carry irreparable consequences. At best it will take extreme care and much study to restore the case to a semblance of order for the correct prescription to follow.

If no aggravation occurs in a vigorous constitution, it is likely the remedy was only partially similar; and it may require several other partially similar remedies to affect the cure.

At times it is observed a patient has an amelioration of symptoms over a sufficient interval of time to bring curative results, but they fail to manifest; that is, the patient does not gain in strength and well being commensurate with the amelioration of symptoms. Such cases are incurable because of pathologic changes in vital organs: heart, kidney, lungs or somewhere in the deep nervous system.

When a greater number of new symptoms appear after the prescription it will generally prove unfavorable. This is especially true if the new symptoms are not old forgotten ones returning (which sometimes happens). In these cases the remedy was not truly homeopathic.

---

1. Kent ibid Lecture XXXV. - Editor.

When many old symptoms re-appear, the remedy is homeopathic and the case is curable.

Is is sometimes noted where symptoms take the wrong direction that is travel from the extremity toward the centers as a case of rheumatic fever where swollen painful joints may be much relieved after the remedy, but serious heart symptoms may come up; when such things happen, the remedy must be antidoted immediately before pathologic changes take place in the vital centers. Often the antidote to a faulty prescription will prove the curative remedy in the case. But sometimes it is not sufficient, and another carefully selected remedy will be needed. Regarding the repetition of the remedy much controversy obtains among many of our good prescribers.

Dr. Kent who devoted much thought on the philosophic aspect of things homeopathic stated that at times in a seriously sick diptheric patient with a weak constitution a repetition of the dose will kill. He admitted he did not know the principle behind the phenomenon other that the weakness or strength of the patient's vital reserve or constitution, which lies in the realm of the inheritable. And he also stated that in febrile conditions, as typhoid occuring in vigorous constitutions, he frequently repeated the remedy dissolved in water every few hours until the fever declined or left, thus often cutting short the usual course of the fever.

Hahnemann repeated the dose at times, giving it in a slightly higher potency in water. Some of our good prescribers give three doses of the potentized remedy two hours apart at the start of every case and claim excellents results.

But are the results any better than those obtained by the single dose?[1] After all it is a matter of the homeopathicity of the prescription. Repetition of dose and the potency required may be important in certain cases, but they are secondary in value and depend on other factors in the case outside the symptom picture. Cases where much pathology occurs in vital organs will be aggravated by a too high potency. And then the repetition of the dose may be more frequent for palliation, because in many cases cure is not possible. They are the incurables which Hahnemann speaks of in the Organon. We must know what is

---

1. Most of the homeopathic physicians were unacquainted with the SIXTH edition of the Organon and especially §§246, 247, 248 with their respective footnotes 132, 133, 134 where Hahnemann taught the repetition of the doses in both acute and chronic diseases. - Editor.

curable in both remedies and sick patients in order to obtain our best success.[1]

Experiments in the bio-electric field show some interesting reactions in the patient's blood. In a blood specimen that is positive the similimum selected out of a negative group of remedies will change that positive blood to the normal negative point always found in the state of health. And when such a selected remedy is given the patient, his reactions are instantly restored to the negative state. This statement is proven by a subsequent test of the patient's blood immediately following the intake of the selective remedy which then will show all disease reactions obliterated, with the vital wave at the maximum height and the polarity at the normal negative point. From the behavior of this phenomenon in relation to homeopathic remedies we can actually see the change from disorder to order, and that state of order will continue for days or weeks until the effect of the remedy is exhausted and a repetition is needed to restore and maintain the flow of vital forces of the stream of harmony.

These things confirm the theory of Hahnemann concerning the vital force as being the fundamental factor in health or sickness. In sickness the vital force is disturbed first, and then chemical changes are set up of the destructive or unbalanced nature soon to be followed by changes in tissue (pathology). When the correct remedy is administered, the above processes are reversed; and the vital force flows in order, restoring the body chemistry to normal then repairing the tissues (replacing pathologic cells with normal histologic cells, thereby completing the cycle of recovery).

If the above observations are true, it is evident that too soon a repetition of the dose of even the right remedy might easily disturb the flow of the vital harmony and interfere with recovery. Clinical observations of hundreds of our most successful prescribers from Hahnemann's time to the present remind us that as long as improvement continues (after the remedy is taken), repetition is not indicated.

---

1. §3 - Editor.

THE VALUE OF MENTAL SYMPTOMS IN HOMEOPATHIC PRESCRIBING[1]

Every homeopathic prescriber from Hahnemann down to the Masters of the present time stress the importance of mental and emotional symptoms for the selection of the similimum.

Many interesting and instructive cases from Hering's book entitled The Symptoms of the Mind[2] afford abundant proof of the use and value of such symptoms. A few illustrations which follow are illuminating and well woth study.

Page numbers in the following section refer to Hering's book. A case, (pg. 134) given by G. F. Muller and called by Hering a model cure: "Talking nonsense in her sleep at four o'clock in the morning; disturbed look, stares at people; head hot, carotids throbbing; flushed and bloated face; eyes fixed, pupils dilated; frequent pulse; hair moist, the rest of the body burning hot; great anxiety; singing followed by weeping and loud screaming, with gasping for breath; beating headache, especially in the vertex; tearing stitches in the brain; crawling in hands and feet; as if they were numb; great thirst, with coated tongue." HYPER. cured, though many BELL. symptoms were present.

Another case, (pg. 135) from M. Muller: "Talks almost continually about fanciful things or such as have really occured, of faithless love, of her teachers and school days; laughs, sings, dances, weeps, makes grimaces and gesticulates with her hands. Clings obstinately to her ideas, without, however, growing angry about it. Face distorted, eyes fixed, no desire to eat or drink, things offered her are hastily dispatched." PLAT. was the remedy that cured. Only a master prescriber would select this remedy.

Another case cited by Th. Ruckert, (pg. 139): "After vexation, mental depression; she is in constant dread, with palpitation of the heart, is afraid of everybody, considers everyone her enemy, despairs of everything, cries easily, trusts no one. At the same time pale earthy complexion with dim, desponding look. No appetite, much thirst, limbs feel as if asleep; is weary, weak, cannot sleep at night on account of fear and

---

1. JOURNAL OF THE AMERICAN INSTITUTE OF HOMEOPATHY, Vol. 40, No. 2, February, 1947, p. 37.
2. This book initially appeared as ANALYTICAL THERAPEUTICS, Vol. 1; it seems that the suceeding volume or volumes never appeared and the title of the book was changed to THE SYMPTOMS OF THE MIND. The American Homeopathic Publishing Society, J.M. Stoddart & Co., Philadelphia, 1881. - Editor.

dread." PULS. was the curative remedy in spite of the thirst present; Puls is more often thirstless.

Model cure reported by Sonnenburg, (pg. 122): "Fear and mistrust of everyone, great anxiety by day and night, no rest in any place, seeks to fly. Her only pleasure is to look into the sun or the fire. She fled into a forest, built a large fire and remained there four or five days without nourishment. Seeks to be alone, flees society; when alone she cuts up queer antics, screws her mouth in all directions, throws money out of the window. Tactiturn; after repeated questioning she screams her answer loudly and angrily." BELL. cured. It is the only proven remedy in melancholy and mania with longing to look in the sun and the fire.

Another model cure by Sztarovcszky, (pg. 124): "Throbbing pain in the brain, dimness of vision, as if he looked through a sieve; frightful visions appear to him when in the dark, or when closing his eyes; he strikes at them and holds the cross up to them." PULS. cured. PULS. has frightful visions in the dark or on closing the eyes.[1]

Quoting Hahnemann in the fifth edition of the Organon, paragraph 253: "The condition of the mind and general behaviour of the patient are to be counted among the most certain and intelligible signs (not visible to everyone) of a slight beginning of improvement or of aggravation in all diseases, especially the acute ones. The signs of incipient improvement, however slight, are: an increased sensation of comfort, greater tranquilitiy and freedom of mind, the heightened courage. The patient experiences, as it were a return of naturalness. The signs of aggravation, however slight, are the opposite of the foregoing: an embarrased, helpless state of mind and disposition, where the behavior, attitude and actions of the patient appeal to our sympathy. This condition is readily seen and appreciated by a careful observer, but not to be described in so many words."

Any experienced physician may note in the patient's face, his eyes, and the coloring and expressions which mirror the thoughts, fears and emotions in no uncertain way, that present sure indications for the selection of the homeopathic remedy.

Hering classified a group of "Bodily symptoms connected with the Mind" that is helpful to the physician and student alike:

1. Ailments from emotions and from exertion of the mind, such as: Happy surprise. Complaints after laughing. Fright and fear. Shock

---

1. KR - p,. 134R. - Editor.

of injury. Ailments owing to fear. After anxiety. Homesickness, Nostalgia. Love pangs. Jealousy. Grief and Sorrow. Better in company and Better when alone, (Will not be looked at. Dislikes to be spoken to. Worse from friendly persuasion). From talking to others. Mortification. Vexation. Anger. Emotions and Excitement in general. Worse when thinking about his condition, better when thinking about something else. Complaints after speaking. Headaches from exertions of mind or intellectual work. Complaints from thinking or meditating. Ailings from over exertion of mind and body.

Happy Surprise[1]

Under Happy surprises, such as excessive joy, a small group of remedies are given: *Acon.*, caust., COFF., croc., cycl., nat-c., *op.* and *puls*. In the remedies not italicized: caust., croc., cycl. and nat-c., the symptoms were observed only in incompletely proved remedies or infrequently met with. In the *italicized* remedies the symptoms both occured in the proving and were cured in the sick: Acon., op. and puls. The remedy COFF. ALL CAPITALS has frequently and persistantly produced the condition in the proving and verified by many cured of the sick.[2]

Where the joy has startled or struck so hard that trembling, crying, weeping, sobbing or fainting away, even apparent death, particularly in children and women, COFF. is the only remedy.

Stunned by it, laughing and crying: Hyos.

Talkative with sudden changing of the subject: Lach.

Merry madness, with headache, blindness or pale face: Croc.

Fainting: Acon., coff.

Headaches after mental exhilaration: Coca, Coff.; glowing red cheeks: Merc.; following such or other excitement: Scut.

After it mouth was suddenly filled with bright blood: Chin.

---

1. Hering ibid p. 71. The remedies that Hering wrote in all CAPITALS were written by Kent in bold so they would jump out of the page at the reader. Kent continued to keep the italicised and ordinary Roman type as Hering had done with the same definitions. In this article we have used Hering's style of all CAPITALS. - Editor.
2. Currim, Ahmed N., Guide to Kent's Repertory, Hahnemann Institute, 1996, pages 9 - 12. This was Kent's method; KLHP lectures XXXII and XXXIII. - Editor.

Gagging or vomituritio: Kali-c.

Diarrhoea: Acon., Gels.

Metritis: Coff.

Weeping, coughing, trembling: Acon., Merc.

Chilly as of chills running over him: Gels.

Shivering flitting sensation: Acon., Kali-c.

Unusually excited by joyous news toward evening: Aloe

If Aml-ns. is inhaled the same conditions obtain that result from sudden emotions, with crimson flushing of the cheeks and quickened pulse. Roth recommends it as homeopathic to the effect of emotions.

COMPLAINTS AFTER LAUGHING[1]

Mind: Easily depressed; Form.; sadness following: Phos.; as of her body were borne upon wings, Thuj.

HEADACHE: Ars-met., croc., iris, phos., tong., zinc., zing.; throbbing: Lyc.; beating in the head mostly after sitting too long: Phos.; deep shooting in right side: Tong.; head internally hot, confused and heavy: Ther.; tearing in right side occiput: Zinc.

EYES: Obscuration of sight, dilatation of pupils: Croc.; shedding tears: Form.; weeping: Lyc.

EAR: Drawing stitch from stomach into ear: Mang.

FACE: Heat and redness of cheeks: Verat.; paleness: Croc.; stiff jaws: Form.; jerking stitches from lower jaw to region above temple: Mang.; toothache in upper molar, afternoons: Tong.

ABDOMEN: Stitches around ribs in the left side: Acon.; in right side of abdomen like a fine jerking: Kali-c.; digging and rooting around the navel, also when exhaling: Coloc.; pain in the belly: Con.; digging rooting colic: Coloc.; sore pain, also with coughing: Ars.; aching pressure in the region of the hernia: Sep.; stitches in the mammae: Laur.

CHEST: Slime in windpipe and cough: Arg-met.; asthma: ARS., aur., cupr., bry., lach., lyc., plb.; dyspnea: Ars., aur., cupr., lach., lyc., plb.; cough: Arg-met., ars., bry., chin., cupr., dros., lach., kali-c., mur-ac., nit-ac., phos., stann., zinc. Pressing like from a piece of wood, in left side of chest: plb.; stitch: mez.; pressing: plat.; pain: laur., lyc., mez., mur-ac., plb., stann.

---

1. Hering - ibid p. 71 - Editor.

LIMBS: Hot hands: Verat.; weakness of muscles of arms and hands: carb-v.

GENERALS: Relaxation: calc., con.; great debility, prostration, collapse: croc.; does not sleep: Verat.; worse in open air: nux-m.; stitches in the ulcer: hep.

FRIGHT AND FEAR[1]

Fright and fear excite many mental and physical states of disease; sometimes long lasting and chronic conditions follow such emotions. Following are some of the symptoms of remedies needed to meet and cure a surprising number of ailments produced by fright and fear as recorded by Hering in the volume on *Symptoms of the Mind* (pg. 72).

Every little surprise frightens; trembling and glowing red cheeks: Merc.; fright with vexation: ACON., *bell.*, calc., cocc., cupr., gels., IGN., nat-c., *nux-v., op.*, petr., *phos., plat., puls.*, samb., sep., sulph., zinc. Terror: Gels., nux-v., op., sil., verat.; after sudden noises, as if thunderstruck, unconscious, convulsions, twitching around mouth, hot red face, feces pass involuntarily: Op.; incessant screaming after a heavy thunder clap: Gels.; often cries without cause: Rhus-t.

AFTER FRIGHT: Soon: Op.; later: Acon.; fear remaining: Merc., nat-m., bell., *verat.*; fear: Op., samb.; fear and anger: Acon.; fear and anxiety: Lyc.; sorrow: Ign. Long remaining anxiousness: Bell., lach., merc., samb., sil. -, and weakness, cannot sleep from frightful visions, night full of complaints, wants to go out doors far away: Merc. -, timidity and nightly complaints: Merc. -, and loss of reason, frightful visions, wants to run away, rush of blood to head, headache rising from neck up, widened pupils: Bell.

MIND: Insanity following fear or fright: Bell., lach., merc., plat., stram.; raving madness: Bell., stram.; loss of reason, talks confusedly as if insane, pain going through the neck up into the head, widened pupils, red burning hot face, or pale and moist, nose dry, neck and throat sore to the touch, fears things he sees: BELL.

Talking, preaching, telling stories, greatest sensitiveness of throat or other parts to the touch even of light clothing: Lach.; often cries out without a cause: Rhus-t.; maniacal notions, starting in sleep, laughing in sleep, convulsions in sleep, spasmodic cough: Hyos.; insanity with laughable jests: Bell.; loss of reason, things appear smaller, sadness in the evening or haughtiness, things appear larger: Plat.; delirium with

---

1. Hering - ibid p. 72 - Editor.

fearful visions: Bell., samb.; delusions of the imagination: Bell.; imagines people find fault with her: Rhus-t.; indifference or contempt of others, fear of the near approach of death, very sad, mostly in the evening: Plat.; melancholy: Stram.; horror, full of apprehension, lamed: Nat-m.; fearful imaginations, particularly at night, cannot bear the warmth of the bed, wants to run away, travel; quarrels with family, complaints about others: Merc.; despair of eternal salvation of soul: Stram.; crying, howling and getting beside himself: Coff.; children weep and move arms about: Samb.; very much dejected and lachrymose, particularly in the evening: Plat.; pride and contempt of others: Plat.; discontent, complains of everything in the whole world: Merc.; disposition to quarrel: Merc.; tries to escape in the night: Bell., merc., hyos.

SENSORIUM: Over sensitiveness of the organs of the senses: Coff.; unconsciousness: Op.; stupor: Bell.; stupor with internal heat: Op.; fainting: Acon., Coff.; apparent death, neither pulse nor breathing perceptible, after a pain in the heart from fright with grief: Lach.

HEAD: Rush of blood to the head: Opium; later: Acon.; still later: Bell.; beating in temple if head is in a low position: Rhus-t.; heat in it: Bell.; heat with stupor: Op.; hot with twitching about the mouth: Op.; pain in forehead: Op.; heavy feeling: Rhus-t.; pain passes into the head through the nape of the neck: Bell.; stitches in the left side of head: Cic.

EYES: Objects around him appear smaller: Plat.; eyes dim, shunning the light: Rhus-t.; cannot see, twitches and starts: Op., glon.; loss of sight, relaxed, sinking together, deadly pale: Glon.; enlarged pupils: Bell.; and darkening of sight: Op.; squinting and rolling of eyes: Hyos.

NOSE: Dryness of nose: Bell.; fluent coryza: Merc.

FACE: Red: Plat.; and burning: Bell., op.; glowing red cheeks: Merc.; after trouble a glowing heat rises in the right cheek - it swells and turns bluish red for two hours, followed by restlessness and shaking chill: Merc.; red, turns deadly pale in sitting up: Acon.; red in bed, getting up instantly pale: Verat.; bluish, bloated with snoring: Op.; - with wheezing: Samb.; changing pale and red, rising headache, looses sight, sinking, relaxed, twitching, fingers or toes spread out: Glon.; twitching around the mouth: Glon., op.; foam at the mouth: Hyos.

DIARRHEA: Op., gels., verat.; returning with every new fear: Acon.; returning at twilight: Puls.; often at night, painless, much wind: Ign.; with tenesmus: Merc.; outer coldness, inner heat without thirst: Puls.;

involuntary escape of stool: Op.; after it very cold: Rhus-t.; with icy coldness of the body: Verat.; retention of stool: Bell.

URINE: Frequent and great discharge: Samb.; involuntary escape of urine and stool: Hyos.; retention: Bell., op.

SEXUAL ORGANS: Metritis: Op.; catamenia too soon and too copious: Plat.; too late and too weak: Puls.; to prevent suppression: Acon.; amenorrhea: Acon., lyc.; displacement of uterus: Op.; during pregnancy diarrhea: Op.; hemorrhage: Sec.; threatened abortion: Acon., gels., op.; suppression of labor pains: Op.; of lochia: Ign., op.; chorea returning in child-bed: Stram.; spasms: Sec.

SUFFOCATION with anxiety: Op.; after vomiting coughing: Samb.; with violent pains in stomach and scrobiculum: Acon.; convulsive choking spells in the night, with crying and grasping about: Samb.; struggle for breath, points to pit of stomach; after Op.: Acon.; suffocation after vomiting or some coughing, bluish puffed-up face, anxious trembling and whining, gasping, heat without thirst: Samb.; bluish face in morning: Op.; ice-cold chest: Verat.; looses breath with even a little cough: Samb.; dry spasmodic cough: Bell.; in the night: Hyos.; whooping cough: Acon., ign., stram.; coughs when lying down, with stitches in pit of stomach: Rhus-t.; ebullitions of blood with trembling of limbs: Samb.; trembling of heart, palpitation: Nux-m.; violent and anxious: Bell.; most in the evening and when sitting: Puls.

CONVULSIONS: Bell., hyos., ign., op., stram., sulph.; with a loud scream: Op.

TREMBLING: *Coff.*, glon., ign., merc., op.; and difficult breathing: Glon., ign., op.; after slight exertions: Merc.

SLEEP: Prevented by fearful visions: Merc.; goes to sleep late in evening, and is restless during the night: Puls.; stuporlike somnolence with snoring: Op.; coma vigil: Hyos.; snoring: Op.; wheezing: Samb.; laughing: Hyos.; starting: Hyos.; worse at night, anxiety and other complaints: Merc.; worse in the evening: Bell., puls.

PAINS: Unbearable, as if driving to distraction: Coff. An ulcer on the hand appeared after Lach., was aggravated by fright and cured by Sil. Genteel, timid and lachrymose disposition: Puls.; if a sudden fright interrupts the good effects of other medicines: Lach.

The foregoing symptoms and conditions produced by fright and fear and cured by our proven remedies is convincing proof of the need for a full knowledge of the mental spheres of the remedies in sickness. This knowledge is also valuable in the study of disease cause and is closely related to the phenomena and claims of psychology and psychatry.

One more model cure is here presented because of the remedy that cured, (p. 84).: Feels the greatest anguish in the head with a whirling before the eyes every day, from 5 a.m. until 5. p.m., since two years. He walks up and down the room, wringing his hands, and moaning continually, "Oh, such anguish! Oh, such anguish!" Only when he takes his meals he ceases moaning. His appetite is good: Psor. William Gross.

SHOCK OF INJURY[1]

MIND: Injury followed by one fixed and anxious idea of impending death or other dire misfortune: Acon.; anxiety as from conscious danger of death: Caps.; anguish: Nux-v.; with great distress and oppression, despairs of life: Verat.; anxious manner: Chin.; after fright: Op.; afterwards: Acon.; after sudden, unexpected severe injury: Camph.; fear of injury: Gels.; afraid of the surgeon: Coff.; of being hurt by persons walking towards him: Arn.; overpowering fear, with fatigue: Gels.; terror: Verat.; intolerance of impressions and of oppositions: Acon.; - of all manipulations, they cause great agitation, which interferes with treatment: Coff.; not to be pacified: Acon.; rather quiet when left alone: Coff.; great forgetfulness: Stront.; weeping over his bad luck: Puls.; preoccupied with lamentations: Cham.; delirium, will dress himself to go home: Cupr.; unconscious muttering of anxious sort: Gels.; nervous anxiety, mingled with stupefaction of mind: Camph.; increasing stupor: Lach.; hardly yielding to any stimuli: Carb-v.

SENSORIUM: Unconsciousness: Arn., chlf., op.; stupefied and cold: Camph.; apopletic dreaminess: Nux-m.; faintness: Sulph.; from slight causes: Nux-v.; from a little pain, is preceded by vertigo: Hep.; syncope immediately after great hemorrhage: Calam.; long lasting syncope: Hydr-ac.; headache after fainting: Hep.

HEAD: Chronic effects after an injury of the head, such as headache, relieved by sweating: Nat-m.; paralysis of brain, with symptoms of collapse: Cupr.

EYES: Loss of vision and hearing: Carb-v.; pupils dialated: Hydr-ac., ip.; inactive: Dig.; eyes fixed unequally: Op.; eyelids paralyzed: Hydr-ac.; dark areola around: Lach.; sunken with dark margins: Sulph.

FACE: Distorted features: Hydr-ac.; wretched expression: Sulph.; motionless features: Chlf.; pallor: Arn., op., ip.; pale and sick and languid: Gels.; bluish paleness: Dig.

---

1. Hering - ibid p. 76 - Editor.

APPETITE: Vomiting: Ip., verat.; copious, easy, gushing: Phos.; especially on moving, better after moving: Tab.; vomits drink instantly after swallowing: Ars.; as soon as it gets warm in stomach: Phos.; vomiting is a good sign after Arn.

STOMACH: Deathly feeling behind ensiform cartilage: Cupr.

STOOL: Diarrhea: Ip., nux-m., verat.; very watery, even involuntary: Sec.; colliquative, cadaverous odor: Carb-v.; visceral hemorrhage: Verat.

URINE: Shuddering all over with desire to urinate: Hyper.; retention: Hyper.; suppression: Sec.

CHEST: In gunshot wounds of chest or lung: Am-caust.

PULSE: Pulse slow and small: Dig., sec., - and weak: Arn., merc., - and feeble and irregular: Tab.; intermitting: Nat-m.; by regular intermission every other beat, apparently slow: *Dig.*; pulse feeble: Camph.; as if dying: Chlf.; feeble and thready: Ars.; feeble and frequent: Cupr.; feeble and tense: Acon.; dying away: Lach.; almost imperceptible: Caps.; weak, slow, scarcely perceptible: Verat.; failing: Chin.; frequent and scarcely perceptible: Carb-v.; nearly extinct: Hydr-ac.

BACK: Injuries to vertebral region: Hyper.

POSITION: Wants to lie with head low: Arn.

COLLAPSE: Tendency to collapse as in cholera: Ars.; threatened collapse, with intermitting pulse and great thirst: Nat-m.; impending death by it: Op. (one dose high); from progress of inflammatory lesion: Op. (repeated lower doses).

TISSUES: Hemorrhage: Arn.; of bright blood: Ip., phos.; of dark blood: Chin., nux-v.; sequelae of hemorrhage: Stront.; emanciation: Stront.; when nervous tissues are mainly concerned: Hyos.; tissues of organic life: Am-caust.; injuries of the tissue of animal life generally, of the feet, the hands, etc.: Hyper.

Remedies against homesickness, love pangs, jealousy, and grief are often needed by the homeopathic physician, to cure stubborn mental illness.

HOMESICKNESS, NOSTALGIA[1]

Silent ill humor: Nit-ac., *ph-ac.*; indifference to everything: Bell.; complains of everything: Merc.; whimsical and sensitive: Caps.; longing: Merc.; after his friends: Ign.; sighing and moaning: Hell.; sorrowful feeling, as if left alone: Carb-an.; loneliness: Mag-m.; anxiousness:

---

1. Hering - ibid p. 84 - Editor.

Merc.; anxious lowness of spirits: Nit-ac.; inconsolable: Carb-an.; cheerful faces increase his woe: Hell.; whining, sorrowful, as if alone: Mag-m.; lachrymose: Ph-ac.; frequent weeping: Caps., mag-m.; melancholy: Aur.; inward grief: Ign.; thoughtless stammering: Ign.; quiet: Sep.; headache, as if bursting when moving: Caps.; redness of cheeks: Caps.; hunger, with weak digestion: Merc.; want of appetite: Ph-ac.; thirst and chilliness: Caps.; insipid, watery taste of all food: Ign.; after eating, burning in stomach: Caps.; with emaciation: Ph-ac.; diarrhoea: Ph-ac.; with tenesmus: Caps., merc.; short, hacking morning cough, lasting for thirty minutes: Caps., dros.; violent cough in evening and night: Caps.; frequent palpitation of heart: Nit-ac.; violent palpitation: Aur.; wants to run away, inquietude, wants to travel: Merc.; weak and trembling after slight exertion: Merc.; averse to moving: Caps.; feels homesick when at home with her family: Eup-pur.; night sweats: Merc.

Love Pangs[1]

Some sickness, or love pangs, so often looked upon lightly and singled out, may be quite serious and produce severe illness in its helpless victims that may require good homeopathic prescribing to straighten them out and restore them back to normal living. A few of the leading remedies and their indications follow:

Unhappy love, disposed to weep, desires to take his life; despair, sudden anger; quarrelsome or melancholy, with longing for death; alternating joyful and sorrowful; congestion of blood to the head, sparks before the eyes, rushing in the ears; putrid odor from the mouth, excessive hunger and thirst; congestion of blood to the chest, and anxious beating of the heart: Aur.; with jealousy, vehemence and confused talking quarrelsome: Hyos.; indigation about undeserved mortification, pushing things away from him: Staph.; with jealous suspicious despair, weary of life: Lach.; with silent grief, one cheek red: Ign.; not inclined to talk, hectic, red cheeks, sleepiness, morning sweats, emaciation: Ph-ac.; pain in heart, fainting, apparent death: Lach.; complaints of girls for grief about faithless lovers: Ars., calc-p., hyos., ign.

Jealousy[2]

Effects of jealousy often need the homeopathic remedy to restore the normal state.

---

1. Hering ibid p. 85 - Editor.
2. Hering ibid - p. 86 - Editor.

Quarrelsome, eager, vehement, with delirious, incoherent speech, rage, mania: Hyos.; with anger, desire to kill; torments others; running about; worse in day-time, mostly women: Apis; with mistrust, suspicion, worse towards evening: Lach.; with excessive nervousness, spasmodic attacks, hectic fever, sleeplessness: Hyos.; jealous thoughts rise in his mind: Camph.; during pregnancy: Lach.

Another short model cure presented by E. Stapf (pg. 86):

A very irritable lady, suffering under the most violent and threatening nervous symptoms, even spasms; had hectic fever, sleepless nights, and her mind was nearly deranged; disturbed by unfounded jealousy. After one dose of Hyos., 30 cent.; she soon was well and remained so.

GRIEF AND SORROW[1]

Grief and sorrow bring on many troubles that can be righted with the correct homeopathic remedy.

MIND: Mental derangement from grief: Ars., bell.; sad, indifferent; aversion to everything; full of fears: Ign.; grief with fear at night, disposition to quarrel, complaining of his relations and surroundings: Merc.; with apprehensions for the future: Staph.; absorbed in his own thoughts, silent ill-humor; indifference; aversion to speaking; absent minded and dullness of mind: Ip.; grief and sorrow with shame; suppressed internal vexation, which continues: Ign.

SENSORIUM: Vertigo: Ign.; in evening: Ph-ac.

ABDOMEN: Long-lasting after-taste, food often thrown up: Ph-ac.; pressing pain in stomach: Ign.

STOOL: Looseness: *Coloc., gels.,* ph-ac.; involuntary: Op.; with tenesmus: Merc.

SEXUAL PARTS: Weakening pollutions: Ph-ac.; amenorrhea: Ign.; in pregnancy, chorea: Ign., stram.; labor pains mostly in back: Caust.; fainting during parturition: Ign.

CHEST: Whooping-cough: Phos.; weakness of chest causes inability to speak long: Ph-ac.

SPASMS: Attacks like epilepsy: Op., ph-ac.; fits: Ign.

TISSUES: Emaciation: Ph-ac.; after suppressed mental sufferings; seems to be weighed down; broods over imaginary trouble: Ign.; chronic complaints after long-lasting grief or sorrow: Caust., lach., lyc., NAT-M. (Kent). After weeping, nose bleeds: Nit-ac.; throat contracted:

---

1. Hering ibid - p. 86 - Editor.

Lact.; cough, with children: Arn., asar., cham.; moving arms and hands about: Samb.

CONCLUSION

The foregoing comments on remedies for mental states and symptoms, makes only a beginning of this absorbing and useful subject. Nothing short of a sizeable volume would suffice to do justice to it. If the writer can help promote the interest and attention of homeopathic physicians to the advantage in prescribing, that a wide knowledge of mental and emotional symptoms bring, he will be happy, for the cause of Homeopathy will then advance with many difficult cures to its credit.

Homeopathically treated, many of the mentally sick, the insane, the victims of bad psychology and environment since childhood, with a bad inheritance to start their ill-starred journey of life, could be made useful and happy citizens instead of inmates of institutions and prisons. Crime and bad mental hygiene are inevitable associates, unbridled passions, unholy desires, unrestrained appetites are phases of sickness that only the homeopathic system can cope with.

What a contrast, Homeopathy, with its gentle certain way, presents to modern scientific methods of shock and violence. The pitiable victims of mental and emotional unbalance and insufficiency are better dead than victims of a terrorizing, torturing, endless experimentation that leads but to mental chaos and death. Verily the world sorely needs the God given balm of the homeopathic philosophy and law of the healing of the nations.

THINGS THAT INTERFERE WITH THE HOMEOPATHIC PRESCRIPTION[1]

The homeopathic physician must work hard and carefully on all his cases if he wishes to cure them.

First, obtaining a full and complete case history requires much time and labor. Then the chase through repertory and materia medica for the most similar remedy uses up more time and labor. When that precious talisman, the similimum, is found and administered, the doctor, with a sense of duty well-performed, relaxes and is content to wait for anticipated reports of desirable changes for the better in his patient on his next visit. For do we not all know the power of cure residing in that similimum once it is obtained? Have we not many times seen the proof of "the law" in cures that had defied other medical means?

What mingled feelings of doubt and disappointment overwhelms the doctor, when after long and laborious study and effort, a classical case is worked to the one remedy that alone most completely covers the symptoms and history of the case, and the remedy is administered with supreme confidence that a prompt and gentle restoration to health in the suffering patient will soon come. Then, after the prescribed time, the patient returns, not with joyous news of beginning cure, but that he is either no better or even worse than before the remedy was taken. Such an experience as this is enough to shake the faith of the strongest, and sometimes confuse the wisdom of the wisest.

What about the vaunted Law, and the miraculous power of the similimum? What is wrong? Whence have they vanished? After all the work and study with the acquired knowledge of remedies and all the courageous faith comes failure, dismal failure like an evil omen to blight the promise of glorious success held out to all those who have the energy to work and the faith to study and apply the great Law of cure. Is the Law then but an illusion? Or a subtle and deceptive force, a changeling in a changing world to bring the joy of a cure here and the gloom of defeat there? No, the Law is immutable and perfect; it needs but free and uninterrupted scope to perform its wonders.

The physician has failed in one respect in spite of all his learning and knowledge of remedies. In spite of his laborious energy and painstaking care, he has failed to instruct his patient in the many things that can

---

1. JOURNAL OF THE AMERICAN INSTITUTE OF HOMEOPATHY, Vol. 40, No. 12, Dec, 1947, p. 423.

nullify a good prescription or cut short a remedy's action and efficiency.

Outside of proper social, psychological, dietary and hygenic conditions which every physician should insist upon having for his patient along with the remedy administered, there are many things in common use among the laity that will inhibit and antidote the action of the homeopathic remedy.

The most frequent and noxious of these things that have occured in my practice during the last forty years, to harass and embarrass me and to plunge me deep into gloom and doubt from time to time will be mentioned in the course of this paper. Nothing is so valuable or vital to the homeopathic course and the doctors who practice Homeopathy than this knowledge of the interferring forces that work against the life force of humanity and thus nullify the harmony and power of curative forces. Never in the history of man has life been so complex, so beset by forces that destroy at every turn. From the time of the tiny babe in the crib all through flowering youth into the pride and strength of maturity, and down to a hasty and premature old age, the evil genies of dissolution hold sway, and this, in spite of, and much of it because of a so-called scientific advance and progress, especially in things medical.

There are so many things that interfere with the action of the homeopathic remedy, it is so hard to know just where to begin. Perhaps the most important of the common antidotes to homeopathic drugs is camphor and camphor compounds, synthetic compounds of menthol contained in moth balls and in innumerable salves, rubs and ointments. Linaments and inhalents such as Vick's Vapor Rub are very pernicious things, as they not only antidote curative remedies, but they have a depressing effect upon the life forces on the body. Many a good homeopathic action has been cut short by a whiff from the garments reeking with the vile odor of moth balls and kindred things.

Many pneumonia cures have been hampered and even prevented by the zeal of a nurse ignorant of the harmfulness of camphorated oil and grease rubbed on the patient's chest and back. Myriads of common colds that break-up in twenty-four hours under the uninterrupted action of the homeopathic remedy will linger for weeks because of the camphorated nose unction or nose drops of menthol, argyole and other powerful chemicals applied as inhalents, rubs or lozenges. This is one of the things the homeopathic doctor will do well both for himself and his patient to warn most strongly against the use of these things when using homeopathic remedies.

Another very common and most vicious class of interferring agents are the many coal tar drugs, derivatives of coal tar with complex chemical formulas. These drugs come under many trade names from Bromo-Selzer, one of the most harmful with its load of acentanilide, to the phenobarbital series and many others too numerous to name such as midol, aspirin, anacin etc. Every physician knows they are all depressants and blood destroying agents producing great and lasting evil effects on the organism.

Another common interferring agent obstructing homeopathic action is the common use of suppressive salves and lotions that deodorize and suppress underarm prespiration. These things drive back into the blood stream toxic material that nature throws off through the natural outlets of the body created for that purpose. The deodorants contain poisonious metallic ingredients, zinc and alumina compounds, that in themselves are toxic to the body and which together with the effete matter they drive back into the blood, render the work of establishing harmony in the play of the body physiologic forces difficult and tedious, sometimes entirely destroying the action of the curative remedies.

To the aforementioned things may be added cough drops containing codeine and other analgesics, dentifrices, mouth, throat washes and gargles laden with antiseptic substances, all more or less toxic and hindering the action of curative processes.

All these products are advertized loudly and constantly by radio and T.V. and in printed sketches which laud their wonders to a gullible public, and they are so easily obtained that their use has become almost universal. The physicians do not warn the public against their uses, either through ignorance or from selfish interests. The physician of today is not only guilty of sins of omission in failing to condemn the unbridled and unguided use of toxic and habit forming drugs, but they are constantly committing serious acts against individual and public health by the wholesale injection of serums, vaccines[1] and numerous animal gland extracts together with the excessive use of drugs so toxic (the sulpha drugs) that the United States Army was obliged to discontinue their use, because the harm done exceeded the benefits accom-

---

1. The evils of vaccination have been exposed by many doctors. These vaccines are among the factors contributing to serious chronic illness including cancer, diabetes, AIDS, disease of the cns, mental illness, SIDS etc. See Coulter, Harris: 1) AIDS, and Syphilis, The Hidden Link, Jain, New Delih, 1989; 2) DPT, A shot in the Dark, Harcourt Brace Jovanovich, 1985; 3) Vaccination, Social violence, and Criminality - The Medical Assault on the American Brain, North Atlantic Books, 1990 - Editor.

plished. This flood of sick making material is given to the very young as well as those older in an unending stream; from the cradle to the grave it flows while disease mounts in alarming proportions on every hand. Insanity, heart and kidney disease as well as cancer are all increasing as never before in the world's history.

It is true that sanitation, hygiene and improved dietetics have restricted epidemics of acute disease. Alexis Carrel observed in his book Man the Unknown that we have reduced infant mortality and restrained epidemics of acute sickness, but more people are dying of degenerative diseases in early middle life, the time of man's most productive and intellectual period than occured formerly. The exception to this statement prevailed in those nations and times when warfare was continuous as occured during the Roman Empire; then the death rate among young male adults was very high so that only a limited percentage reached middle life. In the last few decades, the increase of death from heart and kidney disease, with cancer a close second has been noted by insurance companies and other sources of vital statistics.

Unless physicians awake to the present serious health threat and make an intelligent and concerted effort to educate and guide the public away from the unrestricted use of toxic drugs and animal extracts of various sorts there will be little worthwhile left for humanity to exist for. The only redeeming thing in such a state of affairs as universal broken health is that the fear of atomic warfare will give little, if any, concern; and progress in every way will fail and die.

Of course, there are many cases as every doctor knows that reach an incurable state before any kind of therapy is applied, but even in these the homeopathic remedy is still more efficient in palliation if it be permitted to act without interference than all other known therapeutic measures. As the homeopathic physician grows wise in practice among the sick, he becomes more of a teacher than ever a healer. Instruction in the laws of life; right thinking and right living are mighty factors in the building of better health. The knowledge of the avoidance of all those things that injure and impair health or break down resistance renders the action of the curative remedy more certain and durable. Thus by the union of healing and teaching will Homeopathy grow and prosper and live to bless our children and their children.

THINGS THAT PREVENT THE CURATIVE ACTION OF WELL SELECTED REMEDIES[1]

When the homeopathic doctor has thoroughly and completely taken his case after the Hahnemannian method and gathered in an orderly way an array of therapeutic facts and then proceeded with the laborious task of selecting the one most similar homeopathic remedy for that case, he has every reason to expect prompt curative action from such a remedy.

Almost invariably there is response to the remedy selected from the totality symptom image of a well taken case. When there is no response or only a short acting one, or prolonged aggravation of the symptoms and no beneficial relief following such a painstaking procedure, the homeopathic physician knows there is some deep seated vital cause operating in the patient's life force or that he is the victim of faulty living habits or that there is something drastically wrong in his environment.

Many times unhappy and disappointing results follow a truly homeopathic prescription in these days of universal drugging, processed and adulterated foods, poisoned water supplies (chlorine, flourine, etc.), polluted air (carbon dioxide and monoxide gases from automobile engines,[2] poisonous and noxious wastes from manufacturing and chemical plants of all kinds, etc.), to say nothing of the latest menace to the inhabitants of the world from the atomic radiations that have already impregnated the atmosphere of the earth from the explosions of the atomic and hydrogen bombs set of by the United States and Soviet Russia.

One of the most vital and urgent needs of today for the good of all is a complete and friendly understanding and agreement between the United States and Russia to discontinue the explosions of these deadly inventions, even for experimental purposes, in order to save all mankind from the known and unknown future cumulative effects of this irremediable force. The world should petition them to control and develop this power for the good, not for the destruction of humanity.

Even though Homeopathy has the better weapons and antidotes against this subtle and terribel poison (PHOS. in potency being one of

---

1. This article was written in October, 1955. - Editor.
2. Today other additives in gasoline have already been recorded to cause both respiratory and CNS disease. - Editor.

the best) we should all use our united influence and logic in an effort to bring about a universal protest against this wide-spread evil that it may be turned to use in healing and power for the good of all. In a general way the things just mentioned are among the hinderances to the action of the homeopathic remedy and are often difficult to control or antidote. In recent months in my practice I have found remedies like Phos., Rad-br. and X-ray in potency, more frequently indicated and very helpful in clearing the cases and paving the way for complimentary remedies that may be needed to complete the cure. It seems that radiation influences are already at work.[1]

One of our most frequent and very powerful obstructions to the action of the well selected remedy in recent years is the toxemia caused by aluminum which has become almost a universal poison. Aluminum cooking utensils, aluminum foil (used in cooking meats and baking and in wrapping pastries and other foods), water softened by aluminum chloride, sprays with aluminium products to suppress perspiration in deodorants are among the common sources of this poison.

Aluminum is a slow and subtle toxin corresponding to the action and nature of chronic disease. We need but peruse our Materia Medica and consult the provings of this drug to note its likeness to deep constitutional disease ultimating in serious tissue changes in vital organs. Its first action manifests on the mucous membranes of the body especially those lining the gastro-alimentary tract and producing stasis and paralytic states, especially the bowel elimination which is impaired, making it difficult for the victim to void even a soft stool; and urinary function is also slowed down and difficult. The blood soon becomes impoverished and looses some of its essential elements ending in severe nerve weakness and pain and often the brain and spinal cord become involved, producing symptoms simulating locomotor ataxia and other spinal and cerebral conditions. Convulsions and epileptic states may also be produced. Marked mental depression and melancholy with suicidal tendency develop as a result of the continued intake of this slowly creeping and insidious poison. Almost any chronic sickness known, including cancer, may be whipped into activity in those constitutions of inherited weakness and with tendencies to develop these disease con-

---

1. When Dr. Grimmer first wrote this arcticle in October, 1955, he obeserved that the unhealthy environment caused by pollution, both chemical and radioactive, had already considerably poisoned man. Thus the need for such remedies as Phos., Rad-br, and X-ray in potency. How much more this is the case today is hard to imagine. - Editor.

ditions. For the whole being is changed, physically, mentally and emotionally, slowly, subtlely but surely under the fateful impact of this unrecognized insidious poison. Aside from the drastic power of its sick-making effects it produces an inhibiting effect on the curative action of the selected homeopathic remedy.

A patient suffering with the toxins of alumina to the saturation point seems unable to respond to any remedy not antidotal to alumina. Too frequently in these times we get but short acting action, if any at all, from our best selected remedies because this toxemia acts much like the miasms of Hahnemann, (psora, syphilis and sycosis) and often a remedy must be given to eradicate the predominant miasmatic force that is interfering with curative processes.

In treating chronic diseases where there is a definite evidence of the aluminum toxemia present and the best selected medicine fails to produce the desired results, I give a potency of CADM-O. and obtain surprising and sometimes startling results in cure, often without the need for a complimentary remedy. But if the symptoms of the patient indicate the need for another remedy, it will act quickly and satisfactorily after CADM-O. has done its work. In the treatment of chronic disease in these times our drug antidotes are a powerful asset to homeopathic success.

Camphor and mentholated concoctions must be strictly avoided by the patient, or the curative processes will be short lasting and inadequate. Where reactions are slow and feeble in patients who have been too long under these substances, a dose of CARB-V. 10M will bring about better reactive power in the patient. CARB-V. also antidotes most of the coal tar drugs effectively.

For those cases that are left weak and languid after too much penicillin, CARB-V. has served me most often. For the acute severe skin manifestations following penicillin RHUS-V. cures promptly and permanently. CARB-V., MAG-P. and OP. have been the big three in my book to antidote the coal tars and the antibiotics and bring back the patient's reactive responses that have been weakened by these depressants. THUJ. and MALAND. are the best antidotes against the bad effects of small pox vaccination. ARS. antidotes the evils of yellow fever shots, MAG-P. is a joy for the suffering that often follows the tetanus shots. BAPT. effectively antidotes typhoid and typhus innoculations. DIPH. and MERC-CY. antidote the diptheria shots and are also top curative remedies for the cure and prevention of the disease itself. APIS is useful against the meningitis disease; and BELL., PHYT. and AIL. are useful for the streptococcus strains of scarlet fever.

These observations are brought to the homeopathic profession in order to improve our effectiveness in prescribing, that we may obtain the maximum results in cure.

In the ORGANON, paragraph three, sixth edition, we are told that "when the physician knows in each case the obstacles in the way of recovery and how to remove them, he is prepared to act thoroughly and to the purpose, as a true master of the art of healing". And in paragraph four "He is at the same time a preserver of health when he knows the causes that disturb health, that produce and maintain disease, and when he knows how to remove them from healthy persons". Paragraph five "The physician in curing derives assistance from the knowledge of facts concerning the most probable cause of acute disease, as well as from the most significant points in the entire history of a case of chronic disease. Aided by such knowledge he is enabled to discover the primary cause of the latter depending mostly on a chronic miasm. In connection with this, the bodily constitution of a patient (particularly if he has a chronic disease), the character of his mind and temperament, his occupation, his mode of living and habits, his social and domestic relations, his age and sexual functions, etc., are to be taken into consideration".

These quotations from the ORGANON indicate the necessity of knowing sick-making causes, especially those produced by drugs and chemical poisons as well as the need for the knowledge that can antidote and eradicate such evils and their consequences.

Paragraph seventy-five "Instances of ruined health resulting from allopathic treatment are very common in modern times, (early 1800). They constitute the most pitable and incurable chronic diseases, and it is to be feared that remedies will probably never be found or invented for the cure of such conditions when they have reached a certain degree of severity."

Here Hahnemann speaks as if he were with us today in 1955. With the overwhelming influx of drastic drugs, coal tar derivatives, antibiotics and chemical poisons that deluge us from all sides with their widespread extravagant, misleading, commercialized claims constantly and forcefully fed to the public, is it any wonder that the race is sick with dread new diseases, difficult to combat and cure? Insanity, mental and emotional incompetencies are more wide spread than ever before and are increasing at alarming rates and affect people of all ages and classes.

If Hahnemann found the bad effects of simpler poisons of his day hard to cope with, can the modern homeopathic physician of today be blamed for finding his way to cure blocked by numerous forces and interferences nullifying the satisfactory action of the indicated remedy?

In spite of these fearful obstacles homeopathy can successfully cope with the most drastic and terrifying sickness of these trying times of today. The homeopathic physician armed with the might of the law and faithful to its principles and philosophic techniques stands unafraid and firm, a stalwart knight of healing before the onslaught of destroying disease in all its forms. In his courage born of faith and intelligence he becomes the chosen instrument of Divine Law to bring back the bloom of health to the worn and suffering and restore hope again in sick minds and bring back strength and security and well being in place of weakness and ravage of disease.

No new or unknown disease can baffle the well-trained, experienced homeopathic physician because the law and the philosophy is expanding to meet new and constantly changing situations. New and more potent remedies are being discovered, proved and developed by the homeopathic science as more adequate weapons adapted to destroy the new and more serious types of disease spinging up in the world today as the sequence of the abusive application of the antibiotics and the numerous coal tar drugs.

One hopeful sign looms in the horizon of the medical world; recently men of all schools of medical thought are sounding warning notes of the dangers to universal health from the abuse and the excessive unguided use of these pernicious things.

The world needs a program of public education to teach of the dangers and the serious menace to health that result from self-medication which has been so extensively encouraged by the manufacturing vendors of patent and proprietary medical firms, operating for profit only, regardless of the harm inflicted on a suffering but gullible public.

There is a vital need for a co-ordinated program made up from representatives of all schools of medical thought to warn the public of the serious menace to health and life from the numerous forms of drug abuse operating in the world today. Self-medication should be especially condemned as a pernicious source of evil because it is too fequently unguided by adequate knowledge either of the illness treated or of the remedy employed for its cure.

Far too many people depend upon the patent and proprietary medicine advertised so blatantly and universally by radio, television and the printed word for their medical knowledge and supplies to meet their medical needs.

This type of medicine is unscientific and harmful beyond measure. It is created solely for profit regardless of consequences and must be curtailed and regulated by competent authority that can teach a misinformed public the danger and folly that all types of medication can bring, when not directed by those trained to know both the good and evil properties existing in medicine. Only with such scientific knowledge can evil effects be avoided and curative results be obtained. Only with a competent board of educators made up of united organized groups of all schools of medical thought can the world be saved from a deluge of new and terrible mental and physical diseases that will be most difficult to cope with.

One of the marvels in nature is the autonomic nervous system wherein certain fibres of the motor nerves operate independently of the brain and spinal cord to produce responses to various stimuli likely vibratory in character. Allergies and susceptibilities of the body organism to disease-producing forces are first noted by their impact on this system, and here it is that our potentized remedies begin their action to rally the organism's defensive mechanism to action. From this center the defensive powers of the body get their first summons to respond in its defense. The polarity of the electo-magnetic currents of the body change to modify and change the blood chemistry and to stimulate the activity of the endocrine glands, producing antibodies and all the essential elements needed to meet the requirements of any conditions presented in life's changing processes. Here also in this vital center so essential to life and health is where the irreparable harm of drastic drugging is produced.

When will medical men learn to put more trust in the power for good of the Divine Creator's protective handiwork than they do in the uncertain weapons of puny and often misguided man (who when depending on his own guidance unassisted by natural law looses his way in a labyrinth of confusion and doubt)? Whatever comes as the result of law is good and abiding because it is the result of the Creative Fiat that creates, govens and sustains universal order. Homeopathy is law and order in the processes of the healing act; and because this is so, it will abide as long as there are sick mortals languishing for its care and so long as its practitioners and adherents are true to its teaching and principles.

INTERFERENCE AND DISAPPOINTMENTS[1]

The homeopathic physician must work harder and study more than his colleagues of the old school to obtain success because the homeopath must measure his success in results of cure and not just palliation of disease.

To effect cures requires accuracy in the selection of the curative remedy and that necessitates never ending study of the Materia Medica, as well as skill in applying the homeopathic philosophy to every case.

Prior to the prescription comes the careful, painstaking job of obtaining an accurate history of the individual and his family inheritances and tendencies. After the data is gathered and the study is completed by repertory and other means the prescription is made and the reactions of the patient to it is awaited.

The reactions that follow a homeopathic prescription are often most significant and vital to both physician and patient. The aggravation or amelioration of symptoms, the return of old or suppressed symptoms, the uplift or depression of the patient's general condition are some of the many responses that follow the homeopathic prescription. These all have some expressive meaning for the physician.

If none of these responses are noted, and if the patient experiences no change in symptoms or well being, or if he is in every way worse then one of three things are present in the case. First; the remedy was wrongly selected. Second; the case is incurable. Third; the remedy was interfered with and nullified by some other influence operating in the patient's life and environment. In most cases the third assumption is the correct answer to the phenomenon. Because at this time in the march of science and inventive ingenuity we are beset with a multiplicity of pernicious health destroying agents born in avarice and dedicated to the amassing of many inflated dollars for the coffers of the manufacturing chemists who are the vendors of these things.

Camphorated and mentholated preparations given in rubs and inhalants not only antidote the action of homeopathic remedies but depress the organism and suppress symptoms of disease, leaving the patient a victim of both the disease and the preparations. These preparations are so commonly used that they are really hard to avoid, at least by inhalation.

---

1. THE BULLETIN a journal edited by A. Dwight Smith M.D. in California, vol. and date unknown, approx. date 1945. - Editor.

Pain killing drugs of the coal tar derivatives such as aspirin, midol, anacin, phenobarbital, etc. are all nearly universally used on every pretext, even some in alcoholic beverages. Bromo seltzer is one of the most vicious of these drugs. They are all vital depressants and render the vital force of the body less sensitive to the reaction of curative remedies.

Another deleterious substance which is advertised extensively in a very subtle and effective manner by way of magazine, radio and television are the numerous under arm suppressants guaranteed to stop perspiration and its consequent odors. Any salve that stops perspiration turns back into the economy effete matter that nature is getting rid of by the only means available, the numerous and very active pores in the axilla. Suppressed perspiration by cold and artificial means has produced serious illness simulating tuberculosis in a severe form and this may well inhibit the action of curative remedies.

Dentifrices, mouth washes, gargles, nose drops, face creams, hair treatments, soaps, etc. may and many of them do contain interfering elements to the prescription. To all of these may be added the evil effects of devitalized, processed and adulterated foods and foods vitiated by aluminium toxins from the cooking utensils in which it was prepared. This last named toxin will render a homeopathic cure impossible until it is entirely eradicated from the blood stream by the proper antidote and the best and most certain of these is a potency of CADM-o., and the refraining from any food prepared in aluminium cooking ware.

Another source of aluminium poison can be in the drinking water treated with aluminium chloride used to soften the water. Food prepared in such water contains toxic doses of aluminium which is a cumulative poison building up insidious and slow drastic changes in the blood and nervous system. Every homeopath knows what aluminium even in potency can do to the healthy organism but it is so slow and insidious in its pace of action that great changes may take place in the economy before the victim realizes he is sick.

Speaking of drinking water, the municipal health guardians have added other health wrecking chemicals in the form of chlorine and fluorine and forced it on a gullible public in spite of its wishes, so that the individual must take the poison or go thirsty, and even then his food and beverages are all polluted with the poison insuring him of his share of sick making elements which he can hardly avoid.

With these artificial things in mind added to the natural causes of disease is it any wonder we meet with so much illness? It is not at all strange that we often get little if any response to our best chosen remedies when these agents are acting against us.

Doctors, we must become teachers if we would obtain a good percentage of cures. We must insist on our patients refraining from all interfering agencies to our remedies and their health.

Teach them to think right, to live right and then with the application of the homeopathic remedy we can accomplish what no other system of healing can and bring great happiness to many and much satisfaction to ourselves.

Hindrances to the Homeopathic Prescription[1]

This subject has been brought before you many times, but it is of such vital importance to the success of homeopathic procedures that constant repetition can not be too much.

When the homeopathic doctor has given much time and labor with taking the case history, which is the first great essential in every good prescription, and then devoted more time and labor with repertory study and research through the Materia Medica, he cannot afford to have such a prescription spoiled or interfered with by some foolish external action of the patient, which may nullify the expected results of all the pysician's painstaking efforts and leave both physician and patient disappointed and discouraged.

With these facts in mind, it behooves the physician to instruct his patient emphatically that he must refrain from taking all other drugs such as pain killers, cathartics, camphor or menthol in any form, and most important of all he must refrain from food prepared and cooked in aluminum ware and its alloys.

These injunctions are as important as are the instructions for a proper diet and the correct amount of drinking water, proper ventilation of fresh air, and hygienic living, both mentally and physically.

The control of the mind and emotions is far more important than the average physician realizes. Many a fine prescription has had its curative action stopped by a sudden, violent, emotional upset; shock, grief, anger and fright are often responsible for the shortacting relief of a good prescription that for awhile was doing very satisfying work toward cure.

We have been told by many doctors who consider themselves first-class Homeopaths that they have seen very few, if any, of the reactions supposed to follow the administration of the homeopathic remedy. In most of their cases if the selected remedy acted for them, it was only in a benefical way. They have never seen the return of old symptoms or the sharp aggravation followed by a long period of well being on the patient's part. These same men have voiced disappointment with many cases from which they expected brilliant results from the prescriptions that was made. They had taken the case carefully and fully, repertoired them as well as referred to the Materia Medica for a confirmation of the

---

1. The Homeopothic Recorder, Vol. LXVIII, No. 7, January, 1953, p. 195, and also in The Layman Speaks, Vol. VI, No. 7, July, 1953, p. 239.

selected remedy. The final conclusion was that the time and labor spent in making a homeopathic prescription for the uncertain results obtained did not reimburse them for such time and effort. Many of us have had too many such experiences because we failed to take note of all the factors and elements in the case and either through ignorance or laziness neglected to instruct our patients properly so the remedy might act smoothly and uninterruptedly.

The most pernicious of these interruptables is the aluminum toxins that enter the human system by way of aluminum cooking utensils and by water polluted with aluminum chloride which is used to soften hard water. This toxins acts much like one of the miasms, and it must be eradicated from the system before a cure of the patients is possible. The most certain, rapid antidote for it is CADM-O. in potency, and of course the source of intake of the toxin must be discontinued. After the poison is removed by the CADM-O., the remaining symptoms and conditions of the patient may be successfully attacked by the remedy that is indicated by the totality of the remaining symptoms.

Other interferring agents that are very prevalent today are the numerous coal tar drugs, such as aspirin, anacin, phenobarbital and numerous others of a similar nature which do not require a physician's prescription to obtain them. The four best general antidotes to the coal tar drugs are ARN., CARB-V., LACH., and MAG-P. to be given according to the symptoms present in each individual case.

One more important source of interference to the homeopathic remedy is the wide-spread use of serums and vaccines as protective agents against acute disease. The reaction of these products of disease are often long lasting in their effects and leave the victims of this practice sick and suffering. THUJ. is one of our best, if not the very best, and most effective antidote against these agents, and it helps to restore the patient to a state of approximate order where other complimentary remedies given according to their indications can finish the case in a complete cure.

From the preceeding observations it is clear that the homeopathic physician must be a teacher if he would be a successful healer. His responsibilities are great, and his work tedious and unending as the study of remedies in itself is stupendous. Without the qualities of tireless energy and a devoted faith in his work for the good of his fellows, he cannot succeed in the realm of cure. If and when he does obtain the stature of a master prescriber, he will humbly give thanks to a merciful Providence for the rare privilege of serving in the cause of true healing.

MATERIA MEDICA STUDY[1]

When methodically and logically studied, the homeopathic materia medica becomes a vast reservoir of useful knowledge in the science and art of healing.

Each proven remedy presents its own distinctive blue print or likeness of sickness in the symptoms and changes it brings about in those healthy humans who partake of its potential substance.

Remedies, like diseases, have their pace of action, their periods of aggravation and relief, and are influenced alike by changes of environment such as temperature, weather, time, and circumstances. In the proving of remedies we may note and observe the depature from normal health, with its harmonious play of vital processes, throughout the mental, emotional and physical planes to a more or less disturbed state of the whole being.

The great number of sick people in the world with the vast number and variety of diseased conditions met with require a great array of medical substances to meet the need of sick humanity. Hence the reason for our ever growing and expanded materia medica. To the novice beginning the study of the homeopathic materia medica, its vastness seems appalling, and the multitudinous variety of symptoms bring only confusion and despair. For no memory, however retentive and great it be, can cope successfully enough to master the magnitude of intricacies, synonyms and apparent contradictions found in the materia medica.

And because of these conditions our great masters who preceeded us in the work endeavored to bring order out of chaos. They classified and arranged symptoms according to their relative value for prescribing purposes. Guernsey, Allen and others by long and painstaking study and labor developed a system of valuable keynotes that simplified the study and search for the needed remedy and led to many spectacular cures. Keynotes, for the most part are symptoms of proven remedies that are more or less unusual, rare and peculiar, belong to certain remedies and quite distinctive of those remedies alone. When such symptoms are found in patients and are distictive of their complaints, that remedy will generally prove efficacious in cure. Keynotes like repertories are good as far as they go, but they are too limited in scope to meet all the needs of

---

1. From the handwritten manuscript of Dr. Grimmer, exact date unknown. - Editor.

sickness in the world, and we must experience too many failures in the realm of cure.

Repertories are more valuable than keynotes because we have the choice of larger groups of remedies to select the needed one for the individual case. But even an unabridged repertory, like Kent's is limited largely to our more fully proven polycrests with added fragments of provings from other remedies. Hence there still is much to be desired and added to this already extensive work.

Hahnemann taught that the mental and emotional symptoms of patients and of provings are most valuable and more certain to produce curative action. This teaching has been confirmed by all the great masters and teachers that followed him. And a progressive branch of our old school followers, the advocates of psychosomatic medicine, are now telling us how fear, anger, hate, frustration, and suppression ultimate in pathologic diseases of body and mind. Arthritis, cancer, epilepsy, insanity and in fact all chronic manifestations of sickness stem from mental and emotional strain over a more or less period of time. All of which confirms the incomparable genius of Hahnemann, the Father of Homeopathy, who lived nearly two centuries ago.

Our profession owes much to the concept of materia medica study evolved by Dr. J. T. Kent. This study envisioned each proven remedy as a sick entity with its life function disturbed and presenting a picture of likeness, distinctive and peculiar to itself.

Thus the student could see the ACON. patient with its sudden violence its fear of death its restlessness which in its entirety is not found exactly in any other remedy. ARS. has death, fear and terrible restlessness; but it is cold and weak, and great changes are noted in the blood and tissues which readily distinguishes it apart from ACON. RHUS-T. is restless and is better of its aches and tribulations by motion; but the sudden onset and deadly fear of ACON. is not present, nor is the weakness of ARS. found. BRY. is tired and averse to motion, and if compelled to move, becomes cross. BELL. is averse to motion because of extreme sensitiveness to jar, light, noise, etc. and the mentals of BELL. sets it apart from BRY. GELS. is averse to motion, but it is because of the great relaxation and utter prostration that makes it a GELS. case, and it is thirstless even with fever while BRY. has thirst for large amounts at rather lengthened intervals. BELL. has burning thirst to quench the dry parched throat. Such was Kent's method of teaching materia medica, and no better one has ever been devised. One learns to know one's remedies as one knows one's friends. One recognizes each of them equally well when one has studied each remedy as a seperate distinct entity, each with its own features, correspondances, pace of action, periodicity, etc. To become a master homeopathic prescriber, one must expend much time and labor in study both of the materia medica and the homeopathic philosophy, for both are a unit and cannot function apart.

When the genius of homeopathic philosophy is understood, we can lessen our labor and increase our proficiency with the intelligent use of keynotes and repertories. The more one uses and applies the materia medica to the needs of the sick, the greater becomes the skill in the selection of the curative remedy with a minimum amount of labor and time needed.

Our wonderful predecessors who built the materia medica and the philosophy piece by piece from foundation to superstructure, over the years, with incessant labor and sacrifice are deserving of our everlasting gatitude, for they blazed a path and a highway to spread the healing balm of Homeopathy for the afflicted and the sick of all lands over the earth. It was but to preserve that precious heritage and to add new adornments and attainments in the implements of cure, so that future generations may be freer of sickness and find happiness and efficacy to meet all life's problems.

There is a new factor to aid in the selection of the homeopathic remedy, and that is the electro-magnetic side of life. The cosmos of which we are but a fractional part exists and operates in accordance with electro-magnetic fields and forces that are universal and all-compelling in their activity. The changing seasons and the unchanging swing of the planets in their courses operate through and by this mechanism. All minerals, chemicals, plant, and animal life on the globe come into being and are regulated and controlled by this same law.

There are four well known groups of polarity forces in the world: viz. positive, negative, bi-polar, and neutral. Every substance of earth falls into one of these four groups, including remedial substances and human and animal blood. Those whose blood is positive require a negative curative agent to restore the balance; those whose blood is over negative need a positive agent to restore equilibrium and health. Those with a bi-polar blood need a bi-polar reagent to restore balance, and those of neutral blood must have a neutral reagent for curative purposes.

Thus, when the patient's blood polarity is known, three-fourths of the medical substances may be eliminated for remedy selection, as only that group belonging to the curative polarity group need be considered or studied for the individual remedy; thus much time and labor can be saved, and greater accuracy in prescribing is obtained with the use of this new approach.

Here let it be emphasized that the use of this new method does not eliminate the study of symptomatology and philosophy, for without them Homeopathy would fail. We need to know all that has been given by so much labor and sacrifice; it is for us to carry on and add our mite of information that came because of the work that preceded us. As our horizons are broadened and increased, we will go on to greater things in the realm of healing under God, the giver of all truth and goodness.

THE RELATION OF SURGERY TO HOMEOPATHY[1]

Homeopathy relates to things dynamic, fitting the dynamics of the remedy to the dynamics of the body organism and opposing the dynamic action of morbific agents that are the disturbing factors in the rhythm of health.

Surgery has to do with things mechanical, with the end results of disease or with injury to the material body or its parts. And because Homeopathy is basic in its curative processes, if its aid can be invoked in time surgical procedures will not be required, excepting such as may be needed in cases of injury to the body machine or in other rare instances of congenital physical defects. Much of surgery is but palliative, at best, because it deals with the end results of disease without having the ability to expel chronic inherited toxemias that are behind all disorderly life processes.

Surgery when indicated is like the indicated remedy, a great blessing, and often saves lives and relieves suffering. The evacuation of pus from deep abcesses, and those hidden away in closed cavities of the body, the extraction of ulcerated teeth, the removal of obstructions and stenosed channels and ducts and even the excision of benign growths pressing on important structures are some of the many valuable things that surgery best accomplishes; because when these hindrances and obstructions are removed, the life force of the organism can better carry on its many and complex life functions even though the morbific agent that caused these slow-forming mechanical end results remains unchanged.[2]

However, the extirpation of malignant growths by surgery or radium can result only in increased suffering and loss of vitality to the patient, to say nothing of the material losses involved, because such procedures hamper the already overburdened life force still more by scapping and depressing the vitality and in no way opposes the morbific cause of the disease which is rapidly destructive in its nature.

The intelligent surgeon must trust to this same life force to seal his surgical wounds with or without the aid of one of our homeopathic surgical remedies. And here let it be said without fear of successful contradiction that our specific remedies are of amazing benefit to the surgical

---

1. From the handwritten manuscript of Dr. Grimmer, exact date unknown. - Editor.
2. "It is not necessary to say that every intelligent physician would remove first this exciting or maintaining cause (causa occasionalis) where it exists; the indispotion thereupon generally ceases spontaneaously." Hahnemann, Samuel: Organon, §7 - Editor.

patient. Not only are the tissues healed quicker and better, but the life processes of the whole organism are speeded up and harmonized under the action of this benign power of the indicated remedy.

Post-operative adhesions, one of the bugbears of surgery, will not form if the correct remedy is given a patient after the operation. Many of the immediate sufferings such as shock[1], nausea and vomiting from the effects of the anesthetic[2] can be lessened or entirely prevented by a good homeopathic prescription.

Broken bones that refuse to heal, because of some deficiency magically respond to the impulse of the indicated remedy as has been proven myriads of times with such remedies as SYMPH., SIL., CALC-P., RUTA and others; and who has not seen the restoring power of ARN. and HYPER. in brain and spinal concussions?

In the realm of the gynecologist there is a splendid opportunity for the exhibition of the indicated remedy, and its action far excells routine treatment so largely prevailing at this day. In cases of hemorrhage not due to lacerated arteries the homeopathic specific is all sufficient. For the progress, safety and relative comfort of labor itself, Homeopathy has never been equaled. The danger of infection is hardly possible; or, if it occurs, it is quickly controlled under the influence of the needed remedy. And what a boon to the unborn child, whose destiny brings him a real homeopathic prescriber during the formative processes of his inter-uterine life. A harmonized life force will produce a normal mind enshrined in a perfect body, free of so-called congenital defects.

Surgery has achieved many spectacular results in the saving of human life and the relief of suffering. But with the recognition and use of the power that resides in the indicated remedy, these achievements of the past can be multiplied many fold. And, on the other hand, the light of Homeopathy will shine brighter and farther by bringing to her aid, at the council table, when needed the splendid force of good intelligent surgery.

As physicians whose sole duty is to heal the sick, we cannot afford to ignore intelligent help from any source so long as this aid available is

---

1. Cf., Kent, James Tyler: LECTURES ON HOMEOPATHIC MATERIA MEDICA, Fouth Edition, Boericke and Tafel, Philadelphia, 1956, especially the lectures on CARB-V., HYPER. where CARB-V. and STRONT-C. are indicated. - Editor.
2. Ibid., especially the lectures on PHOS. and HYPER., where PHOS. is indicated, also for the effects of chloroform or anesthesia. However, PHOS. is not the only remedy, and modern anesthetics may call for another remedy to be selected on the basis of the symptoms of each individual case. - Editor.

based on law and common sense. If we are guided by the fundamental principles involved in the homeopathic philosophy, we may employ surgery and mechanical measures with tremendous good to our patients, with increased credit and to the homeopathic cause itself.

From this angle, we see two distinct types of surgical procedure, namely constructive and destructive. The first type fits in perfectly with the doctrines of Homeopathy because it conserves organs and parts of the body organism and aids in the maintenance of the perfect rhythm of the whole life force.

And in this sphere, I wish to mention something of great use that has too long been hidden from the members of our school. One of our honored members, now gone to his reward, Dr. Banning, teacher, writer, lecturer and inventor has left us a contrivance of incalculable good. Subtle and gentle, yet forceful as the homeopathic remedy itself in its action and constructed in accordance with anatomical and physiologic laws, this beneficial contrivance used in conjunction with the homeopathic remedy will help the homeopathic doctor prevent abnormal defects of the spinal vertebrae and even correct them when they have ultimated as a result of disease for in such cases as these, the homeopathic remedy unaided by proper mechanical means is impotent to correct them. No one ever cured a spinal curvature with the remedy alone. And for ptosed viscera, not bound down by adhesions, this same instrument is of inestimable value. With this valuable device, used in conjunction with the indicated remedy, thousands of children now doomed to go through life more or less deformed and crippled could be restored and saved. Any further knowledge pertaining to this amazing instrument can be furnished by Dr. John Panos of Dayton, Ohio, Dr. Banning's protege, and the only man living that can apply this benefic help correctly, because it is homeopathic in the sense that it must be fitted to each individual case. I have mentioned this device for two reasons: first, because the homeopathic profession needs its uncomparable service, and second because of the work it does along the special lines for which it is adapted.

I have only briefly touched on the possibilities of constructive surgical and mechanical measures used in unison with good homeopathic prescribing. Before closing, a brief comment on the destructive type of surgery which antagonizes the concept of homeopathic philosophy might bring fourth some valuable discussion, if nothing else. The wanton destruction of the tonsils of children, the removal of ovaries and of the thyroid and other essential glands of the body, the excision of cancerous growths and the tissues in which they are seated are among some of the pernicious things that destructive surgery indulges in, much to the detriment of its hapless victims. Such measures are unhomeopathic because they destroy part of the organism's defense and in no way correct the disease cause (disturbed life force). All of the above-mentioned conditions are amenable to the correct homeopathic remedy if it be allowed to operate without interference and over a time sufficient to accomplish the necessary changes that must supervene in the curative processes, taking place under remedy action.

If we accept the homeopathic concept of life, of health and disease, we are compelled to admit the great value of surgery when it functions in accordance and in co-operation with the formula of the universal law of similars. Homeopathy is fundamental. Surgery is subsidiary.

THE LAW OF SIMILARS[1]

All laws regulating and governing the Cosmos are relative and complimentary, only differing in each law's specific scope or sphere of action.

Physics (including in its vast field of activities gravitation, electromagnetism, vibration), chemistry, physiology, toxicology and anatomy structure and function, one related to the other, gives us a concrete expression of the material universe. And mathematical law is the measuring rod that builds with precision and regulates accurately both the function and structure of phenomenal nature.

The Law of Similars operating in the realms of physics produces many varied and vital changes in man and in the world about him. Chief of which is the phenomenon of cure and the restoration of the sick to health by the employment of a force or dynamic similar in nature to the sick-making energy of the disease, one force expelling the other from the organism, leaving the vital force of the body free to function unencumbered to perform its function in rhythmic harmony which alone brings health. Thus the law of similars acts like the universal force of electro-magnetism, two similars repelling and dispelling each other which leaves the magnetic field clear for other forces to operate freely.

In the phenomenal aspect of nature, Similars act in divergent paths, showing two manifestations of the same law.

In electro-magnetics, therapeutics and chemistry similar forces repel, all these operate on the material plane. In chemistry two acids or two alkalies will not unite, only a mixture will result.

In the mental, emotional and desire band of nature similars attract and hold together. Love begets love, as the lover finds and cherishes his mate. Species and races everywhere in the world seek their kind and remain in union to form societies and nations. Hence the trite saying about "birds of a feather flock together."

Where love is perverted and turned by selfish desire into envy and hate the repelling power of similars obtains, and hate and envy destroy themselves. This is true of all evil which carries in its nature the seeds of self-destruction and obliteration; leaving the realm free for the all prevailing force of love to operate and rule. Slowly but surely, the potent power of love is gaining control over warring nature. But the way

---

1. Journal of the American Institute of Homeopathy, Vol. 44, No. 7, July 1951, p. 159.

is long and hard and beset with many obstacles, yet not insurmountable for evolution in time will achieve a better order for all.

Man's environment and station in the social order is largely influenced by similars; religiously and politically, hence the existence of political parties and religious sects, creeds and cults.

Also different medical views and methods of treatment obey the same compelling law of similar. Allopaths are indifferent to the claims of the homeopathic law. Homeopathy can not enthuse over the claims of the ever-changing empiric method of therapeutics known as allopathy.

And believe it or not, democrats will not attend a republican gathering but would prefer to vote for a mangy dog if it be labeled democrat. Republicans in their turn cannot see any virtue in anything democratic unless it is dead.

Pet peeves and critical views exist in all the sects of Christians even though they are all heading and working for the same and under the teaching and leadership of Jesus Christ. The deep prejudices of the jew and gentile while regretable is still with us here in the United States of America, leader in freedom and equality for all in the year 1950.[1]

From the aformentioned facts and observations we note that the law of similars operates in two ways, viz; separatively and in a unifying way.

First it unites people into groups, creeds etc. and then seperates the groups as opposing units until such times as the greater law of love and understanding shall bring them together in orderly harmony for their common good. In the lives of individuals as well as in societies and nations, Similar plays a most important role, for likes are attracted by likes. The votary of moral law will not seek his life mate among the frequenters of brothels. Those who joy in the ways of crime and degradation are not attracted to places where spiritual truths are dispensed.

Humanity's evolution to better states of being is largely brought about by this same law of similars; thus we see that outside the sphere of theraputics this law is a potent influence in the affairs and lives of men everywhere and for all time.

From the preceeding statements of self-evident facts, it is safe to deduce that the Law of Similars is indubitably a law of nature, unalterable and eternal.

This law will operate for the benefit of man and all earth life in ever-widening spirals on developing and evolving man and all life below

---

1.   and even in 1995. - Editor.

him, until that time spoken of by the prophets, the millennium shall arrive. In that time love and understanding will prevail; prejudice, envy, hatred and selfish desires will be unknown. Then indeed may the lion and the lamb lie down together with the lamb still on the outside. Rabbi Goldberg may enjoy a pork sandwich at Father O'Grandy's wedding feast. Democrats and republicans may vote for the same canditate running on a communist ticket and allopathic and homeopathic doctors will heal the sick together all for the good of a united world, under the brotherhood of man and Fatherhood of God.

THE LAW OF SIMILARS AND EMPIRICISM[1]

Physicians who follow the Law of Similars, treat the patient as a unit, and the totality of symptoms is what composes that unit. The Law may be divided into two parts, namely: the science and the art, the art being superior to the science because the art is what enables us to apply the science.

As Hahnemann experimented on the Peruvian bark, from which quinie is obtained, he found that when the bark was taken in potency it produced many of the symptoms pertaining to malaria. From that beginning, and after much experimentation, he anounced the Law of Similars, or that "likes are cured by likes." After 160 years of practice in the hands of many physicians in many lands, this law has been fully confirmed. Hahnemann was not the first to announce this law. Hippocrates, the Father of Medicine, speaks of the Law of Similars and the Law of Contraries, but in practice it is found that symptoms when relieved by the Law of Contraries, express palliative and suppressive action of the law, rather than a curative action.

Hahnemann spent twelve years in research and observation in the search for the cause of human sickness. He concluded from the evidence of his findings, that certain inherited venereal toxins plus what he called psora (which is a lighter form of leprosy) are the causative factors. He called these chronic constitutional states miasms and named them syphilis, sycosis and psora.

Empiricism, or the method of working by trial and error, has given the world of medicine much that is good and useful. We need but cite the wonderful advance in surgical procedures which have enabled physicians to cure many cases that would not otherwise respond to known remedies. Those using the empirical method base their prescription largely on the diagnosis of the case. Years ago, in the Massachusetts General Hospital, researchers found that about 50% of the diagnoses were wrong according to postmortem examinations, although we can not say how much progress has been made in the art of diagnosing since that time.

Outside the field of medicine, there have been great advances in technical methods that have given the world many useful products. Thomas Edison, inventor of the incandescent light, where in the whole

---

1. JOURNAL OF AMERICAN INSTITUTE OF HOMEOPATHY, Vol. 59, Nos. 11 and 12, Nov. - Dec., 1966, p. nos. unknown. - Editor.

world has been enlightened; Charles Kitchner, inventor of the electric starter for the automobile, and Georg Washington Carver, teacher and chemist, all achieved their results by the method of trial and error. Hahnemann too was aided by the same method of trial and error in the discovery of the Law of Similars. Hahnemann advises in his Organon "Prove all things and hold fast to that which is true".

As one who has followed the Law of Similars for the past sixty years, I find the successes have far exeeded the failures. I believe this experience has been shared by thousands of physicians who have practiced the same law. When a homeopathic remedy fails, it is not the law that has failed, but that the prescriber has failed to find the best remedy. In fact, the one great objection voiced by many who use the law is that it is difficult, tedious and consumes much time and energy to prescribe for each case of sickness. This fact easily accounts for the reason why so few students are taking up the practice of Homeopathy.

There are certain reactions that may follow, or should follow, the action of the curative remedy:

First: There may be a slight initial aggravation of the symptoms of the case which is generally followed by improvement of the patient.

Second: Symptoms should depart in the reverse order to their coming and disappear from the more vital parts to the less vital parts, from above downward, and from within outward. Frequently, old symptoms which have been suppressed, such as skin eruptions, return with relief of the patient's acute symptoms. Old catarrhal symptoms which have been suppressed by local treatments and malarial symptoms which have been suppressed by quinine belong to this group.

From this we see the frightful harm that suppression of certain conditions brings about in the patient. We recognize the terrible suffering that comes from the suppression instead of the curing of the symptoms. Many of the troubles that the advocates of the Law of Similars are called upon to treat are the results of suppression. Those who follow the law build up a confidence and faith in their method, not only for the physician, but also, for his patients. We are taught by Hahnemann, and the masters who followed him, that we must allow sufficient time for a remedy to work before repeating the remedy, changing the potency or giving a different remedy.

We should remember the wonderful healing mechanism with which the Creator has endowed us. This mechanism enables the organism to furnish its own antibodies and vaccines and build up protection against infections, allergies and injuries, stimulating growth and repair. He tells us that as long as the vital force of the organism is flowing in order, we are well; sickness only comes when that flow is in disorder or is disarranged. Remembering these things should increase our faith in the curative power of the organism. Because of these facts, we can wait longer for the actions of our remedies to do their work and not change the potency or the remedy too soon. The sensitive patient tends to prove the remedy rather than demonstrate its curative action.

In the selection of the remedy, there are several factors to be considered:

FIRST

Symptoms are not of equal importance, but there is a relative value of the symptoms to be used in prescribing. Symptoms are divided into four types: 1) Mentals, 2) Generals, 3) Particulars, and 4) Strange, Rare and Peculiar. These are tested in the descending order of value although it also depends on how strong the symptom is that you are evaluating.

MENTALS

Those symptoms pertaining to the mind and the emotions are the most valuable. Resentment, self-pity, and hatred (perverted love) are among those mentals which undermine the resistance and vitality of the patient and render him susceptible to all kinds of infections and allergies.

GENERALS

Those symptoms pertaining to the reactions of the physical body are next in importance. Examples include reactions to heat and cold and environmental influences of all kinds. Abnormalities of the sexual sphere, the character of the various discharge of the body (color, consistency, odor, amount, acidity), which includes hemorrhages, catarrhal discharges form the orificies of the body, perspiration and discharges from abscesses.

PARTICULARS

Those symptoms referrable to the parts of the organism are next. The various types of pain (burning, shooting piercing, etc.) are among the high grade Particulars.

Strange, Rare And Peculiar:

Those symptoms not found in the proving of many remedies are placed last, but sometimes are the most helpful in choosing a remedy.

For example: aversion to those whom he should love most, (Fl-ac.; Hell., Phos., Sep.).

Second

In taking the case, it is important that no direct question be asked. First let the patient tell this story without interruption; then you can question him about those things which seem essential.

Third

We are told by Hahnemann that we must be without prejudice in treating our patients; that we must not be predisposed to certain remedies without due consideration to the total symptom picture which the patient presents.[1]

Fourth

Careful physical examination with constitutional factors and pathologic lesions noted, indicated laboratory tests, and accurate diagnosis help to complete the picture.

We have not mentioned the question of potency. This bitter controversy divided the American Institute of Homeopathy into two antagonistic sections for over half a century. We now know that both the low and high potencies are necessary in obtaining the best results in homeopathic prescribing. Any potency may be of use and needed in any given case of sickness we may be called upon to treat.

In the homeopathic armamentarium of remedies, are found specific remedies useful in conditions that arise in the course of human lives. These are often listed under causation. For example: Canth. for burns; Staph. for cuts and post-operative healing; Symph. for broken bones; Arn. for bruises of the soft tissues; Hyper. for injuries of sentient nerves, such as the ends of the fingers and the eye; Symph. and Asar. for severe eye injuries, or pain in the eyes post-operatively; Arn., Bell-p., Con. for injuries to the breasts; Ham. for injuries to blood vessels; Lyss. for dog bites; Cocc. and Petr. for motion sickness; Nat-s. for old head injuries. For the sensitive case when too many remedies have been given in too short a time, Teucr. is very effective in clearing the case. Cadm-met. and other Cadmium salts are antidotes to the Aluminum toxemia so prevalent in our civilization. Remedies that antidote the fall-out from atomic radiations are: Stront-c., Rad-br., Phos. and Kali-p.

---

1. §257, 258 - Editor.

The fall-out is one reason why our remedies are often ineffective or have a short action, and this must be antidoted before the constitutional remedy can do its work.

We know that medicine alone is not enough. The patient needs adequate exercise, rest and the right food with the proper proportions of minerals, vitamins and other nutrients to help restore his balance. The laws of hygiene, cleanliness of mind and body are necessary adjuvants to healthful living. Through our experiences and sufferings, we grow in expressing our spiritual selves.

To those of us who have been in practice a number of years, this is nothing new, but it might be taken as a refresher course. To the younger physician just starting his practice, it may be of some use in helping him decide the kind of medical practice he will want to pursue.

Philosophy Versus Empiricism[1]

Philosophy as defined by Webster's Dictionary has several definitions. First: "The knowledge of phenomena as explained by, and resolved into, causes and reasons, powers and laws." Second: "A systematic body of general conceptions or principles ordinarily with implication of their practical application as a philosophy of life." Third: "Practical wisdom, calmness of temper and judgement, equanimity." Fourth: "A treatise on philosophy."

Empiricism defined by the same author gives first: "Method or practice of an empiric especially in medicine, hence quackery." Second: "The philosophical theory which attributes the origin of all our knowledge to experience."

From the above expressed dictums we can see that those who work along with philosophic principles and laws are able to arrive at definite conclusions and results which make for satisfaction and success because it prevents accidents and errors. While those who follow the empiric practice along the thorny road of "trial and error" with no law or principle to guide them on their way must meet mostly disappointment and chagrin. All progress made by the race has come by the light of philosophical laws.

No science can grow or expand without a sound philosophy as its foundation. How far would the neophyte and student in chemistry get in an amply supplied laboratory without the guidance that comes from a knowledge of the chemical affinities governing the union of the elements? Trial and error or empiricism would soon bring him to grief if not destruction. In medicine more than in any other field is the need for philosophic approach most urgent, because medicines are agents fraught with power for good or evil according to the method of their preparation and application. If they are given in a too crude or toxic form, and in an empirical way or on the theory of producing some specific effect in the organism such as cathartic, diuretic or analgesic action, or if given in ignorance or regardless of what may come to the patient as a sequela remaining long after the specific action has past for which the medicine was given, then the agents under such conditions are forces of evil and destruction. Most of the so-called wonder drugs fall into this class, highly specific to overcome certain conditions but

---

1. THE HOMEOPATHIC RECORDER, Vol. LXV, No. 3, September, 1949.

leaving a train of weakness and broken health as a sequela lasting over a considerable period of time.

Experience may teach that the analgesic coal tar drugs, barbiturates etc. can dull the sense of pain for a time; while the philosophic science of Homeopathy knows that such action is not curative but harmful and suppressive leaving in the wake of their administration suffering and weakness and even more or less serious changes in the normal elements of the blood.

Toxicology, the science of classifying and treating poisons, may enable us to avoid the dangers attendant upon the use of these things.

But Homeopathy will teach us how to use for the benign purpose of cure these same death-dealing agents that toxicology warns us against. Homeopathy has proven that drugs can cure when applied by homeopathic technique and principles, the same symptoms and conditions they produce on the well when given in the crude toxic form.

This is philosophic law versus empiricism in action. Man may gather facts from many observations over long periods of time and in many places, but until he arranges and classifies and corelates them and traces their origin back to their causation he will obtain little good from such observations and gleaned facts. When such knowledge is classified and co-ordinated and traced to causes, the results become science, which can be employed with certainty for man's use and benefit. The poet Tennyson says "Knowledge comes but wisdom lingers." Knowledge expresses empiricism or experience. Wisdom expresses philosophy, the gathering together and the scientific explication of such knowledge for uses and development.

Thus we observe the contrast of empiricism versus philosophy in the application of drugs in the treatment of the sick. Then there are other differences to be noted more striking than what has gone before. The concepts of sickness itself are important and fundamental. Empiricism from the remotest times to the present has had changing views of sickness and its origin. In earlier times apart from physical injuries, infestations of devils and evil spirits were considered the cause of disease, and methods for their removal were more or less varied and efficient talismans, philters and repulsive concoctions of filth of all kinds were among the common means employed. Even today among Tibetans and other Asiatic tribes as well as those in Africa and the aborigines of North and South America these concepts and methods are still practiced with fluctuating degrees of success.

In the enlightened glow of the twentieth century, empiricism substitutes germs, microbes, bacteria, virus and allergies as disease causes and invokes the power of toxic drugs and laboratory filth in the form of disease-laden serums and vacines to restore the bloom of health with more or less financial success in the healing process.

Following the night of empiricism dawns the golden morning of philosophy in medicine with its rational concept of sickness and health. Disease is not a material thing or an entity to be cut, burnt or driven away with any material thing or drug. Disease is but a change of state occurring in a normal well human being to a deranged or abnormal state of existence. Disease affects first the internal life forces and processes, the physiologic activities, before chemical and tissue changes begin in the physical body.

The remedies against disease must be as simple and subtle as is disease itself. They need only contain the vibratory forces corresponding to the vibratory rates inherent in the sick-making power. The intelligent application of the sick-producing force to the sick individual body forces will bring equilibrium and health to the individual as his life processes are activated and harmonized. Of course, these processes take place in the unseen realm of physics where all causation of material ultimates has its inception.

It is known that every particle of matter in the universe, organic or inorganic, conscious or non-conscious, from the mightest sun to the smallest electron is inherently magnetic and consequently is governed and sustained by magnetic law. It is also known that when the human entity is sick there is a change in the flow of the magnetic force; it fluctuates from the normal magnetic polarities of the healing body back to abnormal rates of disease, the state of health with changes in unison with the direction and flow of the magnetic current.

The homeopathic remedy carries a charge of magnetism of a specific nature which can change the abnormal polarity of the deranged life force back to its normal state and action. When the magnetic forces of the organism flow in harmony with Cosmic order, then health is present. Anything that interrupts or changes the direction of that force brings about disease.

These forces manifest on the unseen etheric plane of nature where all chemical changes in the blood begin; and the blood is the common carrier of all the attributes and ingredients of life, the solar force, the magnetism and electricity, the oxygen and other gases essential to life and the mineral elements needed for the growth, sustenance and repair of the physical body all are carried from the deepest centers to the remotest externals of the organism by this vital fluid; the blood.

The homeopathic potencies are subtle forces catalytic in nature and impelled by powerful affinities and endowed with unlimited expansion and diffusibility to bring about their astounding results in cure. From these facts we can see the ways and means by which homeopathic cures are obtained and how the homeopathic law of cure fits into the frame work of Cosmic law of which it is but a part. Knowing these things, the physician can meet the problems pertaining to sickness of all kinds with confidence and faith which ensures success and diminishes the possibility of error and failure because he works in tune to the march of the Infinite.

PHILOSOPHY VERSUS EMPIRICISM IN MEDICINE[1]

Philosophy is defined by Webster as "the knowledge of the causes of all phenomena both of mind and matter; a particular philosophic system; and calmness of temper". The same authority defines empiricism as "an observation or practical experience apart from scientific knowledge; the practice of medicine without the usual medical training or qualifications; quackery".

In the realm of healing, Homeopathy is the only therapy that is based upon natural law and that has evolved a comprehensive philosophy that governs every step in the application of drugs for the relief and cure of human sickness. The homeopathic concept of life in relation to growth, development, health and disease on all the planes of nature (spiritual, emotional, mental and physical) stamps it as complete in the knowledge of health and the causes of its decline and loss, together with the means and methods to restore such loss back to normal states.

Perhaps in medicine, more than in any other human endeavor, must action and progress depend on philosophic procedures. Socially, economically and scientifically there is also need of the guidance of philosophic thought to insure success and progress. Man reaches his highest state of development under the philosophic urge. A social order or a therapeutic system built upon the tenents of empiricism is unstable and inadequate for satisfactory accomplishment. It involves too much of the trial and error formulas wherein error prevails preponderately over success.

Empiricism in medicine has produced more harm than good to the race. One so-called miracle drug after another has been tossed at the world in a constant stream to be tried on myriads of hapless human guinea pigs and then discarded as dangerous or unsatisfactory. Long after the dispensers of such drugs have discontinued their future use, the public remains free to purchase and abuse them to the most dangerous degree. Only after much harm and even tragedy has occurred are any warnings from medical experts sounded or legal steps taken to prevent wholesale poisonings.

Empirical medicine is closely allied with commercial medicine. Annually large profits are amassed-millions of dollars - at the expense of a gullible public both from the standpoint of wealth and health.

The physician must know the causes of disease as well as the means to remove them. Since the realm of cause operates on the unseen

---

1. THE HOMEOPATHIC RECORDER, Vol. LX, No. 12, June, 1945, p. 355.

planes of nature only, a philosophic approach alone will insure success in the restoration of health to the sick individual. Also, if the causes of illness are known, the physician through the processes of laws discovered and known to him will be able to prevent a great deal of illness, thereby dispensing with the necessity of cure.

Empiricism may observe and learn some facts relating to life and occasionally produce some happy result; but where one such result is accomplished, many other experiments turn out failures and disappointments. In the world of mechanics the trial and error routine while expensive may lead to an occasional success with the expenditure of much time and energy. Certain good effects in medicine may be accomplished only to be offset or neutralized by the evil results produced by the remedy used in the treatment.

To illustrate: The frequency of long-lasting sufferings that follow immunizing doses of serums and vaccines are a matter of record. We need cite only the recent wholesale cases of sickness and death produced in the army recruiting centers after the yellow fever shots administered for yellow fever prophylaxis, given without the consent and against the wishes of many of the soldiers and sailors, who were compelled to submit to such unscientific and pure empirical methods.

Also, we may note that the so-called curative effects produced by the sulpha drugs against infections are too often followed by blood changes and prolonged weakness and devitalization. The destructive effects of x-ray and radium therapy for the treatment of cancer and other growths together with many forms of skin disease are among the common things met with every day and all to no purpose because such agents, allopathically and empirically applied, never produce cure. The suppression of malaria chills with quinine and its derivatives and synthetic substitutes not only fail to cure, but complicate and aggravate the malarial patient with the development of liver, spleen and blood diseases as sequelae which are more difficult to cope with than the non-complicated malaria infection.

In the treatment of syphilis, empirical medicine has traveled from mercury to kalium iodatum, thence to the arsenicals through the series from 606 to 909, thence to bismuth and the very latest, penicillin. They are still looking with long eyes for the perfect specific that will cure all cases without complication or sequential effects by way of the ideal anti-syphilitic that only exists in the imaginations of earth-bound empirical specialists who proceed by a common patron always in circles like lost wanderers with no compass or guide, no philosophic chart or habit of thought, no plan to show the way, only a blind incoherent haphazard march in search of the magic myth, a specific remedy for all in a given disease. The bitter irony of it all is the fact that for the past one hundred and fifty years they have trampled upon and kicked aside the very object of their long arduous and illusive search. Like worn weary prospectors searching for virgin gold who have crossed and recrossed over the sought-for prize, but because they failed to recognize its presence in a strange though common form, they lost it and are destined to go on forever in a vain searching, destitute and hopeless, doomed to perpetual failure.

Homeopathic philosophy holds that magic key that unlocks the armamentarium of all specific medicine, as each individual case of sickness, regardless of its diagnostic name, receives its own specific remedy, based upon unchanging law, confirmed by numerous cures wrought by many physicians from many lands and upon peoples of all races, who have suffered with every kind of sickness known and named by medical lore. The homeopathic physician obtains his knowledge of the action of drugs by proving such drugs on healthy individuals of both sexes. These provings or symptoms produced make up the *Homeopathic Materia Medica*, a veritable store-house of medical knowledge for the healing of the nations.

The proven *Law of Similars* is the basic foundation upon which the superstructure of homeopathic philosophy is erected to give to the world an edifice of great beauty and use. Every well-proven remedy - that is every remedy tested on many individuals - constitutes an image of sickness; and in that image is reflected the power of that remedy to cure a like picture of sickness to be met in the field of disease. It is necessary to give that remedy in a potentized or attenuated form where cure is desired because if given in the crude or toxic form that produces sickness in the healthy, a severe aggravation or even serious harm may come before cure is obtained. This method precludes all experiments on the sick and eliminates all consequential drug effects that almost invariably follow empirical medical procedures. For how can one measure and harmonize the reactions in the test tube with those of the human organism? Or how can the sufferings, emotional, mental and physical of the guinea pig be known or applied to human needs? Surely not by the pathological end results known only after killing the guinea pig.

By and through the constant application of the homeopathic law of cure to many cases of sickness treated by master prescribers and keen observers through the years, has the homeopathic philosophy been built and expanded from time to time. Without the knowledge of this philosophy the physician might often be confused and fail to cure certain very chronic and difficult cases of sickness.

Sickness has an order of procedure, a direction in its symptomatology and a pace of action, all of which helps determine its nature, acute or chronic, relapsing, periodic, etc. In the same way must the provings of our remedies be studied to ascertain their relation and application by their similarity to disease states and conditions. One of the most valuable observations to remember is the fact that the last symptoms to appear in any sickness are the first to disappear under the action of the indicated remedy; that symptoms get well in the inverse order of their coming. Another observation many times confirmed that patients get well of their symptoms and complaints from center to circumference, from within out and from above downwards, from more vital to less vital parts (Hering's Law).

Whenever disease and symptoms take the opposite direction, there is suppression and danger for the patient. An eruption suppressed by powerful ointments or x-ray or radium applications often is followed by alarming asthmatic states or violent inflammations of the gastro-intestinal tract or congestive headaches, and violent neuralgias may supervene. Sometimes after rubbing powerful linaments to rheumatic joints, there is serious cardiac involvement with pain and dysponea.

Who can measure the stupendous harm that is now here and will increase in the future from the unlimited taking of the myriads of coal-tar drugs to mention but a few - the barbitals, the aspirins, the anacins, the sulpha drugs, the acetanilids, pyramidons and innumerable others that flood social life by way of radio, T.V., newspaper and magazine advertisements where the public without hindrance or medical advice may procure unlimited amounts of these insidious poisons for the relief of pains of all kinds, insomia and infections of every sort. Is it any wonder that heart and kidney disease together with cancer and many forms of mental and nervous diseases are increasing as never before?

And what does empirical medicine say about these things? Nothing, because if it did, it would undermine its own very shaky position. It can not condemn the very methods it employs for the treatment of the sick. As long as millions of dollars are made by these harmful nefarious means, there will be no criticism from those who profit by such methods. And so long as commercialized medicine maintains its position in the world, Homeopathy will be opposed and ostracized by the dominant school. With them the sacred precincts of the profit system in medicine must not be invaded or hampered. But in spite of opposition and selfish greed, Homeopathy will stay and contend for the right and true. Human progress has always come only through sacrifice and contention. Only those souls who love and value truth better than material things are the instruments chosen to carry the standards of progress to the citadels of a better order in the world.

The homeopathic physician is such an instrument in the divine scheme of things. Touched by the power of the love of healing, no work is too tedious or difficult for him, no sacrifice too much if it but sustains and perpetuates the principles of his art and science. If need be, he stands alone, unafraid and resolute in the face of ridicule and calumny.

If medicine ever progesses above the traditions and superstitions of the dark ages, it will come by the light of the homeopahic philosophy. The simple knowledge and application of the law of similars apart from the philosophy built up around it can do only simple and acute work; it can never fathom the complexities and persistance of chronic disease. We have seen several phases of the law practiced under other names without the philosophic complement, and they are far from complete.

Bier's irritation theory of disease and its cure and McDonald's hydration concept of disease, while doing more good and less harm than regular medicine, do not approach the possibility of cure that obtains with the complete homeopathic concept of sickness and its law of cure. Those of us who have dedicated our lives to the divine attribute of healing through the medium of the law and the philosophy of Homeopathy want our children and their children to be born and reared under the benign power of homeopathic healing. In no other way can a more healthy and better race with ideals and intelligence to banish from the earth the scourge of war and universal disease be brought into being. The homeopathic potencies properly applied have the inherent power of touching and turning into harmony the deepest centers of the human organism, and they bring back the light of healing from the darkness of disease.

To rationalize and control the emotions, to banish fear and instill hope - thereby purifying the life force of the whole being that will enable it to build and sustain a more perfect physical body to perform better uses in a suffering world - is reason enough for our united efforts of Homeopathy's perpetuation in the archives of medicine. And our efforts are only exceeded by an abiding faith that this benign doctrine of healing must live and grow with other great truths of nature in the hearts of men through time and eternity.

Two Philosophies of Medicine[1]

Before the time of Hahnemann, medicine was without a philosophic approach either in theory or practice. No fixed principles or laws were known that could be a guide for the practice of the medical art[2]. The experience and observation of the individual physician together with traditional precepts, coming down from antiquity, served in place of law to decide the course of treatment needed. Not enough was known of the basic science of anatomy, physiology, hygiene and diagnosis to be of much use in prescribing. Hence much was left to the whims, prejudices and pre-conceived opinions of the prescriber. Many theories were rampant on how to treat the sick. One of the common concepts of that beknighted time was that the patient either had too much blood or that his blood was pernicious with toxins and needed to be drained from the body. This was done, and often the patient mercifully expired from exsanguination. Today in a more enlightened age the reverse of this procedure exists. The patient is given transfusions of other people's blood at a fancy price; however, it is with less serious immediate results, though not all that might be desired occurs from this procedure.

The numerous theories and practices that were in vogue are so well known to all that we omit to mention them. It is enough to know that before the time of Hahnemann the practice of medicine was a hodge-podge affair and too frequently was an affliction and a menace fraught with suffering and danger to the patient. The case of George Washington, the father of our country, who was attacked with a simple case of tonsilitis and who was so weakened by repeated blood letting that he died an easy victim to the combined effects of medical science and disease, is an example of the old practices. Lord Byron's departure from this mundane sphere at thirty-six years of age was largely due to the same cause, the loss of too much blood taken by his physician in his attempt to cure malaria, from which Byron was suffering.

With Hahnemann came the first semblance of law and philosophy to guide the practitioners of medicine. With the establishment of the Law of Similars medicine took its first step upward from the deep abyss of ignorance and superstition. The second step upward came with the discovery and application of potentized remedies, and the third step into the sunshine of enlightenment came with the creation of the homeopathic philosophy.

---

1. From the handwritten manuscript of Dr. Grimmer, written in October 1955. - Editor.
2. See also Kent, LECTURES ON HOMEOPATHIC PHILOSOPHY, Lecture I, paragraph 1, 2, 3. - Editor.

This philosophy is based on the observations of Hahnemann and thousands of his trained disciples and followers in the past hundred and sixty years, applying the law of cure with potentized medicine. Observing the reactions and the ultimate cure of millions of patients make up the foundation and structure of the homeopathic philosophy.

No one can deny the influence of this philosophy on the advance of general medicine. It now accepts and practices a crude type of homeopathy in the application of its vaccine therapy; and when it accepts and applies the Hahnemannian method of potentization to dilute its toxic remedies instead of using the blood or serum of animals, it will attain much better curative results with no consequential side effects to embarrass the doctors or their patients. The single dose, or shot or application of the selected remedy is now a quite common practice among many prominent physicians of the regular school; and the dosage of medicine is getting smaller and smaller with each passing year because of the so-called side effects of larger doses of drugs.

Homeopathic philosophy emphasizes the necessity of a thorough and careful case history obtained by a judicial procedure of questioning and observation to obtain the facts in the case, then fitting the most similar remedy of the Materia Medica, by way of repertory and Materia Medica study, to the symptoms making up the case history, then giving the selected remedy in potentized form in a single dose. The physician then watches the reactions in the patient as the processes of cure unfold and point toward recovery bringing the patient to a state of order and comfort. After the similar remedy is given a sick patient, his reactions are a reliable guide in the process of his recovery to health. The curative remedy causes symptoms to depart in the inverse order of their coming, the last to come being the first to go. Symptoms leave from above downward and from within outward, and often a case of suppressed eruptions will reappear under the remedy with a complete cure of a severe asthma. Symptoms go from the vital centers and organs to the periphery of the economy. Such are some of the cardinal features of the philosophy. In chronic disease, where the remedy needs repeating only after the recovery processes have ceased, these are shown by the signs and symptoms of the patient.

Regular medicine can hardly claim a philosophy even in these times of advancement and discovery. Much of their effort and achievement have been along the lines of better diagnosis. This is laudable and good, but it is inadequate for the prescribing of remedies for the sick, because no two blood chemistries are alike as the experience and technique of transfusions prove. While the science of diagnosis is improving, it is still far from seventy-five percent correct; and the basing of a prescription on the diagnosis entails a large percent of error to start off with. Even were it one hundred percent accurate, prescriptions based on it alone would prove disappointing in a large number of cases because different patients react differently to the same toxin, infection, or drug. Each patient is an individual with his individual blood type and chemistry with his own peculiar nervous, mental, emotional and physical symptoms responding to the stimuli of environment. Much of the procedure of regular medicine is empirical and based on trial and error which is expensive and often uncertain. Until laws are discovered and applied in any branch of human endeavor and the principals formulated into a science, there can be no success or progress made. Regular medicine is vast and somewhat chaotic for the need of order and law. It needs the homeopathic approach to solve many of the medical problems confronting the world today.

The new young science of genetics especially that section treating of the "black" genes, the purveyors of pathological cell development, sustains the homeopathic claims of the transmission of inherited disease from generation to generation. The homeopathic potency is the only known force in nature, subtle enough and at the same time potent enough, when attuned by a selective law to reach and modify the activity of those tiny arbitrators of human destiny, the genes.

The advance in the science of physics, chemistry and genetics are opening the portals of knowledge to reveal the subtle truths of homeopathic law. Infinitesimal doses of medicine no longer appear to be mysterious in action or power. The known specific effects of bacteria and viruses, on the organism of man and animals, are additional proof of the power packed into minute organisms and things that can cause illness and even death when lodged in a susceptible soil and under certain special conditions and circumstances.

What better weapon can be found to cope with those tiny but destructive entities than the homeopathic potency of the attuned remedy adapted to each specific type and variation of disease-producing cause? Those who have seen the action and reaction of these subtle forces nullify each other to leave the host and rest, free from all semblance of disease, can only give thanks to a benign Creator for the wonder of His work and the illumed instrumentalities He gave His children for their welfare and growth.

PSORA[1]

The history and advent of Psora dates back to the beginning of man, from time immemorial. The tireless and unremitting labor, the keen observation and profound logic pertaining to related facts, appearing and operating in sequential order was Hahnemann's equipment that enabled him to perceive the true nature and cause of all human sickness, both physical and mental[2].

Hahnemann's achievement in the realm of cure, together with the philosophy upon which it is based, is best and most lucidly described by Dr. James Tyler Kent in his incomparable course of Lectures on Homeopathic Philosophy. As this work of Kent's is all embracing and is expressed so clearly and perfectly, one can best convey to your consciousness the import and magnitude of this subject by quoting freely from it in the course of this talk[3].

Hahnemann devoted twelve years proving remedies, amassing facts from his observations on patients prescribed for, before he discovered the nature and cause of all human sickness in the world. With the remedies he and his disciples had proven he was able to make many satisfactory cures in acute cases of disease, but after twelve years of treatment many patients were still sick with recurring manifestations of disease, stubborn eruptions returned and became more difficult to eradicate, severe attacks of asthma persisted with little or no palliation of the suffering, painful rheumatic states and many types of nervous complaints were more and more resistant to the seemingly best indicated remedies.

A man of lesser faith and courage would have ceased to struggle against such unpromising odds as faced him after years of painstaking effort; but Hahnemann had caught a glimpse of truth in the newly discovered, or revised, Law of Similars and his soul was inspired to go on over rough and unchartered seas. For the needs of sick humanity were great and medical treatment was steeped in ignorance and superstition, devoid of any semblance of reason or logic and destitute of technique or law to guide or lighten the way to palliation or cure.

---

1. THE LAYMAN SPEAKS. Vol. X, No. 6, June 1957, p. no. unknown. - Editor.
2. Hahnemann, S. THE CHRONIC DISEASES, Translated from the second enlarged german edition of 1835 by Prof. Louis H. Tafel, Boericke & Tafel, Philadelphia, 1896 - Editor.
3. Kent, James T.: LECTURES ON HOMEOPATHIC PHILOSOPHY, Lectures XVIII, XIX. - Editor.

During this long struggle in the quest of help for the sick, Hahnemann and his dependents were harassed with hardships and privations as a result of a poverty stricken environment; his meager earnings were inadequate to meet his and his family's needs and hunger and cold were persistant companions in this journey after truth for the good of his fellow. But in spite of these obstacles and discouragements he made noteworthy progress in the solution of these deep medical problems; only a soul driven and inspired by dire need and with an abiding faith in the goodness of Divine Providence could accomplish such results against such odds.

During these busy harrowing times Hahnemann made several interesting and important observations from which he was able to deduce the cause of illness and trace them back to their origin or beginnings.

First was the direction disease takes under the urge of the vital force both when operating in its normal natural state and when operating under the influence of drugs both in crude and potentized form. To illustrate: patients, who have had skin eruptions suppressed or driven into the inner skin or mucous membranes lining the internal vital organs, such as lungs, heart, kidneys and gastro intestinal tract by powerful metallic ointments developed severe attacks of asthma or ulceration and inflammation of the intestine or kidneys of a serious type. When the right homeopathic remedy was given these conditions, resulting from suppression, were restored to health and order with the reappearance of the suppressed skin eruption.

This observation established the fact that the chronic Psoric disease gets well under the curative remedy from within outward, from center to circumference, and the last symptoms to appear are the first to depart under the remedy. The progress of disease, unassisted by the curative remedy, travels from without inwards and involving deeper and more vital tissues on its way inward.

These and other observations made by Hahnemann enabled him to perceive that there is a basic universal toxin or miasm that takes on many forms and manifestations of disease, both acute and chronic, and that ramifies throughout the organism embracing the mental, emotional and physical aspects of sickness.

Another observation made was that after a patient recovered from severe and acute manifestations of diseases such as typhoid, smallpox, etc. many severe chronic diseases were much mitigated in their ravages and better general health in the patient prevailed with greater resisting power against all sickness thereafter. This was especially true when recoveries occurred under the impact of the homeopathic remedy.

As many manifestations of disease, especially severe forms of skin eruptions and implacable types of catarrhal and asthmatic types of sickness occurred in the newborn infants the conclusion and inference could only be that such expressions of illness were transmitted and inherited from the parents. Hundreds of such cases were studied and their family histories were checked and this was found to be true and thus was established the wide spread universal racial aspect of all sickness.

Then Hahnemann set to work to prove remedies whose symptoms, nature and pace of action, corresponded to the Psora with its many manifestations of chronic forms of sickness. Such remedies as SULPH., CALC., LYC., GRAPH., MEZ., KALI-C., CARB-V., PETR. and later PSOR. were proven and classified by Hahnemann and Boeninghausen (one of his best pupils).

These deeper remedies proved Hahnemann's concept of the cause of human sickness, for with them he was able to cure permanently many cases of intractable chronic illness, that before the advent and development of these deep antipsoric medicines could only be palliated for a time but without a cure, as recurrence came on more frequently and severly while the patients remained sick until the Psoric miasm or taint in the blood stream was eradicated by the suitable remedy. This is but a brief and meager outline of the tremendous contribution of this great and good man to the everlasting cause of true science.

But the science of Homeopathy, as conceived and developed by Hahnemann, Hering and Kent, is much more than science. It contains and includes the doctrine of a faith in Divine Law and Goodness, hence the abiding power to heal through time and eternity. Material science as the world knows it today is not inspired and activated by Spiritual things that are the real permanent and ruling forces of the Cosmos. Hence the shifting changing aspect of theories and unstable conclusions, and this is more pronounced in the realm of general medicine than anywhere else.

That I may bring to you a clearer picture of Psora, I can do no better than quote some pages from Dr. Kent's Lecture of Psora, in his homeopathic philosophy. Lecture XVIII, where-in he states: "Psora is the beginning of all physical sickness. Had psora never been established as a miasm upon the human race, the other two chronic diseases would have been impossible, and susceptibility to acute diseases would have been impossible. All the diseases of man are built upon psora; hence it is the foundation of sickness; all other sicknessess came afterward."

"Psora is the underlying cause, and the primitive or primary disorder of the human race. It is a disordered state of the internal economy of the human race. This state expresses itself in the forms of varying chronic diseases, or chronic manifestations. If the human race had remained in a state of perfect order, psora could not have existed. The susceptibility to psora opens out a question altogether too broad to study among the sciences in a medical college. It is altogether too extensive, for it goes to the very primitive wrong of the human race, the very first sickness of the human race, that is the spiritual sickness, from which first state the race progressed into what may be called the true susceptibility to psora, which in turn laid the foundation for other diseases. If we regard Psora as synonymous with itch, we fail to understand, and fail to express thereby, anything like the original intention of Hahnemann. The itch is commonly supposed to be a limited thing, something superficial, caused by a little tiny bit of a mite that is supposed to have life, and when the little itch mite is destroyed, the cause of the itch is said to have been removed. What a folly!"

"From a small beginning with wonderful progress, psora spreads out into its underlying states and manifests itself in the large portion of chronic diseases upon the human race. It embraces epilepsy, insanity, the malignant diseases, tumors, ulcers, catarrhs and a great proportion of the eruptions. It progresses from simple states to the very highest degree of complexity, not always alone by itself, but often by the villainous aid of drugging during generation after generation; for the physician has endeavored with all his power to drive it from the surface, and has thereby caused it to root itself deeper, to become more dense and invisible, until the human race is almost threatened with extinction. Look at the number of the population upon the face of the earth and notice how few arrive at the age of maturity. It is appalling to think of the number of infants that die, and these largely from the outgrowths, or outcomings of psora. We see little ones born who have not sufficient vitality to live. The congenital debility, and marasmus, and varying diseases of a chronic character that carry off the little ones, have for their underlying cause the chronic miasms. The principal underlying cause is psora, next syphilis and next sycosis."

From all of this we wonder why the race continues to exist; and it would not, but for the fact that the Divine Creator endowed man and all his creatures of the lower order with a most effective and unique defensive mechanism. For the preservation of his physical life and body, man also constantly receives an influx from the sun, (called prana by the eastern savants, but it is really the vital force described by Hahnemann and emanating directly from the Creative source).

To quote Kent further, Lecture XIX. "In the work on "Chronic Diseases" Hahnemann refers to psora as the oldest most universal and most pernicious chronic miasmatic disease, yet it has been misappropriated more than any other. Psora is the oldest miamsmatic chronic disease known. The oldest history of the oldest nation does not reach its origin. Psora is just as tedious as syphilis and sycosis, and is, moreover hydra-headed. Unless it is thoroughly cured, it lasts until the last breath of the longest life. Not even the most robust constitution, by its own unaided efforts, is able to annihilate or extinguish psora."

"The three chronic miasma, psora, syphilis and sycosis, are all contagious. In each instance there is something prior to the manifestations which we call disease. We speak of the signs and symptoms of a disease, we speak of the outcroppings of the symptoms when we speak of syphilis, but remember there is a state prior to syphilis or syphilis would not exist. It could not come upon man except for a condition suitable to its development. In like manner psora could not exist except for a condition in mankind suitable for its development."

"Psora being the first and the other two coming later, it is proper for us to inquire into that state of the human race that would be suitable for the development of psora. There must have been a state of the human race suitable to the development of psora; it could not have come upon a perfectly healthy race, and it would not exist in a perfectly healthy race. There must have been some sickness prior to this state which we recognize as the chronic miasm of psora; some state of disorder, some state that it would be perfectly rational and proper for man to undertake to solve as to its cause, as to its history, and as to its nature. Some will say, but if we undertake to do this we will have to accept the work of God as historical, as relating to the beginning, because there is no other going so far back. There is no harm in reasoning from that and I hope you will so accept it, not only as history, but as divine revelation, not that I wish to quote from or refer to it, because I never do so in my teachings. If we look upon syphilis we will see that man's own act leads him to the place where he comes in contact with syphilis, it is the result of action."

"Syphilis is that disease which corresponds to the effect of impure coition, of going where syphilis is, of coming in contact with those who have it. It is an action; it is not so with psora, Man does not seek it, he does not go where it is, he does not associate with those necessarily that have it. He may be exposed; but syphilis is the result of his own action, which is an impure fornication or adulteration which he knows better than to seek, and knows enough from his intelligence to avoid. Syphilis then is a result of action although after once ultimated it may be perpetuated by accident. There is always a state and condition of man that precedes his action, and if syphilis corresponds to man's action, and there is a state prior to it, a diseased condition that precedes, that state must correspond to that which precedes action, which is thinking and willing."

"Thinking and willing establishes a state in man that identifies the condition he is in. As long as man continued to think that which was true and held that which was good to the neighbor, that which was uprightness and justice, so long man remained upon earth free from the susceptibility to disease, because that was the state in which he was created. So long as he remained in that state and perserved his integrity he was not susceptible to disease and he gave forth no aura that could cause contagion; but when man began to will the things that were the outcome of his false thinking then he entered a state which was the perfect correspondence of his interior. As are the will and the understanding so will be the external of man. As the life of man or as the will of man, so is the body of man, and as the two make one in this world, there is evolved from him an aura which is vicious in proportion to his departure from virtue and justice into evils."

It is amazing to contemplate the fact, that this philosophy of medicine so beautifully perceived and expressed by both Hahnemann and Kent, (the former nearly two centuries ago) is now being verified (by an advanced group of medical thinkers) and is now referred to as the psychosomatic concept of disease and its cure. This group of medical scientists now prove by modern laboratory methods and technique that the impact of emotional stress, including hate, anger, fear, grief and unholy selfish desires are causative factors in blood and endocrine secretions changing them from their normal life preserving qualities to a toxic disease producing state, thereby inducing many forms of serious chronic disease such as malignancies, intractable forms of arthritis and mental incomptency of various forms and degrees.

And the new physics with its advanced knowledge concerning the relationship of the interchange of matter and energy explains the power and energy inherent in potentized drugs; the quips and the sarcastic shafts of ridicule relative to small doses of medicine no longer carry weight. And finally the new science of genetics furnish the most convincing proof of Hahnemann's theory regarding the inheritability of psora and all forms of chronic disease.

Thus we see that the vanguard of modern science is only now beginning to rediscover the truths in nature perceived and formulated into a workable pattern for the benefit of mankind, one hundred and seventy years ago. Hail to Hahnemann, the torch bearer who dissipated the darkness of ignorance and superstition with the light of spiritual insight, sustained by faith in Divine Providence against the many forces of evil that beset his pathway through life. And hail to Hering and Kent, his two most loyal and effective disciples who gave so much of their lives in the cause they loved and championed. And what of the later followers of these pioneers of the healing art, those of us who have inherited the precious archives of medical knowledge and who have basked in the golden light of their outstanding achievements, built up by unremitting toil and sacrifice of strength and life.

This magnificent edifice of homeopathy resting on the solid foundations of immutable law is showing the corroding marks of time; the brilliance and glamour of its adornments is dimmed and marred by the visitations and calumnies of selfish and greedy agencies who are deaf to the cries of pain and unmoved by the dark gloom of death in its myriad forms, while agony and mental anguish are but the means of profitable ends to those interests the manufacturers and purveyors of habit forming, pain killing and suppressive proprietary drugs. Rank commercialism in its rankest and most pernicious form is the force holding back the progress of an enlightened medical art of healing.

As long as immense sums of money can be made from the manufacture and sale of these pernicious nostrums so long will the advance of medical treatment be curtailed and hindered by paid propaganda and advertisement. This same propaganda extends its interest from reaching the public by means of the news agencies, newspapers, magazines, etc.

Shall we who have inherited so much from our benefactors stay dormant and voiceless and watch Homeopathy fade away and die when the world is in such dire need of healing remedies with no deleterious side effects remaining after cure.

This threatened catastrophe must be prevented. This prevention can only be accomplished by a program of education to counter the noxious propaganda of modern commercialized medicine, and for such a program to be successful means that every individual homeopathic doctor, patient and friend of the homeopathic concept, art and science has a rendezvous with destiny to give his all, in time and means, to attain that desirable end. For not only we of today, but our children and all the children of all the races of the future are benefited and made free of sin and pain, to evolve and flourish in the glow of radiant health, and to build a better world to live in.

THE SCIENTIFIC ASPECT OF HOMEOPATHY[1]

In order to reach correct conclusions relative to the scientific side of homeopathy, we must examine and compare its basic principles together with the results in cure obtained to the contemporary sciences and methods of treatment existing in the common field today.

We must know the nature of sickness as promulgated by Homeopathy as well as the concepts of disease held by other schools of medical thought, together with the advance made by the physicists in the universal realm of matter. Let us measure and compare some of these things and see whither we are led.

Homeopathy envisions disease as primarily disturbed vital function and all chemical physiologic or morbid tissue changes in a sick organism as but resultants of changed organic function.

The remedies Homeopathy employs are such that have been proven on healthy human beings to produce a similar symptom image of illness to that occurring in the individual case to be treated. Homeopathy does not experiment on the sick. Hence the great law, "Similia, Similibus Curantur". And where else than in the homeopathic arcanum of drug pathogenesis can we find such profound and complete knowledge of the action of drugs and their potential possibility in cure? Surely not in the test tubes or the miscroscopes of the pseudo scientists.

A third and most important proposition connected with the healing art is the homeopathic method of drug preparation involving the proceedure of potentization. Pure experimentation indicates that drugs may be given in crude form just short of the toxic dose to produce a change in the individual from that of health to one of disease. Such procedure may constitute a proving if all the changes are noted and recorded, when it will be found that the whole organism of that individual has been more or less affected. In a case of sickness where the organism and the essential cells of the body are more or less reduced in resistance, if such crude doses be given, the effect is much more drastic and in many cases alarming, especially if the drug administered was homeopathic (similar) to the illness of the subject. Hence, Hahnemann was compelled to give more and more attenuated doses of the needed remedy up to the 30th potency in order to avoid what he termed the homeopathic aggravation. With the attenuated potentized doses, he not only avoided the drug aggravation of symptoms but the cures were

---

1. From the handwritten manuscript of Dr. Grimmer, exact date unknown. - Editor.

quicker and longer lasting than those accomplished by the crude drugs. For the explanation of this phenomenon see Beir's matchless paper on "The Irritational Theory of Disease and Its Cure."[1]

Up until very recently the dominate school of medical thought has held decidely material ideas of disease and its cause. But recently the heretofore universally accepted germ theory of disease has received quite a jolt in the findings of the Mayo clinic where the mutability of disease germs changing from one species (streptococcus) to another (pneumococcus) was demonstrated. Further experiments will no doubt show these feared micro-organisms are useful scavengers created to aid in the elimination of toxins and possible reagents in the manufacture of antibodies against the very diseases they were supposed to cause. Similar experiments will prove the wide spread use of serums and vaccines far more efficacious and infinitely less harmful if administered in the attenuations of homeopathic proportions. Pathologic changes occurring in the tissues and organs of the sick have long been held by our friends of the old school to be the disease and its eradication by surgery or other physical means as the necessary proceedure to cure. But clinical evidence proves their concept of disease and methods of cure to be wrong.

The exact value of a philosophy or its tenets can only be known by the results obtained in its practical application. We will first discuss the merits and results obtained in cure under modern accepted methods of treatment.

In the realm of chronic disease we find the best criterion is to test methods of practice for results, because chronic diseases are not self-limited, but go on to end in death unless the intervention of curative measures can be invoked.

Cancer is regarded by the majority of old school authorities as purely local at least in its beginning; and surgery, x-ray, radium and other destructive methods are applied as logical weapons to vanquish the scourge; but the results are far more disastrous to the patient than to the neoplasm; excised from one part of the body it reappears elsewhere in a more virulent form; metastasis is the scientific term used to camouflage their failure of treatment. It is stated by Dudly that ninety-five percent of cancer victims who are operated die the first two years after operation.

---

1. Source unknown. - Editor.

Homeopathy regards cancer as a systemic constitutional disease that must be attacked through the blood stream by the properly indicated remedy for each specific case; by such methods the morbid processes of life are changed to normal vital action, resulting in better metabolism and normal cell growth. The results, in cures obtained, are better than fifty percent; and most of the fatal cases have their lives prolonged and are in comparative comfort without the use of opiates or coal tar derivatives until death.

Epilepsy is never cured by modern scientific methods because its cause is never considered or touched; all efforts are directed to stopping the convulsions either with increasing doses of bromides or luminol[1]. If the convulsions are suppressed, the patient soon goes down to imbecility and ends in some institution for the insane.

Homeopathy cures not less than seventy-five percent of these unfortunates, and by cure we mean the patient as a whole and not just the epileptic seizures that were but the expression of deranged life force.

Right here is the great dividing line of the two concepts. Allopathy sees only the material tissues and chemical constituents of the man arranged as an automatic perpetual motion machine which alone must be repaired. Homeopathy recognizes the mechanical and material body as an instrument and expression or outgrowth of a dominating life principle that is the internal or true man.

When this life force flows in order or harmony, health results; when any morbid influence affects the organism, the life force is first altered or interrupted and disease ensues.[2]

Of course, in cases of violence or accident any injury to the body or machine impairs the flow of life force; and mechanical or surgical measures are indicated and needed to restore order.[3]

Likewise in late cases of disease when organs are partly destroyed or morbid processes impinge on important nerves or vessels, mechanical measures are needed to correct faulty mechanics. But that by itself is often insufficient or unsuccessful (without the needed remedy) to bring about a harmonious play of vital function and orderly repair. Also, the cause of the morbid process is never removed with the knife, for that exists only in the disturbed life force; and remedies alone can change or modify that mysterious energy.

---

1. Today by drugs such as phenobarbital, dilantin and tegretol etc. - Editor.
2. Hahnemann, Samuel: Organon, Paragraphs 9 - 12. - Editor.
3. Together with a remedy to catalyze the repair. - Editor.

At this point it might be well to contract the instruments used by the two schools of medical thought. Each one's armamentarium is consistent with the concept held by each. Allopathy deals with material doses of powerful poisonous drugs to produce a so-called physiological action which is really a toxicological effect that always impairs healthy cells and tissues without repairing the diseased cells for they are overwhelmed by the drug action. Homeopathy employs drugs more or less attenuated; and because of their specific affinity for the diseased cells, the healthy cells of the organism remain untouched while the sick ones are simply spurred to increased activity and cure by the lightest touch, as it were, of the specific remedy.[1]

The various infections are looked upon as merely local points that can be cut or burned out for the most part by the self-styled scientific branch of medicine. Such treatment, however, sooner or later is followed by a more serious change in other body cells more vital than the first. To illustrate, the removal of the tonsils in children[2] is often followed by either chronic bronchitis, tuberculosis, appendicitis, mastoiditis and even asthma as well as heart and kidney inflammations of a serious nature. For the past decade, health departments and, I might add, the majority of physicians have made increasing and vigorous warfare on the tonsils of children. Few have escaped the mutilation of a God-given defense for the organism's protection. And what is the answer in vital statistics? An alarming increase in heart affections among children. Under homeopathic treatment most cases of diseased tonsils are as easily restored to normal as any of the so-called self-limiting acute diseases. In the treatment of chronic skin diseases such as eczema, psoriasis etc., our old school friends employ only local measures; and if they effect any change; it is one for the worse - suppression, which then manifests as chronic asthma or some serious gastro-intestinal disorder, ulcers etc.; even forms of Bright's disease have been caused by the suppression of chronic skin diseases with metallic salves.

In acute sickness the difference in methods and results is even more startling. What of pneumonia and other acute infections of the respiratory tract? Under the scientific ministrations of the old school, the patient is first weakened by cathartics to insure elimination; his fever is forced down by coal tars and salicylates; and then when the over-bur-

---

1. Cf. Beir; ibid.
2. Under hompeopathic treatment most cases of diseased tonsils are as easily restored to normal as any of the so-called self-limiting diseases.

dened heart begins to flag and loose its rhythm, strychnin or digitalis, according to the condition present, is given in heroic doses. Soon the undertaker is called in, to cover up the results of scientific medicine, for its losses are only short of appalling in these conditions. Pneumonia has no terrors to homeopaths, for only cases that have weakened hearts or kidneys, or those weakened by diseases like diabetes prior to the pneumonia die. And how wonderful and quick the indicated remedy changes the pneumonic process to a state of health, rest and warmth; and the indicated remedy is all sufficient for flu and pneumonia.

In migraine headaches, neuritis pains of various sorts and types, what a difference in the effects of treatment and what it all means to millions.

Under allopathic treatment opium or coal-tar drugs are used to stop the pain and force rest for only a brief period and then follows increased suffering and weakness with numerous so-called complications arising (that are often incurable).

These drastic drugs are the answer not only to the startling increase in heart and kidney diseases that recently have alarmed the statisticians; but because of the weakening of body resistance with the breaking down of vital organs by such measures, cancer and insanity are growing by leaps and bounds. And to think of it and know that all such cases before they are slugged and maimed by insane methods could be quickly and surely turned back to health and usefulness by the administration of remedies under the glorious law of similars. Is it any wonder then that men of the Ossler type become medical nihilists and prefer to trust the patient's chances to God and a competent nurse?

However, not all the old school medical men belong to either of the above mentioned extreme groups. Some are doing constructive work that is leading them on to the homeopathic concept of disease and its cure. Dr. Crile in his wonderful work, THE BIPOLAR THEORY OF LIVING PROCESSES,[1] envisages man as an electric man, a great storage battery with his 28 trillion bipolar electric cells which carry on all the multitudinous problems of life and present a self-regulating, self-repairing appartus of amazing parts. The numerous cells arranged into groups, organs and systems are separate units dominated by the organism as a whole to command co-operative work for the body's needs and preservation. This concept of man created and goverened, after the electric

---

1. Crile, George W.: A BIPOLAR THEORY OF LIVING PROCESSES, The Macmillan Co., New York, 1926. - Editor.

laws of the universe of which he is but a miniature prototype, acted on by and reacting to environmental forces of nature, approaches in character the heaven-endowed vital man (of Hahnemann) whose God-given vital force is alone sufficient to respond to the needed stimulus capable of restoring order and health to his sick organs[1].

Science has recently demonstrated that every form of life from the greatest sun in remote space to the tiniest bacterium of the ultra-microscope is endowed with electrical energy and is responsive to surrounding electric forces. Hence the universal law of polarity regulating and controlling every phenomenon in nature in health and in disease, all the affinities, the attractions and repulsions, that mark the growth and development of species and forms through out the mineral, animal and vegetable kingdom. And even the stupendous array of innumerable suns and universes, marshalled in an orderly march throughout the eternity of time and across the immeasurable vastness of boundless space swing in rhythmic tune to the play of this mighty mysterious force of life and being.

And as the horizon of our vision is extended in the field of electronics by the work of the physicists and scientists, we see more clearly the scientific aspects of Homeopathy shining resplendent and bright. The law of Similia consistent with the affinities of chemistry and tuned to the need of each individual patient; speaking a language of unmistakable meaning to guide the intelligent physician unerringly to the one needed medicant for each specific case. And the unique and peculiarly adaptable agents of cure Homeopathy employs, the potentized remedies, are the most amazing and suitable forces conceivable - pure electrolytes of measured and specific charges, that are drawn by their affinities to the cells and centers of disease, whereby equilibrium and order is established and the flow of vital processes resumed in the ruddy glow of health and well being.

---

1. Hahnemann, IBID.

GEMS OF HOMEOPATHIC THOUGHT FROM THE MASTERS[1]

There is more to be gained by a review of cardinal aphorisms based on the observations of some of our outstanding leaders of Homeopathic practice than I can give in a brief paper, and especially when there are no new or original statements to be added to the volumes of valuable knowledge already written and amassed concerning Homeopathic philosophy. It is a great asset to the Homeopathic profession of the world to have this fund of useful knowledge at its disposal to meet everyday needs in practice. A refresher course in Homeopathic philosophy even for those of us who are old and long in practice will repay us well, bringing sharper prescribing and improved end results of more cures.

Without a well ordered Homeopathic philosophic technique in the application of the similimum, the great law of Similia would loose much of its potentiality for cure. Many chronic cases started on the road to cure by the correct prescription have been aborted or spoiled because of an inadequate knowledge of the philosophy in the subsequent management of the case, such as prescribing another remedy or repeating the correct one too soon before the cycle of its action was complete.

Those versed in the philosophy may know by the reactions produced on the patient by the prescription, what to expect in terms of cure. The pace and direction of symptoms, the return of old conditions and symptoms, the appearance of the new symptoms and states are all sure indications of the processes of cure or the reverse that can come from an exact or an inexact prescription.

Perhaps the most important aspect of the philosophy is that pertaining to the taking of the history of the case after the manner originated by Hahnemann himself and followed so closely by Kent and other leaders and teachers of our art. The essentials of the instructions laid down in the ORGANON are as follows:[2] first to let the patient tell his story uninterrupted unless he diverges from the subject. After the history is written down, the physician may make specific inquires in quest of more information, but every question put to the patient must be an indirect one, that it may not suggest symptoms that do not belong to the patient's case; hence the answers cannot be answered yes or no;

---

1. From the handwritten manuscript of Dr. Grimmer, written in June 1956. - Editor.
2. §82 - 99. - Editor.

such answers are of doubtful value and should not be included in the array of positive facts in the symptoms gathered and relating to the sickness. Next the physician may consult relatives and close friends concerning their observations of the patient's illness, and finally the physician himself alerts all his senses and his observing powers in his search for symptoms and deviations from the normal state. When a case is fully taken after these methods, the search for the similar remedy begins. H. C. Allen, one of the illustrious prescribers and teachers of the past, remarked that a case properly and fully taken constituted one half the work required to make a successful prescription. In fact, without an accurate and complete history a successful prescription could hardly be made.

To grasp the spirit as well as the letter of the Homeopathic philosophy and to perceive the true origin of human sickness and its cure, one must read and incorporate into his whole being the first thirty six paragraphs of the ORGANON.

§1: The physician's highest and only calling is to restore health to the sick, which is called healing.

§2: The highest aim of healing is the speedy, gentle and permanent restoration of health, or alleviation and obliteration of disease in its entire extent in the shortest, most reliable and safest manner, according to clearly intelligible reasons.

§3: The physician should distinctly understand the following conditions: what is curable in disease in general, and in each individual case in particular, that is the recognition of disease (indication). He should clearly comprehend what is curative in drugs in general, and in each drug in particular; that is, he should possess a perfect knowledge of medicinal powers. He should be governed by distinct reasons, in order to insure recovery, by adapting what is curative in medicines to what he has recognized as undoubtedly morbid in a patient; that is to say, he should adapt it so that the case is met by a remedy well matched with regard to its kind of action (selection of the remedy indication) its necessary preparation and quantity (proper dose) and the proper time of its repetition. Finally when the physician knows in each case the obstacles in the way of recovery and how to remove them, he is prepared to act thoroughly, and to the purpose, as a true master of the art of healing.

§4: He is at the same time a preserver of health when he knows the causes that disturb health, that produce and maintain disease, and when he knows how to remove them from healthy persons.

§5: The physician in curing derives assistance from the knowledge of facts concerning the most probable cause of acute disease, as well as from the most significant points in the entire history of a case of chronic disease; aided by such knowledge, he is enabled to discover the primary cause of the latter, dependent mostly on a chronic miasm. In connection with this the bodily constitution of a patient (particularly if he has a chronic disease), the character of his mind and temperament, his occupation, his mode of living and habits, his social and domestic relations his age and sexual function, etc., are to be taken into consideration.

In these five paragraphs are contained the requirements and modes of action needed to be a Homeopathic physician. §9 through §12 impart the true but subtle and mysterious nature of man's sickness.

In §9 one reads: During the healthy condition of man his spirit-like force autocracy animating the material body (organism) rules supreme as dynamis. By it all parts are maintained wonderfully in harmonious vital process, both in feelings and functions in order that our intelligent mind may be free to make the living healthy body, a medium subservient to the higher purposes of our being.

We learn in §10: That the material organism without vital force is incapable of feeling activity or self preservation. This immaterial being (vital force) alone, animating the organism in the state of sickness and of health imparts the faculty of feeling and controls the functions of life.

§11: In sickness this spirit-like, self-acting (automatic) vital force, omnipresent in the organism, is alone primarily deranged by the dynamic influence of some morbific agency inimical to life. Only this abnormally modified vital force can excite morbid sensations in the organism, and determine the abnormal functional activity which we call disease. This force, itself invisible, becomes perceptible only through its effects upon the organism, makes known, and has no other way of making known its morbid disturbance to the observer and physician than by the manifestations of morbid feelings and functions, that is, by symptoms of disease in the whole material organism.

§12: Diseases are produced only by the morbidly disturbed vital force; hence the manifestations of disease discernible by our senses, at the same time represent every internal change (i.e. the entire morbid disturbance of the dyanamis, and expose to view, so to speak the whole disease). It follows that after the cure of such manifestations of disease, and all discoverable aberrations from healthy vital functions, their disappearance must necessarily and with equal certainty be presumed to result in, and to determine the restoration of the integrity of vital force, and the return of health of the entire organism.

From the facts presented in these opening paragraphs of the Organon we perceive the subtle occult aspects of life itself and the sickness to which it is subjected during its earthly journey and the nature of the curative force required to correct the evil.

Kent, one of the greatest aspostles of Hahnemann and a forceful teacher of the art and science of Homeopathy, defined the life force in common with all materials in the physical and phenomenal sides of nature as *simple substance*, the basic material from whence all force and forms in the Cosmos have their origin. Modern physics practically confirms this claim in the proven fact that all energy and matter are interchangeable and ultimately made up of tiny electric charges, positive and negative, neutral and bipolar in nature, electrons, protons, neutrons, etc. Thus we see that true science is beginning to prove some of the basic contents of Homeopathic science.

One more great name in American Homeopathy should be mentioned before closing this paper and that is Constantine Hering, author of the Guiding Symptoms, and many homeopathic works. He was a master prescriber, teacher, fearless explorer and the one who developed the great remedy LACH., at the risk of losing his life. Sent to repudiate the claims of Homeopathy his searching investigations led him by the force of truth and logic to espouse the cause and to become one of its staunchest and most effective champions. In his farwell address to the Graduating Class he gave the world of medicine an epic making fund of esoteric knowledge relating to the blood in health and in sickness that stands unrivaled.

The blood is the life, yes it is the man in solution, it carries nutrition to the remotest parts of the organism. It constantly purifies and revivifies the system in the wonderous exchange of gases, oxygen and carbon dioxide. Lastly it is the medium whereby the individual lives by direct contact with the Creator through the agency of the solar power which is known as prana by the wise men of the east. With the progress of true, not psuedo-science, Homeopathic truth will expand over the world in spite of every selfish effort to prevent its growth.

But we do have great need of more and younger homeopathic physicians to fill the ranks of the older men now passing. We must put forth a united effort to bring to the world more Homeopathic doctors to meet the needs of future generations. We have the foundations and groundwork engendered by the untiring labors of the Masters who have gone to their reward, leaving a rich heritage of philosophic truth. Shall we let all that fade away and be lost to the needs of the children of the future? Are we too tired and indifferent to salvage and save this precious gift of healing? The answer is near at hand and with us all.

FLASHES OF MEDICAL WISDOM[1]

Tennyson, the great English poet and philosopher, said, "Knowledge comes but wisdom lingers". And in the realm of medicine more than elsewhere is this most patent fact true. The public is deluged with an ever increasing flood of medical knowledge through the medium of the press and radio. Most of this knowledge is commercialized propaganda designed to increase the revenue of drug manufacturers and dispensers. These unscrupulous racketeers of public health urge all those who suffer from any form of pain or headache or sleeplessness, regardless of the causative factors, and without a physician consultation, to take large and continuous doses of pernicious, blood-destroying, coal-tar drugs for the relief of their sufferings. When nerves are wrecked and the blood stream vitiated and impaired, they then advise large and larger doses of vitamins and so-called tonics, ostensibly to rebuild wrecked constitutions but really to fatten the already plethoric coffers of the drug vendors. That this medical knowledge comes from the journals of regular and accepted medicine and is endorsed by the majority of old school physicians in no way lessens the evil; in fact it tends to increase the evil because of the stamp of authority carried by such origin and endorsement.

The current medical machine of empiricism is constantly grinding out new so-called discoveries in medicine, new germs and viruses, new serums, vaccines and drugs, from the germ of stale beer (which is said to be much more efficient against the streptococcus than even the sulpha miracle drugs) to the recent drug, calcium pantothenate, guaranteed to turn the gray heads of tottering age back to the luxurious hues of perennial youth. All this mass of ever expanding knowledge announced and given the public by allopathic medicine especially in its application to the sick is long on propaganda for selfish reasons, and short of any true wisdom.

But as we journey along the highway of medical history, we find here and there along the way a flash of medical genius or a pearl of wisdom nestled in the mire of superstition and ignorance.

Without doubt the most potent and fundamental discovery in medicine is the *Law of Similars* given the world by Samuel Hahnemann. The influence of this discovery is universal and eternal. It is the greatest single stroke of medical genius the world has ever known; and the wisdom

---

1. "Editorial" in THE HOMEOPATHIC RECORDER, Vol. LVIII, No. 1, July, 1942, p. 49.

of this knowledge may be summed up in the first paragraph of the Organon: "The physician's high and only mission is to restore the sick to health, to cure, as it is termed".[1] No better guide was ever given as a working formula for the men of medicine than this simple yet complete statement.

Who can ever measure or calculate the full worth of Harvey's discovery of the circulation of the blood at that time in the then barren field of medicine, begetting the sciences of physiology, anatomy and surgery to add to man's knowledge and benefit him in his afflictions? And these benefits grew, and continue to grow with the wisdom of the application of that knowledge.

Certain physiologic experiments prove that great danger attends the injection of foreign proteins and other substances in the blood stream; yet, in the face of these dangers, some medical empirists attempt to promote health by violating the logic of proven facts and inject not one but a multitude of serums and vaccines into the blood stream of all who will or can be forced to submit to such illogical and dangerous procedures. Clinical observation in numerous cases thus treated reveals serious symptoms of complex and chronic disease lasting, in some instances, a life time.

Traditional medicine, from the time of ancient Egypt to the present, consists of many dividing sections known as specialities. It is interesting and enlightening to know what one of the greatest scientists in medicine of modern times, Alexis Carrel, has to say concerning specialists in medicine. A brief quotation from his recent book, Man The Unknown, is truly illuminating. It is regrettable that Dr. Morris Fishbein, the man of minimum practice and maximum theory, did not have recourse to the wisdom found in this book before he wrote his treatise on "Medical Follies", wherein he displayed a most pitiful ignorance concerning the philosophy and practice of homeopathy. Could he, Dr. Fishbein, have availed himself of the brief knowledge concerning specialists so lucidly given by Dr. Carrel, it is doubtful if the attack on homeopathy would have been made. "Man cannot be separated into parts. He would cease to exist if his organs were isolated from one another."[2] This is consistent with Hahnemann's concept of the totality of the symptoms. "Still more harm is caused by the extreme specialization of the physicians.

---

1. Hahnemann Samuel: ORGANON OF MEDICINE, Sixth Edition, translated by W. Boericke, 1921. §1. - Editor.
2. Carrell, Alexis (1873 - 1944): MAN THE UNKNOWN, Harper, 31st ed., 1935, p. 44.

Medicine has separated the sick human being into small fragments and each fragment has its specialist. When a specialist from the beginning of his career confines himself to a minute part of the body, his knowledge of the rest is so rudimentary that he is incapable of thoroughly understanding even that part in which he specializes."[1] These statements are self-evident to every homeopath, but old school physicians in civil and military life bounce the hapless patient from specialist to specialist as long as life and finances hold out. Why can they not learn the simple truth that man is *greater* than any of his parts and equal to the sum of all his parts?

One more quotation to illustrate the valueless and uncertain or misleading knowledge, especially relating to medicine, coming from the daily press. "The daily press often gives us the dubious benefit of the sociological, economic, and scientific opinions of manufacturers, bankers, lawyers, professors, physicians, whose highly specialized minds are incapable of apprehending in their breadth the momentous problems of our time." How aptly this tells us that what we get from the daily press is largely the opinion of men divorced from the underlying laws relating to the subjects discussed. Hence, only the statements that are based on discovered laws are logical and acceptable to the real thinker, who, like the alchemist of old, transmuted his base knowledge into nuggets of golden wisdom. If one would obtain a clear, logical, and comprehensive view of medicine, be he physician or layman, he would find it well worth while to read and reread that wonderful book, Man the Unknown, written by Dr. Alexis Carrel.

One of the injunctions of Hahnemann in his Organon, §4 and §5, is that the physician should know the causes of sickness and remove them. Among the most frequent causes of illness of our present time is the wholesale and injudicious use of pain-allaying and sleep-producing drugs, all blood destroying and nerve-wrecking agents. Therefore, it is the urgent duty of every physician, regardless of his medical affiliation, to condemn this wholesale propaganda for the universal use of all toxic drugs for the general public without competent medical advice. It likewise becomes the physician's duty to instruct his patients and the public of the dangers to life and health existing in the ignorant use of all the myriad drugs advertised as pain and sleep palliatives, via radio, magazines and newspapers. This commercialized evil is fast undermining the nation's health and stamina; and it is strictly up to the physicians of our

1.   Carrell, Alexis: ibid, p. 46.

land, but more especially those physicians who are in authority, to correct such serious conditions by education and guidance. This is a splendid opening for the "Society For the Prevention of Heart Disease" to do some real constructive work; up to the present, no word of disapproval of the dangers lurking in the coal tar drugs to heart sufferers has come from this organization. It surely cannot be that the sacred precincts of commercial greed would be permitted to inhibit the usefulness of a society organized for purposes of disease prevention and the elimination of exciting or other causes.

Diet and Health[1]

Basic needs

The most essential ingredient in the life of the whole animal world is food; without it there can be no growth or repair of the waste resulting from the metabolic changes incidental to life's multitudinous and complex processes.

Primitive men, like animals and the insects, obtained their food raw and unprepared or processed direct from their environment. And these simple foods contained all the elements essential to the needs of life throughout generations of evolving species. Man alone has departed from the natural methods of obtaining his food in his evolution of growth and intelligence toward a higher plane of life.

But by refining and processing his food, many of the essential vitamins and minerals have been lost or greatly reduced to produce weakness, disease and abnormal growth (pathology) in his body, in place of health and normal cell growth, which obtains with the use of a normal diet replete with all the essential vitamins and minerals needed for body growth and repair.

In the study of nutrition and food we must include a sufficient water intake as part of the nutritional substances or food, for the body is roughly composed of three-fouths water and one-fourth solid material. Another aspect of nutrition, often lost sight of, is that of oxygen supplied by the intake of sufficient pure air by way of the lungs to expel the waste carbon dioxide and replace it with life-giving oxygen to purify the blood. And to produce all these subtle but necessary functions prepared by the autonomic nervous system which takes care of all the involuntary functions of the body organism, such as respiration, heart beat, circulation of the blood, endocrine activity, digestion of foods and all the processes of elimination of waste material from the body. These processes are produced by oxidation action to engender the electric waves and currents in the organism that furnish the motive and nerve force necessary for the consumation of the organisms multiplicities of automatic functions.

From the foregoing we see that a healthy body, to continue to exist and function in the world of matter, must have first, a proper supply of pure air to cleanse the blood stream of chemical poisons, and to furnish

---

1. From the handwritten manuscript of Dr. Grimmer, exact date unknown. - Editor.

the electric force in the body that enables it to perform those subtle and amazing processes for its preservation and growth[1]. We can exist only a short time without oxygen.

The second need in the nutritional plan is a sufficient amount of pure water to aid in the solution and distribution of salts and minerals and in the circulation of blood and lymph and other fluids throughout the body organism as well as aiding in the elimination of waste and toxins from the body. The human being can exist only a few days without water.

The third need in nutrition is that of food proper coming in its various forms such as fruits, vegetables, dairy products, cereals and the flesh of animals all of which may be classified into specific groups as follows: fats, starches, and sugars, and proteins.

Fats, starches, and sugar furnish the body with heat and energy, and tend to build up the fatty tissue of the body as a store of energy. The proteins build up the muscle cells and tissues in the body. The fruits, vegetables, dairy products and cereals furnish the necessary vitamins and minerals needed by the body's assimilative system.

For the best results in nutrition all the elements and varieties of food so far mentioned must be given in their pure and unaduterated form.

POLLUTION

In this time of so-called scientific progress we find our processed food deprived of much of its essential mineral and vitamin contents. Other foods are adulterated with harmful preservatives, and still other foods, such as vegetables and fruits, are poisoned by poison sprays which enter the body by continuous minute doses eventually building into toxic amounts to produce disease and suffering and to nullify the nutritional value of the food.

Today many of our large cities including Chicago are forced to supply their citizens with a water supply poisoned with fluorine and chlorine. This unhappy state of affairs was forced upon the public in spite of organized protests from large representative groups. Much ill health will result from such high-handed dictatorship of a few willful men jeopardizing the health and ignoring the vested rights of millions. The constant intake of poisoned water will inevitably weaken the resistance of many people against disease contamination and many forms of dis-

---

1. Crile, George W.: A BIPOLAR THEORY OF LIVING PROCESSES, The Macmillan Co., New York, 1926. - Editor.

ease may be activated, thereby fanning the seeds of chronic disease into activity. Of course, after much suffering and financial loss, this will be repudiated and changed in the future; in fact, such is already taking place in many localities that pursued the irrational action of poisoning the water supply under the unproven pretext of preventing children's teeth from decay upon an unsuspecting citizenship.

Last but not least of the nutritional elements of food is pure air. Polluted air causes severe types of respiratory disease and a poisoned blood stream to usher in a host of other sick-making evils that result from impoverished blood, and diseases of nerves.

DIET DURING DIFFERENT PERIODS OF LIFE

Certain foods are applicable to certain periods in life. By the careful selection of diet re-enforced by the homeopathicaly indicated remedy, the steps of "Father Time" himself can be slowed to a creep holding back the aging process in an amazing way. Those in middle life and past need to exert special care in selecting only the purest of natural foods composed largely of fruits and green vegetables free of poison sprays; pure uncontaminated and unprocessed dairy products are next in order with moderate amounts of cereals and nuts to re-enforce small amounts of meat proteins. Eggs, cheese, avocados, pears are good proteins and can substitute for excess of meat which is so loaded with uric acid - one of the aging agents. Fats and egg yolks tend to be causative factors with aging process because of their cholesterol content.

Abundance of pure water is not only nutritional but a great aid in the elimination of toxic material from the body through the kidneys, bowels, and sweat glands of the skin.

By far the most urgent and important sustenance in the maintaince of life is the vitalizing oxygen coming to us by way of the air through the medium of the lungs. Remember we can exist but a few minutes without this God-given ingredient of life. Atmospheric air is made up of a mixture of oxygen and nitrogen with a few other rare gases in very small amounts. Just why nitrogen and oxygen are free and uncombined in the air we breathe and live in I have never heard explained; we only know these elements have been properly blended for our needs by a benign Providence. We also know that the magical formula of atmospheric air is the first and most potent sustainer of life throughout all creation.

The other extreme of life, the very young, requires a very simple but highly nutritious type of food best expressed in the formulas that nearest approach that of Mother's milk, which is rightly named the milk of human kindness, but in these foxy times it is more properly named the milk of bovine kindness since so much of it comes from that source. With growth and development, the simple diet of the infant progressively changes with the pace of that growth.

DIET IN SPECIFIC DISEASES

Certain types of human beings as the over corpulent have need of a specific diet to meet their individual needs; generally a diet rich in proteins and reduced fats and starches, interspaced with fruits and green vegetables.

On the other hand, those who are under weight require a diet rich in starches, cereals, fats, etc., and enough of the fruits and vegetables to furnish a rich vitamin content and plenty of milk products for the necessary calcium.

Such sicknesses as anemia require organic iron contained in specific food such as the livers and flesh of animals and certain fruits such as raisins, figs, prunes and dates together with numerous greens.

Diabetics must avoid sugars and starches or cut them down to a minimum amount; only limited amounts of natural uncooked sweets such as honey and the juices and pulp of fruits are permitted to add energy increase without raising the sugar content of the blood too high.

Persons suffering from liver and gallbladder disease must avoid excess of fats and sugars in order to restore normal liver functions.

Those who suffer from arthritic and catarrhal conditions must limit their starches and sugars as well as the excess of meat proteins and also limit their intake of tea and coffee to extremely limited amounts to more readily free the blood stream acid excess. Organic calcium found in milk and cereals together with potassium found in plants, green vegetables and fruits are most important factors in maintaining the health of the organism by maintaining the alkalinity of the blood, and aiding the repair of injuries to bones, glands, and tissues of the body organism.

Many special tables and diet lists have been produced by experts for those suffering from certain disease conditions, but not altogether satisfactory, because these experts lost sight of the ever-present fact that each individual is a law unto himself with his own individual blood chemistry, his own peculiar food desires and aversions, and his own idiosyncrasies, sensitivities and allergies.

To obtain the best results in dietary science each patient should have a special diet selected for him as his homeopathic remedies are selected to fit his individual needs.

Homeopathic doctors have long observed that patients under the action of certain drugs are sensitive to certain types of food.

Thus, the Lyc. patient is sensitive to coffee which he craves, and to onions and tomatoes to which he is averse. Thuj. also is aggravated by onions. Sil. and Lac-d. are averse to and aggravated by milk and many of its products. Carb-v. and Puls. are averse and aggravated by fats, pork, etc. Puls. craves butter which aggravates if too much is taken.

Children who eat lead pencils and chalk need Calc-p., Graph., Nit-ac., Sil. Ars., Nit-ac. and Nux-v. craves fats, and they agree except in the case of Ars. Nux-v. craves spices, peppers and highly seasoned foods. Nat-m., Phos. and Carb-v. crave salt and salty things. Lyc. and Carb-v. crave sweets and sugars; Ars. and Graph. are averse to them.

Thus we see that the individual patient needs a specific list of foods compatible to him alone as much as he needs the one indicated remedy which alone is suited to his case.

CURE VERSUS SUPPRESSION[1]

All are familiar with the definition and meaning of cure. To cure is to restore a sick person to health and to remove all the bad effects of disease. When this is done the vital processes are normalized and the defensive mechanism of the body is operating to bring up the body resistance against all sick making forces such as infections, allergies, emotional stress, etc.

Suppression, on the other hand, depresses the vital process and lowers body resistance to sick making influences. Invariably suppression is the direct result of palliation of disease in many of its manifestations. Pains of various types, headache, neuralgias, arthritis, etc. are too often relieved by pain killing analgesic drugs such as aspirin, anacin, barbiturates and many other forms of drugs derived from the coal-tar elements.

These things are not only, not curative, but they are harmful toxic agents that stop pain by depriving the organism of its sensitivity to pain and to all feeling as well. They are known as depressants. They disturb the rhythm of the autonomic nervous system, that system which unites our etheric and physical bodies to bring us in contact with the causative forces of the Cosmos which reach us by influx from the sun and the higher planes of being. These vibratory forces are the sustaining and regenerating forces of life; without them there would be no life.

This intimate relationship[2] between the physical body with the deeper unseen forces and planes of he Cosmos is the reason that drugs and various poisons can harm and even destroy the physical body. The sustaining forces of life are inhibited or cut off from the life force of the body which soon ends in deterioration and death of the body organism.

A still deeper and more pernicious forms of suppression exists on the emotional sphere of those unfortunate humans who have been poisoned with the mood drugs and the sleep producers. These things bring temporary relief which soon passes and leaves the patient helpless and hopeless with no possibility of help outside the scope of Homeopathy.

And the homeopathic physician's task is made very difficult in the face of a drug disease added to the natural original ailment of the patient. First the drug miasm must be eradicated and that often takes

1. From the handwritten manuscript of Dr. Grimmer, exact date unknown. - Editor.
2. via the autonomic nervous system. - Editor.

much time and patience on the part of both patient and physician, before the natural sickness can be treated and cured. But with courage, intelligence, and faith in Divine goodness on the part of both a complete cure can be achieved.

Other forms of suppression are those relating to the skin and mucous membranes. On the skin eruptions like an eczema may be driven inward and suppressed by powerful salves or ointments, or by the intensive application of ultra violet and X-rays. When this is done the patient will soon suffer with severe attacks of asthma which will be with him until his dying day if the suppression is not brought back to its original site on the skin through the medium of the internal homeopathic remedy. Many cases of chronic asthma date back to the suppression of a constitutional rash in early childhood lasting into late adulthood. For such a sufferer, only the restoration of that rash by means of Homeopathy can cure their asthmatic suffering.

In the suppression of catarrhal discharges from mucous membranes, especially the sycotic type, these victims of medical ignorance will suffer from severe types of neuralgias and rheumatoid pains and inflammations until the suppressed discharge is reproduced under the influence of the homeopathic remedy.[1]

A lack of philosophic knowledge concerning the nature and causes of disease on the part of the physician, together with his inadequate understanding of the inherent power of drugs for either good or evil according to the way in which they are prepared and applied is the main factor in the ever increasing virulency and malignancy of disease in the human race today. And this evil will grow as long as a soulless commercialism prevails in the ranks of medicine. So long as vast amounts of money can be made in the manufacture and sale of drugs and vaccines whose values are uncertain or unknown these afflictions will exist. Only a campaign of universal enlightenment can correct these evils which aggravate and prolong the suffering of the sick. Such a task is almost impossible in the face of vast and intensive propaganda of selfish interests that constantly bombards the public by way of radio, television and the printed page with plausible and enticing accounts of the numerous ever increasing nostrums of empirical commercialized medicine. These things grow and increase like noxious toadstools in a malarial swamp.

---

1. All suppressions that return under the indicated remedy eventually vanish to leave behind perfect health. - Editor.

Only when the men of medicine again become imbued with the glorious traditions and ideals that prevailed in the realm and time of Hippocrates, aptly called the father of medicine, can we hope to see a better nobler practice of medicine in vogue.

Outside of surgery there has been no real advance in the practice of medicine since the dark ages when the intellectual light of the world was dimmed so long. General and so called scientific medicine is without a guiding philosophy, the supposed science which guides it is but a fragmentary array of empirical procedures adjusted to suit the whims of individual experimenters. Its so called code of ethics is but a means to enable a few to reap a harvest in wealth and position, while the many must be content to thrive on the leftover crumbs of the banquet table. Without a guiding philosophy or an inspiring program of ideals concerning human sympathy and understanding, no system of healing can long endure.

In closing I wish to dwell on the fact, that Homeopathy, with its science based on proven law and its tried and proved philosophic concept of disease cause and its cure, is the one force left in the world, that under the guidance of Divine Providence can restore the practice of medicine again to the high and honored place it once held in the days of ancient Greece when duty and sacrifice were the guiding lights that illumined the pathway of the votaries of the healing art. May the radiance of those lights soar again, ultimate the ranks of modern medicine and all its fractions to enable them to free themselves from the deadly thralldom of commercialized medicine steeped in the dregs of avarice.

50 Millesimal Potencies[1]

To Homeopaths, the 6th Edition of the Organon of Medicine is of great interest for the reason that it gives the Master's last words based on his lifelong experience. During the last years of his life, Hahnemann was deeply engaged in his research for finding ways of effecting cure more quickly but without any risk of aggravation. 50 Millesimal Potencies are the fruits of his invaluable efforts.

What They are and How Denoted

50 Millesimals are Homeopathic potencies prepared in the 1:50,000 scale as distinct from the Centesimal (1:100) and the Decimal (1:10) scales. He would prepare **ALL** remedies by **TRITURATION** up to the 3C scale (1:100) and would dilute this in purified alcohol, taking then only **one drop** of this basic preparation to impregnate **500** of the No. 10 very small granules of globules. After drying them upon a white blotter paper, one of these tiny little globules was dissolved in a drop of distilled water, and to this drop 99 drops of 95% alcohol were added, a proportion that would establish the 50 Millesimal scale. This step would constitute the o/1 fifty millesimal potency. Preparation of these potencies has been advocated and explained by the Master in §270 of the 6th Edition of his Organon, and the potencies are denoted by a "o" prefix as follows: o/1, o/2, o/3, o/4, ... o/40, etc. The prefix "o" used as a symbol of a small globule to differentiate from a drop used for the other scales.

Although the manuscript of the **6th** German edition of the Organon was completed by the Master in 1842, for reasons not worthwhile mentioning here, it was withheld from the profession and could not be translated into English and published before 1922 in spite of repeated efforts by his worthy disciples and followers. Even after it was published only a few (like Dr. Pahud of Lausanne) took notice of the great changes advocated by Hahnemann therein till they were able and very forcefully brought to light by Dr. Pierre Schmidt, M.D. of Geneva, in an article entitled, "The Hidden Treasures of the Last Organon" published in the July-October 1954 issue of the British Homeopathic Journal.

Since then these potencies have been tested at the bedside with tremendous success, so much so that in an article entitled, "The Need for What They Are and How Denoted" addition of the o/30 potency of

---

1. From the handwritten manuscript of Dr. Grimmer, exact date unknown. - Editor.

What They are and How Denoted ...

the new scale seems to have been much more powerful than the CM of the Centesimal.

Their Advantages Over the Centesimal and Decimal Scales

1. **Highest development of power.** For Hahnemann recommended giving **100** forceful succussions to each potency instead of the 2 to 10 that had been suggested for the Centesimal scale.

2. **Mildest reaction.** Can be safely used even in desperate cases without fear of a dangerous aggravation.

3. **Frequent repetition permissible.** Even medicines of a long continued action may be repeated every hour or oftener in urgent acute cases, daily or every other day in chronic cases.[1]

4. **Quick cure of chronic cases.** The period of treatment may be diminished to one-half, one-quarter, or even still less. By repeated deviated doses (at least one step higher), the duration of suffering of the patient is amazingly shortened and cure strikingly enhanced.[2]

Excerpts from Organon, 6th Edition

"What I said in the 5th Edition of the Organon, in a long note to this paragraph, in order to prevent these undesirable reactions of the vital energy, was all that the experience I then had justified. But during the last four or five years, however, all these difficulties are wholly solved by my new altered but perfected method. The same carefully selected medicine may now be given daily and for months, if necessary in this way, namely, after the lower degree of potency has been used for one or two weeks in the treatment of chronic diseases, advance is made in the same way to higher degrees (beginning according to the new dynamization method, taught here with the use of the lower degrees)." Footnote, §246, ... "it must be a matter of great importance to the physician as well as to the patient that were it possible, this period should be diminished to a half, one-quarter, and even still less so that a much more rapid cure might be obtained. And this may be very happily effected, as recent and often-repeated observations have taught me under the following conditions:

---

1. Organon §248. - Editor.
2. Organon §246. - Editor.

EXCERPTS FROM ORGANON, 6TH EDITION ...

1) If the medicine selected with the utmost care was perfectly homeopathic;

2) If it is highly potentized, dissolved in water and given in proper small dose that experience has taught as the most suitable in definite intervals for the quickest accomplishment of cure,

3) But with the precaution **that the degree of every dose deviate somewhat from the preceding and the following**, in order that the vital principle which is to be altered by the similar medicinal effect be not aroused to untoward reactions and revolt as is always the case with unmodified and especially rapidly repeated doses." §246.

"It is impractical to repeat the same unchanged dose of a remedy once, not to mention its frequent repetition. But if the succeeding dose is changed slightly everytime, namely potentized somewhat higher, (§269, §270) then the vital principle may be altered without difficulty by the same medicine, (the sensation of natural disease diminishing) and thus the cure brought nearer." §247.

"Such a globule, placed dry upon the tongue, is one of the smallest doses for a moderated recent case of illness. Here but few nerves are touched by the medicine. A similar globule, crushed with some sugar of milk and dissolved in a good deal of water (Footnote to §247) and stirred well before every administration will produce a far more powerful medicine for the use of several days. Every dose, no matter how minute, touches, on the contrary, many nerves." §272.

"For this purpose, we potentize anew the medical solution (with perhaps 8, 10, 12 successions) from which we give the patient one or (increasingly) several teaspoonful doses, in long lasting diseases daily or every second day, in acute disease every two to six hours and in very urgent cases every hour or oftener. Thus in chronic diseases, every correctly chosen homeopathic medicine, even one whose action is of long duration, may be repeated daily for months with ever increasing success. If the solution is used up (in seven to fifteen days) it is necessary to add to the next solution of the same medicine, if still indicated, one or (though rarely) several pellets of a higher potency with which we continue so long as the patient experiences continued improvement without encountering one or another complaint that he never had in his life. For if this happens, if the balance of the disease appears in a **group of**

altered symptoms then another, one more homeopathically related medicine must be chosen in place of the last, and administered in the same repeated doses[1] mindful, however, of modifying the solution of every dose with thorough, vigorous succussions, thus changing its degree of potency and increasing it somewhat." §248.

---

1. Organon §176 - §184 and especially §183. - Editor.

Clinical Cases

A Few Clinical Cases

Clinical Cases

Homeopathic Confirmations

A Case of Coronary Insufficiency

Homeopathy Versus the Specialist

Clinical Failures

Some Clinical Cases

Typical Clinical Versus Atypical Cases

Cases from Practice

Homeopathic Clinical Cases

A few Clinical Cases[1]

The things we learn from a review of clinical cases are valuable, not only in confirming the law of cure but in developing and extending the philosophy of homeopathy; and in that way prescribers grow in knowledge and efficiency in the administration of both the Art and Science of their chosen profession.

Uterine Tumor Mrs. B. B. age 50

April 15, 1952. has a persistant uterine bleeding since last September, 1951. Flow bright red and not many clots. Good general health, married twenty-four years, never pregnant. No knowledge of family history except father had epilepsy and died of uremic poisoning. Mother living at 75. One brother mentally defective and sick all his life. Three sisters living; one had thrombosis. Patient flowed heavily at periods all her life.

There is little to prescribe on here, mostly common symptoms and those of pathology being present. An electro-magnetic blood test revealed the presence of cystic tumor in the pelvis and toxemia of aluminum in the system.

As I have stated many times before, one will get but little beneficial action with the indicated remedy in these cases until he has removed the source of the toxin and the toxin itself from the system. This toxin acts much like one of the miasms of Hahnemann in preventing the cure of the case until the patient is free of the inhibiting miasm. Cadm-o. is the most certain antidote in my experience against aluminum toxins in the blood, and I generally prescribe this drug at first in all these cases.

But this case was covered best by Calc-ox. 1M; it was given, and the patient advised to discard her aluminum cooking utensils.

May 8, 1952. Better after a week's aggravation. Had two days of headache after remedy. Hot sun aggravated headache. Weighs 126.5 lbs.; Calc-ox. 1M.

June 5, 1952. Had a prolonged aggravation but better last few days. Weighs 136 lbs., a ten pound gain. Is taking a trip to Europe for some months. Calc-ox. 10M.

October 2, 1952. Back from Europe. Has been better until recently. Weight 138. Calc-ox. 10M.

---

1. The Homeopathic Recorder, Vol. LXIX, No. 9, March, 1954, p. 240.

Uterine Tumor Mrs. B. B. age 50 ...

November 7, 1952. Had had a great increase of hemorrhage with aching in legs preventing sleep. Has drunk hawthorn tea. Flow bright red with clots and copious flow worse when lying down. This symptom is characteristic of Mag-c.[1] Is worried over her condition. Mag-c. 10M.

November 17, 1952. Bleeding very slight, but examination reveals a large uterine cyst filling the upper vaginal tract. Continued on Sacch-l.

December 19, 1952. Hemorrhage better but has distressing burning sensation. Mag-c. 10M.

January 29, 1953. Bleeding worse the last few days but had two weeks of freedom from hemorrhage. Mag-c. 50M.

February 9, 1953. Has a number of infected and very painful teeth needing extraction. Heat relieves the pain. Hemorrhage much less. Some chilliness with constant pain in teeth. Sil. 10M.

April 13, 1953. Improved with all tooth pain gone. Sil. 50M.

May 22, 1953. No hemorrhage, no pain in teeth. Has had no extractions. Sil. 50M.

The patient feels and looks well and is free of symptoms. I have not checked the cyst yet by re-examination, but I am confident that it is gone or is on the way out.

Uterine Cancer Mrs. S. S. B. 50 years old

April 24, 1934. Treated recently with radium for persistant uterine flow. Diagnosis is uterine cancer. Since radium treatment, hemorrhage is less but has a very sore necrotic uterus. Cadm-i. and Phos. are antidotes to radium burns. Cadm-i. 10M.

May 7, 1934. Now suffering more from bladder irritation and frequency. Sabal. 10M.

July 30, 1935. Better except a soreness of right knee. Cadm-i. 50M.

March 1, 1936. Cadm-i. 50M.

1.　C.M. Boger gives the symptom: Menses only when lying: Mag-c. on p. 452 of this Repertory.
   - Editor

UTERINE CANCER MRS. S. S. B. 50 YEARS OLD ...

December 14, 1936. Knee swelling and painful again, uterus not bothering her. CADM-I. 50M.

March 11, 1937. Constipated but is some better. CALC-F. 10M.

April 24, 1937. Constipation some better. CALC-F. 10M.

July 16, 1937. CALC-F. 10M.

November 5, 1937. Constipation persists. CALC-F. CM.

October 25, 1938. Has been very well in every way. CALC-F. CM.

December 6, 1939. CALC-F. CM.

November 7, 1940. Return of urinary disturbance and frequency. SABAL. 50M.

May 24, 1941. Right side of nape stiff and sore on turning head. Heat seems to aggravate, cervical glands swollen and sore. A little uterine discharge. GRAPH. 10M.

January 6, 1943. Has had only slight colds and minor complaints for which she took homeopathic remedies on her own. CADM-I. CM.

February 10, 1943. Pain in left hip is leaving hip and going to ankle. Has great heat flashes. Continued on SACCH-L.

March 22, 1943. Headache bothers a great deal (old symptom). Continued on SACCH-L.

November 4, 1943. Pain in knee better but now has pain in left arm. Headaches are lighter. CADM-I. CM.

December 30, 1943. Digestive upset from dietary indiscretion. CARB-V. 10M.

June 5, 1943. Fills up too easily. LYC. 10M.

January 10, 1944. Heat flashes. LACH. 1M.

April 21, 1944. More and constant nausea. CADM-S. 30.

October 2, 1944. Copious appetite. LYC. 10M.

November 4, 1947. Bowels sluggish, bad taste, some nausea at times. CADM-I. 10M.

Uterine Cancer Mrs. S. S. B. 50 years old ...

December 30, 1947. Severe flu, cold (coryza) with chills and fever. Restless, exhausted, copious diarrhea, vomiting, swelling in right side liver region. Very apprehensive. Ars. 10M.

May 11, 1948. Cadm-i. 10M.

September 14, 1948. Had gall bladder removed. Last January had a severe burn followed by loss of strength and weight. No pain but nauseated and poor appetite, some jaundice, likes warm sunshine. Feet cold at night, no thirst, sleeps well but wakens too early, constipated. Sep. 10M.

September 20, 1948. Cadm-met. 10M.

December 20, 1948. Better. Continued on Sacch-l.

January 6, 1949. Some nausea at times. Cadm-met. 10M.

February 11, 1949. Cadm-met. 10M.

March 17, 1949. Cadm-met. 50M.

April 28, 1949. Better. Cadm-met. 50M.

June 6, 1949. Better until she caught cold. Cadm-met. 50M.

August 29, 1949. Weighs 145 1/2 lbs. Feeling well. Continued with Sacch-l.

September 27, 1949. Cadm-met. CM.

October 27, 1949. Pain right arm very painful and better at rest. Continued.

November 4, 1949. Persistant pain in right arm, neuritis. Caust. 10M.

November 21, 1949. For pain in kidney region. Thuj. 10M.

In 1950 this patient had a kidney removed and returned to my care.

November 19, 1951. Got along well after kidney removed. No urinary frequency, appetite good, sleeps well. Blood test brought in Kali-c. 10M.

December 10, 1952. Old bilious headache and retention of urine. Return of old symptoms. Continued on Sacch-l.

December 20, 1951. Cadm-o. 200.

Uterine Cancer Mrs. S. S. B. 50 years old ...

April 27, 1952. Loosing appetite and weight, some shoulder pain, kidney working well, bowels fair. Cadm-o. 1M.

July 7, 1952. Some better but extremely weak. Cadm-o. 1M.

September 22, 1952. Very tired from strain but is sleeping much better after last remedy. Cadm-o. 10M.

December 22, 1952. Cadm-o. 10M.

December 26, 1952. Much better after last remedy. Continued on Sacch-l.

April 3, 1953. Better until she injured her knee. Cadm-o. 10M.

This is a case of uterine cancer, diagnosis from biopsy, that has endured the strain of living for twenty years. She raised her family, nursed her husband through a long illness which ended in his death and passed through two major operations when the gall bladder and kidney were removed. Now at seventy she carries on more comfortably than the average person of her age, thanks to the homeopathic remedies.

This case is not presented as a cure but as evidence of the tremendous possibilities that the persistant, and intelligent application of the homeopathic remedy can obtain.[1]

Carcinoma of Uterus Mrs. R.C. W. age 48

Another case of uterine cancer who did not have radium, X-ray or surgicial intervention.

In the menopause period, had a rapidly growing uterine tumor with a constant flow of dark blood, at times considerable pain. Was weak and cachectic. Biopsy diagnosis was carcinoma.

November 10, 1947. Cadm-met. 10M.

December 9, 1947. Cadm-met. 10M.

December 14, 1947. Less hemorrhage, generally feeling better. Continued on Sacch-l.

---

1. This case is an example of Observation No. 7 discussed by Kent in Lecture XXXV, Prognosis after Observing the Action of the Remedy, Lectures on Homeopathic Philosophy. However Dr. Grimmer, by his persistent and thoughtful prescriptions has done wonderful healing for this patient. - Editor.

CARCINOMA OF UTERUS MRS. R.C. W. AGE 48 ...

December 29, 1947. CADM-MET. 50M.

January 23, 1948. CADM-MET. 50M.

February 27, 1948. CADM-MET. CM.

April 5, 1948. CADM-MET. CM.

June 5, 1948. CADM-MET. CM.

November 9, 1948. Much better every way. Pelvic findings normal. CADM-MET. CM.

September 15, 1949. CADM-MET. 200.

September 26, 1950. CADM-MET. 30.

Nothing further was heard from this patient except continued reports of good health. Then in May, 1951, patient reported frequency of menses without pain or other adverse symptoms. CALC-S. 10M was sufficient to correct this condition.

In two years by a series of potencies of a single remedy, CADM-MET.; this patient was restored to normal and remains so four years later. homeopathy speaks for itself, and it brings joy to patient and physician alike. Thus far, no other system of healing can compare with the gentleness and certainty of the homeopathic law.

Clinical Cases [1]

Epilepsy

Epilepsy in a girl fourteen. Always in good health, no serious sickness; even the childhood diseases were always mild and soon passed. No injuries to head or spine; normal birth. The attacks are always at night and are proceeded by jerking of the arms several days before attacks. The mother thought her daughter had been suffering several months before she was aware of the nature of the illness.

On September 8, 1954, the patient had a convulsion in the morning soon after getting up; her arms had been jerking periodically for some months, but it had not been called to the mother's attention. A doctor was called in for diagnosis, and he checked his conclusions with a brain specialist; an encephalogram was made, and from its findings epilepsy was confirmed, and a course of treatment instituted with the usual drugs employed by traditional medicine.

In spite of the treatment neither attacks nor the jerking of the arms was modified or prevented. The patient had severe spells of depression, crying hard for hours at a time without apparent cause. First menses came shortly after twelfth birthday. Attacks are not affected by the monthly periods. The family history shows no case of epilepsy on either parent's side for several generations back.

Like many of these cases who come to the homeopath after the employment of anti-spasmodic and tranquilizing drugs, there are few - if any - symptoms of therapeutic value. Only those common to the disease are present.

The one outstanding symptom and condition was the time aggravation on onset of the attacks during sleep at night. The other symptoms were common to the disease and partly from the effects of drugs.

A narrow rubric in the repertory (KR 1355L); Convulsions during sleep was chosen because the whole case was there. *Caust., Cupr., Hyos., Ign., Kali-c., Lach., Op., Sec., Sil.* and *Stram.*

The polarity of the patient's blood was neutral[2], and only Sil. and Op. of this group were neutral. But they did not react as the needed

---

1. These cases are taken from the following sources: 1) The Homeopathic Recorder, Vol. LXXII, Nos. 7 - 9, January - March, 1957, p. 74; 2) The Homeopathic Recorder, Vol. LXVII, No. 8, February 1952, p. 244; 3) handwritten manuscriptts of uncertain date. - Editor.
2. See see article "Recent Concepts and New Formulas in Medicine" on page 679 ff. and see article "Importance of Electronic Reactions to Future Medicine" on page 683 ff.. - Editor.

Epilepsy ...

remedy; that is, though neutral they failed to restore the patient's normal polarity. Lach., a likely remedy, is bi-polar therefore not applicable; but Naja, another snake poison, is neutral and did satisfy all blood reactions by restoring the normal polarity of health; and Naja has been curative in epilepsy.

December 2, 1954. No Change. Naja 10M.

March 7, 1955. Naja 10M.

April 7, 1955. Fewer attacks. Naja 50M.

July 26, 1955. Improved. Naja 50M.

September 2, 1955. Patient has been exposed to polio and had headache and stiff muscles of neck and back. Lath. 10M.

September 26, 1955. Extremely severe menstrual cramps. Mag-p. 10M.

November 22, 1955. Menstrual cramps have been better, and attacks about the same. Mag-p. 50M

December 15, 1955. Mag-p. CM.

February 7, 1956. Better every way. Mag-p. CM.

February 23, 1956. Attacks more frequently and severe. Nauseated after attacks. Attacks are now worse around and after the period. Severe backaches. Has a slightly adherent clitoris. A second blood test brought change of polarity and the remedy was Kali-c. 10M. Both symptoms and polarity of remedy and patient's blood are acceptable.

March 27, 1956. Last attack March 17, 1956, after being up late with loss of much sleep. Kali-c. 10M.

April 30, 1956. Fewer attacks. Kali-c. 50M.

June 4, 1956. No attacks. Kali-c. 50M.

June 26, 1956. No attacks and patient is happy and much encouraged.

Epilepsy is one of the most difficult types of sickness to cure; but given sufficient time with strict adherence to rules of health, diet, etc. the homeopathic physician can score brilliantly in a large number of these cases leaving them in a normal state, something that cannot be done with suppressive drugging.

CONGENITAL MALFORMATION OF INTESTINES

Is interesting because of its pathological aspects, said to be congenital and also because of the unexpected response to the homeopathic remedy which was selected chiefly on one unusual symptom. This case was referred to me by Dr. W. J. Gier of San Diego, California. It is that of a young college student of abdominal pain and bowel disfunction, occurring about every week to ten days since early life, but the attacks are gradually becoming more severe and more frequent.

The patient is fond of meat and it agrees; coffee aggravates. Desires sweets, no thirst for water. No serious disease in his lifetime. Father is living at fifty-one, but has a stomach ulcer. Mother living at forty-seven is anemic. X-ray of intestines shows a congenital malformation of intestinal tract. Not much affected by temperature changes; sleeps well and is rested after sleep.

Any prescription based on the symptoms, findings and history of this case would insure little change to find a curative remedy. On taking the patient's blood for testing the patient fainted and fell to the floor. When he regained his composure, he said that the sight of even a little blood always made him faint; this was the key to the remedy. SYPH. 10M was given, and the blood was tested only to confirm the correctness of the prescription which was proved to be the case. The remedy was given on July 11, 1955.

July 26, 1955. Patient reportet improvement, and the remedy was continued.

September 15, 1955. SYPH. 10M.

October 13, 1955. Better until recently. SYPH. 50M.

December 15, 1955. Better except for a great deal of gas. SYPH. CM.

February 10, 1956. SYPH. CM.

April 24, 1956. Continued on SACCH-L.

June 19, 1956. Always perspired profusely in hot weather. LYC. 10M.

At times even while eating he fills up and is satiated. Specific indications like gas and distension and easy satiety with sensitiveness to hot weather mark LYC. a sure winner in intestinal and nutritional troubles.

SYPH. in ascending potencies helped and strengthened the patient in a wonderful way, but finally there was needed the deep anti-psoric LYC. to complete the cure of an apparently surgical case without the need for surgery.

CONGENITAL MALFORMATION OF INTESTINES ...

Many of our master prescribers have observed that a nosode rarely completes a cure of a chronic case; but, on the other hand, I believe we would fail to cure some cases without the searching and unfolding power of these subtle specifics.

Included in this essay are the x-ray findings and reports from the University Hospital at Ann Arbor, Michigan; with their diagnosis and recommendations for surgery.

It is cases like these that should interest physicians from every school of medical thought. Such cases illustrate perfectly the certain working of the law of cure when that law is guided and directed by the technique developed so fully by the homeopathic philosophy built up with one hundred and sixty years of laborious observation and work of thousands of homeopathic physicians, performing their unceasing rounds of duty in the healing art all over the world.

BLINDNESS FROM EYE INJURY

Adi Desai, twelve years old. Case referred by Dr. N. N. Mehta, Bombay, India. This boy healthy and with no symptoms of disease and an unusually good family and personal history, free of constitutional disease. Was struck in right eye with a tennis ball, followed by almost complete loss of sight, being able to distinguish large objects dimly and not farther than ten yards away. LED. 1M, SYMPH. 200 and EUPHR. 1M failed to help.

The patient's blood was sent to me to find the needed remedy indicated over the blood.[1]

January 29, 1949. CON. 10M was given.

May 20, 1949. Repeated, with some slight improvement in vision.

August 10, 1949. CON. 50M.

November 15, 1949. CON. 50M.

February 23, 1950. CON. CM.

June 8, 1950. KALI-BI. 10M.

September 7, 1950. KALI-BI. 10M.

January 4, 1951. KALI-BI. 50M.

---

1. See see article "Recent Concepts and New Formulas in Medicine" on page 679 ff. and see article "Importance of Electronic Reactions to Future Medicine" on page 683 ff.. - Editor.

BLINDNESS FROM EYE INJURY ...

May 17, 1951. THUJ. 10M (2 doses, six weeks apart).

September 27, 1951. THUJ. 50M.

January 2, 1952. THUJ. CM (2 doses, three month apart). All these and successive prescriptions were prescribed from the blood.

May 27, 1952, CALC-SIL. 10M.

September 5, 1952. CALC-SIL. 50M. (2 doses, six weeks apart).

January 16, 1953. CALC-SIL. CM (2 doses, three months apart).

Eye sight improving, patient developing well both mentally and physically.

August 18, 1953. CALC-SIL. CM.

November 26, 1953. CALC-SIL. CM.

August 31, 1954. CALC-SIL. DM Constant improvement.

January 4, 1955. CALC-SIL. DM.

April 25, 1955. CALC-SIL. DM.

June 5, 1956. CALC-SIL. 200. At a standstill.

June 19, 1956. Continued. Improvement in sight of injured eye.

Patient reads fairly large type from a distance of ten inches. Small type can be read from a short distance, if the letters forming the words are widely spaced.

Consider the extent of eye damage, with vision almost entirely gone and even though it took eight years to get these splendid results it was all worth while.

Here again we see what faith in the homeopathic law on the part of the patient and doctor can achieve. In this case we note how well the homeopath's philosophic technique is vindicated by not leaving one remedy for another while improvement in the patient and his symptoms continue. Also may be noted the steady though oft times slow improvement under the steady impact of the remedy given in progressively ascending potencies.

ECZEMA

A young unmarried woman in the twenties had suffered since a baby with a severe type of eczema of hands, wrists, and arms. Much local treatment by salves and ointments only seemed to aggravate the condi-

Eczema ...

tion. her general health was always excellent; her only complaint was severe menstrual cramps.

After several years of careful homeopathic prescribing, this patient was no better much to her disappointment as well as her physician's embarrassment as she was an assistant in the doctor's office.

She was a heavy smoker and was unable or unwilling to stop the habit. She had been given on meager indications the following remedies: Graph., Petr., Mez., Cadm-s., Crot-t., Sul-i., Sil., Sep., Psor., Tub., and the good old anti-psoric Sulph. These remedies were given at properly spaced intervals and brought in and confirmed by blood tests, but their benefits and relief were all short lasting, and many times there was no appreciable relief.

The patient was worse under local treatments and for that reason was willing to keep on with homeopathic remedies prescribed over the blood. She had few symptoms, and they were only common ones and of little therapeutic value. Through the blood tests an unproven, unknown remedy was found that produced the miracle of cure. The beautiful flowering climbing scrub, Bougenville, was tested in the crude state and placed in its proper polarity group and potentized by Ehrhart and Karl. This was the magic balm given in potencies of 30, 200, and 1M at properly spaced intervals that accomplished the cure of a most baffling case. This young lady has not ceased her cigarette smoking nor changed her mode of living anyway.

This case teaches us there is a curative remedy for every sick case, if we have the faith, the intelligence and the energy to persist in our quest till we find it and apply it properly.

Two cases of Facial Neuralgia or Tic Douloureux

Case No. 1: Mrs. E. F. G.

Fifty-seven and one-half years of age. Severe attacks of right sided facial pain off and on for some years. Has used coal tar drugs such as Aspirin, Anacin, etc., until they no longer helped. Painful attacks start in early morning, awakening from sleep about 4 a.m., and pain continues till bed time. Weather changes, especially cold. Very sensitive to touch, pressure, jar and motion. Weeping with the pain. Appetite indifferent, has no food desires or aversions. Modest thirst. Dietary and other living habits are good. Hysterectomy many years ago. Has a discharge of light colored blood from nipple of right breast almost contin-

Two cases of Facial Neuralgia or Tic Douloureux ...

Case No. 1 ...

ually. No pain. No erosion or retraction of nipple. No lumps or swelling of the breast. No glandular enlargement in axilla or elsewhere the body. The appearance of the face is dusky red and almost mottled at times.

July 5, 1948. Kali-cy. 10M.

August 19, 1948. Kali-cy. 10M. Patient had a return of blood from nipple after it had stopped. Is better generally.

September 14, 1948. Remedy continued. Less facial pain and fatigue.

October 14, 1948. Kali-cy. 10M. Nipple healed, facial pain slight after it had ceased

November 9, 1949. Remedy continued, better every way.

December 3, 1948. Kali-cy. 50M.

January 13, 1949. Kali-cy. 50M.

January 27, 1949. Had a very severe attack of intermittent pain in the face for past few days. Pain is relieved by pressure and heat. Mag-p. 10M.

February 22, 1949. Nipple has not discharged blood. has a severe spot of pain in gum on affected side. Sleeping well. Very sensitive to heat and a closed room. Puls. 10M.

March 18, 1949. Puls. 10M.

April 22, 1949. Puls. 50M.

May 27, 1949. Puls. 50M. Still has some facial pain.

June 17, 1949. Remedy continued. Has been some better. Vision impaired, focus is slow. Some show of blood from nipple.

July 28, 1949. Severe pain in face and gums, wakens her in early morning. Weakness of the knees with a sense of shortening of hamstring muscles back of the knee. Caust. 10M.

September 16, 1949. Caust. 10M. More blood from nipple, pain in gums. Better for awhile. (Caust. was not a good prescription. The patient should have been put back on Kali-cy. after Puls. did its work. In all likelihood Puls. would have been better left out also.)

Two cases of Facial Neuralgia or Tic Douloureux ...

Case No. 1 ...

October 5, 1949. A severe head and laryngeal cold cleared up under Carb-v. 10M.

November 11, 1949. Neuralgic pain right side of face. Wakens her in early morning. Pulsation in right ear. Oozing of blood from nipple seems past. Numbness of right hand this morning. Kali-cy. 10M.

December 9, 1949. No relief of neuralgia. Confined to a small area. Patient never chilly. Prefers cool places to warm places. Arg-met. 10M.

January 6, 1950. Bleeding dark brown blood from right nipple. This comes on while bathing. Feels better in the open air and from cold bathing. Kali-cy. 10M.

February 2, 1950. Pain in the right sciatic region, (old symptom). Face pain about the same. Nipple better. Kali-cy. 50M.

March 2, 1950. Kali-cy. 50M.

May 1, 1950. Kali-cy. 50M. Face pain better but very tired from least effort. Sleeps fairly well. A spot of shingles appeared on right breast.

May 29, 1950. Remedy continued; has over worked and was told by another doctor she had indications of cancer and should have her breast removed. Feels very depressed and frightened about it. Patient was assured she need have no fear of cancer.

June 16, 1950. Remedy continued. Much better every way.

July 28, 1950. Hands numb much of the time. Kali-cy. 50M.

August 25, 1950. Slight return of bleeding and face pain. Kali-cy. 50M.

September 22, 1950. After relief, return of symptoms. Kali-cy. 50M.

October 20, 1950. Remedy continued. Better.

November 28, 1950. Better generally, but sore nerve point in face wakens her about 4 a.m. Kali-cy. CM.

January 11, 1951. Nerve in face still bothers in early morning. Kali-cy. CM.

Two cases of Facial Neuralgia or Tic Douloureux ...

Case No. 1 ...

February 12, 1951. Pain persists, not too bad. Kali-cy. CM.

February 13, 1951. Remedy continued. Bleeding from nipple stopped. Pain persists around nose which is swollen and hot. Cold applications > heat < .

March 13, 1951. Kali-cy. 10M.

April 12, 1951. Kali-cy. 10M.

April 26, 1951. Kali-cy. 50M. Pain in face much better. Only comes when rubbing face hard. Nipple discharge gone.

June 8, 1951. Last two weeks has had some slight facial pain and some show of blood from nipple, but the patient looks and feels well and is able to work without fatigue. Kali-cy. 50M.

This patient should in a short time be entirely cured. She may need several super-high potencies viz: the CM and MM before this is accomplished; if symptoms remain after these extreme potencies have acted, we will drop down to the 12 or 30. There can be no doubt about this remedy being her specific.

We are not at all proud of the handling of this case. It is likely that had we never broken in on the rhythm of the remedy with other remedies, even though they seemed indicated for some of the acute and changing manifestations of sickness evolving under the similimum, our patient would have been nearer a cure today. We feel lucky that we did not entirely spoil our case by breaking in with a seemingly needed remedy.

We well know that there are cases that one remedy seems unable to do more than start the patient toward a cure and a complimentary remedy is needed to finish the work.

Or as Kent states, at times a remedy corresponding to one miasm in chronic conditions may need to be followed by another remedy to meet another complicating miasm in the system. Such examples come up often in the treatment of cancer and other degenative diseases.

Case No. 2:

The second case seems simpler - Mrs. G. W. Fifty-two years of age. Neuralgia of face since last October. Teeth X-rayed and declared nega-

Two cases of Facial Neuralgia or Tic Douloureux ...

Case No. 2: ...

tive. Good general health, but always more or less nervous. Pressure and applied heat ameliorate the pain. Uses no tobacco. Coffee and tea moderately. Had no menstrual troubles. Is subject to hay fever. Wind aggravates the pain. Has taken much Aspirin and other pain-killing drugs; they no longer help the pain. She sleeps well, better at rest. Appetite for little food at night. No thirst. Feet always cold. Requires lots of clothing to keep warm. Bowels move without drugs. Pains come and go suddenly (intermittant). Even though pressure ameliorates when the pain is on, the face is sensitive to touch. Any tyro in homeopathy would have given this patient Mag-p., and that is what she got in the 200th potency.

May 23, 1951, Mag-p. 200.

June 6, 1951, Mag-p. 10M. Patient reports less frequent attacks of pain, and it is much more endurable. The patient states it is quite light.

Mag-p. was Dr. Kent's choice of an antidote for aspirin and similar drugs.

There can be no doubt about the speedy cure of this case with the one remedy, indicated by the symptoms and history of the case.

Let us hear from others about remedies used in this most painful and often obstinate ailment which often culminates in nerve infections or cutting of the nerve leaving at best a paralyzed face and often the shifting of the trouble to deeper centers with disastrous results.

Cancer

Mr. G. J. S. In May, 1925, this patient then about thirty-five years of age came to consult me with a large irregular-shaped leg ulcer[1] discharging offensive pus and blood; there was more soreness than pain. His trouble had been about six months standing. Personal history was good having had no serious or infectious disease in his life up to that time. The routine examinations and tests were all negative, and the patient was organically sound and appeared in excellent health.

But his family history told a different story. His entire family consisted of parents, three sisters and a brother. The brother had been a

---

1. Probably a squamous cell epithelioma. - Editor.

CANCER ...

prominent homeopathic physician, well known to the older homeopathic doctors still living. This entire family had died of cancer. A
biopsy revealed this patient's trouble to be cancer, and radio active tests
of his blood confirmed this.

CADM-MET. 10M was given, and the patient was told to report in a
month. Along with the remedy a diet composed mostly of fruits and
vegetables was prescribed and adhered to.

At first the ulcer spread over much of the anterior and lateral surfaces
of the leg. The remedy acted for three months as the ulceration took on
healing and repair. For a period of five years a dose of the remedy was
given in ascending potencies up to the MM potency at intervals of
from six weeks to three months given on the indications shown in the
blood tests.[1] As long as the patient's blood remained negative, each
dose of the remedy was permitted to act; and when the polarity of the
blood changed to positive, another dose was given. At the end of five
years the leg was entirely healed leaving a large brownish indented scar
over the entire surface of the leg.

For three years this patient was well and required no further medication although he kept on his diet adding some starches and dairy products but no meat. Soon after the three-year period of health had passed,
the patient returned with an ulcerated area on his back.

The same remedy, CADM-MET. 30 was given, and it slowly took up
the healing process. Repetition of the remedy was given in ascending
potencies until again the MM was reached and the back healed with the
same characteristic brownish scars remaining and another seven years
glided by. From that time on as much as a year and sometime two
passed by before we would get a request for medicine.

All that remains at the present time is a small ulcerated area at the
base of the large scar on his leg near the place where the first ulcer
started. There is a small shallow area no larger than a lead pencil oozing
a tiny amount of serum. The patient is well and robust and appears
twenty years younger than he actually is. He has continued with his
work and carried on without interruption for twenty-five years. He is
married and the father of several grown children. They are all healthy,
and one daughter is married and the mother of a fine healthy baby.

---

1.   See see article "Recent Concepts and New Formulas in Medicine" on page 679 ff. and see article
     "Importance of Electronic Reactions to Future Medicine" on page 683 ff.. - Editor.

CANCER ...

This case proves the power of the homeopathic remedy to restore the sick to health when it can be found and administered in the proper dosage and timing or spacing in order to promote and maintain the uniform even flow of the life forces in harmony with the rhythm of the cosmos.

This case illustrates not only the inverse order of the symptoms but of the disease as well, "the first to come, the last to go".[1] The last of the ulceration healed very close to the point where the ulceration first began. It also confirms the observation of from center to circumference.[2] The remedies aided the vital force to keep the manifestations and action of the disease at the surface of the skin, thus enabling the vital organs to remain intact and function in perfection and harmony; health being the result.

BRONCHIAL ASTHMA

Bonchial asthma in an infant, three years old. The blood of this little patient was sent by Dr. Florence Santoro with the following brief account of the case; "Dear Dr. Grimmer: This child came to me today for the first time, September 28, 1949. It looks like bronchial asthma. Does not speak well. Mother says she has had twenty different doctors, and each gave the child ten or fifteen penicillin shots. One doctor gave him penicillin every day for thirty-two days, poor baby."

Yes he needed pity and intelligent help, for he suffered with continuous shortness of breath and a cough. No other symptoms were obtained and given; but through the polarity of the patient's blood.[3] The remedy brought unerring but rather slow yet continuous relief. The remedy, an unusual one and only fragmentarily proven, was ARAL. 10M. It has in its brief proving the heavy asthmatic breathing.

The results to date have been most gratifying. The patient has been free of attacks for long intervals, and a repetition of the dose has brought additional strength and relief of suffering. The last dose, a 50M, was given April 27, 1950; the child is practically well and developing nicely.

---

1. Hering's Law - Editor.
2. Hering's Law - Editor.
3. See see article "Recent Concepts and New Formulas in Medicine" on page 679 ff. and see article "Importance of Electronic Reactions to Future Medicine" on page 683 ff.. - Editor.

BRONCHIAL ASTHMA ...

The various forms of asthma are often a difficult malady to relieve let alone cure, but the homeopathic remedy not only relieves promptly but also cures permanently.

WEAK HEART AND EPILEPSY

Weak heart and epilepsy in a five-year-old boy whose blood was also sent by Dr. Santoro for a remedy.[1] This child was given PARTH. 200 the first week in March, 1949, which helped until September, 1949. Then a second test brought ANT-AR. 10M which improved the heart function but failed to help the frequent epileptic convulsions. On October 26, 1949, STRAM. 10M came through on a third test; and from that time on there has been a steady gain in the heart condition and a greatly decreased frequency of the convulsions which have been lighter in nature. To date this patient has had two 10M and two 50M potencies of STRAM., the last given May 15, 1950. This case, while not cured, gives every promise of being so in the not too distant future.

Epilepsy in a young child with a weak heart offers a rather grave prognosis as either one of these complaints by itself can be plenty tough in the way of relief and cure.

These three cases of chronic disease are not self limiting as are the acute manifestations of sickness. Chronic states go on to terminate in death unless cured by the homeopathic similimum.

It might be truly said that the many palliative treatments coming from traditional medicine complicate the chronic sickness and render cure more difficult.

---

1. See see article "Recent Concepts and New Formulas in Medicine" on page 679 ff. and see article "Importance of Electronic Reactions to Future Medicine" on page 683 ff.. - Editor.

HOMEOPATHIC CONFIMATIONS[1]

Among the common things that the homeopathic physician is called on to treat is constipation, and unless the similimum is given many cases will not be cured, and the patient will leave the doctor in disappointment and voice a sour note for Homeopathy. There are cases where inveterate constipation goes on for years no matter how the diet and living conditions may be changed. These are the cases where the exact homeopathic remedy must be given to effect a cure. The main reason the needed remedy is difficult to find for this condition is the large number of proven remedies found useful in the various forms of constipation. Hence, the physician must use his power of analysis to differentiate between many similar remedies for the one needed for each individual.

A case in point, that of a man who had been a victim of constipation for years. He had tried many doctors and taken many cathartics on his own account and on the advice of friends and advertisers and all to no avail. He used coffee in excess and considerable tobacco and alcohol in various forms. He was fond of pepper, spices and condiments. He was thin, highly irritable and very sensitive to noise and drafts of air. His bowels would move only after taking a drastic compound cathartic and then only with severe pain in the bowels with great straining in the rectal region to pass a small stool of mucous and watery matter, which produces some relief of the cramps until the next cathartic was taken. Any homeopath would give this man Nux-v., and that remedy in a single dose of the 10M effected a permanent cure with relief in twenty-four hours and made it unnecessary to resort to any more cathartics.

This same type of patient without any desire for stool (no peristaltic action of the intestine) would make one study two other remedies, Alum. and Bry. If the stool was dry as if burnt and the patient had considerable thirst at intervals, Bry. would be the choice. Alum. has external weakness and inertia of the rectal muscles of expulsion. Such is the way Homeopathy must proceed.

In women who suffer with severe bearing-down pelvic pains extending to the rectum with the ineffectual urge to pass the stool, Sep. would be the most likely remedy to cure.

In bronchial and respiratory troubles, including asthma of infants we have two very reliable remedies, Ant-t. and Carb-v. In those cases

---

1. The Homeopathic Recorder, Vol. LXVIII, No. 3, September, 1952, p. 67.

whose bronchial tubes are loaded with mucous which coughing does not loosen or dissipate, ANT-T. will rarely fail to give quick relief and cure. CARB-V. will be needed in cases where the voice shows involvement in hoarseness and huskiness with more or less severe paroxysms of cough. These remedies run together in the cyanosis, weakness, coldness and lack of thirst. ANT-T. may have more drowsiness in the picture, and in the beginning there may be a dry incessant cough.

An observation concerning DULC. over a period of many years has been confirmed repeatedly in its power to cure almost any case of impetigo contagiosa characterized by quickly forming yellow crusts that soon take on a brownish hue. These lesions clear up quickly after the remedy, and we all know how persistent and difficult this condition is under regular, routine treatment.

Another remedy with a peculiar characteristic is LAC-C. This peculiarity that has been confirmed by many prescribers is its tendency to have complaints that alternate sides; a tonsilitis may alternate or shift from side to side; the same may be true of neuritis or arthritis. These conditions have been cured by the remedy Lac-c. many times, as confirmatory proof of the great law of cure.

Nearly every spring and fall, the homeopathic physician will meet with epidemics of sore throats more or less severe in nature. It is surprising how frequently one of the following seven remedies will prove curative, quickly and permanently. FERR-P., HEP., LACH., LYC., LAC-C., NIT-AC. and PHYT. Still more surprisingly are the few slight points of differentiation needed to select the curative remedy from this group, and rarely is a second prescription required. The following points of difference have been used to decide our choice of remedy over many years with highly satisfactory results.

Where the right side is chiefly affected, FERR-P., LYC., and PHYT. are first choices for further study. Where there is worse by swallowing hot and better swallowing cold drinks, PHYT. becomes the remedy. Where there is great thirst with worse from empty swallowing, FERR-P. is the prescription, and where better by hot drinks with little thirst or none for cold, then LYC. is the remedy. Strictly left-sides cases are best covered by LACH. although LAC-C. has the same symptom, but the latter tends to soon shift to the other side. These remedies are both relieved by cold drinks. NIT-AC. has extreme sore, burning, shooting pain with a feeling of great dryness in the throat, worse by any attempt to swallow, especially fluids. HEP. has very sharp, splinter-like pains, generally right sided. Better by swallowing hot drinks like LYC., but HEP. sweats easily and profusely without relief and is extremely sensitive to cold air. Lyc. desires the fresh air. There is no chance of confusion between these two drugs.

It is true these are rather meager indications for the selection of the similimum, but years of successful clinical practice justifies them. Especially when the doctor has on an average of forty to fifty phone calls a day and the aforementioned cases are largely by way of telephone and the remedy must be sent or called for; to these phone calls are added thirty to forty patients to be seen in a day as well as some to be prescribed for by mail. Thus it becomes necessary to conserve time if all the day's work be accomplished.

These facts are mentioned to show that with experience the doctor will develop an awareness of the great resources of the Materia Medica and find the key to rapid and accurate prescribing by persistent study and use of its vast storehouse of knowledge. I am sure every busy homeopathic physician could add a great many more simple but useful applications of our remedies to every class of disease both acute and chronic as the Materia Medica contains within its covers everything needed for the relief and cure of suffering humanity. No matter how many times we see them or how simple they may be, we all are always delighted and interested in beholding confirmations of cure brought about by the action of the homeopathic remedy. I will close this little paper with an apology to my learned colleagues for taking up their time listening to a primary account of remedy action. I am sure this could be transcended by any one of them with accounts of difficult and unusual cures much more interesting and instructive to both the profession and laity.

A Case of Coronary Insufficiency[1]

Many physicians believe that the homeopathic remedy is less efficient in curative action for heart disease in general and in the coronary cases in particular. But years of practical experience of many good homeopathic prescribers have left a splendid record in palliation and cure that has not been equalled by other systems of healing.

The following case illustrates a somewhat atypical case of coronary disease: A man in the early sixties had been treated for a poorly functioning liver and gall bladder. He was mentally depressed, with irregular bowel action, alternation of constipation and diarrhea and complaints of a difficult, slow starting of the urine with a feeble stream. Very drowsy and tired. Marked tendency to catch colds which settled in the sinus and resulted in severe headaches.

Gradually under homeopathic prescribing and corrective living routine such as care in diet, adequate rest, moderate exercise in the open air and walking, this patient attained a better state of health and felt better and stronger for quite a period with most of his symptoms gone.

However, some months after this general improvement, this patient began to have severe chest pain, left and right side, extending to arms with marked shortness of breath. This was accompanied with a return of digestive symptoms stemming from a gall bladder condition, some jaundice being present, with large amounts of gas in stomach and bowel not relieved by belching. There was considerable weakness and anxiety. Chin. 10M. brought immediate relief of all symptoms except the dyspnea which came from only a short walk. Heart sounds were apparently normal, but as the chest pain returned and the dyspnea persisted, an electro-cardiogram was made and pronounced positive for coronary disease.

In sickness with much pathology present and especially in vital organs like the heart, lungs and kidneys, experienced prescribers have found it best not to use too high potencies of the needed remedy because of the severe aggravations that are often produced and not followed by the usual improvement expected after such action. This is likely because most of these conditions are incurable, and the best that can be hoped for is palliation and prolongation of life. Hence, drugs should be given low or in tincture depending on the nature of the remedy needed; in this way severe aggravations do not occur, and the

---

1. From handwritten manuscript, exact date unknown. - Editor..

homeopathic remedy will surely relieve suffering and prolong life even in incurable cases. If good curative action is obtained by the lower potencies, then the higher ones can follow with marked and permanent results.

Because of the tumultuous, vigorous action of the heart and pulse, marked palpitation and dyspnea with general muscular weakness, STROPH. 6X was given, three powders to be taken twelve hours apart and no other medicine for a week (This patient understands the efficacy and philosophy of the single dose). STROPH. in ascending potencies up to the 1M brought about astonishing results in restoring the well being of this man over a period of six months, enabling him to walk quite a distance with no pain or dyspnea.

Improvement was interrupted by a violent digestive upset brought on by indiscretion in diet and over exertion for which CARB-V. 10M was given with rapid relief of all symptoms, but the patient failed to have curative action any longer with STROPH. in any potency or even the tincture which was given for a short time.

As the patient was at a standstill, very irritable and depressed with difficult, slow-starting urine and violently sensitive to cold drafts, KALI-SULA. 10M was given; this remedy was partially selected over the patient's blood.[1] In comparison chiefly between KALI-SULA. and HEP. the first mentioned remedy registered stronger reactions.

KALI-SULA. in infrequent doses from the 10M up to the CM put the patient back in a state of symptomatic health and comfort, but the cardiogram still gave evidence of coronary disease. This covered a period from *April 25, 1952,* to *December 6, 1952.*

December 6, 1952. The patient was profoundly depressed mentally, even suicidal as he felt it was a case of incurability and a gradual oncoming state of physical incompetency and uselessness. He was worried that he would become a burden, and the symptoms of dyspnea and pain were returning from the least exertion. At this time AUR-I. 10M was given because of the typical mental states associated with the cardiac conditions.

January 8, 1953. Mentals improved, sleep fair, feels exhausted, heart sounds are good. Pressure 140/100. AUR-I. 10M.

---

1. See see article "Recent Concepts and New Formulas in Medicine" on page 679 ff. and see article "Importance of Electronic Reactions to Future Medicine" on page 683 ff.. - Editor.

February 16, 1953. Has been more constipated but sleeps better. Electrocardiogram negative. Aur-i. 50M.

March 20, 1953. Extremely tired, digestion better, severe aching in cervical glands. Aur-i. 50M.

May 4, 1953. Had a severe attack of indigestion, cleared up without any medication, very irritable, but mental depression much less. Aur-i.. CM.

June 6, 1953. Patient looks and feels better than in years. Heart sounds good. Pressure 140/100. No more pain in chest or dyspnea on walking or exertion. Negative cardiogram.

We feel justified in claiming a cure for this case.[1]

---

1. There are no further notes available for the editor. The remaining mild to moderate hypertension BP 140/100 presumably was treated, but Dr. Grimmer's seconds were not available to pursue this matter further. However the choice of remedies and their sequence: Chin., Stroph., Carb-v., Hep-s-k. and Aur-i. is very interesting. - Editor.

Homeopathy Versus the Specialist[1]

Many years ago, when I was younger and less experienced in the practice of medicine, and while I still held over from college days a strong feeling of awe and admiration for the wisdom that is supposed to repose in the cerebral centers of the widely heralded specialist, there came to my office a little patient totally blind as a result of congenital syphilis.

He had been treated by several eminent specialists, one at the clinic of the North Western Medical School. His parents were told that his case was past all help, as the scars from the extensive corneal ulceration had completely covered the pupils in spite of the most skilled treatment in the hands of one of the world's greatest eye doctors.

Why this case was brought to a young general practitioner of medicine, after the failure of the great specialist, may seem strange to the innocent by-stander. It was more than strange to me; it was a shock to ask me to help in such a case. It was agreed, however, that I would take the case and do the best I could with no promise of any kind.

Kali-bi. 10M, 50M and CM in single doses at intervals of from one to three month apart completely restored that child's vision although the little fellow is not robust. And subsequent to the treatment for his eyes, he had other very serious troubles. Once the parents submitted to the advice of the school doctor to have enlarged cervical glands cut out, which left him with a running wound in his neck for over a year, and that was finally cured by the homeopathic remedy Tub. Some years later this little patient developed a very severe case of osteomyelitis in both legs, for which Merc-k-i. was given in a series of potencies from 10M to CM; this remedy cured after Hep., Sil., Syph. and Toxi. had only slightly helped or failed to give any permanent relief.

This apparent miracle of cure did much to rout the inferiority complex of the general practitioner toward the specialist. The veneration of college days gave way to the clear light of reason; the lesson gained by following the great therapeutic law brought forth a faith based on absolute knowledge that no sneering illusion of pseudo-science could ever shake.

Some years later a lady, who had been my patient off and on for a long time, came to me with a badly inflamed eye discharging thick yellow pus which was worse in the morning. A microscopic test showed a

---

1. The Homeopathic Recorder, Vol. XLVIV, No. 2, Second Quarter, p. 59 ff.

gonorrheal infection. Still remembering some of the college aphorisms and injunctions of the danger to the vision from this infection, I promptly referred this patient to an eye specialist of good reputation and standing. After month of local treatment and much suffering and expense, the eye was pronounced cured; its pus discharge was gone, but it still remained red, painful and very sensitive to light with weakened vision. Again the homeopathic prescriber of an internal remedy was invoked to try to improve on the results obtained by the specialist. NAT-M., PULS. and THUJ. given at considerable intervals apart restored first the discharge that had been suppressed, not cured, by argyrol drops with atrophine to keep the pupils dilated so adhesions would not form, and then cured the chronic inflammatory condition and restored the vision to normal clearness. NAT-M. antidoted the mischief wrought by the specialist, and PULS. and THUJ. took care of the natural infection in its unfoldment and gradual decline until health was restored.

The patient, while grateful for these results, was much incensed to think of the time, suffering and money expended with the specialist, when Homeopathy could have handled it better in every way from the start and brought the patient and her eye through quicker, gentler and with far less expense. Comparisons are often odious especially to the ones not flattered by them. Needless to say, the specialist, in my eye, no longer stood on the pedestal of superior power to heal and save, however much special knowledge he might claim to have.

Again, a few years back another patient whose blood registered a 4 plus Wasserman reaction came in with a corneal ulcer for treatment. This man had been cured by Homeopathy of periodical headaches of a severe nature which had been pronounced migraine by a nerve specialist of good reputation.

Not wishing to shoulder the full responsibility as the possible loss of an eye, the prescriber sent the patient to a homeopathic eye specialist of national reputation and a high potency prescriber, not for treatment, but to watch the remedy action and to act as counselor in case of need. The prescriber after numerous experiences of like nature had developed a faith in the power of the homeopathic remedy that may have made him appear egoistic in the presence of specialists, but results obtained could not be other than convincing from both ends of the riddle; namely the great and uniform success of Homeopathy and the lamentable failures of the specialists in serious eye cases. Theoretically this last case should have proven an ideal one from every point of view, but alas the homeopathic prescriber was doomed to another cerebral shock.

This time our homeopathic specialist (the others were men of the old school) lost faith or his nerve, as he told the patient he could not afford to risk the loss of eye sight for the ideals of Homeopathy, and he proceeded to treat this patient with atrophine drops for the prevention of adhesions without consulting the prescriber. After several days the patient came back in a worse condition with more pain and redness and the ulcer spreading; he also told the patient he would assume full responsibility and relieve the specialists of both his fears and of the patient.

The patient was informed that the homeopathic remedy action had been aborted by the local irritation of the treatments and that a greater number of successes in the past (after specialists had failed to help and had actually injured a number of cases) was the best guarantee for the saving of his sight.

A very unusual remedy brought in over his blood[1], cured the ulcers of the eye in a surprisingly short while. The remedy was CARBN-S. in the 10M and 50M potencies. All local measures were interdicted.

I regret I cannot bring all these patients to you that you may hear the testimony from their own lips. I will endeavor if it can be arranged for one or two of them to be presented after this paper is read. One more case will conclude this paper.

September, 1929, the widow of a homeopathic physician and the mother of a young allopathic doctor, recently graduated, came in with a badly inflamed eye, resulting from the lodgement of a grain of sand in the corneal coat; the sand had been removed and the patient sent home to apply to hot boric acid compression. But the eye remained sore and inflamed, and for this condition, SIL. 10M was given.

As the condition did not improve as fast as the young doctor son thought it should, he insisted on his mother seeing one of Chicago's leading eye specialists and receiving treatment from him. Many months elapsed, and this patient came back. The inflammation and pain were gone, but the eye was sightless with a thick film covering the whole outer coat. The specialist had proposed the removal of this so-called dead eye in order to save the well eye. This advice was concurred with by one of our homeopathic eye specialists, but the patient decided to consult her doctor again before taking such a step.

---

1. See see article "Recent Concepts and New Formulas in Medicine" on page 679 ff. and see article "Importance of Electronic Reactions to Future Medicine" on page 683 ff.. - Editor.

The doctor could see no reason for such an operation; it is true the sight had been destroyed probably more by the severe argyrol applications and the atrophine drops to prevent adhesions over the pupil than from the ravages of the infection itself. GRAPH. was prescribed for the extensive scar tissue and given in several doses at long intervals with no appreciable results after three month had elapsed. KALI-BI. 10M was given, and after thirty days a slight improvement in the color of the eye was noted. KALI-BI. in a succession of potencies up to the CM was given with amazing results after two years had elapsed; the deadly white of the eye had given way to the natural blue color, the thick tough film that covered the whole eye had become thin and so transparent that the patient could distinguish objects, faintly at first, but steadily improving as time and the action of the remedy went on. Today there is every indication that this pronounced dead eye will be absolutely restored to normal appearance and vision by the homeopathic similimum.

Such cases as those mentioned are but commonplace experiences in the life of every good homeopathic prescriber, and until we are able to contrast the results obtained with those of the specialists, whose only technique is to wash, scrape, burn or cut, we are not cognizant of the vast superiority of homeopathic law.

One thing more in closing, and that is the much greater advantage the specialist has over the general practitioner in so much that he may fail to help and even injure by his technique and treatment, and yet be absolved from all blame or responsibility in the matter because a successful propaganda over the mass of humanity has established his claims for greatness. While the general practitioner failing in matters that seemingly belong exclusively to the specialist is in danger of a suit for damages and malpractice, thanks to the same propaganda that brands all who differ with them, quacks and charlatans. "But verily, by their works shall ye know them". Who are the quacks and tricksters and who are the apostles of light and wisdom? Only the afflicted ones, who have experienced the ministrations from both systems of treatment can give the true answer.

Clinical Failures[1]

Case 1

One case in early practice lingers in my memory: A man somewhat past middle life, but of vigorous constitution and excellent habits of living, wealthy and (most priceless boon) happily married, was suddenly stricken with lobar pneumonia. He delayed calling the doctor until twelve hours after the chill, thinking he was suffering from a slight cold.

The symptoms were typical of Bryonia no other remedy even competing:
- Right lower and middle lobes involved;
- < from motion, jar, inspiration,
- > lying on painful side, etc.
- Thirsty for copious drafts of water.

Bry. 10M was given.

Twenty-four hours later, cough and pleuritic plains were better and even some of the jaundice, which was quite marked, had cleared up; the fever had advanced one degree.

The patient was better, but his fever was up - and he was impatient to return to very pressing business. I was over-anxious to hasten results and made the fatal mistake of changing the remedy without definite symptoms to justify it.

Sulph. 10M was given, with expectation of returning to Bry. in broken doses in another day; but instead, the death certificate was signed. Just twenty-four hours after Sulph. was given that great, strong, good man lay lifeless: for his trusted physician had, in a moment of weakness, violated the tenet of homeopathic law.

It is not possible to tell all the processes or changes that occurred in this case after Sulph. was given; some things we do know: The benign curative action of Bry. was checked by the deeper remedy - was antidoted - and the disease was permitted to develop at a rapid rate. The whole right lung became consolidated and the right side of the heart dilated. There was much fat about the heart and the heartmuscle was flabby; the organ was unable to support the strain of severe illness - especially such strain as pneumonia imposes.

---

1. The Homeopathician, Vol. VI, No. 1, January - March 1916, p. 14. This article shows the greatness and humility of Dr. Grimmer for writing of his mistakes and furthermore of analyzing how to correct them. Each of us may be so inspired by him to give ourselves freely to introspection of ourselves. - Editor.

CASE 1 ...

The result was not from ignorance nor from lack of training: I was of the fortunate ones who had the best of training. Somewhere I had read that SULPH. was always good, in any case or at any stage of pneumonia, to hasten the progress of resolution... This was among my most bitter experiences in medicine; after a period of shock and grief I began to see that this awful sacrifice would serve as warning ever to hold me unswerving from the rules of practice under the law: *I would never again change the remedy so long as my patient was improving*; all the masters and teachers have announced this as the only proper mode of procedure: If improvement lapses, give the remedy in a higher potency, or if it is an acute case: give it in repeated doses until the fever begins to fall. If after this the patient does not react, a re-study of the case is in order, and the symptoms alone can guide to the needed remedy.

Many times since I have given SULPH. in pneumonia - but only under the proper indications - and with perfect success. It is a wonderful medicine and frequently needed; but by very reason of its power it is capable of setting up most violent reactions, which may kill a weak patient. Its power in antidoting similar curative medicines is indicated by the result in the case here cited.

CASE 2

This was a case of malignant diphtheria, the only case of that disease I ever lost. Not because of mistake in prescribing; that was highly successful: the hemorrhages, the swelling of the throat, and the very extensive and putrid membrane entirely cleared up under LACH. But a week of incessant nursing, together with the attendant anxiety, exhausted the mother completely. The family was desperately poor and friendless, so that a nurse was out of the question; the weather was extremely hot, and trying to the slowly convalescing patient.

Though urgently warned against permitting the child even to sit up in bed, the mother, exhausted and worn to the limit of endurance, so soon as the acute strain had passed, relaxed her vigil awhile and fell asleep. The child-patient, unable to waken her mother, for some purpose started to get out of bed and fell to the floor fainting. When the mother roused, she found her child dying from cardiac weakness.

I am sure this child could have been saved, had her physician been sufficiently alive to the situation and performed his full duty by obtaining the necessary help to insure quiet and comfort to his patient. It has

CASE 2 ...

always since been a source of keen regret that I did not, for even a night, put a nurse on that case until the mother might have obtained a little rest. It would have been a sacrifice then - for this was an incident of my early practice, and money was about the scarcest thing I knew.

CASE 3

A young married woman, who was a chronic sufferer from asthma, had had many physicians and varieties of treatment, under which she steadily grew worse. Under homeopathic remedies she improved rapidly for some six month, when a severe cold was contracted - a bronchitis - and her asthma returned with violence and persistence in spite of my efforts to find a curative remedy. As the patient resided about fifteen miles distant it was difficult for me to see her as often as she wished, and after several days of suffering without relief her husband decided to change to another doctor, in spite of his wife's wish to remain under homeopathic treatment.

An allopath was called and the usual hypodermic of morphine was administered, which afforded relief for a few hours for her breathing; but lobar pneumonia followed, the outcome of which I have not learned, but of which, from the nature of things, I have grave fear.

This case illustrates the harm of suppression by crude drugs: especially the danger from masking symptoms through palliation by opiates. It is trying - to see suffering, especially in those we love - but we must have the moral stamina to be unmoved by human suffering, if we would save human life. The first impulse of the regular is to stop the cry of pain, regardless of the subsequent cost; the homeopath, from his knowledge of symptoms and their significance, is aware that a great deal of suffering must sometimes be borne by patients before their cure may be effected. It is always well to take time and explain this to such patients, since they are better prepared to bear their trials. This is especially true after allopathic suppressions.

CASE 4

Young, refined, beautiful and everyway happy, a six-months bride had quite rapidly, after her marriage, developed typical Graves disease. Symptoms called for Lyc. which was given in 10M potency, and she returned to her home, some fifty miles from Chicago, with instruction

CASE 4 ...

to remain very quiet, to avoid all excitement, and to report in two weeks time.

Three days after the remedy came a violent aggravation of the heart-symptoms, ending in syncope.

The young husband, crazed with excitement and fear, sent for a local doctor who condemned and ridiculed the idea of homeopathic treatment for such cases; he advised for and insisted upon the necessity for immediate operation of the goitre, as in his learned opinion that was the whole cause of the patient's trouble. The goitre was successfully removed; but the patient never recovered consciousness.

My mistake was in failing to keep her in Chicago for the first week, until after the period of remedy-aggravation had passed. Had I been able to observe the developments as they arose, I believe that a beautiful and useful life would have been preserved.

The homeopathic physician must be constantly alert; not only must he be trained in the law and in the mode of its application, but outside the realm of prescribing he must use judgement in many other matters. His sympathy should be broad and deep, but it must be tempered with firmness, as of steel, against temptations to deviate from exact methods of practice.

DISCUSSION

Dr. Dienst: You say that (Case 1) SULPH. 10M killed the patient?

Dr. Grimmer: BRY. was holding him; SULPH. not only antidoted the curative medicine but also struck the heart and interfered with its action. I'm satisfied that SULPH. killed the man.

Dr. Schwartz: It appears as though his constitutional state was SULPH., and giving the higher potency caused too much reaction?

Dr. Dienst: SULPH. has marked affinity for the heart; it pumped the heart so fast that the veins could not take care of the blood, and the heart began to dilate.

Some Clinical Cases[1]

Sarcoma of Mouth and Gums - L. D. A. - age 50 years

June 27, 1938: Sarcoma of mouth and gums following a tooth extraction, diagnosis from biopsy and clinical aspects.

Not only were the gums ulcerated and swollen, but the whole affected side of the face was enormously swollen presenting the well-known frog face appearance; the cervical and sublingual glands were enlarged; and the patient could, with great difficulty, open his mouth the space of a lead pencil.

The family history was good and in no way significant; he had always enjoyed good health having always been free of infections and venereal disease.

There was no definite symptomatology to base a homeopathic prescription on, unless the recent surgical injury following extraction with curettement and scraping of the bony processes of the jaw might be used as an irritating factor.

Radium and x-ray were advised with possibly more extensive surgery by the dental specialist who attended the case. But this was refused by the patient on the advice of his family physician who, having no therapeutic symptomatology to prescribe on, sent him to me for a remedy to be selected over the patient's blood.[2] Symph. came through, and that remedy given in the 10M and 50M potencies at well-spaced intervals of from one to three months apart cured this case completely in the space of a year.

This case continues to report to me at intervals for a sinus condition of a rather mild catarrah nature for which Carb-v. had been prescribed since September 11, 1939, to the present time.

The same intervals of time have elapsed in a series of potencies of Carb-v. from the 10M to the CM which was given in April 1, 1940. He will now be turned back to the physician who sent him to me, cured entirely within the space of two years.

This case presents a classical cure with the single remedy given in a series of potencies at properly spaced intervals. Unfortunately we see relatively few cases showing such happy action of cure in cancer with one single remedy.[3]

---

1. The Homeopathic Recorder, Vol. LVI, No. 2, February 1941, p. 73.
2. See see article "Recent Concepts and New Formulas in Medicine" on page 679 ff. and see article "Importance of Electronic Reactions to Future Medicine" on page 683 ff.. - Editor.

CARCINOMA OF BREAST - MISS D.

August 12, 1929. Carcinoma of breast two years standing; diagnosis confirmed by biopsy. Has been under good homeopathic treatment, but the breast is about one-third ulcerated away; and the patient has lost weight and color, but has suffered little pain. Under continuous treatment by remedies selected over the blood[1] (this also is a case referred from another homeopathic physician), this patient has carried on actively for eleven years. Her breast is healed, but her bones are weakened and break very easily; x-ray now shows bone cancerous. Under the action of a number of remedies chief of which were CADM-I. and CADM-MET., SAMARSKITE, ALUM-SIL., GRAPH. and the last remedy KALI-THIO-CYAN., the patient's breast has entirely healed, and she remains without pain; but because of the weakened bones, she must now be kept very quiet and avoid physical exertion of all kinds.

This is a case of advanced cancer where deep changes in the blood and tissues have ultimated; rarely - if ever - do we find one remedy sufficient to cope with such conditions; generally a series of deep homeopathic constitutional remedies are required, and those can be best selected over the blood of the patient.

The more I see of cancer, the more convinced I become that our greatest use must come in the field of prevention; treating the pre-cancer stage by careful homeopathic prescribing especially in the children and young adults.

One thing more that must strike every Homeopath is the wonderful advantage that must accrue to the race where three successive generations could be blessed with real homeopathic treatment. Not only cancer but the groundwork on which cancer grows, tuberculosis, could be entirely eradicated with three generations of consecutive homeopathic treatment. One of the things we might do with great profit for the future of the race is to organize our patients into a group looking ahead to the time and with the object of having homeopaths uniting with homeopaths that better and happier healthier children may be born into the world.

---

3. see case below. - Editor.
1. See see article "Recent Concepts and New Formulas in Medicine" on page 679 ff. and see article "Importance of Electronic Reactions to Future Medicine" on page 683 ff.. - Editor.

Typical Clinical Versus Atypical Cases [1]

When the homeopathic physician meets a case of sickness with symptoms simulating the typical classified symptoms of the Materia Medica which have been produced in provings on healthy humans and confirmed by clinical cures, his work is much lighter, and the prospects for curative action are more certain. This especially is true in acute conditions where nature unassisted is able to limit the extent of the trouble and often terminate it. The homeopathic remedy will enable nature to do this quickly and gently, saving time and suffering.

In chronic troubles the physician's work is beset with many difficult problems requiring study and patience and unlimited faith in the power of the similimum; and these are the cases where we rarely find the typical expression of one proving; they are always more or less atypical. In recent years chronic disease has been deeply complicated and confused by the universal abuse of the numerous and ever-increasing coal tar and antibiotic drugs that deluge the human race today. These drastic poisons and chemicals depress the life forces of the organism, destroy elements in the blood, enervate the central nervous system, suppress many natural expressions of disease and leave in the wake of their use myriads of human wrecks, victims of heart and kidney disease, anemia, leukemia, cancer and insanity. All these afflictions have increased in a most alarming way during the past ten years. To the disastrous effects of universal drugging is added the deleterious action of processed and adulterated foods; vegetables and fruits contaminated with poison sprays, drinking water everywhere polluted with harmful chemicals, cooking utensils made of aluminium which slowly but surely build up a pathological residue in the organism that results in many forms of degenerative disease. All these destructive elements not only depress life forces but inhibit the action of homeopathic remedies. Hence the increased obstacles in the way of successful homeopathic prescribing. Patients chronically poisoned with aluminum will not respond to seemingly indicated remedies until that toxemia is removed by CADM-MET. in potency.[2]

A few examples from practice will suffice to illustrate typical versus atypical cases.

---

1. Taken from handwirtten manuscript, written in May, 1952 for the Bureau of Clinical Medicine, Illinois Homeopathic Medical Association, never published. - Editor.
2. or CADM-O. - Editor.

Cough

A two-year-old infant girl, with fever, harsh cough and restless irritability was quickly cured after several other remedies failed by SENEG. 10M, one dose, when it was noted that the cough ended with or rather was followed by sneezing and was markedly worse on beginning to eat.

Tetanus

A four-year-old boy in tetanic convulsions resulting from a sliver from an old barn yard in the palm of his right hand some seven or eight days before. He was free of convulsions and asleep in an hour after MAG-P. 10M was given. No more convulsions ensued, and good health remains to this day. The patient is now a man thirty years of age. Why was MAG-P. chosen? The regular intermittency of the convulsions and the relief of the paroxysms by holding the little patient firmly and tightly in the mother's arms; intermitting and better from pressure are typical MAG-P. provings.

Cough

A lady of sixty subject to taking cold from the least exposure to cold air. Suffering from a nagging, tickling cough at throat pit with coryza, worse by cold air and in the early morning hours from 3 to 4 a.m., cough with copious, thin expectoration. Aggravated by inhaling air, pressure on throat and lying down at night. RUMX. 10M covered the symptoms and modalities perfectly and cured promptly.

Bronchitis, Tonsilitis, Nasal Blocking and Sleep Apnea

An infant boy, eighteen months old, suffering from nasal blocking and large inflammed tonsils with rattling of loose mucous in bronchial tubes. Wakened from sleep suffocating and gasping and cyanotic. Neither LACH. nor OP. were given (KR pg. 763R). Why? Because during sleep his skin was dry, and soon after waking he was bathed in profuse sweat (KR pg. 1293R). SAMB. soon relieved and saved that child's life, my own son who is now a hardy six footer of twenty.

Any busy homeopathician could multiply such cases by the hundred over the years of his practice, for these are typical cases exhibiting striking similiarity to the symptoms of the Materia Medica. In the treatment of infants the homeopathic physician has tremendous advantage over the routine prescribing of so-called regular medicine, and the chances for recovery in serious forms of illness of the little sufferers are vastly greater.

A few cases of chronic disease from practice show little but common symptoms to choose a remedy.

CHOLECYSTITIS

Very frequently the homeopath is presented with a case of gall bladder trouble with or without stones. It is said one third of the population of the United States past thirty years of age suffers with gall bladder and liver trouble. Most of these cases have had old-school treatment and advice, and surgery is always recommended.

The following is a typical one; but from homeopathic therapeutics it is quite atypical, having only common symptoms of the disease to prescribe on.

August 17, 1951. J. R. age 46. Has had recurring gall stones and colic since January last. X-ray shows stones. Appetite poor and easily satisfied. Bowel elimination fair without drugs; good general health, but complexion is jaundiced. Had bronchitis in 1927. Operated for appendicitis a year ago. Now on a fat-free diet. Teeth are in good condition and cared for. No vomiting with attacks but has a bitter taste. Not affected by weather changes. Not thirsty. Often belches before attack. Uses no tobacco or alcohol, drinks one cup of coffee per day. Sleep varies, good at times. Although only common symptoms make up the study, the easy satiety, bitter taste and tendency to belch, with thirstlessness, jaundice not marked and no marked sensitiveness to cold are best covered by LYC., and that remedy was given in the 10M potency.

September 17, 1951. A month later patient reported having more gas and broken sleep. LYC. 10M.

October 10, 1951. Had a headache for 3 days (old symptoms), otherwise feeling better; the remedy was continued.[1]

October 24, 1951. Better. Remedy continued.

November 29, 1951. Better until recently. LYC. 50M.

January 9, 1952. Had a light attack. LYC. 50M.

February 1, 1952. Better every way. Remedy continued.

---

1. "Remedy continued" means no remedy given or SACCH-L. - Editor.

CHOLECYSTITIS ...

February 20, 1952. Had a severe headache and took an aspirin. LYC. 50M.

April 17, 1952. Better but some jaundice remains. LYC. CM.

May 9, 1952. The patient feels he is well, and all jaundice and symptoms are gone. We have advised another x-ray be taken of the gall bladder to note what changes, if any, there are in the stones. But it looks like this patient is well without surgical intervention.

CHRONIC ASTHMA

Among the most resistant diseases to cure is chronic asthma.

October 4, 1939. Dr. J.A.R. had suffered with asthma all his life. Now 45 years old. Has had every treatment known to medicine, both homeopathic and allopathic; and despite the continuous use of adrenalin in increasing dosage, he continued to grow worse, not only in the asthmatic paroxysms but is generally weaker and thinner.

Under a series of remedies brought in over his blood[1] the patient was able to get away from adrenalin and other drastic palliatives to improve in general health with lighter attacks of coughing and asthma in the space of seven years.

May 27, 1947. SOLANUM INTEGRI (the wild tomato) in the 30th potency produced a month of almost complete freedom from asthma. He wrote at that time, "I had a month of the most comfortable time I ever knew before in my life". From that time till the present day, this patient experiences only slight and short-lasting attacks of asthma. A series of potencies of SOLANUM INTETGRI up to the 50M was followed by a deeper remedy CALC-SIL. 10M brought in over his blood. He has been under this remedy since April 17, 1951, and is in better health and more comfortable than he ever remotely hoped to be.

More and more often the homeopathic physician is called on to treat not only intractable but incurable and painful conditions like cancer in

---

1. See see article "Recent Concepts and New Formulas in Medicine" on page 679 ff. and see article "Importance of Electronic Reactions to Future Medicine" on page 683 ff.. - Editor.

its terminal stage. Such things are now possible by means of a knowledge of the polarities of remedies and diseases and by changing the polarity and chemistry of the sick patient's blood to a normal state by means of the properly selected homeopathic remedy placed in the circuit with the blood specimen.

The following case deemed hopeless by every standard of medical lore proves the power of the exact homeopathic remedy in the realm of cure.

CANCER OF BREAST

August 17, 1951. Dr. M.B.S. of middle life was stricken with breast cancer about seven years ago. After biopsy, an early operation was performed. Two years later a severe and painful ulceration appeared in the surgical scar of the amputated breast. X-ray, radium and various old-school remedies administered hypodermically were tried with a constantly increasing painful destruction of tissue and a progressive weakness and anemia and marked mental depression. Later on many homeopathic prescriptions were made with some degree of relief, but no definite improvement in the general state of the patient. About August 9, 1951, this patient received a dose of HIPPOZ. 10M which is the nosode of glanders, a malignant disease of the horse. This remedy repeated about six weeks apart in the 10M and 50M produced most unusual and spectacular results in the condition of the patient. Healing began in the injured parts, and the general strength and well being of the patient improved. On January 14, 1952, another remedy was required over the blood viz, STREPTOM. 1M. This was taken several days later. The latter part of March, I had the privilege of seeing this unusual patient and found her well and cheerful, doing her household duties; and the ulceration on the ulcerated area was almost entirely healed with only a slight scab remaining.

These last two cases are beyond the scope of the usual homeopathic procedure for the selection of remedies and are presented for the sole purpose of proving the possibility of cure when the similimum can be found, thus bringing hope to thousands who languish in the gloom of black despair.

CASES FROM PRACTICE[1]

The homeopathic physician must be an optimist, chiefly because by training and philosophy he has developed a concept of life, health and disease, vastly different to that held by old-school medical thought. The homeopathist works with the processes of proven laws, and with instrumentalities as subtle as the mysterious force of life itself. Disease in all its ugly aspects and material changes brings to the homeopath only the message of inharmony and distunement in the play of vital forces. And as if by White Magic, the homeopathic potion is sufficient to re-establish harmony and order in vital function, and to banish suffering and replace it with comfort and well being and radiant health.

So it is not strange that the homeopathic doctor welcomes a type of sickness that the practicians of the old school seek to avoid by referring all such to various specialists or by sending them away to other climates and environment.

We are told by competent medical authorities that ninety per cent of acute illness will get well without medical aid by the so-called self-limiting nature of acute diseases. And it can be stated without fear of contradiction that most acute illnesses recover quicker and better if only left to nature's powers unhampered by empirical medicine.

In the realm of chronic disease we hear another story. Cancer, epilepsy, diabetes, asthma, tuberculosis and many forms of chronic dermatitis are listed as incurable, and the majority of of old-school doctors prefer not to treat them other than in a palliative way. Homeopathy alone offers encouragement, hope and comfort to these unfortunate victims of chronic disease without mutilation and without financial embarrassment. To the real physician the response of some of these cases to homeopathic treatment is amazing and satisfying beyond the power of language to adequately describe.

CHRONIC PEPTIC AND INTESTINAL ULCERS

The first two cases presented are patients who suffered for years with chronic gastric and intestinal ulcers, diagnosed and treated by old-school doctors after elaborate x-ray and laboratory tests of blood and stomach contents, rendering the diagnosis accurate and complete.

---

1. THE HOMEOPATHIC RECORDER, Vol. LVII, No. 4, October, 1949, p. 161.

Chronic Peptic and Intestinal Ulcers ...

Case 1 Mr. F. W. T. age 29

December 18, 1939: Since 1935 has suffered with gastric and intestinal distress. X-ray at that time revealed duodenal ulcer; was given milk diet with alkaline powders and relieved for awhile. About two years ago had a protracted dizzy attack resulted in fainting accompanied by very low blood pressure. Never had any hemorrhage or vomiting. Has lost some weight because of the restricted diet. His work confines him to much desk work and intense mental application. He has periodic neuralgic headaches. There is no marked response to heat or cold. Is a good water drinker, wants it fairly cold. Sleeps well if digestive pains are not present. Recent test of urine negative. Mental strain and hurry aggravate. Rarely has any preceptible gas. Bowel elimination regular. Very sensitive to a closed hot room. No food desires or aversions. Arg-n. 10M. Had facial acne cured by x-ray treatment before his stomach trouble.

December 24, 1939: First few days were better, but for the last week there is more pain especially when stomach is empty. Graph. 10M.

January 3, 1940: More pain than he has had in a long time; pain awakened him several hours after he went to sleep. Mezer. 10M.

February 21, 1940: No relief until the last two days. Continued on Sacch-l.

March 8, 1940: More acidity and pain; must drink milk every hour for relief. Pains awaken him too early in the a.m. Graph. CM.

March 27, 1940: Improved. Continued on Sacch-l.

May 15, 1940: Much more pain again lately, some tenderness in appendix region. Pains occur two to three hours after eating. Burning acid pain but no nausea; cold things feel better in his stomach. Phos. 1M.

July 17, 1940: Has been much better but some slight return of symptoms. Phos. 10M.

June 1, 1941: A report from him through a friend says he is in perfect health and enjoys all kinds of food with no distress. He feels that he is cured.

Chronic Peptic and Intestinal Ulcers ...

Case 1 Mr. F. W. T. age 29 ...

This case presented few therapeutic symptoms, hence the application of a number or remedies, some of which were of doubtful value. It is interesting to note that Phos. is one of the best antidotes for the therapeutic abuse of x-ray and radium; but as no recurrence of acne occurred, we can hardly call this one of suppression, although the effects of the x-ray might well be a causative factor in the case. I would be grateful for any observations relative to the effects of x-ray radiations for treatment purposes from other members of our society.

Case 2 O. P. Age 45

October 23, 1940: Ulcer of cardiac end of stomach - recent x-ray diagnosis. Old school treatment, liquid diet and alkaline pills. Has little thirst. Has lost considerable weight, now weighs 132 lbs. Bowels normal; some night frequency. No nausea or vomiting. Not affected by weather changes. Lumbar pains extend from back to stomach. Generally better when resting. Mutton tallow in the stomach gives the most relief. Nit-ac. 10M.

November 13, 1940: Bowels better; weighs 135 lbs. with heavier clothes. Seems generally better. Continued Sacch-l.

December 4, 1940: Had an accident; lost a finger at his work. Nit-ac. 50M.

December 27, 1940: Improved; gained two pounds. Continued on Sacch-l.

January 17, 1941: Nit-ac. 50 M.

February 12, 1941: Since a cold in chest has had burning in stomach with much gas. Carb-v. 50M.

March 14, 1941: Better, gained a pound. Continued on Sacch-l.

April 2, 1941: Better until he had nervous upset. Carb-v. 50M.

April 30, 1941: Generally better. Continued on Sacch-l.

May 23, 1941: Patient doing well. It would be interesting to have another x-ray examination of both of these cases made, but is difficult to persuade patients to go to expense and trouble when they are well.

Asthma

Asthma is generally considered incurable by old-school authorities; hence their usual procedure is palliation with drastic medication with adrenalin injections and anti-spasmodic drugs which are the chief factors in rendering these unfortunates incurable. Such treatment also is the chief obstacle the homeopathic doctor must overcome in the restoration of the asthmatic patient to health. Hence many of the chronic drug-soaked individuals take long and tedious prescribing with a series of complimentary remedies to produce a cure. Two cases follow:

Case 3 Mrs. C. P. age 47

April 1, 1940: Has had asthmatic attacks for the past ten years with all kinds of treatment and is steadily getting worse. Has always been subject to catarrhal conditions. Gall-bladder removed years ago. Had kidney trouble while carrying her children. Heart sounds are good, but has much gas gurgling in transverse colon. Bowels always regular and has normal movements daily. Headaches only during asthmatic attacks. No unusual thirst. Generally better in warm weather. Walking aggravates asthma also aggravates the back pain. Not sensitive to cold but sensitive to a hot room, wants the fresh air. Heat flashes lasted two or three years. Menses intermittent lately. Sleep is poor, restless and broken. Frequent urination. Irritability increased and more sensitive to noise. Not tearful. Upper teeth are out, but lower teeth are infected. Carb-v. 10M.

April 8, 1940: Has an acute attack. Carb-v. 10M.

April 16, 1940: Has been some better, but wakens with attacks about 5 a.m. Kali-c. 10M.

May 2, 1940: Has been better, but has a light attack. Kali-c. 10M.

June 4, 1940: Better, but feels a cold coming on. Kali-c. 50M.

June 18, 1940: Has an earache (old symptom). Continued on Sacch-l.

July 3, 1940: One attack of asthma and hot flashes; ears are better. Kali-c. 50M.

August 2, 1940: Better every way. Continued on Sacch-l.

September 13, 1940: Kali-c. 50M.

Asthma ...

Case 3 Mrs. C. P. age 47 ...

October 18, 1940: Suffocating sensation in throat, asthma has been better, lost 16 lbs. from 180. There is a slight asthmatic rale in left bronchus, has had a slight cold. Kali-c. CM.

January 15, 1941: Has a slight cold. Kali-c. 10M.

March 22, 1941: Kali-c. 10M.

May 1, 1941: Patient's daughter reports mother well and free of asthma.

Case 4 Miss F. F. age 30

June 13, 1935: Has had asthma and bronchitis all her life. Had several attacks of pleurisy as a child. Always had a marked tendency to catch cold. Constipated tendency. Generally better in warm weather. No menstrual troubles but delayed at times, three or four months. Had a bad nervous breakdown 10 years ago. Mother living, age 55, has diabetes. Father, 64, is in general good health but gets attacks of asthma. Patient sleeps well as a rule. Restless type. Very sensitive to noise. Appetite not keen, has no thirst. Uses a very careful diet of mostly vegetables and fruits. Heart and lungs sounds are normal. Ant-t. 10M.

June 13, 1935 to July 22, 1935: Slightly relieved. Ant-t. 10M.

August 7, 1935: Asthma < damp weather. Nat-s. 10M.

August 19, 1935 to *September 23, 1935*: Asthma better but has had an intolerable nervous crawling in skin as if bugs were crawling which was removed by Coca 10M several doses a month.

October 9, 1935: Has severe cold with hoarseness and spasmodic cough. Carb-v. 10M.

October 16, 1935: No relief of severe spasmodic cough, and asthma is much aggravated. Meph. 10M.

October 23, 1935: Slightly better but asthma is very bad. Meph. 50M.

November 12, 1935: Improved. Continued on Sacch-l.

December 5, 1935: Meph. 50M.

December 26, 1935: Relieved until today. Meph. 50M.

ASTHMA ...

CASE 4 MISS F. F. AGE 30 ...

February 7, 1936: Asthma better but more throat and sinus catarrh. MEPH. 50M.

March 7, 1936: More asthma. MEPH. CM.

April 27, 1936: Has been better but symptoms are coming back. MEPH. CM.

May 11, 1936: Has an attack of asthma which was > after an attack of flu. Continued remedy.

September 1, 1936: Improved; has been continued since last dose until today. MEPH. CM.

September 23, 1936: Catarrh of nose and throat aggravated; but asthma better until recently, very constipated, face sallow. SEP. 10M.

October 3, 1936: Has been better. SEP. 10M.

November 19, 1936: SEP. 50M.

December 3, 1936: Shortness of breath and fullness after a little food. LYC. 10M.

January 16, 1937: Continued on SACCH-L.

February 18, 1937: LYC. 10M.

March 4, 1937: Better until she caught cold. LYC. 50M.

March 25, 1937: LYC. 50M.

April 15, 1937: Better. Continued on SACCH-L.

May 1, 1937: Doing well. Continued on SACCH-L.

May 24, 1937: Better until today. LYC. 50M.

June 30, 1937: LYC. CM.

August 24, 1937: Has been on SACCH-L. and well until now; some return of symptoms LYC. CM.

September 27, 1937: Has been better every way. LYC. CM.

October 25, 1937: LYC. DM.

December 11, 1937: Better until today. LYC. DM.

Asthma ...

Case 4 Miss F. F. age 30 ...

December 24, 1937: Coryza and cold excoriating discharge. Chilly and weak. Ars. 10M.

January 8, 1938: Improved after cold.

January 22, 1938: Another cold with labored breathing and hoarseness. Carb-v. 10M.

April 3, 1938: Improved since last remedy, slight asthma. Carb-v. 10M.

April 30, 1938: Carb-v. 10M.

May 17, 1938: Better until today. Carb-v. 50M.

June 2, 1938: No asthma until recently and attacks much lighter. Carb-v. 50M.

July, 1938 to August 1, 1938: Continued on Sacch-l.

August 30, 1938: Continued on Sacch-l.

September 2, 1938: Better. Carb-v. 50M.

December 17, 1938: Has been better. Carb-v. CM.

March 18, 1939: Has intervals of months without asthma. No medicine until today. Carb-v. CM.

August 15, 1939: No more medicine until today. Carb-v. CM.

January 5, 1940: Carb-v. CM.

March 15, 1940: Asthma has not bothered her for months, but the constipation continues to bother, and the finger nails are thin ridged and brittle, and the teeth show a deficiency of enamel and some acrid eruptions are on face. Calc-f. 10M.

Calc-f. at infrequent doses in gradually increasing potencies from the 10M. to the CM potency has helped the constipation and improved the stamina and appearance of the patient from a life time of suffering and weakness to a future of hope and well-being stretching out before her; but this happy result could only be won by courage and persistent intelligent application of the Hahnemannian law by the patient and the doctor.

ASTHMA ...

CASE 4 MISS F. F. AGE 30 ...

The patient was constitutionally weak with a poor inheritance, and even good remedies failed to hold sufficient intervals to give nature the chance to build better cellular structure. Perhaps a nosode might have simplified and shortened the time required to cure but none stood out in the family history or the symptom complex. The order of the last remedies in sequence Lyc., Carb-v. and Calc-f. is interesting.

ECZEMA

Eczema or chronic dermatitis is among the difficult and discouraging conditions met with today. Most cases coming to the homeopath have been the rounds of allopathic specialists and have had suppressive ointments of metallic poisons etc. and in more recent times x-ray radiations. These pernicious and suppressive treatments either aggravate the skin condition or drive it inward to some vital part of the economy, generally resulting in a bronchial asthma or a chronic enteritis. Such a case coming to the homeopath must be made to understand that the treatment requires time to remove constitutional and inherited causes and that palliative treatment only serves to prevent the cure.

CASE 5 MRS. E. J. AGE 60

December 29, 1939: Dermatitis of the hands for last ten years, sticky itching complaint, mass of dark brownish crusts exuding serum. Recurring off and on. Always < winter and covering hands and fingers extending up to wrists, scattered spots on arms. Good general health. (This is true of the majority of these patients; vitality is sufficient to keep the disease cause from the centers to the surface of the body.) No trouble with bowel elimination. Mother of three healthy children. Had an ulcer of leg following an upset bile, now healed. Drinks 3 or 4 cups of coffee a day. Eats too much pastry and pork. Has had x-ray and ultra-violet radiations on hands and many salves without help. No urinary symptoms. Was told at Billings Clinic they could do nothing for her. GRAPH. 10M. with a corrected diet.

January 20, 1940: Better until recently, has taken cathartics. GRAPH. 10M.

ECZEMA ...

CASE 5 MRS. E. J. AGE 60 ...

February 10, 1940: Since a nervous shock and a cold has not been so well. GRAPH. 50M.

March 6, 1940: Better. Continued on SACCH-L.

April 4, 1940: GRAPH. 50M.

April 11, 1940: Eruptions aggravated again; now scalp is involved with violent itching. Feeling good generally. Continued on SACCH-L.

May 7, 1940: At a stand still. GRAPH. CM.

May 23, 1940: No change. MEZ. 10M.

June 11, 1940: Eruption better, but right leg is swollen. Continued on SACCH-L.

July 11, 1940: Better every way. Continued on SACCH-L.

August 6, 1940: MEZ. 10M.

August 27, 1940: Continued on SACCH-L.

October 3, 1940: Better; but hands rough and sore. MEZ. 50M.

November 7, 1940: Not as well again. MEZ. 50M.

December 16, 1940: Improved. Continued on SACCH-L.

February 20, 1941: Bruised right foot severely. ARN. 10M.

March 4, 1941: Eruptions gone, but there is return of old leg ulcer. CARB-V. 10M.

March 28, 1941: Ulcer healing slowly; this is the spot where eczema began.

May 2, 1941: Ulcer at a standstill. CARB-V. 50M.

May 26, 1941: Ulcer spreading with burning pain. Eczema gone. MEZ. CM.

June 18, 1941: Ulcer healed; no more eczema, skin everywhere smooth and normal.

TUBERCULOSIS

We are told that T. B. is one of the chronic diseases that medical science has made some progress in lessening and controlling. However,

Tuberculosis ...

their chief efforts have been spent in the field of prevention by isolation and control. As for the cured, they are far from definite and uniform. That rest and nourishing diet and abundance of fresh air are strong factors in the combat against the tubercular ravages must be admitted; and the universal operation of pneumothorax is far from satisfactory as far as real cure goes. Under this regime the tubercular patient is either a semi or complete invalid for life. It is stated that about ten in a hundred become immunized against the disease and recover; and the others die in a more or less short period of time.

Homeopathy added to rest, diet and fresh air without pneumo-thorax operation has a much better record in the cure of tubercular sufferers. It is true that it takes persistent and protracted unremitting effort in the way of careful prescribing along with the other things mentioned to make the majority of these affected ones well. But when they are cured by homeopathic prescribing, there are no relapses or any of the so-called sequellae such as weakness, anemia, etc.

Dr. Kent mentions an observation of his, that many of the so-called cures of T. B. by natural methods later in life become insane, an indication of suppression rather than cure, the disease progressing from less to more vital centers.[1]

Case 6 Mrs. H. M. age 25

One case presented to illustrate the certain curative power of the homeopathic remedy when obtained and administered properly. This case, a nurse I never saw, but all the data including x-ray and copies of laboratory reports with history and clinical findings were sent to me. As nothing but common and diagnostic symptoms were sent, the remedy was selected from her blood, specimens of which were obtained at monthly intervals.

July 6, 1937: Films taken at this Sanatorium on July 6, 1937, showed no disease on the right side, and the disease on the left was a diffuse area of clouding in the centre of the first left interspace.

Right lung: Is clear.

E. J. Lehman.
July 6, 1937

---

1. §216 - Organon - Editor.

TUBERCULOSIS ...

CASE 6 MRS. H. M. AGE 25 ...

March 1938: The films taken at Pembroke in March, 1938, showed a definite spread of this disease down into the periphery of the left 2nd. interspace.

The right lung was clear at that time also.

E. J. Lehman
March 2, 1938

December 1939: COPY: REPORT FROM ONTARIO DEPT. OF HEALTH.
Name of Patient: Miss H.M.

Physician referring patient: Dr. Higginson, Pembroke, Ontario.

Contact with Tuberculous Disease: Sister died from Tuberculosis 1933.

No contact. Contact as a nurse.

HISTORY: Has rested 1 1/2 years, feels well at present, some pain in left chest, easily tired, gained in weight. No cough, no sputum. Physical Findings: Temp. 4 p.m. 97. Weight 116 lbs. Development - Fair nutrition.

LUNGS: Some diminished resonance over the apices. Other conditions: Thyroid palpable. Tuberculin reaction - Positive before.

DIAGNOSIS: Pulmonary tuberculosis, minimal, quiescent.

BLOOD REPORT: The blood sedimentation was 7 in the 1st hour which is quite normal.

D. McCallum - Clinician.

X-Ray Report December 1939

Right lung: slight increase of linear markings.

Left lung: There is a cloudy shadowing about the size of a small marble in the first and second interspace. There are a few nodular clouds scattered through the 1st. and 2nd. interspaces. The trunk structures in these inter-spaces are accentuated. There is also some thin mottling within the circle of the first rib. The base of the lung is clear. There is not evidence of cavity.

On the left side, the infiltration in the 1st. and 2nd. interspaces has contracted considerably and has changed from soft exudative clouding to a nodular productive type which has very little sur-

TUBERCULOSIS ...

CASE 6 MRS. H. M. AGE 25 ...

rounding perifocal reaction. While definite improvement has occurred in the left apical lesion, it cannot be classified as healed and maximum benefit has not yet occurred.

Compared with film taken June 6, 1939, there is some improvement within the two interspaces.

Report of Dr. Grimmer:

On December 18, 1938, when first blood specimen was obtained for remedy finding[1], the patient Miss H. M. Age 25, had been undergoing a rest cure for 18 months. The above was the report from Ontario Department of Health (this report came about a year after the homeopathic remedy was given). Also copies of the stereoscopic chest films were sent (for comparison).

The selected remedy in this case, ARS-IOD. 10M. given first on December 21, 1938, was repeated at intervals of from four weeks to several weeks and in successively increasing potencies until the CM was reached and taken February 18, 1941.

X-Ray Report March 10, 1941:

Reports from x-ray taken March 10, 1941, interpreted by Dr. D. McCallum (see above) as being as good as it will ever be.

March 21, 1941: Patient feeling very well and back at hospital on full time duty. Regaining weight; still becomes tired after a heavy day, but on the whole says she is finding it easier each day. Latest report is that she is contemplating marriage.

CARCINOMA OF BREAST

It is only in cases not too far advanced where tissue changes are not too great that a cure can be consummated with a single remedy given in a succession of potencies. Advanced cases frequently require a succession of remedies not too high in potency over much longer periods to effect cures.

---

1. See see article "Recent Concepts and New Formulas in Medicine" on page 679 ff. and see article "Importance of Electronic Reactions to Future Medicine" on page 683 ff.. - Editor.

CARCINOMA OF BREAST ...

I had hoped to present a case of epilepsy and one or two of diabetes, but the paper is already too long for reading before our bureau, but will present an unusual one on breast cancer briefly even though it may not be read for lack of time.

Cancer of the breast cured by the single remedy is not often met with; and when such results are obtained, it almost seems to belong in the realm of the miraculous. From very ancient times down, cancer has been the most mysterious and implacable disease to afflict and baffle the race. When ever its dread presence creeps in on its hapless victim, there dwells tragedy and utter despair with suffering, impoverishment and death as the certain seal of doom. Such is the dismal picture presented by millions in the world today. and modern medical science stands impotent to help.

Yet Homeopathy is curing many of these unfortunates and prolonging life with comparative comfort in many more. And as time passes on, Homeopathy alone will save the race from the evils of these constitutional and inherited diseases transmitted down the generations.

The obvious lessons taught by the numerous and painstaking experiments on rats by Dr. Maud Sly is illuminating to all who are not willfully blind. Cancer may be bred out of rat families and bred into the cancer-free families by selective mating. Men and women by carefully selecting their mates especially along homeopathic lines would rid the world of cancer, tuberculosis, epilepsy and many types of insanities in three generations, if such selections could be reinforced by careful homeopathic prescribing. The afore-mentioned group of diseases are all the product of a common disease soil as all homeopaths know.

CASE 7 MRS. A. M. AGE 30

October 21, 1938: Married, mother of two healthy children; herself in apparent good health, but recently developed a lump the size of a small hen's egg in the left breast, fixed but not painful, although showing a deep red color on the skin covering the growth with a small area of raw surface. This patient lived about a hundred miles from Chicago and had previously consulted her local doctor who, after making a biopsy, advised immediate removal of the breast. The growth was first noticed about two months before her first visit to my office. No symptoms of pain, no functional disturbance of digestion, no abnormal menstrual symptoms could be found.

CARCINOMA OF BREAST ...

CASE 7 MRS. A. M. AGE 30 ...

All vital organs were normal. The only mental symptoms were those of deep concern because of the tumor and its diagnosis with a gloomy prognosis.

The remedy was selected over the patient's blood[1] which confirmed the other physician's findings except that it was found to be of tubercular type and origin. NAJA was the remedy found, and it was given October 23, 1938, in the 50M.

December 16, 1938: The lump of breast red and painful the past week; before this time was much improved. NAJA 50M.

January 3, 1939: Lump in breast opened and discharged serum and blood. Continued on SACCH-L.

January 24, 1939: Is stronger and lump smaller. Continued on SACCH-L.

February 17, 1939: Spot on breast smaller, generally better, weight 116, gained four pounds. NAJA 50M.

April 14, 1939: The remedy continued until today. NAJA CM.

August 8, 1939: NAJA CM. This acted with patient improving in weight and strength with growth diminishing in size.

November 16, 1939: NAJA CM.

February 2, 1940: Breast healed, growth gone, weighs 120 lbs. Menses delayed two weeks, suspects pregnancy.

February 27, 1940: NAJA CM. Is sure of pregnancy; the following November, 1940, gave birth to a healthy baby with no recurrence of breast trouble and had no more medicine until

January 14,1941: NAJA CM.

Has reported perfect health and no breast trouble. March 13, 1941, and last report April 17, 1941, is perfectly well and happy. No more medicine; patient dismissed cured.

---

1. See see article "Recent Concepts and New Formulas in Medicine" on page 679 ff. and see article "Importance of Electronic Reactions to Future Medicine" on page 683 ff.. - Editor.

HOMEOPATHIC CLINICAL CASES[1]

Among the more difficult cases of sickness to cure are those suffering from epilepsy. Such cases are considered incurable by regular medical standards, and only palliative methods are applied or advised to mitigate the convulsive aspects of the disease.

Aside from the Jacksonian form of the disease, where pressure or mechanical conditions exist, causes of other forms of the disease are uncertain or unknown. Surgical intervention sometimes helps these cases of mechanical origin if excessive brain damage has not already occurred. In the idiopathic forms of the disease, the only causative factors present are the constitutional or miasmatic ones described by Hahnemann in his *Chronic Diseases.*

Most of these cases coming to the homeopathic physician have been treated with suppressive drugs, sometimes over a long period, and they present only common symptoms of the disease intermingled with drug symptoms given for the suppression of the convulsions. The family history and the life story of the patient, with all his sicknesses and injuries, are the main guides for the selection of the remedy. Remedies corresponding to the miasms of the patient and his family must be chosen and given in properly spaced doses and in a succession of potencies. Complimentary remedies are often needed to consummate a permanent cure, because as one miasmatic influence is erased from the patient's economy, another comes up to replace it until it in turn is eradicated by the suitable remedy. Thus it frequently requires a series of remedies, often in a succession of ascending potencies to cure such intractable, chronic conditions of epilepsy and the malignancies - all listed by the leading medical authorities as incurable; and indeed they are so unless treated by a master of the Hahnemannian homeopathic art and science.[2]

EPILEPSY

A middle-aged man who had suffered for years with irregular, recurring convulsions, diagnosed by allopathic doctors as epilepsy and given in abundance the classical, routine anti-spasmodic, suppressive drugs for some years with no mitigation of his trouble.

---

1. THE HOMEOPATHIC RECORDER, Vol. LXXIII, Nos. 10 - 12, May and June, 1958, p.106.
2. Dr. Grimmer was a master of the Hahnemannian Homeopathic Art and Science. - Editor.

EPILEPSY ...

On August 13, 1945, the following report was received: "I feel that we have made progress during the last year. The night of July 26 I had a recurrence; attack came as usual during sleeping hours in the early morning. It was the lightest of any in eight years. Was able to go back to work about 10 a.m. Rested well the two nights following the attack; on the third and fourth night was restless but finally overcame the restlessness and slept. Since then I have felt fine, rested well every night and have used medicine per schedule (one powder of SACCH-L. each week). Have not been bothered with backache this time as I was with former attacks. "This change occurred under two doses of KALI-BR. 10M, given six to eight weeks apart, and one dose of KALI-BR. CM on April 1, 1946, and another dose of KALI-BR. CM given on June 13, 1946. On August 6, 1946, NAT-S. 10M was given as KALI-BR. CM held too short a time; and a re-study of the case brought in NAT-S. 10M. This was repeated on September 16, 1946. From this time on until February 22, 1955, NAT-S. in ascending potencies was given at long intervals until NAT-S. DM (second dose) no longer acted. A blood test February 28, 1955, brought through KALI-I. 10M.[1] This blood test revealed the syphilitic miasm (inherited). KALI-I. in ascending potencies to the CM seems to have completed a cure of this very chronic case. In the past year there have been no attacks, and the patient is in excellent health.

This case is an excellent example of Hahnemann's miasmatic concept of chronic disease: First, a series of potencies of the *antipsoric* remedy KALI-BR., followed by the *antisycotic* remedy NAT-S. and lastly the *antisyphilitic* remedy KALI-I. All were required to make a perfect cure of a most resistant condition complicated with drastic drugging from suppressive antispasmodic nostrums

CHRONIC DERMATITIS

Chronic dermatitis is another condition difficult to cure with any treatment outside the homeopathic remedy. A case in point: V. C. age 13. Given CARB-V. 10M on January 17, 1942. A history of dermatitis of arms and hands since early childhood. Has had measles and chickenpox. Gets severe headaches with vomiting at times. There is no tenderness at McBurny's point. Has a hemic heart murmur. Extremely fond of sweets, no desire for salt.

---

1.   See see article "Recent Concepts and New Formulas in Medicine" on page 679 ff. and see article "Importance of Electronic Reactions to Future Medicine" on page 683 ff.. - Editor.

Chronic Dermatitis ...

February 7, 1942: Eruption better, but has had a severe head cold. Carb-v. 10M.

March 2, 1942: Some better. Carb-v. 50M.

March 28, 1942: Improved in every way; continued on Sacch-l.

After this date the patient moved to Florida from Chicago and discontinued homeopathic treatment and placed herself in the hands of a regular physician of the old school. She was given Cortisone internally and had ultra-violet ray treatments on the skin which aggravated not only her skin trouble but impaired her general health. She was also given a weight-reducing drug.

April 12, 1948: the patient returned to Chicago for homeopathic help.

April 26, 1948: Calc-s. 10M.

May 3, 1948: Has a case of athletes foot; Samarskite 10M.

May 10, 1948: Improved; continued on Sacch-l.

June 2, 1948: Skin some better, but menses too soon with a heavy flow; gaining weight fast, does not feel well; perspires too freely and perspiration irritates skin eruption; was given another dose of Samarskite 10M.

June 10, 1948: Skin is better, but is gaining weight too fast; Graph. 10M. From this time until

April 17, 1957, the patient has been on Graph. 10M and 50M in repeated doses of each potency. Her last report on

April 17, 1957, was that her skin has entirely cleared and that she is in better health than ever before.

Cervical Cysts and Swellings

The next case is of interest to the internist because of the amount of pathology involved.

March 29, 1955: Mrs. B. H. E. Married. Age 37. History of profuse irritating vaginal discharge; history of being treated from the preceeding December for an infection of the vaginal canal with severe burning and itching with a putrid odor from the discharge. All this was accompanied with severe backaches and pains extending into

CERVICAL CYSTS AND SWELLINGS ...

both groins and down the thighs, legs and feet. Feet swell when on them too much. Has severe headaches from time to time with nervous irritability. She was given a series of penicillin shots and sent to a gynecologist who advised an operation. She was also suffering from rose and hayfever. Was told she had a small tumor in uterus, but my examination showed extensive swelling and cystic changes in the cervix, the uterus heavy and enlarged with an enlarged cystic left ovary. THUJ. 10M.

May 12, 1955: Has had an attack of rose fever. Last period shorter with backache. Craves sweets, appetite poor, easily satiated. LYC. 10M.

July 14, 1955: Increase of irritating discharge, period improved; LYC. 10M.

August 19, 1955: Increase of irritating discharge, tendency to varicose veins, hay fever attacks recur annually; flow dark but not clotted; LACH. 10M.

SEPTEMBER 22, 1955: Pain in left ovarian region, tired and broken sleep, hard to get to sleep. Full bloated sensation with hunger, feet swollen and sore, no thirst. LACH. 10M.

October 27, 1955: Pain and discharge persist, but is sleeping better; LACH. 50M.

January 10, 1956: Pain in back after resting, no headache at last period, discharge is less, pelvic findings much improved; LACH. 50M.

March 13, 1956: Had two severe headaches. LACH. CM.

May 1, 1956: Continued on SACCH-L.

June 5, 1956: Has had several vomiting attacks with constant pain in left ovarian region. Has lost ten to twelve pounds. Pelvic findings better. Continued on SACCH-L.

July 17, 1956: Had severe vomiting attack a week after period with anxious fear. Sleeping better, pelvic findings improved; LACH. CM.

September 11, 1956: LACH. DM.

October 2, 1956: Flow scanty, headaches are lighter. Continued on SACCH-L.

CERVICAL CYSTS AND SWELLINGS ...

November 13, 1956: Feet swelling again, periods are more regular; continued on SACCH-L.

January 14, 1957: KALI-C. 10M.

February 4, 1957: Menses very scanty. LYC. 50M.

March 12, 1957: No period since last Thanksgiving, breast sore and swollen. Has a slight mitral murmur. Has used fluorinated water; CADMIUM CALCAREA FLUORICUM 10M.[1]

April 12, 1957: Expects a baby this coming September. No headaches and is feeling better in everyway. Continued on SACCH-L.

NERVOUS BREAKDOWN

Still another case. Mr. H.B. Middle aged. Has had repeated nervous breakdowns where fear and suspicion produced prolonged attacks of insomnia ending in a loss of strength and weight with a complete lack of confidence and deep mental depression which is indeed a very gloomy picture.

Perhaps this type of case is as trying and difficult to cure as those suffering from phobia, frustration and resentments with insomnia which so often wind up as so-called nervous breakdowns; and these are the hapless victims of the pain killers, the mood drugs and the sleep producers which are so abundantly advertised on radio and television.

March 13, 1956: For the third time in as many years this man returned for the kind of help he had found on previous occasions under homeopathic care. NAT-S. 50M.

June 22, 1956: NAT-S. 50M.

July 7, 1956: Not able to sleep; MAG-M. 10M.

August 7, 1956: Unrefreshing sleep; LACH. 10M.

August 30, 1956: A blood test brought this new remedy through[2], THUJ. 10M.

---

1. CADMIUM CALCAREA FLUORICUM is one of the Cadmium preparations used by Dr. Grimmer. - Editor.
2. See see article "Recent Concepts and New Formulas in Medicine" on page 679 ff. and see article "Importance of Electronic Reactions to Future Medicine" on page 683 ff.. - Editor.

Nervous Breakdown ...

September 25, 1956: Very suspicious and depressed, is sure he cannot get well; Kali-thio-cyan. 10M.

October 8, 1956: Full of unreasoning fear; Op. 10M.

October 19, 1956: Suicidal and restless; Aur-m. 10M.

October 25, 1956: Slight improvement; continued on Sacch-l.

November 2, 1956: Better on motion, extremely irritable and restless; Kali-i. 10M.

November 16, 1956: No better, Kali-br. 10M.

November 23, 1956: Does not feel he is improving; return of physical symptoms, better in the dark; Hyos. 10M.

November 27, 1956: Syph. 10M.

December 4, 1956: Thuj. 10M.

March 29, 1957: Improved. Has regained nine pounds, weight 166; Thuj. 10M.

The last report on May 15, 1957, found the patient feeling well and full of confidence with regained strength.

Such cases are especially hard to treat homeopathically because so much easy palliation is at hand, and this type of patient will grasp any promised relief with no thought of consequences. And since they have had a little palliation even for a short time, their will to fight and endure for positive cure is lost.

These mental and nervous cases with their severe tensions seem to require more remedies given on their indications and more frequent repetition of remedies to obtain curative results. But cures are possible if no interference with palliative drugs are interjected and enough time is permitted to find the one best drug or the best array of complimentary remedies needed to do the work. This requires much patience and study on the part of the physician as well as immense faith and courage on the patient's part. Only such patients as have been indoctrinated in Homeopathic Philosophy and have experienced the great advantages of homeopathic prescribing are conditioned to cooperate with this method of treatment in the face of the enumerable palliative nostrums confronting him today. But present day palliative treatments only plunge the patient deeper into the mire of despondency and frustration. Homeopathy is the only hope for a real cure for these unfortunate victims.

Special Diseases

A New Medical Approach in the Treatment of Alcoholism

Asiatic Flu

What Not to Do in Flu

Homeopathy in Heart Disease

Homeopathy Psychosomatic Medicine

Mental Disease Cured by Homeopathy

Homeopathic Treatment of Typhoid

Undulant Fever

Homeopathic Success Against Infantile Paralysis

Homeopathic Palliation in Incurables

A New Medical Approach in the Treatment of Alcoholism[1]

Medical science to date makes no claim for the cure of this rapidly spreading disease, already assuming universal proportions, and now a major health problem to the world. The victims of alcoholism are now regarded by doctors of medicine as being very sick people, with little, if any, prospects for a cure.

To date there has been no specific remedy or drug discovered that can cure or cope successfully with this destructive malady. We are told, alcoholics have acquired an allergy to the alcoholic poison in all forms. Even when taken in small amounts it can and does suspend the power of the will to resist an overwhelming urge for more and more of the poison, until the body organism is saturated and rendered helpless, morally, mentally and physically, to become a human wreck floating on the ocean of delusion and oblivion, blown by the self-made winds of adversity into the whirlpools of suffering, degradation and death.

One of the causative factors related to the disease, that has not been sufficiently stressed and on which little, if any, research has been done, is that of heredity. During the last forty years, the world has been afflicted by three major and many minor wars, leaving a harvest of poverty and moral degradation, in which intemperance of all forms has increased to its present alarming proportions. At least three generations have been born and have lived under the impact of alcoholic excess. This was greatly aggravated during and following the prohibition era.

While geneticists are not a unit in recognizing the transmission of inherited allergies, it is fairly well established that among the *black genes* are noted certain types of allergic conditions that are transmissible, such as asthma, and an individual sensitivity to many substances that produce untoward effects, with sick-making powers, that can disturb the human organism.

Alcohol is a poison causing vast, far-reaching changes in the body organism, ultimating in serious pathological changes in the brain, nerves and blood vessels, as well as in the other vital organs of the economy. Since the brain and nervous system are so profoundly affected by the alcoholic poison, it is logical to infer that alcohol in excess, (through several succeeding generations) might produce, by a form of mutation, genes similar to the *black genes* that could transmit

---

1. From handwritten manuscript, written about 1949. - Editor..

allergic sensibilities to alcohol and produce in certain individuals both an intense craving for it and a strong susceptibility to its degenerating effects on the tissues and vital organs of the body.

Whatever the etiological factors may be, it has been quite generally noted that the tendency to the intemperate use of alcohol does run in certain families through succeeding generations. This observation applies especially to the period of the past thirty to forty years. It is true that from most ancient times drunkenness has affected some individuals more or less but never to the extent that is noted at present and the malady is rapidly increasing.

Geneticists have established the fact that many serious, constitutional types of disease, both physical and mental, are transmitted by way of the genes through succeeding generations. To cite a few of the more well known and drastic ones: several forms of cancer, diabetes, epilepsy and many forms of chronic skin disorders difficult to cure, such as psoriasis, keloid, persistent eczema, and lichen. These conditions, along with alcoholism, are listed as incurable by modern medical science.

Nevertheless, many individual patients suffering from these various diseases have been cured by a new medical approach, by using medicines prepared in a special way that will enable them to reach and eradicate the deep hidden causes of human sickness, which are the result of constitutionally inherited states and conditions of disease. These remedies are prepared in such a way as to reduce them by a process of potentization to a state of electromagnetic or electronic energy.

This energy corresponds to the subtleness of the disease energies that afflict mankind and also to the life energy that builds and sustains the physical organism with its innumerable, complex functions that constitute all life's marvelous processes in its ceaseless struggle for existence against disease and environmental stress of all kinds. This is the only type of energy that can cope with the energy of disease, be it chemical, viral, or bacterial, or even the most subtle of inherited toxins, which are the prime cause of all constitutional disease.

When the subtle disease energy operating in the body is brought in contact with a similar drug energy, each energy repels and dissipates the other, to leave the vital energy of the body free to act in its normal way, to control and direct all of its many and various tasks relative to the vital processes of the living organism.

It is by way of the autonomic nervous system, which is an important part of the defensive mechanism of the body organism against disease and hurts of all kinds, that these subtle energies are empowered to act involuntarily, automatically and effectively for the protection and preservation of the whole being.

When we contemplate these marvellous things pertaining to the life side of creation, with all the orderly processes vibrating in sequence and harmony for the perfection of uses, we are appalled with wonder and reverence in this presence of divine order, operating throughout all animated nature. This expression of divine power and goodness behind the form side of the material cosmos, should convince even the most material-minded skeptic of the presence and rulership of a supreme being, who guides and maintains his created universe and its inhabitants by immutable law.

By observing the growth and development of plants, animals and men in the material world and studying the processes and laws that control and regulate these things, we become aware that back of the form side of nature there is the force or causative expression of nature, active though hidden and unapparent. From these observations, we are able to conclude that prior to, and back of, both the material and phenomenal worlds there is the spiritual world where Deity and all causes exist and have their origin. The acceptance of this knowledge and its application, in the realm of healing, brings to the needs of suffering humanity hitherto unknown powers for the restoration of spiritual, mental and physical health against all forms of disease.

To substantiate this statement we need but cite the wonderful work of rehabilitation and cure for the victims of alcoholism by the organized groups known as Alcoholic Anonymous. Hundreds of hopeless human wrecks, who had failed to find help from medical science and psychological therapy or from the spiritual efforts of ministers and religious advisers, have made complete and permanent recoveries through the beneficial program of A.A. From a medical point of view, these recoveries are more than interesting, they can be highly instructive to the physician and psychologist anxious to restore these scientifically acknowledged incurable patients to a state of health, spiritually, mentally and physically with the restoration of their uses to society.

The victims of alcoholism, when through suffering and frustration have been brought to the point of recognizing that human agencies are powerless to aid them, are then conditioned to accept the fact that only a *higher power* whose resources are greater than man's can help them. When these facts are recognized and accepted, there comes to these patient an illumination that completely transforms their nature. The depressed, morbid outlook is dissipated by light of Divine truth and goodness. Love, faith and understanding become a triangle and a talisman in their lives. Love for the Lord and their fellow human beings and faith in the goodness and power of the heavenly Father brings them understanding and compassion for the suffering and misfortune of all others whom they meet along the rugged highways of life.

These victims of alcoholism, who are living by the program outlined in the A. A. category of rules are especially conditioned to receive the benefits that the Homeopathic medical approach can bring to them without in any way interfering with their A. A. program. In this new aspect of medical approach there can be a most effective, complementary, agency to insure the certainty and permanency of cure for those patients who have been conditioned by the highly spiritualized program and unifying influence of A. A. The heavenly Father works by many diverse ways his wonders to perform and he employs those agencies best suited for the work, at the given time and place to accomplish his ends. Hence, it becomes easy to accept all possible and proven means available for such desirable results, as a permanent cure for the victim of alcoholism.

In the extensive scope of the Homeopathic Materia Medica and literature can be found hundreds of cases cured of alcoholism. It is unfortunate that the possibilities for great good along these lines have been too long neglected. With the establishment of clinics for the treatment of alcoholism, at least in our larger cities, or even where one or more Homeopathic prescribers are located, clinics similar to those serviced by Gallavardin of Paris, France, might be formed and serviced for the good of humanity and the advancement and recognition of Homeopathic science.

In Kent's Repertory (pg. 36) we find under MIND the rubric[1]

DIPSOMANIA: ars., bufo, *calc.*, caust., con., hep., lach., mag-c., merc., *nux-v.*, op., petr., puls., staph., *sulph.*

drinking on the sly: sulph.

menses, before: Sel.

Under STOMACH the rubric DESIRES **alcoholic drinks** (page 483), we find 57 remedies. Sel. (in black type) has it occurring before the menses.

---

1. These rubrics have been inserted by the editor.

DESIRES (pg.483) **alcoholic drinks** (57): Acon., aloe, am-c., ant-t., arn., **Ars.**, *ars-i.*, **Asar.**, aster., *aur.*, bov., bry., bufo, calc., *calc-ar.*, calc-s., **Caps.**, carb-an., chin., cic., **Crot-h.**, cub., cupr., fl-ac., gins., hell., *hep., iod., kreos.*, lac-c., **Lach.**, *led., lec., med.*, merc., *mur-ac.*, naja, nat-p., **Nux-v.**, *op., phos.*, plb., *psor., puls., sel.*, sep., sol-t-ae., *spig., staph.*, **Sulph.**, *sul-ac.*, sumb., *syph.*, tab., ter., ther., *tub.*

menses, before: Sel.

ale (3): ferr-p., *med., sulph.*

beer (52): **Acon.**, agar., aloe, am-c., ant-c., arn., ars., asar., *bell., bry.*, calad., calc., camph., carbn-s., *caust.*, chel., chin., *cocc.*, coc-c., *coloc.*, cupr., dig., *graph., kali-bi., lach.*, mang., *merc.*, mosch., nat-ar., *nat-c., nat-m.*, nat-p., *nat-s.*, **Nux-v.**, op., *petr., phel.*, ph-ac., phos., psor., *puls., rhus-t., sabad.*, sep., *spig.*, spong., staph., stram., *stront.*, **Sulph.**, tell., zinc.

brandy (34): acon., ail., arg-n., ars., ars-met., aster., bov., bry., bufo, calc., chin., cic., coca, cub., ferr-p., *hep.*, lach., mosch., mur-ac., **Nux-v.**, olnd., **Op.**, *petr., phos.*, puls., *sel., sep., spig., staph.*, stram., stront., *sulph., sul-ac.*, ther.

whiskey (22): acon., *arn., ars.*, calc., carb-ac., *carb-an.*, chin., cub., fl-ac., hep., **Lac-c.**, *lach.*, merc., nux-v., op., *phos.*, puls., *sel., spig.*, staph., **Sulph.**, ther.

wine (37): *acon., aeth.*, arg-m., *ars.*, asaf., bov., *bry., calc.*, calc-ar., calc-s., chel., chin., chin-a., *cic.*, colch., cub., fl-ac., *hep.*, hyper., kali-bi., kali-br., kali-i., *lach., lec.*, merc., *mez.*, nat-m., **Phos.**, puls., sec., sel., *sep., spig.*, staph., **Sulph.**, *sumb.*, ther.

claret wine (4): calc-s., staph., *sulph.*, ther.

Under GENERALITIES (pg. 1344) we find rubrics for aggravations from alcoholic drinks as follows:

Aggravated by alcoholic stimulants (59) acon., *agar.*, alum., alumn., am-m., anac., *ant-c., arg-n.*, arn., **Ars.**, **Asar.**, **Bar-c.**, *bell.*, bor., bov., cadm-s., *calc., calc-ar.*, carb-an., *carb-s., carb-v.*, caust., *chel., chin.*, chol., cocc., *coff., con., crot-h., dig.*, gels., hep., hyos., *ign.*, kali-bi., **Lach.**, laur., *led., lyc.*, naja, *nat-c., nat-m., nux-m.*, **Nux-v.**, **Op.**, *petr., puls.*, **Ran-b.**, *rhod., rhus-t., ruta*, sabad., *sang.*, **Sel.**, sep., *sil.*, spig., *stram.*, stront., *stroph.*, **Sulph.**, **Sul-ac.**, tab., thuj., verat., zinc.

Aggravated by brandy (25): agar., *ars.*, bell., calc., chin., cocc., hep., hyos., ign., lach., laur., *led.*, **Nux-v.**, **Op.**, puls., *ran-b.*, rhod., *rhus-t.*, ruta, spig., *stram.*, **Sulph.**, sul-ac., verat., zinc.

Aggravated by wine (page 1422) (54): acon., agar., alum., am-m., *ant-c.*, *arn.*, **Ars.**, aur., aur-m., bell., *bor.*, bov., bry., cact., *calc.*, carb-an., carb-v., carbn-s., *chin.*, chol., coc-c., **Coff.**, coloc., *con.*, cor-r., ign., *fl-ac.*, *gels.*, *glon.*, kali-chl., *lach.*, *led.*, **Lyc.**, *naja*, nat-ar., nat-c., *nat-m.*, *nux-m.*, **Nux-v.**, **Op.**, ox-ac., petr., puls., **Ran-b.**, *Rhod.*, rhus-t., ruta, *sabad.*, *sel.*, **Sil.**, stront., thuj., verat., **Zinc.**

Aggravated by sour wine (6): **Ant-c.**, ant-t., ars., ferr., sep., sulph.

Combining the rubrics of Desires alcoholic drinks and Aggravated by alcoholic stimulants we get the following rubric:

Desires alcoholic drinks and aggravated by them (24): Acon., arn., **Ars.**, **Asar.**, bov., *calc.*, *calc-ar.*, carb-an., *chin.*, **Crot-h.**, *hep.*, **Lach.**, *led.*, *lyc.*, naja, **Nux-v.**, **Op.**, *puls.*, **Sel.**, *sep.*, *spig.*, **Sulph.**, **Sul-ac.**, tab.

Eighteen of the twenty-four are in high type, and thus a most important group of remedies for individual study in the treatment of alcoholism until further clinical experience in treating the disease will enable us to add other remedies to this list from time to time. This important group of remedies does not prevent the study of any other discoverable remedy in our vast materia medica and there are many others that have symptoms to indicate their use in such condition. This group of clinically proven remedies is one place to start the search for the individual remedy needed for each case.

ARSENICUM ALBUM

The first remedy of the group for individual study is Ars.. The patient needing Ars. is far on his way to the place of deterioration. Pathological changes are tearing at his vital organs; the brain and nervous system are impaired and faulty; the memory and mental equipment are disturbed and unreliable and the moral nature confused and befogged or obliterated. Profound depression and despair with uncontrollable restlessness and anxiety, alternate with fits of apathy and indifference, or, at times, with irritability and resentment.

All the senses are more impressionable to the vibrations of sound, light, touch, etc. causing painful annoyance and an irritable state of

Arsenicum album ...

mind, with bitter complaining, anguish, tears, and despair. With the deepest melancholy comes unreasoning fears of death, misfortune and an extreme dread of being alone. The moods are changeable and often alternating; the mental states may range from a super alertness to impressions to one of dullness and stupidity with extreme weakness of memory and a lack of ability to concentrate on mental activities. Delirium, with a great flow of ideas full of fears, ghosts, specters, robbers, malcontents, wild animals, poisonous insects, snakes, etc. is often present. There may be loss of consciousness and sensation, often imbecility. Religious complaints of the most depressing types, loss of faith and hope in God and also in his fellow human beings are common symptoms.

The Ars. patient is weak, faint, cold and exhausted. His appearance is either bloated and besotted or emaciated and cachetic; in the lowest states of sickness a cadaveric [1]appearance often is noted.

Ars. pains are burning and severe, yet for the most part, relieved by warmth; the head pains being one exception. There is a marked tendency to ulceration and even gangrene of the tissues, both internally and externally. The time aggravations are after midnight until two or three a.m. This is the time when the tides of life are at their lowest.

This brief sketch of Ars. presents a picture of the victim of alcoholism in all its worst aspects. Fearful, weak, hopeless, anguished, anxious, restless, but unable to rest, alone in the gloom of despair, a human wreck on the verge of a bottomless abyss, beyond the power of any human agency to save. Only the influx from the source of all goodness and power, God, can dispel the thick enveloping darkness surrounding those lost ones, the victims of alcoholism. In the depth of their hopelessness and agony, they now are ready to reach out, seek and accept, the help of a power surpassing all human agencies that have proven powerless to help or mitigate them in all their long past suffering and misfortune.

When this mysterious contact with the spiritual influx is consummated, a marked change takes place in these lost beings, with an equally mysterious change in their lives, minds and bodies, rendering them susceptible to all the finer forces and instincts vibrating throughout the realm of nature in all its planes, physical, etheric, mental, and spiritual.

---

1. i.e. hippocratic. - Editor.

Arsenicum album ...

It is then, that the fine, specifically selected drug force of the Homeopathic remedy, can insure the permanency of cure in these intractable and relapsing cases. Better yet, it can, if applied early enough, prevent many incipient stages of the disease from reaching the terminal stage of pathological destruction.

Asarum europeum

Asar. will be found more useful in the incipient stages of the disease before pathologic changes in tissues and organs have developed. It has three main spheres of action, mental and nervous system, the digestive tract and conditions involving the eyes.

In an oversensitive nervous system the slightest noise, such as scratching with the finger nail on linen or silk cloth, is unbearable. Exaltation of the senses, shivers from any emotion, a gradual vanishing of ideas, imagines he is hovering in the air like a spirit when walking in the open air; vertigo as if drunk when rising from a seat and severe compressive headaches are symptoms of the mind and nervous systems.

The eyes are the seat of much trouble; such as inflamed red eyes, obscuration of sight when reading, very sensitive to light, sunshine and cool air aggravates yet cold bathing relieves. Asar. is valuable in post surgical operations and after painful and lacerating injuries to the eye.

General relief in damp wet weather is an uncommon and valuable indication (Aur-m.). Frequent eructations; empty, sour, setting teeth on edge. Violent empty retching which increases all symptome but relieves stupid feeling in head. Nausea (with clean tongue) < eating. Nausea and fainting, vomiting with great anguish; a horrible sensation at the epigastrium on waking in drunkards are the main symptoms relative to the digestive tract. With the retching and vomiting pain and anguish, there is an unquenchable longing for alcohol.

Calcareas

The Calcarea preparations, Calc., Calc-ar., Calc-p., and Calc-s. are useful and effective remedies in this disease. Their indications are found along the constitutional and general aspects of the provings but we will add a few distinctive symptoms of each preparation that may prove helpful in the selection of the specific remedy needed for each individual case.

CALCAREAS ...

CALC.: Craves eggs, salt things, wine and thirsts for cold drinks; he is a chilly patient yet sweats profusely around the head and feet. The perspiration is sour as are most of the body secretions (HEP.). There is a great weakness of the digestion and acid eructations. It is one of the remedies craving indigestable things such as chalk, coal, etc. (GRAPH. and NIT-AC.).

CALC-AR.: Consists of symptoms of the two components of which the remedy is composed. It meets those cases where pathology tends to ultimate in the *liver* and *pancreas*, hence, cancer in the pancreas and cirrhosis of the liver with hypertrophy.

CALC-S.: Much like HEP., but is sensitive to heat. This remedy combines the power of the two great antipsorics SULPH. and CALC. especially in its power to meet many of the states and symptoms pertaining to alcoholism.

SNAKE POISONS

The SNAKE POISONS are especially useful in the treatment of this disease. CROT-H. and LACH. are two most prominent. The disorganizing effects on the blood produced by these remedies is the marked feature of their action. Next in importance is the tendency of shock to the nervous system they cause and can cure.

The CROT-H. case is one of a broken down constitution, brought on from the toxins of typhoid or malaria as well as from the ravages of the chronic symptoms arising from alcoholic excess. There is a great tendency to hemorrhagic symptoms, bleeding from all the orifices of the body (even the perspiration is bloody). The patient is mentally depressed, tearful and despondent. Mental perception is clouded and confused. There is great craving of stimulants with the pain; weakness, nausea and vomiting of black blood, coffee ground vomit, vomiting of uncoagulated blood, black stools and jaundice. Symptoms and conditions are *right sided*, (LACH. usually is left sided). Both remedies crave stimulants such as wine and other alcoholic beverages. They both, in common with all serpent poisons, are aggravated during and after sleep. The mental symptoms of CROT-H. are more clouded and obscured, stupidity and confusion with inability to concentrate mentally. In LACH. the senses are more acute and active, great loquacity is present. Both remedies have profound depression with anguish and despair.

LYCOPODIUM

LYC., like SULPH. and the CALCAREAS, must be used on the basis of the deep constitutional symptoms and conditions. There are a number of general and characteristic symptoms that will enable the alert prescriber to recognize the need for the individual patient presenting LYC. characteristics. Clarke observes that LYC. is one of the pivotal remedies of the Materia Medica and an intimate acquaintance with its properties and relations is essential to a proper understanding of the Materia Medica as a whole.

Fear of being alone, of men, of his own shadow, apprehensiveness, susceptible to mental causes, fear which makes a profound impression of bodily organs especially the liver. Mental states resulting from fear, profound sadness an inclination to weep, consolation aggravates, forgetful, avaricious, imperiousness, miserly, difficult concentration, general aggravation 4 to 8 p.m. are strong in the LYC. drug picture.

Easy satiety, distention and discomfort with loss of appetite, after the least amount of food or drink, canine hunger followed by satiety, belching of much gas which relieves, sensitive to light, noise and jar. Emaciation from above downwards, marked irritability, many symptoms and conditions are brought on or made worse by anger.

LYC. is right sided, symptoms travel from right to left especially the symptoms of the throat and ovaries. General aggravation from heat and becoming heated, relief in the fresh open air, double vision, opthalmia, falling of hair, severe neuralgias and other forms of nerve and rheumatic pains, the pains come on suddenly and depart suddenly. LYC. frequently causes severe aggravations and should not be given at first in too high a potency and the indications for its use should be clear cut.

MEDORRHINUM[1]

This remedy corresponding so intimately with inherited and suppressed sycosis which universally affects humanity may well be a frequently needed remedy for alcoholism, especially if complicated with diabetes.

Forgetfulness of names, words, and even letters. Dazed feeling. Far off sensation as though things done today occurred a week ago; looses constantly the trend of her talk; seems to herself to make wrong state-

---

1. This text here is from the articles MEDORRHINUM by E.W. Berridge; TRANSACTIONS OF THE INTERNATIONAL HAHNEMANN ASSOCIATION 1889, p. 221 and corrections of this article by the same author in the IHA TRANSACTION 1892, p. 152. - Editor.

MEDORRHINUM ...

ments because she does not know what to say. Difficult concentration of thoughts. Thinks someone is behind her, hears whisperings; sees large people in the room and large rats running, felt a delicate hand smoothing her head from front to back. Is sure she is going to die; all life seems unreal like a dream; wild and desperate feeling as of incipient insanity; cannot speak without crying; suicidal; hurried, becomes fatigued from hurry; weighed down with gloom; dread of the dark. Feeling as if he had committed the unpardonable sin and was going to hell. Feels most matters sensitively before they occur, generally correctly; clairvoyance. Violent headaches with sensitiveness to sound, light and jar. Great selfishness and impatience. Burning soles, wants them fanned, swollen painful soles.

NUX VOMICA

The alcoholic patient needing NUX-V. is one whose special senses are acute and even exaggerated; sight, hearing, touch, smell and taste. Even a slight disturbance from light touch and noise may cause convulsions and extreme pain; hypochrondical, peevish, stubborn and irritability of mind; anger and bad effects from it; debauchery, masturbation, sexual excesses and perversions.

Those who have wrecked their health from excesses and brought on mental incompetency associated with deep melancholy and even despair, and whose digestive organs are greatly impaired, often end in malnutrition and weakness mentally and physically. This gives a brief general picture of the NUX-V. sickness and the indications for the use of the remedy. IGN. must be compared, especially in those cases where the long lasting effects of grief is a causative factor.

OPIUM

OP. is to be thought of in cases of threatened apoplexy and paralytic weakness in those who have been subject to shock, fright and severe tensions, long lasting effects from fright. Patients whose vitality is so low they cannot react to well selected remedies. Carelessness, great anxiety and uneasiness; inconstancy and fickleness; strong tendency to take alarm; timorous character or rash and inconsiderate boldness; alternating states; stupidity and imbecility; great flow of ideas, with gaiety and disposition to indulge in sublime and profound reflections; vivid imagination; mania; delirium and confusion; loquaciousness; visions of

Opium ...

mice, scorpions, etc.; mendacity; kleptomania; lying disposition; loss of moral senses are some of the mental symptoms that strongly point to Op.

Psorinum

Psor. is needed in deeply psoric constitutions where these manifestations persist through several generations, especially those conditions pertaining to the skin, respiratory and digestive systems. Cold weak patients with feeble reactions to well selected remedies; depressed suicidal subjects; loathing of life; all is dark and hopeless; offensive body odors and discharges are strong indications in this patient, who often craves stimulants. All the nosodes are useful remedies when given on the strict indications calling for their use.

Selenium

Sel. will fit some cases of alcoholism in rather chronic or advanced states. Among the key symptoms for its use is that of profound weakness of body and mind, extreme sense of fatigue. It acts strongly on the male sexual sphere and the larynx. It has cured incipient tubercular laryngitis; prostatitis and impotency; lascivious ideas; pollutions with flaccidity of penis; discharge of semen drop by drop during sleep; lascivious dreams with emissions, followed by weakness and lameness of the back; during coition feeble erection and too quick emission; long continued voluptuous thrill. Debility and weakness after coition.

Extreme craving for alcoholic stimulants especially brandy, which aggravates the symptoms. In women, strong craving for alcohol at the menses.

Reveries of a religious and melancholic character; great loquacity; excessive forgetfulness, especially in matters of business; great forgetfulness when awake with distinct recollection during half sleep; stammering; uses syllables and words in wrong connections. Mental labor fatigues him; dread of society.

Causation: alcohol, tea, sugar, salt, lemonade, debauchery, walking, exertion, masturbation, loss of fluids. The above is only a brief aspect of the patient needing Sel.

Sepia

Sep. may be needed in women suffering from alcoholism. Women relaxed with weak ptosed organs as uterus, bladder, intestines, kidneys,

Sepia ...

etc. Women become averse to their husbands without any known cause even to themselves; women never well since the birth of a child, with pelvic pathology and symptoms; weak women who crave stimulants.

Sulphur

The symptomatology of Sulph. covers every type of disease acute and chronic afflicting the human race. It stands at the head of the anti-psoric group of remedies. The typical Sulph. case is unkempt, dirty, and abhors bathing. He has been called the ragged philosopher perhaps because he is content in an environment of filth and disorder. This character readily becomes a victim of the alcohol habit. Cases whose ailments date back to some form of suppression: either a skin disease driven inward to the vital centers by powerful medical topical agents, or by powerful radiation therapy; or a discharge from mucous membranes lining the orifices of the body, (such as catarrhal or gonorrheal discharges) suppressed by powerful medicants which has no affirmity with the processes of cure. In patients of feeble reaction to the best selected remedies.

Patients whose family history is deeply psoric, patients sensitive to temperature changes of every variety, sad and depressed with loathing of life; dwells on religious or philosophic speculations; despair of eternal salvation; fears he has committed the unpardonable sin. Egotistic, indifference to the lot of others, dwells on past unhappy events, self pity, vexations. Hypochondrical and full of morbid ideas, irritable and hurried, weeping, sad and frightened are some of the long array of mental states associated with Sulph.

This remedy is most successful when given on the broad general indications that call for its use.

Sulphuric acid

Sul-ac., like Sulph., is one of the most valuable and effective remedies for alcoholic sufferers. It, like Sulph., has many skin manifestations but in the acid the conditions are more drastic, tending to ulceration and destruction of tissues. Extreme irritability and excitement of mind is strangely characteristic, ulceration and hemorrhages may occur from mucous membranes internally or externally from gangrenous ulceration of the skin and deeper underlying tissues.

TUBERCULINUM

TUB. may be needed in those cases whose family and personal history may be the leading indication for its use, as a result of suppression of tubercular manifestations from generation to generation.

Stepped up nutritional measures, surgical removal of tubercular glands, collapsing of affected lugs, remedies that suppress cough without curing the constitutional cause, living in the open air, are palliations only. Suppressive drugs may be seemingly helpful and seemingly prolong life, but unless the constitutional and miasmatic causes are removed the tubercular sickness only changes its form and intensity. Many cases of tuberculosis apparently cured in early life later suffer mental and nervous diseases, even insanity. Other cases in later years show cancerous involvement of the lungs, glands, bones, skin, etc.

At this time the race seems to have developed another miasm, namely the tubercular miasm; hence this nosode is becoming more frequently used either as an intercurrent or complementary remedy to the other miasmatic remedies or as a direct agent against the tubercular disease.

Before closing I will mention a brief study of a few more homeopathic remedies whose proving and nature correspond to the nature and aspects of alcoholism verified by clinical application.

CADMIUM SULPHURICUM

CADM-S. has been curative in drunkards who have developed stomach and intestinal ulcerations with severe gastric pains and vomiting of dark blood; they are chilly, weak, emaciating patients. Clarke states it is a notable anti-psoric.

CAPSICUM

CAPS. is effective in delirium tremens given in dram doses. The patient's face presents a dusky redness which is cold to the touch, plethoric type of lax fiber. Alternating states of mind, home sickness, easily enraged, capricious, bewildered, severe burning lung pains, internally and externally. In males atrophy of testicle has been noted. They are flabby patients who have gangrenous, slowly healing ulcerations and crave coffee and beer.

HYDRASTIS

Clarke lists HYDR. as a remedy for alcoholism. Because of its drastic action of the gastro-intestinal tract and liver with its marked tendency to malignancy, this is a valuable remedy for serious study.

STROPHANTHUS

STROPH. given in two to ten drop doses of the tincture three times a day cured a dipsomaniac sixty-three years of age. Two other cases cited by Clarke were cured of the alcohol habit. The marked action on the heart and stomach is well known. This remedy needs a more complete homeopathic proving which might well place it high in the list of effective remedies for the treatment of alcoholism.

CONCLUSION

This paper embraces only a fraction of the likely remedies of our Materia Medica that could be useful in the treatment of the alcoholic disease, it does give those remedies and their candid implication that over the years in many lands have been most effective for this dreadful malady. We trust that this humble beginning will awaken wide spread homeopathic interest for the development and spread of homeopathic effort in this work which might well give homeopathic science a splendid opportunity to prove its worth in the field of medicine, where failure and acknowledged disappointment has been so universally admitted.

Asiatic Flu[1]

Considerable comment is going on concerning Asiatic Flu; and preparation for wholesale vaccination with experimental vaccine is planned by health authorities both for the laity and the armed forces. Homeopaths have been asked what remedies they have to meet a flu epidemic if one should come.

From all accounts, the present epidemic of Asiatic Flu is rather mild in its action with few fatalities. The epidemics of the past, notably the one of 1917 - 18 began in a rather mild way and as the season passed into late fall and winter the disease took on the nature of the severest type and the death toll mounted up to drastically high proportions. The ravages of the disease continued for months with a mounting death rate of from 20% to 40% of the victims contracting the disease.

In the early stages of the epidemic a group of from fifty to seventy-five remedies were needed for study in the search for the similium. As the epidemic went on, fewer and fewer remedies were needed for the selection of the best similar remedy until towards the end a group of less than a dozen remedies were needed for the study.

Ant-t., Ars., Bry., Carb-v., Caust., Gels., Ferr-p., Kali-c., Phos., Puls., Sang., Seneg., and Sep. made up a reliable group for study for several months in that terrible epidemic of the war years 1917 - 18. Not only the civil population but the personnel of the armed forces suffered frightful losses. In some localities as high as 40% losses occurred.

Homeopathy scored great success with a great reduction in the death rate of their treated cases; less than 5% of the cases treated homeopathically died.

What about prophylactic protection? No protection ever developed against all acute diseases can surpass or even equal the homeopathic constitutional treatment, as it not only removes susceptibility to all disease producing agents, including allergies of all kinds, but it harmonizes the play of vital processes and stimulates the body defence mechanism to its highest efficiency and power. These desired ends are accomplished by centralizing the inherited toxins engendered by the chronic miasms stated by Hahnemann, viz: Psora, Sycosis, and Syphilis plus the many artificially produced drug diseases from the abuse of antibiotic and coal-tar derivative drugs.

---

1. Journal of the American Institute of Homeopathy, Vol. 50, 11 - 12, Nov. - Dec., 1957, p. 299.

And for the bad effects following the abuse of coal-tar or other depressive drugs there is a small group of remedies that will antidote these evil agents and restore the weakened defenses of the body organism back to normal function: *Carb-v.*, *Am-c.*, *Lach.*, and *Op.* are a small group from which the best antidote may be found guided by the individual symptoms of the needed single remedy.

The group of remedies required for study in the early stages of the Great Epidemic: *agar.*, ail., all-c., am-c., ant-t., apis, arg-m., **Ars.**, ars-i., arum-t., asc-c., asc-t., bapt., bell., **Bry.**, berb., cact., cadm-s., calc-f., calc-p., calc-s., camph., canth., caps., carb-an., **Carb-v.**, carb-ac., caust., cedr., cham., chel., chin., chin-s., chlol., cimic., cina, coc-c., coff., cor-r., crot-h., crot-t., cupr., cur., dig., dios., dros., dulc., elaps, ery-a., *eup-per.*, *ferr-p.*, form., gels., graph., hell., hep., hydr., hyos., iris, kali-bi., kali-c., kali-cy., kali-s., kalm., lac-c., lach., lachn., laur., led., lept., lob., lyc., lycps., mag-m., *merc-c.*, *merc.*, merc-i-r., mez., *myris.*, naja, *nat-ar.*, nat-m., *nat-s.*, nit-ac., nux-m., nux-v., olnd., op., plb., petr., phos., ph-ac., phyt., podo., puls., psor., pyrog., ran-b., rhod., rhus-r., rhus-t., rhus-v., ruta, *sabad.*, samb., sang., sanic., sarr., sars., senec., seneg., sep., spong., staph., stram., sulph., syph., tarent., ter., ther., thuj., tub., verat., verat-v., zinc.

Different locations required some different remedies during the last great epidemic. Should an epidemic strike, it would be helpful for homeopathic physicians of the various sections of the country to keep in touch and compare their remedies that are frequently indicated in their locality. In that way the true epidemic remedies can be known and used to great advantage.

WHAT NOT TO DO IN FLU[1]

Much has been said about the things to do in the treatment of flu by many eminent physicians, and the advice they give in the main is safe and sound. But the things a patient should not do have been greatly neglected and that is the subject of this talk.

At a recent meeting of the high lights of the Public Health Service of the U.S. it was admitted that the present knowledge of flu, its exact origin and the treatment to be employed was sadly insufficient and unsatisfactory. It is to be regretted that the government is unable to avail itself of the service and knowledge of at least in part homeopathic physicians because the treatment end of the subject is efficiently and satisfactory solved by homeopathic therapeutics. We are told by these learned savants that the exact virus cause of flu has not yet been demonstrated. It is uncertain whether a single organism or a variety of mixed viruses are causative agents in the flu infection.

The good medical advice which all should follow is first: Absolute rest in bed in a warm, well ventilated room. A light nutritious diet of fruit and vegetable juices, with abundance of pure spring or distilled water. Chlorinated water is a positive injury to even the well, hence much more so to the sick. Warm, *not hot*, sponge baths to keep the skin functioning vigorously should be frequently given. All these measures protect the heart and encourage elimination through the kidneys, bowels, and skin, thus aiding nature in her fight against infection while the organism is manufacturing antibodies to overpower the infection.

But often these desirable ends are frustrated by misguided actions and advice of the patient and his friends and that phase of flu and its treatment will be the main part of talk here tonight. The first and worst thing that many people do when they feel the symptoms of cold or flu is to load up on either aspirin or quinine. While the aspirin may reduce the fever by depressing the cardiac function, and benumb the sensibilities to pain, it is a most pernicious and insidious poison that adds an additional burden to the poisoned blood of the flu sufferer[2]. And the reactive powers of the body are weakened by this drug - to a degree greater than that which opium produces. These things pertain in a greater or lesser degree to all the coal-tar deriatives such as acetanilid,

---

1. From handwritten manuscript, exact date unknown. - Editor..
2. Aspirin often is the cause of the HEPATO-RENAL-SYNDROME fraught with all its dangers - Editor.

phenacetin, pyramidon, luminal, veronal, tylenol and others of like nature.

It is repugnant to any thinking individual to give such toxic agents to a sick organism weakened by infection and disease. Another deleterious effect of the coal-tar poisons is the checking of the elimination from the bronchial tubes and lungs. Expectoration often is entirely suppressed adding greatly to the already frightfully over burdened respiratory functions so necessary for oxidation purposes. Is it any wonder we have so much pneumonia accompanying, complicating and following flu? No, it is only the natural sequence of a stupid therapeutic procedure. There is another effect that should not be ignored, and that is the irritated action on the mucous membranes of the gastro-intestinal and genito-urinary tracts. These are but a few of the primary effects of coal-tar drug poisoning.

There is a secondary action on the heart and nervous system that lays a train of many chronic conditions such as gastric and intestinal ulcers, kidney and heart disorders of various forms. In the past decade or two, those coincident with the advent of the coal-tar drugs, there has been an alarming increase in heart and kidney diseases. A society headed by highly advertised medical specialists to prevent heart and kidney disease has never uttered one word of protest against the abuse and almost universal use of these pernicious poisons which confront the public in a multitude of forms and are even recommended by physicians for the relief of pain of every sort regardless as to its causation and origin. While the government is so busy prohibiting, it might just as reasonably and profitably prohibit the unrestricted use of these harmful things. And with such curtailment in their use, and especially if every practicing physician were to put his stamp of disapproval on them and educate the laity regarding the harm done from their universal use we would soon see a drop in the vital statistics death rate from kidney and heart disease.

Why do not some of the leading knights of the profession come out and put the people right on these things? Surely it is not because they are ignorant of the harm that is done by these agents? My guess is that commercialism in medicine as well as in business plays a most stupendous role. Quinine effects primarily may be more severe, but it does not produce the intense and protracted end results observed in the coal-tars, except in its effects on the VIIIth nerve and lining membranes of the ear.

Quinine, like the coar-tars drys up the respiratory secretions of the lungs and predisposes toward pneumonia. Its chronic effects are plugged sinuses and deafness with a long train of neuralgias and nerve suffering. Chronic liver and spleen disease frequently results from the drastic and prolonged intake of Quinine.

A second common mistake laymen make is the application of cathartics to favor what they fondly believe the elimination of poison from the system, but there never was greater medical delusion perpetrated on an unsuspecting public than this because far more toxins are absorbed with the increased peristalsis action of the intestines and the liquefaction of the fecal waste than would take place if this waste remained undisturbed for days, for nature provides against absorption of toxins from fecal waste by covering such waste with a membrane impervious to the passage of gases and toxins. And all cathartics destroy this protecting membrane and favors the absorption of the putrefactant toxins.

A third mistake that is made by physicians as well as laymen is the use of huge doses of baking soda and other alkaline substances in order to maintain what is known as the alkalinity of the blood serum. This blood alkalinity is indeed a necessary condition to maintain the state of health, but the methods employed to obtain such a desirable end are all marked for either success or failure. If the alkalinity of the blood is maintained by the liberal use of fruit juices especially the citrus fruits, there is no harm done and only good accrues to the patient because the mineral balance in the blood is left undisturbed by this process. But if the alkalinity is obtained by the use of large doses of sodium bicarbonate there is an unbalanced calcium and potassium content in the blood stream that may be very inimical to a sufferer of flu or other infection. Besides the danger of over alkalinity from large doses of alkaline salts is a possibility that would prove unfortunate for one suffering from very acute infection.

The use of pure unmineralized spring water is urged for the reasons just mentioned and it is very necessary to avoid all chlorinated water in any state of either acute or chronic sickness if health is to be speedily restored to any sufferer of flu or other acute or even chronic sickness. The action of chlorine on the mucous lining of the lungs and bronchial tubes as an irritant is well known and hence should be avoided if possible. It is an irritant to the digestive and genito-urinary tracts as well. Boiling chlorinated water does not dissipate the chlorine content. Chlorinated water is much more harmful if contained and used for cooking in aluminum vessels. Water or food so kept and prepared contains appreciable doses of aluminum-hydroxide with chloride hydroxide, an active irritating poison.

Another therapeutic error committed by laymen is the use of cough drops or cough syrup containing opium, codeine, or chloroform. Such agents block the secretions by paralyzing the nerve ending in the bronchial mucosa. The use of camphorated or mentholated salves or grease rubbed into the skin of the flu or pneumonia sufferer is another mistake that may end fatally, because the pores of the skin through which many impurities are eliminated are clogged and rendered inefficient in their important function. These pernicious nostrums and drugs are advertised in the public press and in streetcar signs as being specific for flu and colds of all kinds. They are the undertaker's most helpful friends and without their specific influence many victims of flu and pneumonia would recover instead of filling premature graves.

Not withstandig the vicious depressing action of the things mentioned many sick sufferers recover in spite of such application thanks to a wonderful vitality. But really only those in the extremes of life or those afflicted and weakened with organic heart or kidney disease should die from flu or pneumonia under sane and truly scientific treatment. I believe that self medication or lay prescribing of all kinds to be a great mistake except, perhaps in an emergency where expert medical advice cannot be obtained without too much delay. In that case there are a few homeopathic remedies given on their specific indications that can be recommended to abort the dangerous symptoms of flu and pneumonia quickly and gently, that is there will be no consequential drug effects remaining after the infection is overcome.

In the very early stage of a cold following the chill, coming on suddenly and followed by fever and arteriole excitement, a drop of homeopathic tincture of Acon. in one quarter glass of water, the mixture to be given in teaspoon doses two hours apart until the fever breaks when no more medicine is needed as the attack will be broken and only rest and a careful diet is needed to regain health completely in a very short time.[1]

If the coryza is continued and excoriating and accompanied with weakness, chilliness, and severe aching of muscles and bones producing

---

1. Dr. Grimmer suggested use of tinctures because at the time of writing this article (1947 or thereabouts) most pharmacies (not specialized in Homeopathy) sold Homeopathic remedies in tincture form. Of course the better way would be to use the remedies in potency. - Editor.

extreme restlessness, a homeopathic dose of ARs. 30X dilution will soon relieve all suffering and restore to perfect health.

In cases of extreme bone pains, severe headache, and nausea EUP-PER. or the old fashioned bone set. One drop of the homeopathic tincture in one quarter glass of water to be given in teaspoon doses as advised for ACON.

In the bronchial and pleurisy cases where the patient is aggravated by motion and relieved by pressure over the diseased lungs; where every breath causes sharp cutting pains BRY., one drop of the homeopathic tincture given as advised before.

I believe the homeopathic tinctures are superior to the other preparations because the fresh plant is always employed by the homeopathic pharmacist to obtain and prepare their tinctures and attenuations. Be sure to use only spring or distilled water when taking these remedies. The wonderous life force of the body is not strongly enough depended on to restore health to the sick. The influence of homeopathic thought on general medical progress cannot be too greatly stressed.

HOMEOPATHY IN HEART DISEASE[1]

This terrorizing number one killer of our time apparently defies the organized medical effort of our country to curtail or arrest its far-reaching and devastating onslaught on the ever increasing number of its victims. Scientific medicine ascribes much of this deadly increase to the tension and hazzards of our present day social and industrial order. But there must be other more forceful causative factors at work not recognized by the dominate medical science. From the pioneer days up to and beyond the civil war into the eighteen eighties, we were an expanding country whose economy was beset with money panics and industrial crises entailing much greater hardships and tensions than we have today; yet relatively few died of heart disease; in fact all the chronic degenerative diseases were far less marked and rarely occurred until old age came on; today these diseases are rampant among the middle age group in the prime of life; yes even many younger victims are now afflicted.

Between the eighteen eighties and nineties we were visited with raging epidemics of flu or grippe as it was called then. At about this same period the dye industries of Germany produced and gave to the world the drugs derived from the coal tar by-products. Such well known drugs as acetanilid, phenacetin, antifebrin and many others, especially the barbiturates used extensively by physicians and laity alike, flooded our public with a mass of depressing and nerve-destroying drugs whose harvest is heart disease and mental incompetence. From the well known effects of these chemical poisons on the human economy it is only reasonable to cite the coal tar drugs as a strong factor in the increase of heart disease.

A second factor in predisposing to renal and cardiac weakness and disease is the universal poisoning of the nation's water supplies with such chemicals as chlorine; this has been a universal custom in the last twenty-five years, and in that period kidney and heart disease have reached first place as the cause of death in humans. The homeopathic provings of chlorine water made with the 6X potency (one part to a million parts of water) on healthy subjects produced long lasting and serious symptoms affecting the heart and kidneys. The amount of the poison of chlorine infused in the drinking water is said to be approximately about one part to a million, equivalent to our 6X potency.

---

1. From handwritten manuscript, probably written in 1952. - Editor..

When the human body is subjected to the continuous impact of a poison over a long period of time, several things happen; those with weakened hearts and kidneys take on the degenerative disease of their organs, a few of the hardier and less susceptible become immune to the poison. Because of the facts brought out by homeopathic provings on well folks, it is reasonable to conclude that a chlorinated water supply may well be a causative factor in the increase of heart disease; and heart disease has most certainly increased during the time the American public has been subjected to these influences.

In seeking a cure for any disease condition, Homeopathy seeks the causes or etiology inducing or precipitating the sickness; often the mere removal of such factors will not only cure but also prevent the spread of disease. The organization to prevent heart disease by research, etc., has collected large sums of money from the public for the purpose of preventing heart disease and has failed to enlighten the public concerning the dangers inherent in the wide spread use of coal tar drugging and has tacitly endorsed the universal poisoning of our water supply without one sign of protest. The Homeopathic medical profession has long and constantly warned the public of these dangers to the health of the individual and the public of which he is a part. But in spite of these warnings many more people must be sickened and even die before the medical profession at large will see these dangers and be spurred into action to correct the situation by enlightening the public and advising the necessary measures to eradicate the troublesome causes operating so far and wide.

For heart disease in its many forms, Homeopathy has a multitude of remedies each one a specific for a specific case. To get the most certain and satisfactory results in cure, these remedies must be prescribed by a thoroughly trained and competent master prescriber.

There are no specific remedies for disease by name, only remedies for patients suffering with the symptoms and the pathological changes associated with heart disease. Before the homeopathic prescription is made, all adverse elements in the patient's environment are corrected, such as faulty habits of eating and drinking, exercise or lack of the same, with sufficient fresh air and sunshine, proper and adequate rest; all these things are adjuncts and preceed the selection of the Homeopathic remedy, thus causes are removed and success is assured.

Hundreds of clinical pictures of sick patients suffering with some aspect of heart disease could be cited to prove the efficacy of the homeopathic remedy, but time and space demand we be content with relatively few illustrations.

Many serious conditions of heart disease have been cured with the guiding symptom of the case expressed, as if an iron hand were squeezing the heart. This symptom is most marked in the proving of CACT. and that remedy has given relief from suffering and good health to thousands of suffering ones over the years by faithful doctors of the homeopathic faith.

A case of terminal pneumonia complicated with acute nephritis and a failing dilated heart muscle was cured by Dr. Kent on the symptom complex of a weak fast pulse with a subnormal temperature with the remedy PYROG. in the 10M potency; the patient, a Dr. Austin[1] of New York, completely recovered, lived and practiced, a devoted homeopathic physician for over twenty years after what seemed to be a certain fatal illness. Few mortals rise from the portals of the grave to emerge into the sunlight and bloom of health with the great privilege of attaining a useful life devoted to the happy task of healing. Dr. Austin carried on, a devoted champion of Homeopathy, until extreme old age closed the curtains on his labors. Many cases of serious illness, hundreds in fact, with a separation of pulse and temperature as the chief index in their case has found the curative remedy in PYROG.

Many cases of angina pectoris with pain radiating down the left arm and on the verge of complete collapse have been restored and comforted by LAT-M. (the remedy prepared from the virus of the Black Widow Spider).

DIG. cures or mitigates dilated hearts with slow, weak, irregular pulse generally with cyanosis.

CARB-V. in high potency cures dilated hearts where the patient seems dying, bathed in cold sweat yet wants to be fanned.

ARS. cures cases of a similar nature where despite a great weakness and coldness there is an anxious fear of death and restlessness; if the body is too weak to move, a hand, foot or head will be in motion.

ACON. may save a life where the shock from sudden fright has affected the nervous mechanism supplying heart function. ACON. heart conditions are associated with great fear of death and numbness of the hands and fingers.

---

1. Eugene Alonzo Austin M.D. was one of Dr. Kent's star pupils (as was also Dr. Grimmer). Dr. Austin, Dr. Frederica Gladwin were the major preceptors of Pierre Schmidt of Geneva, Switzerland - Editor.

A cardiac asthma relieved by lying flat on the back will be relieved if not cured by the remedy LAUR.

A disturbed runaway pounding heart is frequently cured by the remedy LYCPS.

It is well to remember that the cardinal symptoms or so-called keynotes must be accompanied with the totality of the patient's symptoms. These keynotes are useful and time saving leaders to the study of the whole case; if the nature of the case and the totality of the symptoms agree, successful results are assured.

These illustrations are presented to show how Homeopathy works with its array of one thousand (more or less) proven remedies. Only the polychrests are anywhere near completely proven, but our Materia Medica is vast and still growing. To use this great store of useful knowledge much study of the Materia Medica and Repertory is required to achieve the maximum success in cure.

Any busy Homeopathic physician can submit many interesting case histories of cures in many forms of heart disease and because it is the commonplace to effect more or less dramatic cures of heart disease with the homeopathic remedy, I will submit in brief one interesting case recently occurring in practice.

A busy industrial surgeon in the early fifties about eighty pounds overweight, weight 240 lbs., 5 ft. 7 in. tall, collapsed while operating on a patient. X-rays showed a large dilated heart, and later cardiograms showed coronary insufficiency and a damaged heart muscle. Marked dyspnoea on least exertion, a chronic harsh croupy, dry cough, incessant when lying down, had to be propped up to sitting position to breathe at all. Edema of the extremities and fluid in abdomen completed this dismal picture, the cough relieved by being propped up and with hot drinks, waking out of sleep choking, allowed only a little breath. This case presents few therapeutic symptoms for remedy selection. Practically all symptoms are of a pathological origin and of inferior value for remedy selection. The apparent sleep aggravation at night suggested remedies from Kent's Repertory pg. 1342 in high value.

Ars. Chin. *crot-h. dig.* **Graph. Lach.** *lyc. nux-v.* **Phos. Puls.** *samb. spong.* **Sulph.**

COUGH HOARSE - p. 793: Chin. graph. *lach. lyc.* nux-v. Samb. *spong.*

COUGH DRY AT NIGHT - p. 787: **Phos. Puls. Spong. Sulph.**

COUGH CROUPY - p. 785: **Spong.**

COUGH BETTER WITH WARM FLUIDS - p. 810: Spong., the only remedy running through the selected symptom group.

Wishing to confirm this remedy by a blood test[1] to ascertain the patient's polarity, which was bi-polar, most of the remedies studied are bi-polar, and SPONG. was the only remedy satisfying the blood polarity equation. SPONG. is a rather unusual remedy given in heart complaints even though its symptomatology is rich in heart symptoms. This patient was put to bed and given a specially selected low calorie diet and given SPONG. 10M with amazing beneficial results. Within a few days he was sleeping like a baby, free of dyspnoea and cough. In a month he reduced forty pounds, and his heart findings were within the range of normalcy. This is an ideal cure of a very serious and difficult case.

Homeopathic medical science has much to offer in the world of healing. Not only does it produce ideal cures in the most difficult types of disease, it also stands supreme in the field of disease prevention. From the cradle to the edge of the grave, its ministrations are a God-given boon to suffering humanity. No unhappy and dangerous side effects accompany homeopathic treatment.

Only organized groups of manufacturers of proprietary drugs who are moved by selfish interest alone, through constant studied propaganda to a misinformed public, can keep back the march of the true science of healing for a time of relatively short duration.

New discoveries in physics, biochemistry and genetics are all revealing the truth and power for healing in the laws, principles and techniques of Homeopathic medicine.

---

1. See see article "Recent Concepts and New Formulas in Medicine" on page 679 ff. and see article "Importance of Electronic Reactions to Future Medicine" on page 683 ff.. - Editor.

HOMEOPATHIC PSYCHOSOMATIC MEDICINE[1]

This type of medicine truly began with Hahnemann, the father of Homeopathy. His plea for humane treatment of the insane (before this time they were chained in the gloom and filth of dungeons) emphasized the need of such procedure. Hahnemann was the first to perceive the inseparable unity of mind and body that constitutes the patient as a whole. Sick minds often stem from sick and ill conditioned bodies and vice-versa.[2]

The one great difference between Hahnemann and modern medical scientists is their difference of approach to the end results and the treatment required. Hahnemann perceived the very nature of man as preceding from the spiritual and mental to the physical, hence his stress on the relatively greater importance of the mental and emotional symptoms both as etiological factors of sickness as well their greater value in the selection of the curative remedies. Modern medical scientists have reached similar conclusions in this new aspect of healing by different methods and by the empirical procedure of trial and error.

Laboratory tests of the blood and vital secretions of the human being under the influence of anger, fear, hate, grief, etc., show definite chemical changes from alkaline, which is the normal reaction of the blood and vital secretions of humans in health, to acid which is the abnormal and sick-producing toxin of disease. We are told by these scientists that chronic diseases such as cancer, heart and kidney disease as well as the deforming action of arthritis stem from years of shock, frustrations, anger, grief and fear that permanently change the blood chemistry ending in pathological changes in the cell formation of the body organism. These tests are constantly confirmed by the electro-magnetic tests of the blood demonstrating the processes preceding the chemical changes in the body, viz; there is first a change in the blood polarity which in health is negative in a specific standard of measurement.[3] Any change from that standard polarity indicates the beginning of disease with an immediate change in the blood chemistry.

The factor of most vital interest to the homeopathic physician is the fact that the homeopathic remedy placed in the circuit with a patient's

---

1. From handwritten manuscript, exact date unknown. - Editor..
2. Organon §210, 211. - Editor.
3. See see article "Recent Concepts and New Formulas in Medicine" on page 679 ff. and see article "Importance of Electronic Reactions to Future Medicine" on page 683 ff.. - Editor.

blood will normalize that blood; that is it will render the blood negative to the specific standard found in every case of health. Then if the remedy selected in accordance with the law of polarity be given the patient, his blood stream will become normally negative; and his blood chemistry is also changed to a normal state starting the instant rhythm of normal vital processes in the body organism which leads to harmonious health. When these proven facts are understood, it is easy to perceive how disease starts and grows in intensity until the causative factors cease to operate by eliminating them from the life environment of the patient.

Who can know how much fright and frustrated anxiety started and activated every crippling case of arthritis, and who could measure the degree of shock and nerve tension behind every case of mental aberration and incompetency How much envy or hate or selfish desire was required to start the proliferation of the wild body cell that ultimated in the malignant change called cancer? Who can measure the degree of grief or blighted affection disturbing the normal rhythm and action of the heart to end in organic change behind so many cases of heart disease? What about the paralyzing effect of fear and panic prevailing so widely in the world today? What are these mystic things of evil doing to our subconscious mind? With these disturbed mental states, how can we have blood sufficiently oxygenated and free of toxic poisons to perform its destined function of restoring and revivifying the whole being? Homeopathy alone has the answer to these potent questions because Homeopathy can meet and correct all these causative elements in every individual case.

First, every being subjected to shock, tension, grief, and frustration does not suffer the dire effects of chronic degenerating disease, but too many so exposed do. Those whose life has been free from the debilitating power of the chronic miasms suffer lightly, if at all, from the tensions of environment. It is those of bad inheritance who through ignorance or otherwise could not avail themselves of the positive benign influence of Homeopathy that suffer disastrously from the many mental and emotional tensions of today.

The provings of the homeopathic remedies are rich in perverted and abnormal mental states, showing the power residing in medicines to cure when taken in an attenuated form because of their power to produce aberrations and changes in the healthy when taken in crude or material form.

A few instances of model cures taken from Herring's volume on ANALYTICAL THERAPEUTICS[1] will suffice to illustrate the superiority homeopathic procedure in the realm of cure.

CASE NO. 1.

A very irritable lady suffering under the most violent and threatening nervous symptoms, even spasms, had hectic fever, sleepless nights, mind nearly deranged, disturbed by unfounded jealousy. After one dose of Hyos. 30 was well and remained so. E. Stapf. pg. 86.[2]

CASE NO. 2.

Feels the greatest anguish in the head with a whirling before the eyes every day from 5 a.m. until 5 p.m. for past two years. He walks up and down the room, wringing his hands and moaning continually, "Oh such anguish; oh such anguish". Only when he takes his meals does he cease his moaning. His appetite is good. PSOR. cured. W. Gross. pg. 84.

CASE NO. 3.

Suffering from fear of hydrophobia after dog bite, mad or not without having been bitten. LYSS. pg. 82.

CASE NO. 4.

A child, three years old, apparently well, waked too often from sleep with a scream and continued to cry. The more they tried by persuasion to quiet it, the worse it got. CALC. did not help much. After CALC-P. was given, the spells ceased altogether. Lippe. pg. 90.

CASE NO. 5.

Especially after mental agitation of a vexatious character to which she is very subject (in deficiency of the valves), a trembling and fluttering of the heart with distressing pain in the heart and as far as between the shoulders. It extends upward into the head where it is felt as an equally painful throbbing; at the same time air, on inspiration, seems so cold that it is felt unpleasantly cold even in the lungs. LITH-C. cured. N.N. pg. 95.

---

1. This book initially appeared as ANALYTICAL THERAPEUTICS, Vol. 1; it seems that the suceeding volume or volumes never appeared and the title of the book was changed to THE SYMPTOMS OF THE MIND. The American Homeopathic Publishing Society, J.M. Stoddart & Co., Philadelphia, 1881. - Editor.
2. All page numbers in this article refer to Hering's ANALYTICAL THERAPEUTICS. - Editor.

Grimmer's Work

CASE NO. 6.

Pressing, stupefying pain in forehead, particularly after mental exertion and emotions. Toward evening restless, anxious and fidgety. Sleep disturbed by dreams; twitching of whole body, sits up in bed with anxious gestures; weeps, cries out mournfully and wants to run away. Next morning does not remember what occurred: BELL. Bicking. pg.98.

CASE NO. 7.

After over study, feeling at times of a foreign body under the skull, in vertex; better during reading; worse on going to sleep or from excitement or thinking of the pain, better by touch; the relief during reading seemed to rise from the mind being diverted from the pain. CON. 3M (Jenichen) cured. Berridge. pg.104.

Volumes could be written describing model homeopathic cures of the severest and most intractable types of sickness, but enough is written here to demonstrate the excellence of Homeopathy's success in Psychosomatic Medicine.

One heartening thing about the growth of this advance in old-school medical thought is a near approach to homeopathic fundamentals by at least a portion of our colleagues of the dominate school. Such progress in their ranks brings hope for further great advances along these lines that will eventually lead them into the ample and all sufficient fold of Homeopathy, the crowning glory of medical achievement throughout the ages.

Mental Diseases Cured by Homeopathy[1]

Homeopathic procedures are especially efficacious in the treatment of mental diseases. The literature is rich in numerous abnormal mental symptoms produced by the provings on healthy subjects. So perfectly are the moral, mental and physical states of patients linked up together by homeopathic methods of study that the underlying disease causes involved are more certain of being removed than by other less thorough or scientific methods. A few cases will illustrate the powerful curative agents abounding in the archives of Homeopathy.

Case 1 Insomnia and Depression

Mrs. A.H.J. age 68. Mental trouble came on rather fast almost like a shock; began with insomnia and a general run-down state. This patient had been an active church worker for forty years. Memory poor; time seems too long; complained of very depressive mental states which she accounted for by so-called evil thoughts of a tormenting feeling of guilt. Lascivious thoughts forced themselves before her with obscene visions, these things very contrary to her real life and nature. Impulses to kill her husband of whom she is very fond. She was annoyed and puzzled why she should have such thoughts and impulses because she had been a pious and devoted worker in her church. For all this the impression came to her that there was no forgiveness and that she could no longer pray. A quick repertorial analysis of this case gleaned by four major general groups of mentals, reveals the closely associated remedies needed.

Religious affections (including anxiety, despair etc.) Kent Rep. page 71: *Arg-n., ars., aur., bell., calc., carb-v., cham., chel., graph.,* **Hyos.,** *ign., kali-p.,* **Lach., Lil-t.,** *lyc., med., meli., mez., plat., psor., puls., sep., stram.,* **Sulph., Verat., Zinc.**

Lascivious thoughts: which are contrary to the patient's life and nature and are abhorrent even in her sick state. (Kent Rep., pg. 61) under Lasciviousness. Only those remedies also present in the first rubric are taken.) *Calc., carb-v., graph.,* **Hyos., Lach., Lil-t., Plat.,** *puls., sep., stram., verat.*

Desires to kill (Kent Rep., pg. 60) **Hyos.,** *plat., stram.,* to kill husband of whom she is fond (Kent Rep., pg.60) *merc., nux-v., plat.*

---

1. The Homeopathic Recorder, Vol. LIV, No. 4, April, 1939, p. 3 ff.

CASE 1 INSOMNIA AND DEPRESSION ...

PERSISTENT THOUGHTS (Kent Rep. pg. 87): *stram.*

PRAYING (Kent Rep. pg. 69): *stram.*

The complimentary second remedy needed to clear the case was LACH. which ran pretty well through the first study. The mental symptoms were entirely removed by STRAM. LACH., later followed by CARB-V. was given for incidental physical ailments that developed after. This patient remains well today. Dr. Welsh, a very good homeopath, who referred her to me had given her SEP. with some benefit for the insomnia but with no help for the mental states.

Over a period of thirty years I have seen a number of very serious cases of insanity and mania, some of extreme violence, clear up under STRAM. It is especially efficacious in the puerperal mania of women when indicated, and it frequently is indicated under those conditions.

CASE 2 SUICIDE BY JUMPING

Suicidal mania, especially with the impulses to jump from high places, will find its best remedy in AUR. An interesting case of a young man whose desire to commit suicide by jumping through a window always around the time of the full moon is improving under AUR.

CASE 3 SUICIDE BY HANGING

Another case of a highly nervous business man who has been under the strain, disappointments and hardships incident to the economic ravages of the depression, who has suffered with insomnia for months finally elected to find a way out by hanging. His wife cut him down when he was almost gone and rushed him to the hospital where I attended him. Prior to this episode he had been given PULS., ARS. and other remedies with little help. After this he was given AUR-AR. 200, repeated at intervals of months apart, with a complete restoration of mental and physical health, and with a much better business success under the same disadvantages he had worked before.

CASE 4 INSOMNIA AND DEPRESSION

Another case of a school teacher overworked and under severe strain and worry with a brother afflicted with a depressed mania. This case sleepless, worried and profoundly depressed received some benefit under AUR-M. in several potencies, but made no real or permanent gain until PIC-AC. in the 10M and 50M potencies was given. She is now

Case 4 Insomnia and Depression ...

stronger, happier and well even with the same worries and responsibilities to carry.

These things show us that we need but find the one indicated medicine for the individual case, in order to restore mental health as easily and certainly as nature unassisted restores acute ailments of all sorts.

Nowhere else in the realm of medicine can those afflicted with mental and so-called nervous disease be as certain of cure as that offered by Homeopathy.

HOMEOPATHIC TREATMENT OF TYPHOID[1]

Introductory Note: Typhoid fever and pneumonia are two dread ailments over which Homeopathy has especially triumphed; their periods of illness have been wonderfully shortened and the violence of the sickness much reduced, while the so-called sequelae are almost never manifested. Wherever this method has come into competition with old-school treatment, superiority is demonstrated by the statistical comparative record of a much lower death-rate under Homeopathy.

The present writing relates chiefly to the therapeutics of typhoid. We do not follow the old-school's latest dictum of liberal feeding, as advocated at Johns Hopkins, nor do we use the so-called intestinal antiseptics much in vogue some ten years since but more recently discarded by a majority of old-school leaders. The only adjuvants, if such they may be called, used by the writer are the tepid sponge-bath and the alcohol-rub; both are refreshing, comforting, and in no way change or mask the symptom-image. Stimulants not only are unnecessary, but they are harmful when the patient is under influence of the indicated remedy, which is itself all sufficient to carry the patient to a speedy recovery.

The real homeopathician rarely sees the extreme features of typhoid, if he has been called on the case early. It is aborted with the shorter-acting remedies before the extreme symptoms develop. There are rare exceptions, when, due to some psoric or some constitutional element, the case persists and progresses downward or lapses back after improvement under well-selected remedies; then will the symptoms call for deeper remedies.

Again: the physician may not be called until late in the progress of the case, after some pseudo-scientific bungler has masked or distorted the symptom-image and has weakened the patient's natural resisting-powers by drastic and ill-selected medication. Or the case, even under attendance, may have been left to Nature's sole care - to run its course - and progressed toward death, at the lowest ebb of life. In these belated stages the magic impulse of the indicated remedy is still available.

In any one illness more than others justifies the claims of the Law of Similars, exhibiting the necessity for strict individualization in the selection of the curative medicine - as against routine treatment - it is typhoid. Many of the cases will clear up within a week - even before the Widal reaction can be obtained.

---

1. THE HOMEOPATHICIAN, Vol. V, No. 5 - 6, May - June, 1915, p. 150 ff.

Observe the difference between the symptom-pictures in any typhoid ward: One patient is so restless that he can scarcely be kept in bed; another, sunk in profound stupor, is aroused only with difficulty. One is chilly, even through his fever; another is relieved only by cold bathing and cool air. One has unquenchable thirst, another is thirstless with high fever; and varieties of delirium, in multitude, are manifest. Yet all are labelled typhoid; all suffer with the same micro-organism. If they are under scientific old-school care, all receive the same routine treatment.

Although any remedy containing in its pathogenesis the symptoms and the nature of typhoid may be indicated, the application of the Law of Similars through a period of one hundred and twenty years by many excellent prescribers directs us to a group of remedies which are more frequently indicated that others in this disease.

First let us premise that NO REMEDY WHOSE PROVINGS DO NOT INCLUDE THE NATURE OF TYPHOID - THE CONTINUED TYPE OF FEVER, ETC. - WILL CURE A TYPHOID CASE, even though the other remedy's symptoms be present. BELL. and ACON. can never be really useful, even though some of their symptoms appear.

HYOS. and Stramonium have all the heat and wildness and violence of BELL., and they have more: the continued type of fever, which BELL. has not. RHUS-T. and ARS. are as restless and full of fear as is ACON.; and they have the typhoid type of fever.[1]

LET US CONSIDER (pg. 1284): Apis, arn., **Ars., Arum-t., Bapt., Bry.,** *canth., caps., carb-an.,* **Carb-v., Chin.,** chin-a., chin-s., **Chlor.,** chlol., cocc., **Colch., Crot-h., Gels., Hyos., Lach.,** lyc., *mur-ac., nit-ac., op., ph-ac.,* **Phos.,** *psor., pyrog.,* **Rhus-t.,** *sec., sil.,* **Stram.,** sulph., *sul-ac.*

Viewing these remedies in groups presenting similarities in symptomatology, and omitting the common features of typhoid let us note the things rare, strange and peculiar.

GROUP I: FREQUENTLY INDICATED

APIS (CEREBRAL FORM)

— Confusion depriving patient of realization that he is sick. He says: "I feel fine! Nothing is wrong with me, at all!"
— Children with brain-cry; stupor.
— SENSITIVE ON HEAT; DESIRES TO UNCOVER;

---

1. All page numbers refer to Kent's Repertory III or later editions. - Editior.

GROUP I: FREQUENTLY INDICATED ...

APIS (CEREBRAL FORM) ...

— WANTS COOLING APPLICATIONS
— Abdominal distension.
— Much tenderness. At times intense straining with diarrhoeic stool.
— Thirstless with fever, frequently. Tongue sensation as if wooden[1]; taste lost.

ARNICA

— Confusion depriving patient of realization that he is sick. He says: "I feel fine! Nothing is wrong with me, at all!"
— Stupor; roused only to lapse again.
— BRUISED, BEATEN, SORE PAIN. CHANGES POSITION CONSTANTLY IN BED; NO PLACE GIVES COMFORT THERE. MUCH ECCHYMOSIS. PROSTRATION OFTEN PROMINENT. FREQUENTLY HEAD AND FACE WARM, BODY AND EXTREMITIES COLD.
— Stool involuntary during sleep or during stupor. Urine frequently involuntary; may be retained.
— Tongue dry, almost black; taste putrid, bitter.

ARUM TRIPHYLLUM

— Unconscious, picks at fingers.
— PICKING AT BLEEDING LIPS AND FINGER-TIPS. TINGLING AND NUMBNESS OF FINGERS AND LIPS.

BAPTISIA

— Rapid progress; symptoms due in second week appear in first week (third or fourth day). Early blood changes. Intense stupefaction; speech thickened. Low muttering delirium.
— THINKS LIMBS AND PARTS OF BODY ARE SCATTERED IN BED. BUSILY TRIES TO GET THEM TOGETHER: Cann-i., PETR., PHOS., PULS., SIL., STRAM. (SENSATION OF BEING DIVIDED INTO PARTS.)
— COUNTENANCE BESOTTED; DUSKY RED.

---

1.   i.e. numbness - Editor.

Group I: Frequently Indicated ...

Bryonia

— Delirium, Restless, desires to go home; thinks is away from home. Talks much of business; its worries abound and annoy.
— Desires to lie quiet and rest. < From motion.
— Constipation often present; not diarrhoea.
— Drinks copiously at rather long intervals.
— Asks for things and refuses them when offered.

Colchicum (Abdominal form)

— Wants to be undisturbed because of his weakness.
— Complete loss of perception. Weakness of memory. Excessive mental confusion. No fear; appears unconcerned about condition.
— Sensitive to the smell and thought of food. (Ars., Cocc.)
— Bowel symptoms marked and uncommon. Stools frequent, with mucus, scrapings as from intestines; involuntary stools. Tenesmus.
— Urinating may be involuntary, copious, or suppressed. Frequently scanty, dark.

Cocculus

— (When homeopath not called to patient until second week:) Sleeplessness. Mental sluggishness; gradually sinks into stupor. (Arn., Phos-ac.) Time passes quickly, unnoted. Numbness.
— Extreme irritability of nervous system. Sensitive to noise and jar. Paralytic weakness and stiffness of extremities.
— Intense colicky pains in abdomen, as from sharp stones rubbing together.
— Muttering mumbling speech; clear plain speech impossible.

Gelsemium

— Early relaxation and weakness more prominent than Bryonia; mental confusion deeper. Cerebral congestion with chilliness.
— Brain and spine suffer shock of the poison. Paralytic weakness. Impaired thick speech.
— Frequently involuntary stool. Diarrhoea apt to be worse from fear, excitement or depressing emotions. Frequent, copious, limpid urine relieves the heaviness and pain in the head. Urination involuntary: paralysis of sphincter.

GROUP I: FREQUENTLY INDICATED ...

GELSEMIUM ...

— Thirst slight of absent. Pain along spine. Pulse full flowing; rather soft.

RHUS TOX.

— Symptoms appear early. Delirium of busiest sort; working, going, doing something.
— INTENSE PHYSICAL RESTLESSNESS (Ars., Chlor., Mur-ac., Pyrog., Sec.)
— SENSITIVE TO COLD; BETTER WHEN WARM AND FROM WARM APPLICATIONS.
— Involuntary stool with intense exhaustion. Maybe hemorrhage of black blood from bowels.
— Tongue dry, sore, with red tip; triangular red tip, sometimes cracked; may take imprint of teeth; coated at root. Yellowish white or thick brown mucus except on the edges.

HYOSCYAMUS

— Slower in development than Rhus-t. and Bry. Symptoms appear in second week.
— Persistent but mild muttering delirium. Violence may be present. Keen suspicion and refusal of medicine, as poison. (Apis, Lach., Rhus-t.: less intense.) Alternating with shamelessness and obscenity.
— MANY QUEER AUTOMATIC MOTIONS. WANTS TO UNCOVER; OBSCENE; USES VILE SPEECH. FREQUENTLY BETTER IN THE DARK.
— Speech unintelligible because of parched, thickened, almost useless tongue.

STRAMONIUM

— Many symptoms resemble HYOS., but violence more intense and fever higher. Alternate states; laughs, sings, cries, prays by turns; at times cursing.
— TENDENCY TO STRIKE, BITE AND FIGHT. < IN DARK. IRRITATION OF BRAIN THROUGH VISIONARY CENTERS; YET WANTS LIGHT BURNING DIMLY. < IN DARK.

GROUP II: RESTLESS TYPHOID

Prostration is extreme. These are suitable later in the disorder, often when RHUS-T. has done all for which it is capable; or when RHUS-T. was not early enough administered. Blood-changes have resulted, and the vital forces are about to be overwhelmed.

ARSENICUM

— ARS. and SEC. have symptoms so similar, distinguished with difficulty. Both have withered leathery skin; extreme weakness; foul odor; ulceration; offensive discharges; all symptoms that pertain to extreme cases in their latter stages.

— ARS.: More fear of death. Stupefaction rarely so complete as to overcome the characteristic restlessness.

— ARS.: SENSITIVE TO COLD; CAN SCARCELY GET ENOUGH HEAT.

SECALE

— WANTS TO UNCOVER, EVEN WHEN DEVITALIZED TO THE EXTREME, AND COLD AS DEATH.

— Haemorrhages: blood dark, offensive, thin. (LACH.)

MURIATIC ACID

— Intense cyanosis revealed in lips, ears and finger-nails. Lower jaw hangs down.

— TENDENCY TO ULCERATION IS STRONGER THAN IN OTHERS OF THIS GROUP.

— GROANING MORE OR LESS PERSISTENT THROUGHOUT THE SICKNESS: IN SLEEP, IN DELIRIUM, IN STUPOR. SLIDES DOWN TO FOOT OF BED.

PYROGEN

— Restlessness (Rhus-t.); prostration (Ars.); bruised sore pain in body (Arn., Bapt.); bone-pains (Eup-per.).

— DISCREPANCY BETWEEN PULSE AND TEMPERATURE. SENSATION OF COLDNESS AND WEAKNESS FELT AT THE HEART.

— Cold intense. Chill and heat intermingled. Sometimes vomits water as soon as it is warm in the stomach (Phos.).

GROUP III: HEMORRHAGIC TYPHOID (ACIDS)

PHOSPHORIC ACID

— Sinks gradually to complete stupor; roused only to lapse again. Looks with staring glassy eyes.
— Wants to be alone.
— Affects mental sphere first: stupefaction and mental prostration. Physical weakness appears later (contrast Mur-ac.)
— Diarrhoea may be very profuse and frequent, but at first does not weaken the patient.
— Fever progresses slowly. Thirst at first slight gradually increases to intensity.

NITRIC ACID

— Most irritable and sensitive of all acids.
— NOISE, JAR, ODORS, PAIN ARE ALL UNBEARABLE. WALKING OF OTHERS ACROSS THE ROOM IS INTOLERABLE. PAINS IN ULCERS ARE STITCHING. PRICKING. (HEP.)
— Physical weakness develops with more or less rapidity, and ends in all the toxemia and circulatory changes of the worst cases.

GROUP IV: HEMORRHAGIC TYPHOID

SNAKE POISONS

— The snake poisons are very similar in the profound blood-changes, aggravation from sleep, etc.

CROTALUS HORRIDUS

— More septic.
— Apathy more than in Lach. Aversion to members of the family. Cerebral congestion; even apoplexy may be present. Mental depression. Delusions of hideous animals; of enemies. Constant drowsiness; moaning and groaning. (Mur-ac.)
— HAEMORRHAGES FROM MUCOUS MEMBRANES OF ALL PARTS. PERSPIRATION SOMETIMES BLOODY. BLOOD BLACK, CLOTTED OR THIN. RIGHT SIDED.

LACHESIS

— More excitable.
— Nervous excitement. Fear of poisoning (Hyos., Rhus-t.). Ecstatic

GROUP IV: HAEMORRHAGIC TYPHOID ...

LACHESIS ...

state; clairvoyant visions. Thinks self some one else in hands of higher power. Imagines enemies are pursuing, and tries to escape.
— Sensation of sinking.
— HAEMORRHAGE OF DARK THIN FLUID, OR RESEMBLES CHARRED STRAW; DECOMPOSED BLOOD. NERVOUS EXCITEMENT AND SUSPICIOUS FEAR. SENSITIVENESS TO TOUCH, AROUND THROAT AND ABDOMEN. LEFT-SIDED.

PHOSPHORUS

— Fear of death; of thunder; of being alone; of dark; of surroundings, as though something were creeping out of corners.
— Mental excitability first; later, stupefaction. Wild, crazy delirium. Loquacious. Violent, obscene delirium.
— Craving for ice-cold water; it may or may not be vomited when warmed in the stomach.
— Haemorrhagic tendency with coldness.
— Anus open or sensation of being open.
— Stool frequently profuse, gushing; patient much exhausted afterward. Haemorrhage of bright red blood may occur.

SULPHURIC ACID

— Very irritable. Impulsive. Wants things done in a hurry. Intense mental depression; disheartened; tearful.
— DESIRES FRESH FRUIT; BRANDY-STIMULATION.
— Aversion to odor of coffee. Haemorrhages of dark, thin blood with rapid sinking of vital force.
— Tendency to gangrenous ulceration of skin, and ulceration of mucous membranes. Ecchymosis (Arn.). Without mental stupefaction of Phos-ac. Weakness common to acids.

GROUP V: ADVANCED STAGES

CAPSICUM

— Plethoric individuals despondent; home-sick; sleepless; do not react to well selected remedies.
— Chill with thirst, but drinking aggravates it. Perspiration with fever.

Group V: Advanced Stages ...

Capsicum ...

— Chill especially between the shoulders.[1]
— Restless sleep with dreams and terrors; awakens in dreamful fear. Tenesmus of bladder and rectum.[2]

Cantharis

— Aversion to water, in delirium. Mania with urinary suppression.
— Urinary spasm. Frequent ineffectual desire to void scanty blood urine.
— Nervous difficulty in swallowing fluids.
— Scrapings of intestines (Colch.).

Carbo animalis

— Resembles other carbons.
— Stony hardness of glands in all parts.
— Perspiration profuse, stains the linen brownish yellow (Lach.).

Carbo vegetabilis

— Last stages in collapse.
— Cold, with cold perspiration and blueness, yet wants to be fanned. Craves more oxygen.
— Deficient reaction to remedies. (Caps., Psor., Sulph.)

Opium

— Cerebral form. Unconsciousness with all the indications of intense cerebral congestion. Impending apoplexy. Wild fancies and delusions. Distant noises distinctly heard. Coma vigil.
— Fever very high; desires cooling applications even with copious warm perspiration. Pupils contracted, no reaction to light. Dusky purplish countenance. Stertorous respiration. Extreme image of Op. Intense sleeplessness.

China

— Extreme sensitiveness of all senses: sight, hearing, smell, touch.
— Putrid typhoid condition.

---

1. KR 1263R. Back, between the scapula. - Editor.
2. Rep. 630R. - Editor.

GROUP V: ADVANCED STAGES ...

CHINA ...

— China preparations are frequently needed by patients who have suffered more or less from malarial influence.
— Exhaustion intense, following haemorrhage, loss of vital fluids.
— Diarrhoea leaves patient prostrated. Perspiration copious and debilitating.
— Frequently patient worse every other day.
— Stool frequent, loose, copious, dark, offensive; much flatus.
— Ringing in the ears, with fainting. Aggravation from even a draft of air. Abdomen intensely distended.

CHLORALLUM

— Intense sleeplessness and irritability, melancholy and despair prior to or alternating with stupor.
— Hears voices; holds conversation with imaginary beings, in delirium. Jumps out of bed in dreadful fear, with cold perspiration and screams of terror.
— Corresponds to advanced cases where stupor is complete, ending in cerebral congestion. (Crot-h., Hell., Op., Zinc.) Requires constant fanning (Carb-v.). Face dark scarlet, flushing from roots of hair to neck and chest, persisting under pressure of finger.
— Diarrhoea frequently worse at night.
— Hyperaemia of skin increased by taking small quantity of wine. Fever intense.
— Urticaria form of eruption.

CHININUM ARSENICUM

— Prostration most prominent. Angina and symptoms of cardiac weakness and anxiety. Weakened heart-action. Icy coldness of extremities. (Carb-v.)
— Chilliness in waves. THIRSTLESS with fever (Chin.) Aversion to cold water. Eggs and fish occasion painless diarrhoea.

CHININUM SULPHURICUM

— Predominating high fever and furious delirium, with humming in ears. Despondency and lassitude.

Group V: Advanced Stages ...

Chininum sulphuricum ...

— Periodicity of fever more exact: same hour for each recurrence. Thirst during all stages.
— More thirst than China. Much neuralgic pain in head and various parts of body. Many liver and splenic symptoms.

Group VI: Psoric or Constitutional Remedies

Feeble reaction with scarcity of characterizing symptoms. Predominance of symptoms common to the disease.

Lycopodium

— Many nervous symptoms. Fear of being alone; fear of darkness. (Phos.)
— Sensitive to slight noise, as crackling of paper. Many illusions and delusions. Delirium and stupefaction late in progress.
— Develops slowly. General aggravation 4 to 8 o'clock p.m.
— Easy satiety when eating.
— Red Sand in urine. Sensitive to heat; desires open air.
— Capricious appetite. Craves sweets. Desires warm things in stomach.
— Abdominal distension. Generally thirstless, even during fever.

Psorinum

— Morbidly gloomy. Despair of recovery even after the danger has passed. (Ars. and Calc., each characterized by its peculiar symptoms.)
— Convalescence at a standstill. Offensive discharges. No reaction to remedies.
— Weak and weary; averse to any exertion. Cold.
— Restores to health, strength and hope, such who delay in convalescence from typhoid.

Silica

— Sensitive to cold. Weak patient in whom typhoid condition has developed tendency to suppuration. Abscesses in various parts, even in abdominal cavity.
— Abscess-formation as result when typhoid remedies insufficient to overcome the toxemia.

Group VI: Psoric or constitutional remedies ...

Silica ...

— Especially in last stages or following the termination of the fever.

Sulphur

— Aids in restoration of order in class of deeply psoric individuals with deficient reaction.
— Extremities burning heat; skin dry, with heat. Discharges from all parts of body are offensive and excoriating.
— Emaciation.
— Starts reaction even when symptoms very few; resistance of patient is increased, guiding symptoms appear, and other remedies act better after this remedy is given.

Conclusions

The indications here noted are necessarily meager and incomplete; the one thing sought to be here emphasized is the method of applying the law, fitting the remedy to the patient. As illustrating the possible applicability of any remedy (though not listed for typhoid,) mention may be made of the typhoid case cured by Dr. Nash[1] with Cina. The present writer has used this remedy with success in two cases with children, one having cerebral symptoms predominant.

The success of Homeopathy over this dread malady, typhoid, is but one of the many reasons for the persistence of our school - a justification of our claim for generous support from the public - and appeals for the most scientific, pure application of its principles.

In the name of sick humanity, let us turn from a sloven, soulless routinism originated by the old school and weakly followed by too many of our own. Be homeopaths in heart and soul, as in name: cast aside clumsy, lazy methods of alternation and polypharmacy that end only in disappointment and suffering; pursue the path enlightened by the great law of Hahnemann: administer the single indicated remedy under the accurate life-sustaining methods of truly scientific medicines. So shall we maintain the steady march toward our goal: complete and universal recognition and acceptance of God's best gift of healing to sick mankind - the Law of Similars.

---

1. Nash, E.B., Leaders in Homoeopathic Therapeutics, Sixth Edition, Boericke & Tafel, Philadelphia 1926, p. 359.

Undulant Fever[1]

The original aim of this paper was to report several cases of asthma together with two cases of undulant fever. But a review of the literature of the latter disease shows so much of real interest; and at the same time with a better recognition of this, heretofore considered comparatively rare complaint, indicates that it is by no means as rarely occurring as was generally believed. Also the fact that it is so resistant to treatment, and so much serious sequelae remain behind, which is doubtless the result of the routine treatment as much or more so than from the disease itself, makes a thorough review of the malady something of real value to the general practician. Therefore, we will confine the contents of this paper to undulant fever. For references and data, I am indebted to the Nelson Medical Service.

Undulant fever has many other names describing its processes and habitats. It is found extensively throughout the temperate and torrid zones of the earth, but is most common around the shores of the Mediterranean Sea. Other names by which it is known are Malta fever, Mediterranean fever; Melitococcemia; Bruce's Septicemia; Goat fever; Mountain fever; Slow fever (Texas); Gibraltar fever; Rock fever; Neopolitan fever; Cyprus fever; Munhinyo (Uganda) and Mediterranean Phthisis. It is defined by Aldo-Castellani and Albert J. Chalmers as: A specific fever due to micrococcus melitensis Bruce 1893, characterized by its long undulatitory course, early arthritic symptoms, sweats and increasing anemia and debility.

The history of the clinical features of the disease dates back to 400 years B.C. and perhaps earlier. Hippocrates describes cases of protracted fever that no doubt were undulant. It is known to have existed along the shores of the Mediterranean for many hundreds of years, though it was not until the end of the eighteenth century that attention was drawn to it by the large numbers of cases occurring in Malta. The name Malta fever, by which it is most commonly designated, was originally applied to it at this time. Marston, who suffered from the fever himself, was the first author to give an accurate description of it; writing in 1859, he differentiated it clinically and pathologically from both Typhus and Typhoid and suggested that it should be called either Mediterranean remittant or gastric remittant fever.

---

1. The Homeopathic Recorder, Vol. XLVIII, No. 1, Jan. 15, 1933, p. 3 ff.

Many other writers recognized the disease, but nothing more definite was discovered concerning it until 1886, when Bruce found the causative organism, a micrococcus, which he called micrococcus melitensis and succeeded in reproducing the disease in monkeys by inoculating pure cultures of the organism. From this date the disorder began to be generally accepted as a separate pathological entity. In 1897, Wright and Dougles published the results of experiments undertaken with a view of proving that the disease could be diagnosed by the sero-agglutination method. In the same year, Hughs wrote a detailed history and clinical description of the fever and subsequently published his work in book form with the title of *Mediterranean Fever.*

In 1904, a commission was sent out by the British Admirality and War Office to study the disease in Malta in co-operation with the Civil Government of the island. This body sat until 1907 and issued an exhaustive report on which all present ideas of undulant fever are based. Among other points it elucidated the fact that the germ leaves the body through the medium of the urine and that it continues to live some considerable time after such evacuation; that micrococcus melitensis may frequently be found in the blood of apparently healthy goats, and that in such cases the milk of the goat agglutinates the organism; and that infected goats, whose milk is able to transmit the fever to man, suffer no inconvenience from the presence of the germ in their blood.

In recent years, much further work has been carried out on the etiology, pathology and prevention of the malady; and it has been proved that certain cases of undulant fever may be caused by an organism serologically different from the true micrococcus melitensis, producing what is known as para undulant fever. But as the clinical aspects and course of the disease processes are identical in both undulant and para undulant fevers, though caused by distinctly different micro-organisms, for prescribing purposes, it is not necessary to describe the history and writers of the para undulant type of fever.

Climatically undulant fever is not restricted to any particular zone. In Malta the largest number of cases occur in the hot weather but the disease is present at any time of the year.

The causative agent is found in the spleen, liver, kidneys, lymphatics and salivary glands; in the blood, bile and milk. It may occasionally be isolated from the feces. It does not occur in the expired air, the sweat, saliva, or scrapings from the skin.

The organism is very resistant and has been known to live for as long as eighty days in dust and to survive for a month in water, either fresh or salt.

It has been found possible to infect animals with it experimentally in various ways, but its natural mode of entry in the system is by the mouth.

Micrococcus melitensis is a small coccus or cocco-bacillus, gram negative and non-motile and, not rarely, growing in pairs of short chains. It does not liquify gelatin or redden litmus milk. It may be cultivated on agar at a temperature of about 37^0 C and is of a very slow growth, colonies only appearing as a rule on the third or fourth day after inoculation. The milk of infected animals contains agglutinins for the micro-organism. The goat is the natural host of the organism; but ewes, asses, horses, mules, cows, and monkeys are susceptible to the infection. Fifty percent of goats examined in Malta were infected, and the infected animals appear to have suffered no inconvenience.

The disease is transmitted from one animal to another by mouth from browsing on herbs, contaminated by the urine of infected animals. It is carried to man by way of infected milk to the intestinal tract. In some rare instances the fever may be spread by human carriers, although hospital attendants and others have never been known to acquire the disease by direct contamination.

The four recognized modes of infection are: first, by the alimentary canal (usual); second, by the respiratory system, the inhaling of dust contaminated by goat's urine (rare); third, by the cutaneous system (very rare); fourth, by sexual intercourse (possible). Most authors concur in the opinion that the infection is not transmitted by the bites of mosquitoes, though micrococcus melitensis has been obtained from the stomach of mosquitoes, after the latter had fed upon a patient suffering from undulant fever. Nor do flies, fleas, lice or other insects appear to possess the power of communicating the disease by their bites.

Infection produces a true septicemia accompanied by a characteristic swelling, softening and congestion of the spleen. Examination of the blood of undulant fever patients shows the presence of hemolysis produced by the organism, the formation of agglutinins and specific immune bodies. The agglutinins have been proved to remain in the blood for a very considerable length of time and have been found as late as ten years after recovery. Some writers believe the patient to be immune after one attack of undulant fever, but others think unlimited recurrences possible.

Post-mortem examination reveals an enlarged softened spleen with congestion of the lungs, liver, kidneys, mesenteric glands, large and small intestines may go on to ulceration and hemorrhage in some cases.

The period of incubation varies from ten to fourteen days; the onset is characterized by chills, malaise, cephalalgia, anorexia, dyspepsia, muscular pains, insomnia and depression.

1) In a **typical** case, the temperature rises in step-like gradation reaching a higher point on each successive evening and falling a little every morning. By the fifth day the temperature is usually about 103^0 F. (39.5^0 C) with a pulse running between 80 and 90, the headache and muscular discomfort are more severe, the face haggard, the tongue lightly coated dorsally by showing red tip and edges, and the throat somewhat congested. The patient may complain of a cough, the voice may be husky and there may be signs of a slight bronchitis. The spleen may be tender and is often palpable. Constipation occurs in most cases, but at times there is a slight diarrhea.

Little change occurs in the symptoms for twelve or fourteen days; then the temperature which may have ranged between 103^0 (39.5^0 C) and 105^0 F (40.5^0 C) (in the evening) begins to fall, and by the end of another fortnight may have reached normal, only to mount again in a relapse after two or three days.

During the recurrence of the fever the symptoms of the first attack are approximately reduced; in the apyrexial intervals the patient feels much better, though he is, of course, weakened by each repetition of the attack. The wave-like process of alternating recrudescence and defervescence continues almost indefinitely and may last for a year or even longer. Writers have observed a case lasting for more than two years and another for even three.

As time goes on, there is a marked anemia together with a gastric irritation, palpitation, cardiac murmurs, and painful spleen and often sponginess and bleeding of gums. Lobar pneumonia may develop. The patient frequently becomes very dejected and nervous to the point of hysteria, and may complain of pains all over the body.

Insomnia is a feature of the condition, but delirium is rare or mild. The degree of prostration gradually increases. Profuse perspiration usually accompanies each febrile attack particularly at night, and the sweat often emits a very unpleasant odor. Sudamina may appear, desquamation, prickly heat, boils, bed sores, subcutaneous abscesses, ulcers and even hemorrhages are not rare. The joints, usually hip, knee, ankle or shoulder often become painful and swollen without redness and their arthritic symptoms when they occur are very characteristic of the condition.

Neuritis particularly sciatica is another symptom, which assists diagnosis. Pain in the sacro-iliac region, orchitis and inflammation of the parotid glands may be noted.

Blood changes show a reduction of the corpuscles of from 20 to 40 per cent, a certain amount poikilocytosis and considerable decrease in hemoglobin. The white cell count is normal, but the polymorphonuclears are reduced, while the mononuclears show an increase of 80 per cent in extreme cases. Phagocytosis and the bactericidal power of the blood are dimished according to the writers cited, Basset-Smith, Gabbi and others.

The urine is normal in amount, and the infective organism is commonly to be found in it; its presence has been observed as long as two years after recovery. The reaction is slightly acid, and the deposit usually shows phosphates and urates. Albumin is rarely noted; bile is sometimes present but only in severe cases. A slight albuminuria is not rare and true nephritis may occur; hematuria has been observed.

The average duration of the illness from the onset to convalescence is three months, but cases lasting for a year or longer are not rare. Four varieties are usually described: 1. typical, 2. malignant, 3. intermittent and 4. ambulatory. The typical variety has been described above.

2) The **malignant type** comes suddenly and without warning. The temperature rises to 104^0 F (40^0 C) or higher at a leap with severe headache, acute and generalized muscular pains, vomiting, diarrhea with offensive stools, congestion of the lungs and sometimes basal pneumonia. After a few days a typhoid-like condition supervenes, and death occurs from cardiac failure in one to three weeks after the onset.

3) The **intermittent type** is gradual in its onset and mild in its course. There is low Serotine fever, malaise, slight chills, nervous irritability and night sweats. The condition lasts from a few weeks to several month (six or more). The patient may be quite unaware that he is suffering from anything unusual until successive attacks gradually debilitate him and he begins to feel weak and depressed.

4) The **ambulatory variety** is even more benign than the intermittant type, and the sufferer may show no symptoms at all, while at times he may complain of weakness and may occasionally feel slightly feverish. In such cases though clinical symptoms may be entirely absent, the

organism is present in the blood as proved by hemocultures, and the individuals so affected may have the power of transmitting the infection to others.

The most common complication is orchitis, and pneumonia is not rare. Persistant vomiting, diarrhea and hyperexia may lead to serious consequences. Cardiac failure usually terminates the malignant type of the disease. Ulcers may occur though rarely in both large and small intestines, and may give rise hemorrhage in those cases; it is often difficult to differentiate clinically between undulant fever and typhoid. Periostitis has been occasionally noted.

Sequelae: Neuritis, asthenia, impaired memory and neurasthenia are the most usual. Muscular atrophy and general invalidism also occur; morphinism as the result of the administration of morphia for severe insomnia and pain has been noted.

The type of fever, the clinical aspects before mentioned, the spleen and blood symptoms and the recovery of the specific organism in the urine and blood, microscopically and by the agglutination method will render a diagnosis.

Differential diagnosis; malaria, kala-azar and typhoid. In contrast to malaria, the malady seldom begins suddenly and severe rigors are rare; quinine has no effect and malaria parasites are absent.

In kala-azar the spleen is generally much more enlarged and harder, and the examination of the spleen juice obtain by puncture will reveal the presence of leishmaniae.

The differentiation from typhoid fever may at times be difficult, but the diagnosis is cleared up by the result of agglutination tests and hemocultures.

Prognosis; except when it occurs in the malignant type, undulant fever rarely proves fatal. The death rate does not exceed 2 or 3 per cent normally, though during certain epidemics a much larger mortality has been known. Birt and Lamb attribute a certain amount of prognostic value to the agglutination test and regard persistent low agglutination as a bad omen.

The treatment given by the old school is rest in bed with careful nursing, tepid sponging and a light nutritious diet. The symptoms of pain, insomnia and fever, are met with the various coal tar preparations, morphine and bromides. They have found no drug specific to the disease, and serums and vaccines have proved to be disappointing and without real value, although recommended by some advisers. In cases of severe persistent vomiting, that do not yield to milder remedies, two drops of iodine in one ounce of common water may be tried, and when all else fails, minute doses of cocaine 1/16 gr. in chloroform water may be given and a mustard leaf may be applied to the pit of the stomach. Change of climate is recommended for protracted cases, in a locality of medium altitude, where Malta fever is not endemic.

The following cases, briefly stated, will show the vast difference obtained in clinical results of cure, between the two systems of treatment, the old school, contrasted with that of our own. The time of recovery required less than half of the average patients treated empirically and with no sequelae remaining.

November 20, 1931: I was called in consultation with another homeopathic physician to see a little girl, age six, who had been ill about three weeks with a type of remittant fever and a clinical picture that puzzled the attending physician. The case started like a flu with chills, fever and general muscular pains, which soon localized in one ear, causing acute pain. By ruling out typhoid and flu and because of the peculiar and typical curve of the fever, which ranged as high as 105^0 F, we decided to test for undulant fever. Laboratory tests of the blood and urine confirmed our tentative diagnosis. The physician in charge had given several remedies on more or less uncertain indications and with no result in relief of conditions. BRY., BELL., ARS. and HEP. had been given in low potencies.

The symptom picture and history, at my first visit suggested to me one of the *mercury* preparations. The tongue, flabby and offensive, the copious sweats without relief, and the night aggravations were the prominent features standing out. But which mercury preparation was best? This was decided by testing and comparing not only the mercuries but many other remedies over the blood of the patient[1], which brought MERC-K-I. through as the best remedy reactor. The remedy was given in the *10M. potency* and repeated only when the fever recurred at certain irregular intervals, fever remission coming every 8 to 10 days and each time not rising as high as in the preceeding attack.

All fever remissions were gone 30 days after the first administration of the remedy, but quite a long convalescence followed, a condition where the pulse ran relatively high 90 to 120, although the temperature was constantly normal; this lasted for at least six weeks, during this time the patient was not permitted to be on her feet. At the end of this

---

1. See see article "Recent Concepts and New Formulas in Medicine" on page 679 ff. and see article "Importance of Electronic Reactions to Future Medicine" on page 683 ff.. - Editor.

period the pulse and temperature attained a relatively normal curve and the patient was permitted to gradually resume her usually exercise and diet.

The second case was one of much milder aspect, the fever never reached above 101⁰ F. The diagnosis of this case was also confirmed by laboratory tests of the blood and urine. The same remedy MERC-K-I. given first in the 30th potency, repeated once a week apart and one dose of the 10M given two weeks after the second dose of the 30th, cured the patient in about six weeks time.

Homeopathic Success Against Infantile Paralysis (Polio)[1]

Probably no disease carries so much terror for the parents of children as poliomyelitis does. Hence the so called medical drive against this disease enables the professional propagandists to cash in large dividends garnered from a sympathetic and interested public. So called medical science has spent vast sums of money and slaughtered millions of animals, monkeys, guinea pigs, and rats in an antiquated form of research chasing the delusion of finding the specific remedy and prophylactic for the disease.

If they would follow homeopathic techniques and experiment on healthy humans they would find some very illuminating facts. First they would note the harm done by material doses of serums and vaccines to the human economy. Second they would become aware of the improbability of finding a specific remedy for a disease because of the difference in individual susceptibilities and reactions to drugs, stimuli, and even infections of all kinds. Third, the truth of the law of similars would flash before their materialistic minds as they behold the fact, that only those drugs are capable of curing which can produce similar symptoms (on the healthy) to the pathogenesis of the disease conditions to be cured. And fourth, they would soon learn by the law's application of the **Law of Similars** to the sick, that the same dosage of a drug used to produce symptoms on the healthy would prove harmful, and even dangerous even when indicated if given to the sick. In other words they might be impressed with the vastly increased sensitivity of the sick over the healthy organism to the actions of drugs, serums, vaccines, etc.

For over a hundred years homeopathic treatment has cured thousands of cases of the various forms of paralysis and neuroses afflicting humanity. However it is only in comparatively recent times, twenty-five to thirty years, that epidemics of infantile paralysis (polio) have been more recognized and studied, because of its increasing frequency and virulency, (despite the efforts of the so-called medical science which so loudly advertizes its wares by way of the public press while interdicting from the same forum all other schools or methods which have not the orthodox stamp of the American Medical Association). In the armamentarium of Homeopathy there are many remedies having the power to produce and cure states and symptoms found in the pathogenetic picture of poliomyelitis. Clinical application over a period of years ena-

---

1.   From handwritten manuscript, probably late 1948. - Editor..

bles the keen prescriber to rely on a comparatively small group of remedies that are more frequently indicated in such conditions and diseases.
The group of fifty remedies which follow are by no means the only
ones that may be needed but they are more frequently found indicated
for paralytic states in general.

Acon., **Agar.**, **Alum.**, *anac.*, *arg-n.*, *ars.*, *art-v.*, *bapt.*, *bar-c.*, *bell.*,
bry., **Bufo**, *calc.*, *calc-s.*, **Caust.**, *cic.*, *chin.*, **Cocc.**, *colch.*, *con.*, *crot-c.*,
crot-h., *cupr.*, *cur.*, *dros.*, *dulc.*, *gels.*, *kali-c.*, *kali-p.*, *kalm.*, **Lath.**, *lach.*,
naja, *nat-m.*, *nit-ac.*, *nux-v.*, *olnd.*, *op.*, *phos.*, **Plb.**, **Rhus-t.**, *ruta*, *sep.*,
Sil., *stram.*, **Sulph.**, *tarent.*, *verat.*, *zinc.*

For the acute infective and toxic forms of paralysis including Infantile, I have found a much narrower group of twenty-two remedies sufficient:

Acon., *agar.*, *ars.*, *bell.*, *caust.*, *cocc.*, *cur.*, *dulc.*, *gels.*, *kali-p.*, *kalm.*,
Lath., *lach.*, *naja*, *nat-m.*, *nux-v.*, *op.*, *phos.*, *plb.*, **Rhus-t.**, *stram.*, *zinc.*

For cases that have passed the acute stage and ultimated in chronic
paralysis, thirteen remedies need to be studied.

alum., *bar-c.*, *calc-s.*, *caust.*, *con.*, *cupr.*, *kali-p.*, *nat-m.*, *phos.*, **Plb.**, *sil.*,
sulph., *zinc.*

Some years ago a case was submitted from another doctor where
there was complete and total paralysis with unconsciousness; only common symptoms were presented. A remedy was selected over the
patient's blood[1] not in any of the aforementioned groups and in whose
proving no paralysis has been observed. That remedy NAT-AR. 45M, in
a single dose was given with a rapid and complete cure. No atrophy or
impaired motion or function resulted. The NAT-AR. case is cited to show
with what certainty, alacrity, and completeness, the perfectly attuned
remedy acts. Also to remind us that a remedy never heard of in relation
to a certain case or condition may nevertheless be the curative drug
needed to effect the cure.

The one remedy in our Materia Medica presenting the most striking
picture to typical cases of infantile paralysis symptomatically, pathologically, and clinically is LATH., and for that reason we are justified in pre-
suming it to be a *most effective prophylaxis* against this disease. And
clinical application in many thousands of cases over a period of thirty
years has registered one hundred percent success.

---

1. See see article "Recent Concepts and New Formulas in Medicine" on page 679 ff. and see article
   "Importance of Electronic Reactions to Future Medicine" on page 683 ff.. - Editor.

It is in this phase of the disease (prevention) that Homeopathy has its most golden opportunity to compel recognition from both the public and the medical profession in general. If every homeopathic doctor who reads this will try immunizing the children under his care with a dose of the remedy in the thirtieth or twohundredth potency given about once every three weeks during an epidemic, I am confident he will have no cases of paralysis among those so immunized. Also let them pass it on to their old school doctor friends and soon the world will hear more about Homeopathy and its benign power to heal.

Homeopathic Palliation in Incurables[1]

Incurable cases of sickness are among the most distressing and depressing things a physician meets. To many doctors there is nothing left to do but give enough of some narcotic or pain killing drug to relieve suffering and await the end.

But it is not as simple as that, because after a time these drugs fail to bring relief any longer and to the natural trouble of the patient are added the torments of a drug disease. Many cases of painful arthritis and neuritis will continue to plague the patient for years, gradually impairing his activities to finally end in his being a helpless cripple wracked with pain and in spite of large and increasing amounts of numerous analgesic drugs which eventually add to the patient's misery without even lessening his pain. Of course the most common and difficult of these cases are those suffering with cancer and most of these become narcotic addicts before a merciful death ends their suffering.

To the homeopathist these incurables while presenting a very difficult problem are nevertheless responsive to his prescribing and with infintely happier results than those obtained under the routine of narcotics and other analgesics.

It is true that therapeutic symptoms are meager, and frequently nothing but drug symptoms are present for selecting the homeopathic remedy. But in spite of these handicaps it is surprising and heartening how frequently relief can be given even until the last breath of life is passed.

Remedies may have to be given at short intervals. Sometimes a remedy comforts for only a few hours or days when a new one must be found and given.

Always remember that better results are obtained in these incurables suffering great pain if the potencies range from the 200, 30, and even much lower because the severe reactions of the real high potencies, brought on by the economy's effort to cure in an incurable case, adds agony to the suffering.

At times when tissue changes are very extensive in vital organs a single does of a high potency will bring on euthanasia within 24 to 48 hours.

In cases where cancers attack centers rich in sentient nerves as the optic and other nerves it is amazing the relief that Cod-p. will bring in

---

1. From handwritten manuscript, exact date unknown. - Editor..

the 1X to 3X potency, given disolved in a glass of water in drachm (i.e. small) doses at intervals of every 2 to 3 hours.

BELL. and CHAM. are frequently indicated and effective in the 30th potency in those who have had too much of the opium derivitives and they no longer relieve but must be given to appease the craving of the addict.

Perhaps among the very difficult cases of sufferers to relieve homeopathically are those of chronic asthma who have been loaded with adrenal injections[1]; they are like the cancer cases over treated by X-ray and radium; it is most difficult to find help in this class of cases. I would prefer not to take the responsibility of trying to relieve such cases and advise them to stay with the allopathic methods that brought them to their present state.

Diabetics who have had too much insulin rarely respond to the most carefully selected remedies; it is generally better not to undertake to even palliate them for failure is almost certain and the doctor and Homeopathy will be discredited. No matter how much failure old school methods meet, it is accepted in quiet resignation by the public as the inevitable, because scientific medicine has done everything that could be done. Such is the power of propaganda.

Cases not spoiled by too drastic drugging or by overtreatment of X-ray or radium will respond to careful and painstaking homeopathic prescribing. And no greater reward or real joy can come to the physician whose skill can bring solace and even comfort to these tragic sufferers and their loved ones as well, with the benign touch of Homeopathy. It is all so worthwhile bringing courage and strength, that they might bear their cross lightly down the dark passage to the valley of the shadows till they sink into unconsciousness and earthly oblivion to awaken on the other side, victorious over all the inhibitions of the flesh. A few brief cases picked at random will illustrate the power of Homeopathy to palliate and comfort incurables.

CARCINOMA OF BREAST

CASE 1 MISS C.L.D. A MAIDEN LADY OF 38

February 13, 1932: Reported with a large hard tumor in the right breast and swollen painful axillary glands, also a slight retraction of the nipple. At this time the pain was steady but not severe and the gen-

---

1. and today with steroids-cortisone. - Editor.

CARCINOMA OF BREAST ...

CASE I MISS C.L.D. A MAIDEN LADY OF 38 ...

eral health excellent. CON. 10M was given and repeated at long inervals in a series of potencies. The glands in the axilla receeded and lost their pain; the breast tumor grew smaller and harder but free of pain. This remedy was sufficient to carry the patient along a period of about six years. Part of that time she continued in her usual secretarial work, the latter part was devoted to a trip around the world through Europe, the Middle East, Egypt, India, China, and Japan and back to the U.S.A. As the trip neared the end the patient's condition grew worse: the tumor began to ulcerate and break down with pain and hemorrhage; the latter symptom is always an indication that the degenerative changes are in the ascendency.

This was about *March 15, 1938* when the patient was given CADM-MET. which held until December 1938. The remedy was given in **10M**, **50M**, and **CM** potencies during which time there was a general improvement and the patient was free of pain and hemorrhage. But at the end of December more hemorrhages, very profuse came on to leave the patient weak and somewhat discouraged. The flow was bright red and hot and BELL. brought relief to both pain and hemorrhage. Later in

May, 1939, ACON. in potency for bright red flow with anxious fear of death. This ameliorated for some months.

July 1939: FORMAL. 200 was prescribed. The 200, 1M, and 10M of this remedy ameliorated the patient and her symptoms until October 10, 1939.

November 2, 1939: Coldness, weakness and much flatulence in the bowels required CARB-V. 10M. This prescription was confirmed by the blood prescription; but relief was slight and short lasting.

November 27, 1939: KALI-C. was given for shooting sharp pains in the left chest, interfering with breathing. KALI-C. in a series of potencies from 1M to the 50M held and helped all symptoms from *February 28, 1940* until *February 25, 1941.*

Carcinoma of Breast ...

Case 1 Miss C.L.D. a maiden lady of 38 ...

In this year the patient showed marked decline in health and the local trouble had extensively broken down and spread. This was culminated by one of her worst hemorrhages which was followed for days by a copious discharge of blood and serum.

February 25, 1941: Plb. 1M 10M and 50M relieved symptoms and helped patient until

May 20, 1941: when Durbital[1] 30 to 1M relieved pain and hemorrhage until

July 8, 1941: when there was hemorrhage; thick dark clots: Elaps 10M. This helped until

August 26, 1941: when Chin. 10M for weakness after hemorrhage was given which acted well until

October 9, 1941: When Chin. ceased to act and Sec. 10M was given with benefit until

January 10, 1942: When a letter stating patient was in bed unconscious with a greatly swollen scalp and an erysipelous eruption over scalp and face. A local doctor was called and pronounced the case hopeless, advised local antiseptics and medicine for fever, which was not taken. The family prefered my treatment and so Chin. 10M was sent with plenty of Sacch-l.

From *January 10, 1942* until *February 2, 1942* the patient slowly improved after the eruption went with the discharge of copious amounts of pus from abcess in the scalp.

February 21, 1942: This remarkable patient was put on Nat-thio-cy. 200[2] which was repeated April 1, 1942 and April 21, 1942;

May 8, 1942: Nat-thio-cy. 1M. was given.

June 13, 1942: The last report received this patient was walking around the house dressing her own breast, free of pain and again encouraged and hopeful.

---

1. Durbital, unknown to most homoeopaths, but used by Dr. Grimmer. - Editor.
2. Natrum thiocyanatum (NaCNS), unknown to most homoeopaths, but used by Dr. Grimmer. - Editor.

Chronic ulcer

Case 2 Mr. C.F. G. 86 years

October 1, 1938: Has a chronic ulcerating sore[1] on dorsal aspect of hand of several years standing, oozing a considerable amount of blood, not much pain. CADM-MET. 10M. This remedy helped in ascending potencies; **10M, 50M** and **CM** at rather long intervals until

April 28, 1939: when KALI-THIO-CY. 200 which restrained soreness and bleeding until

October 16, 1939: FORMAL. 200 was given.

November 16, 1939: Was relieved until recently;now much more bleeding. FORMAL. 200. This held well until

January 3, 1940: FORMAL. 10M.

January 26, 1940: FORMAL. 10M. Was better until he hurt the sore hand.

February 26, 1940: More swelling, pain bleeding and odor to the sore. FORMAL. 200 once a week.

April 29, 1940: More or less continuous pain; growth on hand spreading. At this time X-RAY 200. Patient and his sore improved until

June 25, 1940: Slight return of pain. X-RAY 200.

July 3, 1940: X-RAY 200.

October 11, 1940: Remedy not giving the relief: X-RAY 10M.

November 11, 1940: Patient weaker and tumor increasing. X-RAY 10M.

December 13, 1940: Weaker but comfortable. X-RAY 10M.

January 10, 1941: Less pain and no more hemorrhage. X-RAY 10M.

February 9, 1041: Patient died without pain almost 89 years of age.

Advanced breast cancer

Case 3 Miss H. H. age 39

March 14, 1942: In 1939 noticed a small lump in left breast, now the whole breast is ulcerated, with pain and considerable hemorrhage

---

1. Probably a squamous cell epithelioma. - Editor.

Advanced breast cancer ...

Case 3 Miss H. H. age 39 ...

whenever breast is dressed; radiated heat aggravates the breast. No great loss of weight; appetite and digestion good. No menstrual troubles. Recently sleep has been much interfered and skin on right breast is indurated. Lap-a. 1M.

April 9, 1942: Has a dry disturbing cough aggravated at night while lying down. Sang. 10M.

May 2, 1942: Very thirsty, cough gagging with increased breast pain. A blood remedy, Phyt. 10M relieved cough and pain until death ended the tragedy.

Bilateral breast cancer with axillary metastasis

Case 4 Mrs. C in her early fifties

October 27, 1940: Both breasts indurated with small ulcers over whole surface; periodically sharp pains. Glands in axilla enlarged. Patient in good health and appearance. Alum-sil. 10M.

December 13, 1940: Alum-sil. 10M.

January 23, 1941: More pain at times. Alum-sil. 50M.

February 12, 1941: Improved. No medicine.

April 3, 1941: Alum-sil. CM.

April 28, 1941: No pain. No medicine.

May 16, 1941: Alum-sil. CM. This remedy seemed to improve patient and her symptoms until

August 20, 1941: Breast painful and oozing serum. Graph. 10M.

September 23, 1941: Graph. 10M. This helped until

October 21, 1941: Graph. 50M.

November 19, 1941: Breast better.

December 4, 1941: Breast more indurated. Aur-nat-fl.?? 10M (blood remedy).

December 18, 1941: Better.

January 14, 1941: More pain and hardness in breast.

BILATERAL BREAST CANCER WITH AXILLARY METASTASIS ...

CASE 4 MRS. C IN HER EARLY FIFTIES ...

February 6, 1942: Not improved in the last month. NAT-THIO-CY. 30.

March 3, 1942: Some better. No medicine.

March 13, 1942: Very severe breast pains. Reaction. No medicine.

April, 17, 1942: Improving. ENAT-THIO-CY. 200.

May 22, 1942: Symptoms not as well. NAT-THIOCY. 1M.

June 8, 1942: No medicine.

This patient should have many years yet of usefulness and comparative comfort as her general physical condition is good and she is organically sound. Yet in the end she will die of cancer if accident or acute disease does not shorten her span of life.

CONCLUSION

These cases are only typical out of hundreds I have treated in the past twenty-five years, but under Homeopathy much of the terror of the disease as well as the suffering is mitigated and a large number will live and carry on for ten or fifteen years.[1]

Compare these with the mutilation and increased agony and expense of Old School methods and the contrast is striking. In the majority of operated cases life expectancy is from two to five years with crucifixion at the end. X-Ray and radium therapy has proven still more disappointing except perhaps in the suppression of skin leisons which are driven to some vital spot to later take its inevitable toll.

---

1. The above cases defy present day statistics of malignancy and survival. In case 1 the patient survived 10 years, in case 2 three years and in case 4 the end was yet to come. - Editor.

Essays

PRESIDENT'S MESSAGE - AN AUTOBIOGRAPHY[1]

Born in San Jose, California, August 29, 1874, the eldest of nine children, of poor but thrifty and industrious parents. My childhood and playtime was brief in span and broken at frequent intervals in the performance of certain chores incident in the household of every large family not financially able to hire servants.

Up until my sixth year my life existence was care free and mostly given over to rambling through the large fields of tall mustard which grew more than six feet high and so thick and close that it was difficult for a small boy to force his way through the miniature forest, for such it seemed to me.

We lived on the outskirts of the city and at that time the country was sparsely settled and wild game of all kinds were to be found in great number and variety. Even the grizzly bear was frequently killed twenty or thirty miles from the outskirts of the city when they came down from the nearby mountains to raid the stock of the pioneer farmers of that day.

After my sixth birthday my family moved to San Francisco where I attended my first public school. When not in school mornings and evenings I sold papers to help swell the family budget. In pursuing the sale of my papers I covered much of San Francisco, in saloons, restaurants and other public places, and on trolley and cable cars as well, I plied my trade energetically and untiringly with all the enthusiasm of impetuous youth. Two years later we moved to Oakland, California where I spent the happiest years of my youth. There I completed all the primary schooling I was destined to have. When I was twelve years of age my father decided to locate on a hundred and sixty acre piece of Government land in the mountains of Northern California in Lake County, where the quicksilver mines are found.

The twelve years that followed were rugged and adventuresome and beset with many difficulties and tribulations. My father was not a farmer or a pioneer in any sense of the word, and with a large brood of small children to provide for and no money or capital at hand to work with the going was tough, and rations were scant and poor. But game was abundant and wild fruits and berries were plentiful. With a little flour, corn meal, coffee and sugar we were able to survive the first few years of real hardship and privation until we had cleared some land and

---

1. JOURNAL OF THE AMERICAN INSTITUTE OF HOMEOPATHY, Vol. 46, No. 7, p. 216, July 1953.

brought it under cultivation, and were able to procure some chickens and other poultry together with a few hogs and cattle.

We learned to cope with the elements and vicissitudes of the changing seasons. In summer and fall the raging forest fires required courage and ingenuity to meet successfully. In the deep snow and the cold of the winter the stock had to feed on the foliage of certain trees and shrubs to help tide them over until warmer weather, when the snows melted and other food was obtainable for them. We became expert hunters and highly proficient with the axe, the saw and the tool that enabled us to make shingles for the roofs of the buildings built from the hewn logs of the trees that grew on hand.

The second year after our arrival my father suffered severe injuries from a fall off the mountain road. The wagon and the food contents were destroyed, one horse was killed, the other badly injured and cut in numerous places, and my father was left an invalid for the rest of his life.

This unhappy event added new responsibilities on my young shoulders. I was then a lad of fourteen, undersized but unafraid and as tough as whale bone, a heritage from my mother whose tireless energy and unflagging courage stood out like the Rock of Gibraltar as the main factor in the founding and maintenance of a home that for many years to come was to be a haven and a place of security where we came after expeditions and journeys, from work in the mines and the timber lands, and found rest, comfort and recuperation.

Because of my father's accident and consequent physical incompetency I had to leave my mother and younger brothers to care for the home and go in search of work in order to get a little cash to buy the bare necessities needed. My first job was on a large ranch where cattle, grain, hay and wine grapes were raised on a large scale. I earned the munificent sum of eight dollars a month and my board, which sufficed to help meet the needs at home. This job required the milking of sixteen cows night and morning. After eight months dissatisfaction gnawed at my vitals and I sought a new base of operations in the quicksilver mines as a mucker, that is, shoveling the rock and earth dug loose by the miners and bringing it out to the dumps in cars. This job paid me $1.50 a day with board. In a few months I qualified for a regular miner and was paid three big dollars a day for ten hours work; this also included board.

From this time on things became brighter for the Grimmer family, for in a few years three of my younger brothers were able to obtain similiar employment, thus enabling us to add improvements and other comforts to the home such as running water piped to the house and the establishment of a bath tub, which was a real luxury in those times and places.

It is well to state in passing that my father was a highly educated man and his most prized possession was his library. This was made up of a wonderful collection of books on science and literature together with ancient and modern history. I had free access to these books and made the most of the opportunity they presented for acquiring more knowledge. I read long hours every night, whether at home or away, averaging but five hours sleep from the time of my fourteenth year up until my thirty-fourth year. This reading, together with my father's tutoring, enabled me to pass a successful high school examination[1] (Hyde Park School, Chicago) that permitted me to enter Hering Medical College to start my medical education.

It will be interesting to some of my friends to know how I became a homeopath in principle and conviction. My father treated his family with homeopathic remedies by following Johnson's Family Guide, an excellent work, one of the best of its kind, in my opinion. Father had sixty polychrests, a good selection for many homeopathic physicians. By the time I was seven I knew most of the indications of those sixty remedies by heart and at that early age I had the urge to be a homeopathic doctor.

After we had lived six or eight years in the mountains I met Dr. J. E. Hoffman at Healdsburgh, California, the town we had to go to for our supplies. Dr. Hoffman was my real preceptor and never let up telling me I must go to Chicago and enroll under the teaching of Dr. J. T. Kent. He also fired my mother with ambition for me by telling her I was an unusual prospect for a successful homeopathic prescriber. He used to say physicians, like poets, were born, not made, but how he could visualize a great physician in the raw, uncouth youth from the mountains has always been a mystery to me.

At twenty-six years of age I left my mountain home for Chicago and the study of medicine. I had my railroad fare and a few extra dollars in

---

1. In September 1902 when Arthur Grimmer left California to study with Dr. Kent at Hering Medical College, Chicago, he had not attended his highschool (having worked to support his family). However reading books in his father's library together with his father's tutoring had made young Arthur a very keen student. He was allowed to take the highschool exam at Hyde Park School, Chicago, after arriving in Chicago, passed the exam and immediately entered Hering Medical College. - Story told by Audrey Grimmer Winters.

my pocket, not much ammunition for the conquest of a place in the sun, but I was lucky and kind Providence surely guided and protected me in my great adventure toward the fulfillment of my dreams.

In the fullness of time and in company of my colleagues we made the grade and obtained our diplomas. Then came the trial of establishing a practice common to all young graduates.

Forty-seven years of homeopathic practice in the service of my fellows has made my life replete with much joy and few regrets, for the outstanding miracle of cure and deep satisfaction far outweigh the relatively few disappointments that come to those who really follow the law of faith, because faith in the law implies faith in God. Without faith the healer will fail, and without faith the sick will succumb.

Trusting these sketchy highlights of a homeopathic physician's coming and going will not prove too boring to his sure to be indulgent readers, I take this time to express my deep appreciation for the high honor conferred upon me by my election as President of the American Institute of Homeopathy for the year 1953. I appeal to my friends and fellow members for their prayers and aid in the service of the Institute that we may keep it a fit and efficient custodian for the protection and growth of the homeopathic law of cure.

Yours in the true faith.

June 1953

A. H. Grimmer, M.D.

FIFTY SEVEN YEARS IN THE PRACTICE OF HOMEOPATHIC MEDICINE[1]

In early September, 1902, a gangling, uncouth youth left his mountain habitat in California, on horseback, to start on a two thousand mile journey by rail to Chicago, to begin the study of medicine. No visions of grandeur, or dreams of wealth or worldly fame disturbed the even tenure of his way; only a burning desire to qualify for the privilege of becoming a homeopathic physician and serve as a humble healer of the sick and needy inspired his every thought and effort. No sacrifice of time or worldly possessions, which were meager indeed, was too much to give to attain this precious goal set by a longing heart.

Well, he came and saw and conquered, in the language of the great Roman warrior, Julius Caesar. He conquered, not an empire or destroyed armies with their spoils of victory, but he conquered self by the grace of God, to endure privations, loneliness, hardships, temptations, despair and the black form of fear in its numerous aspects; he learned to replace fear with faith and despair with courage and to develop a will that defied obstacles and frustrations. He cultivated the God-sent light of reason and intelligence to lead him on life's stormy highway in preparation for his life's work, the practice of medicine.

Four tedious, painful, but exciting years glided by and graduation day came and the fledgling doctor, with many of his colleagues was born and dedicated to the healing arts.

In June, 1906, at high noon, he hung out his shingle, A.H. Grimmer, M.D., at Twenty-ninth and Groveland Ave., Chicago, to embark on a new career, the practice of medicine. From miner and lumberjack and farmer and "Jack of all trades", laborer, etc. came the sudden, startling transformation to a Doctor of Medicine, this coveted degree was a prize whose worth was priceless; yes, it meant opportunity and prestige and eventual wealth, but it really meant much more, a chance to serve, to comfort and instruct in the restoration of lives, from pain, sickness and sorrow to states of health and happiness. With these desirable boons came a deep sense of responsibility for the custodianship of other lives coming for help and healing and guidance. Many questions loomed, with but vague answers. Was he really prepared to meet the challanges and obligations imposed? Did he have the patience and equipment needed to successfully cope with the numerous trying situations com-

---

1. THE LAYMAN SPEAKS, probably December 1953. - Editor..

ing up in this work? Only if the love of the work and its uses, was strong enough could he be sure of success and happiness in its performance.

Doctors, like poets and artists, are born and inspired from birth for their special work, they are never artificially made.[1] However, training and long application in their chosen occupation can enhance the value of their work greatly by developing greater efficiency and satisfaction in its performance.

With a capital of thirty dollars on that bright June day began the practice of medicine. Full of hope and expectancy, undaunted by lack of funds and a limited credit, the start was made. At the end of the first month sixty dollars in cash was earned and collected, enough to pay rent, laundry, and buy a scant supply of food. Practice gradually increased and the clientele slowly grew in numbers and importance until after a year fortune began to smile on the work with better remuneration. Now, looking back, one can see that it was well that things developed slowly as it gave ample time to study cases and the remedies needed to bring the desired results.

The long and intensive study of remedies for sick patients not only brought success at the time, but laid the foundation for more successful prescribing in the future, when pressures in time and increasing numbers of more baffling and complicated cases piled steadily up, together with increasing house calls from various sections of Chicago, North, South, West, with great distances between and at all hours of the day and night consumed much time and protracted effort. But, the driving interest and love of the work with the sustaining power of Divine Goodness gave the strength of will to carry on without the sense or thought of fatigue, only a few hours sleep sufficed to refresh for a new day. The work was blessed with the joy of success beyond all expectations. Perhaps the bright solar orb on the noon meridian, with the attending Stellium of Planets, Pluto, Jupiter, Venus, Mars and Mercury was symbolic of rapid and far-reaching success in the profession started at that auspicious time. According to Astrologic Law the Midheaven or the tenth house rules the profession or business. The sign Leo rises at my birth, making the Sun ruler of my life.

Be these things law or coincidence, the next few years marked the advent of a large office and general practice, including obstetrics, which in those days meant the delivering of babies mostly in the homes. Also,

---

1. Dr. J.E. Hoffmann's words to young Arthur Grimmer (see article "President's Message - an Autobiography" p. 501 ff.) - Editor.

at that time frequent consultation cases with Homeopathic doctors in neighboring cities and states, especially from Michigan, Indiana, Wisconsin and Iowa. These cases necessitated over-night trips by rail, with the need to be back at ten a.m. for office work. Often only a couple hours sleep could be obtained in the performance of this work, but it was sheer joy and never ending excitement and expectation; for new and unusual types of cases were often met. After twenty-five years of this work the decision to specialize in chronic diseases seemed to offer greater opportunity to do more good to a greater number of patients and thereby help spread the light of Homeopatic healing.

The broad field of chronic diseases presented the chance to really cure people of their inherited miasms which are the prime cause of all sickness. Also, this type of treatment enters greatly into the phase of disease prevention, especially for the younger and middle-aged groups of patients. Here also, the thoroughly trained Homeopathic physician who has developed skill and keen awareness in the prescribing art, by years in the application of the pure Hahnemannian technique will see with constant delight so many cures of cases generally looked upon as incurable, such as cancer in its numerous aspects, crippling arthritis, severe types of nervous and mental disease all in some mysterious and unexpected manner being restored to health under the impact of the Homeopathic remedy. These happy occurrences are Heaven-sent blessings to patient and physician alike and they invoke the spirit of reverence and thanksgiving for the precious gift of Homeopathy.

Fifty-seven years in this work has made me deeply reverent and humble, and illumed my consciousness with the influx of the truth and goodness from Divine Providence for all His children in their needs. These fifty-seven years of service with my brothers and sisters, from all walks of life, all God's children, has brought me more joy than all the world's wealth could give. My soul is thrilled and my heart warmed by the gratitude and love expressed by hundreds of my grateful patients for my humble efforts in their behalf. A bond of mutual love and trust has been forged that transcends any honor the world of men can give. It has been a rare privilege to serve my fellows, under God, who has blest my work so abundantly.

Another delight that gladdens the sunset years of my life is the many students of all ages, throughout these years, to whom it has been my privilege to teach the truths and principles of Homeopathic philosophy and Materia Medica.

Their progress and achievements in the realm of Homeopathic healing are outstanding landmarks that insure the future continuity of Homeopathic medicine to meet the greater needs of humanity in the near future. Homeopathy, in its purity alone can meet the apparent threats of universal radiation sickness, as well as the evil effects from the abuse of drastic drugging, even now undermining mental and physical health, everywhere. Added to all this is the world wide spread of alcoholism with all the admitted hopelessness of cure involved[1].

In times of crises and great need, Divine Providence provides the men and instrumentalities needed to meet the situations and conditions that exist. Because of these facts we believe that Homeopathy will be re-discovered and accepted for the good of the world. In closing I wish to give expression of love and admiration for my many Homeopathic colleagues from all parts of our world, of all countries, and all religious faiths, and of all political alignments, and from all the races of men everywhere in the world because they are all children of our Father in Heaven, as we are, hence our brethren.

Homeopathy is God-inspired and God-sent for the good of all His children, where-over they may dwell, hence it is one of the universal mediums for the spread of love, peace and service.

Finally, let me end with a plea to you, my beloved colleagues and devoted students, and numerous friends, who have known the benefits of Homeopathic medicine, for your support of the ideals and principles of the Homeopathic philosophy, that all the future may be blessed with the gentle, safe, and sure power inherent in the similimum empowered to cure a sick world, by the Grace of God. And may His choicest blessing be with you, my friends, as I bid you a fond farewell.

---

1. And today we have the world wide spread of the numerous recreational drugs and all the evil diseases that ensure therefrom - Editor.

James Tyler Kent[1]

My first meeting with Dr. Kent was in early September, 1902. I had journeyed from California with the sole purpose of availing myself of the great master's teachings and concept of homeopathic philosophy and materia medica. Through the acquaintance and friendship of Dr. J. E. Hoffman of Healdsburg and later of Santa Rosa, California, an admirer and post-graduate student of Kent's, I was familiar with his outstanding achievements and splendid teaching ability.

That I might be privileged to receive instruction from such a fountain of inspired knowledge I made great sacrifices to obtain it, a common occurrence in those days, for many others went through similar experiences for the purpose of better preparations for their chosen life work. If one decided to be a comforter and healer of the sick, the best preparation regardless of cost was not too much.

I was received formally but kindly by the good doctor and given instructions regarding the location of the college and the necessary arrangements I would have to make for my stay in Chicago.

As time went on and I progressed in my work, I was privileged to watch the doctor at his office occasionally and discuss homeopathic principles together with the necessary studies needed by good homeopathic prescribers.

By the time I reached my junior year, I had made such headway in materia medica, case taking, repertory study and philosophy that the doctor appointed me his quiz master, a place held during the rest of my college course. Kent's lectures were given to both juniors and seniors, and my quiz work was accepted in a rather unusual way, much to my gratification and surprise. At this time Dr. Kent was in failing health; he had taken a severe toll from his life energy in the building of the repertory, teaching and carrying on an exhaustive practice at the same time.

His quiz work and part of his lectures together with a large Saturday afternoon clinic in the Hahnemann College of Chicago were turned over to me to do the best I could with it, a real job and a supreme test for a junior student to undertake. The job was done to the satisfaction of Dr. Kent, the college faculty and the student body.

About this time my relations with Dr. Kent grew in great friendliness and mutual satisfaction and sympathy, and I frequently visited him and his gracious wife at their home. The Kents were charming hosts who

---

1. From handwritten manuscript, exact date unknown. - Editor..

lived without show or fanfare in comfortable and orderly surroundings, and those who were fortunate enough to be invited to their circles enjoyed a feast of knowledge and all the niceties of a refined social time.

They dearly loved to gather a few of those students who dedicated themselves to the cause of Homeopathy with all-out enthusiasm. At these gatherings Dr. Kent was at his best with interesting accounts of noticeable and unusual cures with the indicated remedy illustrating the cardinal symptoms that revealed the needed remedy.

After my graduation I continued to teach and lecture in college while starting to practice homeopathic medicine. My second year out, I occupied offices in the same suite with Dr. Kent. This closer association with the great doctor was most beneficial and enjoyable. How to study remedies in their relationship with human illness, to learn to observe the nature and pace of action of remedies and of diseased states and fit one to the other was a revelation that spelled successful prescribing over the many years of homeopathic practice. But my association and friendship with Dr. Kent gave me more than proficiency in the art of homeopathic prescribing; it introduced me to the writings and philosophy of Emanuel Swedenborg, which changed my views of life from that of a doubting agnostic to the more appealing aspects of hope and faith opening up vistas of beauty and use to better meet all the realities of life.

Dr. Kent revered the work and character of Hahnemann with almost a religious fervor. He had little patience with those who deviated from the law, regardless of pretext or excuse. With all his great knowledge and experience in medicine, and having been a practician in all the medical schools - allopathic ecclectic and homeopathic - he had little patience with those who were not sufficiently skilled in homeopathic knowledge and who fell back on allopathic methods to treat their patients when they were unable to find the needed homeopathic remedy. As physician, writer, teacher, and medical philosopher, Dr. Kent will always rank among the foremost. His wonderful repertory is increasingly more used by the homeopathic physicians to render their work of mercy more efficacious, and his treatise of Homeopathic Philosophy is the most potent force in the spread of homeopathic practice and healing ever given the world.

Hahnemann, Hering, and Kent are names synonymous with homeopathic healing. These names are inscribed on the scrolls of time among the benefactors of the race. When the names of the pseudoscientists of our time are lost and forgotten with the myths and the half truths they sponsored, Homeopathy and its votaries will grow and live in an ever expanding service to the world of suffering.

HAHNEMANN IN MEDICINE[1]

Homeopaths who are discouraged at the future prospects of homeopathic doctrines and philosophy need but glance back in the annals of medical history prior to Hahnemann's time, and compare conditions and the status of medical practice then with those of today to find real cause for encouragement for the future of Homeopathy and for medicine in general as well.

From the ignorance and superstition of ancient medicine to the nihilistic medical thought and technique of Osler was a wide gap, but nevertheless a constructive step forward and that step was largely based on the results obtained by homeopathic practice. Osler and his colleagues believed that the homeopathic remedies were equivalent to immaterial nothingness, and that many startling clinical results of brilliant cures of a wide and varied nature might be ascribed to mental suggestion and a good and careful regime of proper diet and good nursing.

Another startling fact is found in the modern treatment and cure of the insane. This is directly the result of Hahnemann's concept that these mental unfortunates were sick individuals and deserved treatment to fit their state. Kindness and more humane and normal surroundings and wherever possible some work to fit the needs of the patients were instituted in place of brutality, chains and dungeons.

Another interesting medical fact is that all case taking in our modern hospitals and clinics is patterned after the methods and technique evolved by Hahnemann.

Perhaps the most outstanding fact that must strike all thinkers both medical and non-medical, is the unchanging stability of the homeopathic doctrines in the face of the most bitter opposition of bigotry and prejudice together with the cupidity of commercialized individuals and groups that ever conspired to destroy a system or philosophy.

For one hundred and forty-five years of unremitting warfare, this benign system of cure has struggled and triumphed by the sheer power of its votaries to cure where other systems had failed. As evidenced by the aforementioned facts we become conscious of the mighty influence exerted by the mind of Hahnemann on the whole field of medical thought down through the years. Only now is modern medical thought colored and directed by the advance of the physicist catching up to grasp the clear vision of truth based on natural law given the world by the master mind of Samuel Hahnemann.

---

1. THE HOMEOPATHIC RECORDER, Vol. LVI, No. 6, June 1941, p. 287 ff.

HOMEOPATHY IN WORLD MEDICINE [1]

At the birth of Homeopathy the world of medicine was just emerging from the shadows and supersitions of the dark ages. The employment of seton and blistering poultices with blood letting and polypharmacy made up of drenching cathartics and sickening emetics, constituted much of the practice of medicine. Anti-sepsis, sanitation and dietetics were unknown. Psychiatry had not even been dreamed of, and the treatment of mental sickness was brutal and not only stupid but unthinkably reprehensive-chains, floggings and dungeons making up the principal instruments of treatments. As a consequence, epidemics of typhus, typhoid, small-pox, diphtheria, scarlet fever and cholera destroyed whole populations. There was no law or guide for systematic prescribing; only hair-brained theories regarding the causes of sickness and the remedies for the removal of the same.

Science and philosophy were only beginning to waken the mental world out of a long slumber. Two centuries before the advent of Homeopathy Sir Francis Bacon had written the wonderful "Organon of Human Reason" teaching men how to think logically and to a purpose. Shakespeare, Goethe, Byron, Shelley the vanguard of prophetic and liberty loving poets had fired the minds and stirred the hearts and souls of men for the struggle from physical bondage and mental shackles.

Sir Isaac Newton had announced the discovery of the law of gravitation and expounded the vision of earthbound denizens to an almost unlimited extent.

The science of chemistry started on a march of developement and accomplishment that was destined to change the whole structure of economic life in the social order of the race and to soon bring about the epoch-making progress in surgery by the discovery of safe anesthesia.

In the midst of all these perturbations and stirrings of the mental spheres, medicine remained a dead and useless mass of nonsense and ignorance until the inspired genius of Hahnemann with the power of inductive reasoning and a tireless energy battered down the age encrusted portals behind which reposed a mass of superstition and ignorance called medical knowledge. The advent of the *Organon of Homeopathic Medicine* was a ferment that stirred medical thought as it had not been stirred in centuries. The announcement of a discovered and proven law, the application of logical thinking in the collection and

---

1. JOURNAL OF THE AMERICAN INSTITUTE OF HOMEOPATHY, Vol. 38, No. 4, April 1945, p. 116.

evaluation of indubitable facts for the establishment of an expanding medical philosophy and a rational technique in the preparation and application of drugs for the relief and cure of disease was stupendous and world shaking and stunning[1].

Medical thought was slower to respond to the impulses of new and awakening knowledge and sciences than other lines of endeavors. Perhaps because then, as today, the selfish power of commercial interests dominated the progress of medicine and hindered any advance that might interfere with the profits of certain powerful individuals or corporate groups.

The pharmacists of that day were among the most bitter opponents of Homeopathy from its very inception. Hahnemann knew they could not be trusted to prepare the homeopathic potencies properly and drug substitution was as common then (as it is in our day providing the motive exits). Hence all homeopathic practicians were taught to prepare and dispense as well as prescribe the remedies they used. This opposition from vested interests against the new medical system was soon carried to the individual physicians really desirous of curing who were converted to the new medical technique. Ostracism, calumny, ridicule and even physical violence were practiced against Hahnemann and his disciples.[2] All social amenties and ethical behaviour were refused them. In spite of these things converts among the enlightened from various parts of the world successfully practiced the new art and science of medicine making brilliant cures where traditional medicine had failed. Soon after Homeopathy was established in most of the western world Dr. Edward Jenner (1749 - 1823) of England announced the discovery of vaccination: the use of cow-pox. This is a homeopathic principal but the method of preparation and administration is incompatible with homeopathic techniques and while immunity against small-pox may be procured it frequently comes at a tremendous cost in health along the lines of chronic disease which often develops into violent and fatal terminations. Clinical observers all over the world report numerous cases of serious chronic illness following small-pox inoculations. The homeopathic preparations of VACCINUM and VARIOLINUM administered by mouth show excellent prophylactic power against small-pox. Without

---

1. It seems that Hahnemann was greatly influenced by the Postulational (Scientific) Method of Sir Isaac Newton who taught that a theory only needs to be accepted as successful if by it we can repeatedly verify the experiments and predict new ones based on this theory. The theory (hypothesis) then becomes a law. - Editor.
2. This is still true today. - Editor.

any acute or chronic manifestation of consequential disease, only slight skin reactions being observed in some cases.

The next medical discovery was the claim of Louis Pasteur. He stated that by inoculations of an attenuated virus from a rabid animal immunity and cure may be produced against the frightful torments of rabies. But prior to Pasteur's claims, the homeopath, Constantine Hering of Philadelphia, had potenized and proved the saliva of the rabid dog (Lyss.) and successfully used the remedy in the treatment of hydrophobia. Pasteur's claims are interesting because of their similarity to homeopathic proceedure even to the attenuation of the virus although crudely accomplished through the blood of several animals as vehicles. Like vaccination it is homeopathic in principal but unhomeopathic in the technique of its preparation and administration.

Later still came the discovery of diphtheria antitoxin with which traditional medicine promised to entirely do away with the diphtheria disease. Here again the toxins of diphtheria are attenuated through the serum of the horse. The proceedure is said to build up anti-bodies against the disease in the body of the horse and this horse serum injected into the human blood furnishes it with the necessary antibodies to fight the disease. But homeopathic potencies of DIPHTERINUM have cured after heavy doses of antitoxins had failed to control the symptoms of the disease and the patient was sinking rapidly toward death. This experience has occured with many homeopathic physicians.

Coming down to more recent times, August Bier, an eminent German surgeon, in a paper read before a large assembly of German physicians asked "What would be their attitude toward Homeopathy?". Bier accepts all three cardinal rules of homeopathic technique; the similiar remedy, the single dose, and the minimum dose and explains the modus operandi of the Law of Similars and the single attenuated dose by what he calls the "Irritational Theory of Disease and it Cure". These conclusions were reached only after extensive clinical application of the law in a large number of difficult cases of diseases resulting in cure. And subsequent to Bier's announcement, McDonald of England had accepted the homeopathic law and technique of administration and was making excellent cures with homeopathic potencies up to the 30. His conclusions and explanation of the working of the homeopathic principal is based on his "Hydration" theory of disease. The above mentioned so called new advances and discoveries in world medicine are positive proof of the extraordinary influence Homeopathy has had on the thought processes of true investigators and truth seekers everywhere.

Further evidences of the homeopathic influence on medical procedure may be found in the almost entire rejection of polypharmacy. Prescriptions are simpler and many contain a single drug. Also there is a tendency to use smaller amounts and less drastic doses.

A new aspect of medicine today, that of the mind and emotions (psychiatry), is now claiming much attention from medical men. The power of thoughts and emotions on the state of health was first stressed in Hahnemann's Organon wherein he states that the mental and emotional symptoms stand highest and most important in the study of remedies for the cure of disease (§211 Organon). Great and constructive work is now being done *without the use of drugs* in restoring the normal mental and emotional balance in the mentally sick by a process of mental hygiene; how to think constructively for the good of the individual and society as a whole.

Hahnemann's influence in case taking and record keeping is everywhere manifest today. Every hospital staff and clinic all over the world follows the Hahnemannian methods of case taking. With this brief summary of historical facts before us we, the homeopaths, may well be heartened concering the future of the Homeopathic concept of disease and its cure.

It is interesting to note in passing the number of pioneer thinkers in the fields of science and philosophy contemporary with Hahnemann (1755 - 1843); Priestly (1733 - 1804), Sir Humphrey Davy (1778 - 1829), and Lavoisier (1743 - 1794) were leaders in the realm of modern chemistry. Goethe (1749 - 1830) Shelly (1793 - 1831) and Byron (1788 - 1824), fiery emissaries of liberty and democracy whose messages stirred nations to revolution and regeneration.

Sir Isaac Newton (1642 - 1727) the great mathematician and physicist opened the vistas of almost limitless horizons to our view. Emanuel Swedenborg (1688 - 1772) scientist, inventor and mystic left a tremendous imprint on the pattern of religious thought as well as able contributions to scientific knowledge.

It is very fitting that Samuel Hahnemann brought into being with such an array of mental giants, should be the instrument, armed with the magnificient mental equipment and flawless courage he had to redeem the ancient status of healing and carry it onward to the dignity of a true science, adorned by a perfect artistry to be used for the good of man everywhere on the earth.

Homeopathy's Place in Medicine[1]

The march of medical progress in the past fifty years has been one of disease prevention rather than cure. The ravages of yellow fever, malaria and typhoid have been greatly restricted, if not entirely overcome, by measures of hygiene and sanitation and mosquite control. Most likely the reduced frequency and virulence of diphteria, scarlet fever and small pox epidemics have been more controlled by the same means than by inoculations of serums and vaccines so universally used and often with deleterious side effects.

The success of preventive medicine has been almost exclusively in the realm of acute disease. Chronic heart and kidney disease, cancer, arthritis, and many forms of nervous and mental disease all have greatly increased during this same period. Even tuberculosis has been only slightly reduced in frequency and virulence.

The antibiotics, which seemed so promising for a time, soon loose their efficacy in acute disease and are worse than useless in chronic trouble because of their drastic side effects.

Because of these facts homeopathic therapeutics provide the best solution to the pressing medical problems today. First, because any curable condition, either acute or chronic, to which sick humanity is subject can be quickly and gently corrected with no consequential side effects by the homeopathic remedy. Second, because of the curative power residing in the similar remedy, the homeopathic system of treatment holds the key to the most efficient prophylactic and preventive medicine even devised by man.

When medical science learns the true nature of sickness, a great step forward in the progress of cure for all human ailments will be attained. Until the Hahnemannian concept of inherited constitutional toxemia is recognized and accepted by medical science as the fundamental cause of all disease, that science will continue to flounder in the quagmire of confusion and error while suffering humanity languishes for succor and relief. By its power to eradicate inherited evils the homeopathic remedy becomes a most potent factor in disease prevention. This is especially true in the chronic forms of disease such as cancer, arthritis, chronic heart and kidney disease about which so little in the way of cure has been accomplished.

---

1. The "President's Message", JOURNAL OF THE AMERICAN INSTITUTE OF HOMEOPATHY, Vol. 47, No. 1, January, 1954. Article with the same title, but different text see p. 519 ff.

More and more it becomes patent that the most certain cure for these things must be found in the field of prevention. Here in this field homeopathy does its most certain and efficient work. All chronic illness in the early stages and beginnings is amenable to cure by cleansing the organism of the causative inherited toxins thus permitting the life forces of the patient to restore the processes of repair.

Because of these time-proven facts, Homeopathy must be taught and practiced until the world can become aware of its power for good in the sorely needed realm of true healing.

So vital to a sick and suffering world in its need is this subject that it becomes a crusade exciting the interest and enlisting the aid of all who value health and well being.

HOMEOPATHY'S PLACE IN MEDICINE[1]

From its beginning, the homeopathic concept has exerted an appreciable and growing influence on medical thought. The single dose of the single remedy is now quite general in use, and the tendency to minute doses and even attenuated ones is coming more in vogue with the passing years. The alkaloids given in very small doses and the colloids of metals are expressions of the smaller doses frequently used in practice. The Law of Similars is also becoming more understood and accepted by doctors of high rank in the old school.

The science of physics with the release of power contained in an atom and the import of vibrations and frequencies no longer make it illogical or difficult to accept the action of high potencies in their role of restoring order in a deranged vital organism.

If things as infinitesimal as a virus, ultra-microscopic in size, can produce serious illness and even death in a susceptible subject, why cannot the infinitesimal homeopathic potency acting on the same plane as the virus, antidote or nullify the action of that virus and restore order in the sick organism? There is overwhelming clinical evidence that such is the case.

The relatively new science of genetics, especially its importance and relationship with hereditary disease, lucidly explains how the homeopathic potency by a mild form of mutation can change pathologic tendencies and processes to a state of normal activity, producing normal histological cell growth instead of abnormal pathologic cell growth.

What can better be conceived to act on those tiny microscopic groups of elements within the cells, the genes, those mystic carriers of heredity, than a homeopathic potency attuned to each individual's special needs? Human genetics is co-related with all other sciences dealing with human beings in health and in disease; hence sociologists, psychologists and physicians, especially that group known as the psychosomatic practitioners and the homeopathic physicians, are deeply interested in the proven conclusions of this new science. Physicians especially need the knowledge pertaining to the existence, nature and activity of the so-called "black genes".

These are the impelling factors of inherited pathologic development of cell growth ultimating in malformation of organs, parts and tissues

---

1. THE JOURNAL OF THE AMERICAN INSTITUTE OF HOMEOPATHY, Vol. 49, No. 5, May 1956, p. 103. Article with same title but different text see p. 517 ff..

in the physical body with an impaired and abnormal function. Blemishes, morbid growths and certain types of cancer are the direct results of these genes; as are brain and nerve degeneration of certain types, producing blindness, paralysis, and idiocy, convulsions and epileptic states. Allergies, diabetes due to pancreatic defect, high blood pressure, arterial hardening, malignant types of cancer of the eye and brain in children, bleeding disease, hemiplegia, defective blood clotting together with abnormal mental states, schizophrenia, various forms of adolescent insanity, mania depressions, etc. are all due to the presence and activity of these "black genes of doom".

Every competent prescriber of the homeopathic art has seen many of these inherited conditions frequently entirely cured or greatly modified and changed in intensity by the homeopathic remedy in potentized form. That no other branch of healing can cope with these things is the chief reason for the perpetuation of Homeopathy in its Hahnemannian purity.

That is why this truly scientific aspect of medical science will soon be recognized and accepted as one of the important adjuncts of general medicine, where its teachings and philosophy and wide clinical uses can be available to all who are unable to get relief for their chronic ailments which cannot be helped with routine methods of prescribing.

With a knowledge and understanding of homeopathic principles and techniques, the researchers of medicine will be able to solve many of the unsolved problems of medicine existing today.

Strange as it may seem to many physicians and laymen alike, Homeopathy has already developed remedies that cure and prevent the polio disease. Thousands of subjects have been immunized against the infection in many epidemics that have occurred during the past forty years.

Why has the public not been informed of this boon to suffering humanity? Because organized medicine, controlled by an inner circle of officials, has been able to establish a working agreement with the associated press to keep all medical knowledge, not censored and vouched for by this inner circle of the American Medical Association, from the American public.

Perhaps the vast and selfish interests of the manufacturing chemists and pharmaceutical firms play an important role in suppressing any information concerning valuable curative agents that might hinder the sales of their routine products extensively and extravagantly advertised for commercial reasons only.

Witness the frequency of one wonder drug after another and numerous antibiotics in constant succession with multitudes of pain-suppressing coal tar drugs advertised by way of newspapers, magazines, radio and television, telling us how to use them without a doctor's advice so that we may be free of pain and able to sleep even with a guilty conscience. Humanity is drugged and poisoned from the cradle to the grave.

How can there be health, happiness or efficiency in thinking or working under such hateful influences? It is not strange that we have so many accidents in industry and travel when minds and senses are dulled with these things. When will medical men wake up to these dangers and evils and sound the alarm against the use of these pernicious agents and help bring on a saner, healthier better social order? With the homeopathic healing system predominating, there would be no need or use for the many depressing and suppressing type of drugs which dull the intellect and lower the moral and physical tone of the whole being.

This is an appeal of reason to the practitioners of every type of medicine to investigate without preconceived prejudice the claims of superior healing through Homeopathy by reading carefully Hahnemann's Organon of medicine. In it, the message of healing balm was given the world over a century and a half ago. Today science is now verifying these truths announced so long ago by that inspired and untiring genius who lived and labored for the good of all mankind.

The time is near at hand when the name of Hahnemann shall be known and revered throughout the world as one of the great benefactors of the race, bringing it a law-directed system of healing - effective yet gentle - that shall do much to advance the happiness and well being of humanity everywhere.

OUR GRATITUDE AND OUR OBLIGATION[1]

How many homeopathic physicians ever stop and try to realize how much successful prescribing depends on the purity and verity of our homeopathic remedies and on the accuracy and painstaking care given in their preparation and manufacture; of what avail the genius and the infinite laborious study, that good prescribers put into their selective work in search of the similimum if the drug selected be adulterated or in any way defective to its proven standards. And our incomparable Materia Medica and repertories produced by so much sacrifice and effort would be worthless junk.

Since the inception of homeopathic science our pharmacists have rendered the profession loyal and outstanding service in their accuracy and care in the preparation of homeopathic remedies, and often with little profit to themselves beyond the satisfaction of doing their job right. Without this loyalty and reliability on the part of our pharmacist the whole super-structure of homeopathic science with its inimitable philosophy would pass away.

Into this picture our friends are harassed between the forces of necessity and loyalty at times. In supplying the physician exclusively at the reasonable, almost generous price asked does not bring much profit for the necessary precise and care-taking work involved. On the other hand a lay clientele would render much greater profit of the work, because of a great increase in sales.

Every physician knows that lay prescribing, especially with the higher potencies may produce more harm and chaos in sick cases than a complete neglect of drug application leaving natural forces to do the healing (free of drug symptoms).

In recent years the reduced number of homeopathic physicians has made it imperative for patients preferring homeopathic prescribing to call on physicians residing at a distance from their home for help. By phone or letter the patient's symptoms are relayed, sometimes with a diagnosis from a local physician and the remedy needed is learned. These patients have availed themselves of a full working set of homeopathic remedies for such specific purpose, never prescribing for themselves or their family without the advice of their chosen doctor. This method provides one item for increased profit to the pharmacist.

---

1. "President's Message" in JOURNAL OF THE AMERICAN INSTITUT OF HOMEOPATHY, exact vol. and p. no. unknown. - Editor..

Another way to help all concerned: Every physician could advise each of his patients to acquire a number of homeopathic remedies in low potencies to meet accidental emergencies such as burns, bruises, sprains, etc., together with those remedies useful in colds and the numerous acute epidemic diseases.[1] These remedies given with their special classical indications will prove helpful in cure, and will prevent the use of harmful proprietory drugging and numerous topical agents of doubtful value and even some of them being inimical to health.

A closer bond and understanding of our physicians and their pharmacists should be formed that the mutual interests of all can be furthered and obtained for the common good of both the profession and the whole homeopathic public.

This brief message to the homeopathic profession is given in the hope that definite action for a constructive program pertaining to this subject may be inaugurated at our coming convention of the American Institute of Homeopathy with the International Hahnemannian Association next July 18, at Makinac. We have many more vital projects to consider at this meeting that mean a great deal to the welfare and growth of Homeopathy in America and because of these vital things we hereby urge every homeopathic physician in our land to attend this great meeting to give their aid in the advancement of an expanding and useful Homeopathy.

---

1. Many homeopathic practitioners today have readily available kits for their patiens. - Editor.

Homeopathy's Future [1]

With the almost certain passage of legislation imposing some form of state or federal medical control over the nation, the practicians of Homeopathy and their numerous patients are faced with the prospect of oblivion and consequent serious loss. There is no protective constitutional edict in behalf of medical liberty as exists in the case of religious freedom.

Therefore, the advocates of medical freedom, of which there is a majority of such if we include the non-medical cults together with many liberal old-school practicians, can all work together to have incorporated into the proposed medical act a restrictive clause protecting the practicians of all methods of healing and insuring them and their patients the privilege of practicing their special forms and acts of healing without interruptions from any source. Indeed, there is urgent need of a constitutional amendment guaranteeing the same sacred rights in the field of medicine and medical practice as exists in favor of religious freedom.

But until such time as a constitutional amendment for the protection of medical freedom and equality can be obtained, there is need for organization and unity among all advocates of medical freedom in order to obtain the right to practice the art of healing of each group in accordance with its education and training and its belief founded on such training and education. Without some specific clause in the body of a nationalized medical act, the homeopathic physician will not be permitted to practice his art; and his patients will be deprived of the specialized medical service that only a trained homeopath can give. Also, many individual physicians of the regular school will be compelled to practice their arts contrary to their better judgment appertaining to a medical practice that is controlled and dictated by a routine standard of practice.

For a state or federal control of medical practice must be reduced to a more or less cut and dried routine denying the individual practicing physician the valuable use of long clinical experience and individual initiative. Such an organization as is contemplated by the advocates of federalized medical control will be purely political in its scope and aim, and as such will be carried on along the lines of the political spoils sys-

---

1. "Editorial" in The Homeopathic Recorder, Vol. LXI, No. 1, July, 1945, p. 29.

tem where graft and special privileges will hamper the smooth and efficient operations of good medical service.

The world of medicine has always been and still is in a constant state of flux and change built on the uncertain foundation of empiricism. That which is good today is soon discarded for something newer and better. This process is never ending, so that the judgment and conscience of the individual experienced physician are safer and sounder things to depend on for real help to the sick than the cold routine edicts of a medico-political clique far from the sick room or its patients.

Organized Homeopathy in conjunction with other organizations and individuals who desire medical freedom and equality can obtain the needed clause in any proposed medical legislation to safe guard the rights of all organizations and individuals.

Unless such organization is put to work to bring before the Congress the facts just mentioned, every medical practician will be only a paid servant taking orders concerning treatment of the sick regardless of whether or not his judgment and conscience approve or endorse the same. The physician will be helpless to appeal to any higher court for correction of mistakes or wrong conclusions or prescriptions he might be forced to make by the routine of a medico-political set up.

There are other things the homeopathic organizations can do with profit. First, we must take steps to strengthen and protect our pharmacists; without their splendid work in our behalf, our cause would suffer almost certain annihilation.

Secondly, each individual homeopathic physician should seek out and train some younger medical graduate or graduates to succeed him in his practice. In that way we will be assured of no further decrease in our numbers, and we could leave young blood to carry on with the cause until such time as the law of Similiars shall be recognized and accepted as an essential part of medicine to be taught to every medical student in all recognized medical institutions.

That the time is near for such recognition at least through the re-discovery of the law by another Hahnemann or scientist is highly probable, because already, many leaders in medical thought are experimenting with the claims of the homeopathic law.

The Need of Public Education in Homeopathic Accomplishment[1]

The world needs a wider and more intimate knowledge of the inherent powers of disease prevention and cure residing in homeopathic principles of medicine. Homeopathy is the medicine of the future, only waiting the time, when through education by way of efficient wide spread publicity, the medical facts of a superior system of healing will make the world cognizant of its value and use in the great field of medicine.

All who have experienced the benign force of the working law applying the potentized remedy need no further proof of its worth. But those unacquainted with the principles and the facts must be reached and taught. To do this requires organization and effort. One of the means to this end may be found in Homeopathic Laymen's Leagues: one of which should be organized in every large city of the nation and in fact wherever a dozen or more homeopathic patrons can meet together to plan and evolve ways and means to instruct the public in the homeopathic concepts of sickness, its cause and its cure. Not only is the cure surer, but it is gentler and safer and really quicker, and with this time saved, and lessened expense or cost involved, a great economic factor in sickness prevails, thus adding to its value and desirability. We have such leagues in Boston, New York, and Chicago now. I hope we may soon have a dozen more, especially from our larger centers such as Cleveland, San Francisco, Los Angeles, Philadelphia, and Seattle.

Along with public education in Homeopathy, the Leagues may build up funds from small donations to give scholarships to worthy medical students indoctrinated with homeopathic tenets to help educate them, thus giving the world more homeopathic doctors to help fill the great need now with us. When we behold the vast sums extracted from the public for research for various disease conditions, such as heart, polio, T.B., cerebral palsy, etc., we are appalled because much of these sums are spent on the personnel of the several organizations requiring high salaries that must come out of the collected funds to perpetuate and maintain these organizations as permanent institutions; when these costs are met not much is left for research which is often tedious and the expected results in cure are frequently disappointing. Homeopathic

---

1. President's Address, JOURNAL OF THE AMERICAN INSTITUTE OF HOMEOPATHY, Vol. 47, No. 4, April 1954.

research is cheaper to maintain and much more effective in terms of cure, because it works from established definite laws and principles, whereas traditional forms of research proceed on the basis of trial and error, and error is costly and disappointing in results obtained. Hence, another function for the united leagues in the future would be that of homeopathic research.

Homeopaths, we must maintain and strengthen our local, state, and national organizations: support and keep up our homeopathic journals and publications and start an intelligent crusade of homeopathic education for a long suffering public needing homeopathic care. In presenting our crusade for superior healing so much needed for the ills of the world, we will not fail to recognize all that is good in the progress of modern medicine and surgery. Many of these newer things are indispensable and we are grateful to have them available for the use of all.

Our chief aim is to have Homeopathy recognized as an important component part of general medicine that can be available to the healers of all schools of medical thought. With this object obtained medical rivalries will cease and the world of suffering will benefit under a less prejudiced and more enlightened medical realm. Out of the bitterness of the past with its antagonizing clash of medical claims and thought will come enlightenment and progress with more tolerance and charity from all sides.

Men of vision in all the schools today are waiting for, and seeking the better things offered everywhere today. Then let us proceed on our way, tolerant and open minded that we may be aware of and respond to the subtler but more potent forces energizing the cosmos. The good book tells us "to seek and we shall find, to knock and the door shall be opened to us".

We homeopaths have sought medical truth for the past one hundred and fifty years and found it. We have knocked at the door, behind which is the reservoir of universal knowledge, and lo, in response to that knock the door opened to reveal the genius of Hahnemann holding in his hands the boon of homeopathic healing for a sick and ailing world. We are told by the same Divine source that "The Truth" shall make us free: and surely, Homeopathic truth when universally accepted will free the world of much of its sickness, its sin, and its misery.

ORGANIZATION AND PUBLIC INSTRUCTION FOR HOMEOPATHY NEEDED[1]

When the congress of states was abolished by the American Institute of Homeopathy a grievous mistake was made. The Institute lost contact with it local adherents everywhere over the country, and they in turn lost interest in a national organization that functioned largely for the edification of a few office holders mostly intent upon perpetuating their tenure in office. Result: our state societies dwindled and passed away leaving weeds and desert waste where once bloomed homeopathic gardens of beauty and use.

And those who had employed homeopathic doctors were gradually compelled to employ other types of curative agents, as the homeopathic forces grew weak. With no replacements from homeopathic ranks there had to be replacements by unhomeopathic methods of cure.

Our most feasible and efficacious medium for public instruction of homeopathic principles is to be had in our Homeopathic Layman's Leagues which the Institute should aid and encourage at every homeopathic center in the country be it large or small. It would be helpful if the Institute appointed a special board to aid in the organization and perpetuation of the various leagues throughout the country. In this way the institute would be brought back in touch with the local and scattered elements of Homeopathy, and its forces would be unified and consolidated for all its efforts in education, for both the laity and members of the healing art everywhere.

Such a consolidation of homeopathic forces staffed by enthusiastic homeopathic leaders would soon bring about astonishing results in the way of growth and public recognition because of the opportunity given to show the world what miracles of cure Homeopathy has for the sick and afflicted.

There are those who think it useless to try to restore homeopathy in the U.S. to its golden era of success that prevailed 1900 - 1920. They are appalled at the oppostion that has developed against us; such as the powerful corporations of drug manufacturers whose interest in the sick is soley commercial; their take from the afflicted ones of the nation

---

1. President's Address, No. 12, in JOURNAL OF THE AMERICAN INSTITUTE OF HOMEOPATHY, exact vol. and p. no. unknown. - Editor.

amounts to many billions annually. But the insatiable greed of these agencies will end in their downfall and rebound to our advantage.

Because the cost of medical care including hospital service is fast becoming prohibitive for the average citizen of our land, Homeopathy gives a more certain and durable type of treatment success at prices within the reach of all while permitting satisfactory remuneration to its physcians as well. We need only intelligence and courage to meet the exigencies of our time by perfecting our organizations and expanding our quota of homeopathic physcians. We still have many places calling for them.

Everywhere outside of the U. S. Homeopathy is growing and thriving; Mexico and Brazil are notable examples. In Europe and India it is recognized and employed extensively. In Buenos Aires, Argentina there is a growing group of very high grade homeopathic physcians that are a credit and an asset to their country and the world. Because of these facts this is a psychological period for us to put forth our best efforts to build an expanding Homeopathy that can serve the needs of our nation effectively and economically

In closing I must ask pardon for putting into verse my sentiments concerning Homeopathy's past and future.

Weep not for the fight that is lost

Refuse to weaken or to yield

Honor's glorious strategic field

Though high and grievious be the cost

In the strife for the cause of truth

Deathless Godess of potent youth

By that sign and by that token

We shall rise again, strong and brave

And see Similia's banners wave

O'er our ranks firm and unbroken

With the healing power in our hands

For the suffering ones of all lands.

NEEDS OF HOMEOPATHY[1]

Mr. Chairman, Friends and Colleagues of the American Institute, I am most grateful for the privilege of addressing you concerning the needs of Homeopathy today and for the future.

Homeopathy's greatest need is more homeopathic physicians to meet the increasing calls from everywhere for homeopathic doctors. To supply this want, we must increase and expand our educational facilities by both correspondence and post-graduate courses. We should contact those men who are competent and worthy practitioners of all schools of healing and acquaint them with the superior results obtained by homeopathic methods of healing which is free of all injurious side effects. In many states of the Union, nonmedical groups are qualifying to practice medicine and surgery. It is among these we will find our most sympathetic prospects for homeopathic physicians. At little cost the Institute could help place new doctors at advantageous and desirable locations for practice. By such means we could soon expand the membership and influence of the Institute for a more effective, organized Homeopathy.

We need permanent committees made up of energetic and enthusiastic men to reorganize our state societies and examining boards. We should have Laymen's Leagues in every city and town in our country; the publicity and true understanding of homeopathic concepts and principles coming this way would be more valuable and effective than thousands of dollars of paid publicity could bring us.

We need close co-operation and understanding with our homeopathic pharmacists that our mutual interests may be strengthened for our common good.

There is a growing segment of medical practice today whose tenets are based on the homeopathic concept of disease cause, viz. the psychosomatic branch of medicine who attach the greatest importance to mental and emotional disturbances and symptoms. From Hahnemann to all the present masters of the homeopathic art, the mental and emotional symptoms have taken first rank as guides in the selection of the curative remedy.

Homeopathic literature is teeming with a great many brilliant cures of even the most serious types of mental incompetency. And our school of medical thought was the first to recognize the truth of these

1. From handwritten manuscript, exact date unknown. - Editor..

modern observations that mental and emotional stresses are causative factors in most of the chronic illness afflicting the race today. Since the homeopathic remedy is the most potent force known to remove the weakness that makes one a victim of worry, fear, frustration, inhibitions, etc., it would be all together fitting and proper to bring these facts to the medical profession and to the world of sick folks as well that all might greatly benefit by this knowledge.

Medical statistics inform us that from sixty to seventy-five percent of sickness has its origin in psychosomatic influences. Because of such facts, the homeopathic profession is better equipped to cope with these types of illness than other branches of medicine; and it should organize its physicians for still further development and advance of this progressive branch of medicine by forming a permanent bureau in the Institute devoted to the study of these various and numerous symptoms and their relation to disease and its cure.

The establishment of such a bureau would sharpen our physicians and render their work more successful in cure; and it would attract the progressive minds from all schools of medical thought, bringing prestige and an expansion of a splendid type of membership to Homeopathy. A bureau of such a nature could soon be developed into a virtual post-graduate course of psychosomatic medicine with the homeopathic approach in treatment, thereby assuring the greatest possible success in terms of cure never before obtainable by the routine methods of the past and present.

Today we live in an unstable world of flux and change politically, economically, and scientifically. As new truths unfold concerning the nature of matter, new concepts and theories regarding life evolve. The whole field of medical thought is in the throes of vast and rapid change. New drugs of great power have been manufactured and exploited, but much of the good accomplished by them has been offset by dangerous side effects that make their continued use prohibitive.

Man is something more than a mass of chemicals; and he lives on other planes with and beyond the physical, though his physical body is nourished from the contents of the earth. His emotional and spiritual bodies are nurtured by forces flowing from the higher planes of existence. Born into the world naked and helpless, a whining, crawling animal, nevertheless by painful and devious ways he finds and follows the spiral stairway leading to the stars and to the abode of the creative center of universal order to bring back to earth the wonders of inventive science and the far-reaching knowledge of the all-embracing gift of mathematics. Also from the same source come all the imagery and beauty of poetry, art and music to stimulate the intellect and delight the soul.

There is in nature and in man an etheric bond or plane wherein the physical and higher and more subtle bodies and forces of our being meet, intermingle and coalesce. In this bond all changes from health to sickness and from sickness back to health take place before any change, chemical or physiologic, is manifest in the tissues of the physical body. That is why the homeopathic potency is such a powerful agent in the process of cure. Its subtle nature is very similiar to vibratory formation of the etheric plane into which it is readily attracted and associated.

The advance of modern physics has done much to explain why the homeopathic potency acts so actively and effectively. The process of all life activity is vibratory. In fact, all the physical phenomena in nature such as light, electricity, magnetism, etc. are the results of certain specific vibratory rates.

The biological scientist has uncovered some interesting facts that explain why homeopathic medicines alone are capable of curing constitutional and inherited disease. That minute group of microscopic cells and atoms forming the genes which carry through time and eternity the specific traits of character and body formation from generation to generation of each species, races and individuals can best be affected by a mild form of mutation, wrought by the administration of the homeopathic potency, thus nullifying the subtle toxin of inherited disease and leaving healthy cells to perform their allotted functions unhampered and imparting to the growing organism a normal physiologic activity. Where normal physiologic process exists, health and normal histologic cell growth result.

In the light of these facts just cited, the homeopathic concept of sickness, its cause and cure is clearly seen and understood. We homeopaths understand and appreciate these things, but the world does not, and it becomes our duty and mission to bring it to the world by every means at hand that we may lessen human suffering and help install a healthier race for the future.

Organized Homeopathy is duty bound to protect its patrons from the evils of poisoned water supplies and foods processed and adulterated with injurious chemicals and preservatives. Even the life-sustaining air we breathe is poisoned and made toxic by death-dealing sprays designed to kill insects, but these activities destroy the balance of nature and defeat the purpose for which they are used while doing great harm to the health of whole communities.

Hahnemann tells us we must know the causes of sickness and remove them as the first step toward health. When these causes are removed, we place man in a better environment wherein the constitutional remedy can accomplish much more in terms of health.

The homeopathic physician is not only a healer but a teacher as well. His patients are taught to avoid the foods and the drugs that are inimical to helath and that interfere with the action of the homeopathic remedy, and they are taught mental and moral as well as physical hygiene. Thus equipped, these patients make unusual and lasting recoveries from illness and build up a powerful resistance to sickness of every kind.

As the importance and value of homeopathic medicine are so great and so much needed in the world today, it becomes the duty of each and every one of us, both doctor and patient, to exert all the means we can muster to advance this worthy cause that our children and their children may obtain the God-sent blessing of homeopathic medication.

With faith, courage, intelligent co-operation and organized effort, we can create a greater Homeopathy than we have ever known and give the general field of medicine a heritage of medical knowledge of countless value. Indeed, organized Homeopathy must go on with the fight until general medicine progresses sufficiently to recognize the great advantages of a truly scientific therapy and accepts it as a part of the great field of medicine.

Homeopathy has the equipment in the law and a well-proven philosophy backed by a literature of wide magnitude and inestimable value. Also the great *Materia Medica* and numerous excellent text books on homeopathic practice together with the time-saving, accuracy-producing repertories all constitute an array of accurate knowledge built up by the genius and unremitting toil of many sacrificing men.

With so many glorious traditions of the past before us and with the magnificent attainments of the great pioneers in Homeopathy that amaze and gladden us, we are inspired to carry on and add our mite of useful knowledge and sacrificial effort for the preservation and advancement of the homeopathic cause. We know this cause is just and benign and sorely needed for the good of God's children, and because of this knowledge our faith is strengthened and our courage is enhanced to meet the needs of these trouble-packed times.

Friends and colleagues, ours is a great privilege. To be a homeopathic healer brings us closer to Divine goodness and power than many others can come, but it also brings us obligations and responsibilities we cannot evade. Then let us stand united and true to our principles and ideals that the cause we love and labor for may go on and abide forever.

Homeopathy's Needs[1]

Friends and colleagues of the American Institute of Homeopathy, it is a great privilege to greet you and to thank you for the high honor you have conferred upon me by permitting me to serve as your president for the coming year. But with this honor goes a heavy responsibility that no one man can carry to success unless he has the sustaining power of the complete membership behind him. Because I realize my own limitations and inadequacy for this important work I am here calling on you all for your help, advice and suggestions for the good of Homeopathy and the Institute.

The Institute is the medium for protection, perpetuation and growth of Homeopathy. It is the representative and the expression of organized Homeopathy in the United States. It is the soul of homeopathic thought and action. Let us keep that soul clean and untarnished that it may function unafraid and strong for the promulgation and defense of homeopathic principles.

There are a few who think our efforts and even our sacrifices are in vain and of little use, but the struggle for the cause of truth is never devoid of use, because there are kindred souls to follow us who will take hold where we had to leave off our unfinished work. All progress in the sciences and the arts are painfully and slowly built up and perfected not by one individual or in one era but by a succession of workers through succeeding periods of time. Each era and each individual worker add their mite of new knowledge and improved skill until the work is completed as a unity of beauty and worth. This work of man is paralleled in nature by the activities of the small sea mites that build through labor and the sacrifice of their lives that vast and wide spread deposits of beautiful coral rising from the ocean floor.

In spite of dwindling numbers and diminishing prestige, there are many vital reasons why Homeopathy and the Institute should continue to live and perform its destined function for the good of all humanity.

We hear much about the progress of medicine these days - one analgesic or pain-killer after another until the number is legion, innumerable shots of drastic blood-polluting specifics, vast numbers of nerve-destroying sleep producers and "goof" pills. Small wonder the world is fast going insane with countless preparation of synthetic vitamins and

---

1. Inaugural Address, A.I.H. Banquet, July 1, 1953. JOURNAL OF THE AMERICAN INSTITUTE OF HOMEOPATHY, Vol. 46, No. 8, August, 1953, p. 238.

so-called tonics and successive crops of "wonder drugs", many of them as malignant in their action as blood destroyers. Terramycin and Chloromycin are examples. The wonder indeed is that any humans are left alive.

The array of health and life destroyers is perpetuated by the insatiable greed of huge commercial interests, the manufacturing chemists and pharmaceutical companies, whose revenue and "take" from the American public runs well into the billions of dollars annually, comparable to what it takes to run our most extravagant government of the United States. Indeed, if all the harmful rubbish in the way of empirical medicine could be discarded and replaced by homeopathic medication not only would the health of all be greatly improved, with cancer, kidney and heart disease vanishing as if by magic, but our vast national debt could at the same time be liquidated by the savings resulting from universal homeopathic treatment.

This is not all together a homeopathic view of the medical situation; a few conscientious doctors of the dominant school have from time to time issued warnings concerning the dangers accruing from the injudicious use of the drugs aforementioned.

Both from health and economic reasons, homeopathic organizations must be maintained until the law of Similia is recognized and taught as part of the curriculum of medicine, a possibility not too remote because science is already proving and accepting portions of the homeopathic concept concerning matter, energy and life.

Even a progressive branch of old school medicine, psychosomatics, is rediscovering some of the cardinal tenets of homeopathic philosophy. Because of these facts one of the urgent duties of the Institute is to find a repository where the writings and essays of the inspired leaders of the past and present may be kept and preserved for the needs of the future. The Institute, working closely with the American Foundation of Homeopathy, must preserve this precious heritage of accumulated knowledge and at the same time develop and maintain post-graduate schools for graduate physicians who become interested in a system of healing based on law. In this way we can justify the need for our existence.

There is much more that can be said and has been said on this important subject by men who preceded me, wiser and more gifted in essential knowledge; why weary you with repetitions. You know as well as I do our needs and goals we seek, not for ourselves alone but for our children and all the future.

Organized Homeopathy is obligated to the public as one of its reasons for existing in its role of teacher and protector of health. In this day of political graft and commercial greed there is a frequent attempt at universal medication by way of public drinking water through the process of fluoridation and chlorination. These experiments are paid for by the tax payers, whether they want it or not, and they must suffer the side effects of poisoning from the prolonged and accumulated action (provings) of these things as well. Those wishing such medications could use these chemicals in their individual drinking water cheaply and with little effort; why poison a whole community for the satisfaction of a few egotists who wish to force their ideas on a suffering public and compel them to pay the bills as well.

Homeopathy must take its stand for the freedom of the individual prescriber that he may always remain untrammeled by any political or scientific group, leaving only the individuals doctor's conscience and intelligence as his guide for the good of his patient. Only by such procedures can real progress be maintained. These are but a few of the cardinal features that seem important for consideration and interest at this time.

But, more important than the things just mentioned, is the imperative need for unity of action among and between all homeopathic organizations in the United States. The Institute, the International, the Southern, and the American Foundation, through their respective representatives, should be welded into a solid unity to give us the solidarity and power needed in the attainment of our goal, viz. the establishment of homeopathic teachings, in their completeness and purity, by precept and scientific proof, into the curriculum of every medical school where men and women are taught to equip themselves to become healers of the sick. And this desired end can be sooner accomplished if every individual homeopath in this great land of ours, physicians and their patients in unison, dedicate a little of themselves in the way of time, effort, and a little of their savings, salvaged from non-essentials in the form of luxuries such as the curtailment of their tobacco and cocktails, together with less bridge, golf and other form of amusement that make up the lesser extravagances of modern life. The proceeds from this source could well furnish us with the sinews of war for our crusade. Such a procedure could hardly be called sacrifice; it would merely fall into the category of little vices eliminated, for which we all would be richer and better physically and spiritually.

In closing, again I plead for help and support from you, all my friends, that I may serve you and our cause faithfully and well. Let us invoke Divine Providence with prayers for strength and wisdom to perform the duties we meet, with justice to all and with charity in our hearts for those who do not share our views.

WORLD'S NEED FOR HOMEOPATHY[1]

Not only the world of men but the world of medicine needs Homeopathy. In spite of the many claims for the progressive achievements of modern medicine, the fact remains that outside of surgery and sanitation, therapeutic medicine is far from satisfactory. The drastic side effects of the antibiotics and the numerous coal tar drugs make these agents more potent for evil results than for good results, while so-called scientific medicine stands baffled and bewildered, impotent to remedy the wrong of their efforts to heal.

A large amount of medical research of recent times has emerged from the laboratories of the large pharmaceutical houses and manufacturers of patented drugs, whose first and most vital concern is entirely commercial. Billions of dollars are made annually from the sale of these various nostrums in the United States. These same institutions are the purveyors of all medical knowledge that is given the American public in overwhelming doses by way of radio, television, newspapers and magazine publications. Highly paid writers and salesmen are employed through these agencies to hypnotize an unthinking, medically ignorant and unsuspecting public with false claims and half truths concerning the efficacious use and value of these baneful products. The doctors of the medical profession itself have been ensnared in an insidious way to help further the commercial ends of these same selfish agencies. By distributing free samples and specially prepared literature, clothed in scientific language, to the doctors to use in experimentation on their patients, they obtain the tacit recognition of their products from these doctors who are too lazy to think for themselves and who find it profitable and easy to dispense these unscientific products.

Every true physician, regardless of what school of medicine he graduated from, must resent the intrusion of any individual or agency that attempts to dictate the methods or remedies he should give his patients, either individually or in groups. He alone is responsible for their welfare and safety, and he is so held by the state that licensed him to practice. For that reason alone he is permitted and expected to select his remedies and treatment in accordance with the dictates of his best judgment and knowledge regardless of the opinions or desires of outside influence.

---

1. From handwritten manuscript, written in 1956. - Editor..

From the foregoing statements it is easy to see how the powerful manufacturers and dispensers of proprietary drugs dominate and control organized medicine with their legal and educational activities, even perverting its highly publicized code of ethics to suit their trade requirements, ruthlessly unmindful of the universal harm perpetrated on a defenseless humanity while they pile up billions of dollars from their nefarious traffic in misery and disease.

Since the wide and extensive use of the coal tar drugs and the numerous antibiotics, cancer and malignant types of blood disease, severe forms of heart disease and drastic states of mental incompetency have all increased to alarming proportions. Competent highgrade medical observers of both the regular and the homeopathic schools of medicine have issued warnings of the dangers concerning these practices, but the propaganda coming from the wholesale drug manufacturers and vendors grows ever louder and more incessant and drowns out the notes of sage advice from men who really know the harmful consequence resulting from the wide-spread dispensation of these harmful products. Those men are true physicians who have the courage to present the true picture of these dangers that are undermining the health and well being of humanity everywhere in the world today.

Hahnemann stated that one of the most important duties of the physician was to find and remove disease cause wherever he meets it. Logic teaches us that disease cannot be cured without removing the cause, and these products we have mentioned are at best palliative and act only for a short time. Their continued use produces dreadful side effects resulting in artificially created diseases that are often difficult to cope with. Because of these facts, the world of men and the world of medicine desperately need the understanding and the application of the Homeopathic Philosophy and practice of medicine to redeem a serious situation in a sick world which is treated by an inadequate and unscientific system of medicine based on strict empiricism without a guiding therapeutic law.

Every physician knows that the blood chemistry of every individual is peculiar to himself alone and differs from that of every other human being; hence the necessity for a remedy suited to each individual rather than a remedy for a disease by name.

The essence of Homeopathy is "one single remedy for each individual patient" discovered by the *Law of Similia*: "Likes are cured by likes". In a crude way general medicine has applied this law since the times of Jenner and Pasteur, but their technique lacked the fine precision and refined adjustment of Hahnemann in potentizing and diluting toxic material in distilled water and dilute alcohol instead of using the blood of animals with all of its unknown qualities for that purpose.

Hahnemann's technique obtained maximum results in cure without the consequential side effects resulting from the allergic action of the crude and insufficiently refined vaccines and serums which contain many unknown inimical qualities peculiar to the animal blood.

Another factor which we have lost sight of is the violation of the physiologic law of injecting directly into the blood stream a foreign protein substance which can and generally does set up a violent reaction throughout the whole body organism, at times terminating fatally.

The selected remedy given by mouth cannot produce such violent effects; the reactions are only sufficient to stimulate the defensive mechanism into activity for the protection of the organism, and in this process the cure of the sick disturbed organism is accomplished gently, quickly and surely and with no morbid product remaining in the bloodstream. There are no side effects or end results, only the normal physiologic processes left to function in a healthy, harmoniously working body organism.

Progressive medical men everywhere are stressing the advantages that can be gained from the application of preventive medicine. If we prevent the possibility of disease, no cure will be needed. Dietary science, hygiene and sanitation are generally recognized methods for successful disease prevention, and these methods are good and successful to the extent that they are applicable. With these methods acute epidemics of disease have vanished, and many lives have been saved. But there are states of chronic sickness in the human race that these methods cannot eradicate.

The mass of piled up inherited toxins stemming down the generations of men are activated and increased by the abuse of drugs, alcohol and tobacco, food and water impurities, polluted air, etc. Only the homeopathic remedy, scientifically administered and permitted to act uninterruptedly over a space of several years, is adequate to cope with these confirmed evils culminating in all kinds of chronic sickness. Hence, Homeopathic Science becomes the most potent weapon in the prevention of all human sickness yet known to man. It is the guided missile that can destroy man's most ancient and implacable foe, chronic disease, which no other system of healing even attempts to oppose; all their efforts are exhausted in attempts to palliate the sufferings and cripplings that are the fruits of chronic sickness.

The science of genetics provides us with the proof of the power of Homeopathy to cure in so-called incurable cases. Cases of certain types of cancer transmitted from generation to generation have been dissipated and cured with the homeopathic remedy, thus breaking the fateful chain of inevitability by a mild process of mutation in the cause-producing genes of the individual sufferer.

It is well known that genes can only be affected and their inherited nature changed by a process of mutation which only happens in nature under the influence of some form of radiation, x-ray, radium, cosmic ray, etc. Changes produced this way tend to produce abnormal growths and deformities. But the mutation that takes place under the impulse of the homeopathic potency is the restoration of normal function and cell growth.

Up until recent years much ridicule from many sources has been hurled against the smallness of the dose of homeopathic remedies. But those who have kept in touch with the modern advance of the science of physics can be reassured of the power and efficacy of homeopathic potencies. In fact, this science gives the answer why and how these instrumentalities of energy can produce the miracles of cure that they do. Physics tells us that matter and energy can produce the miracles of cure that they do. Physics tells us that matter and energy are interchangeable. The power released by the atom, the minutest division of matter known, is a startling witness of the potency of infinitesimals in nature.

Medical men can better appreciate the power of the infinitesimals in the study of viruses, those ultra microscopic organisms that carry disease and death so far and wide and that are immune to the action of the wonder drugs. Hence regular medicine is deprived of its most highly publicized weapon of cure for acute infectious disease, the worst forms of which are virus produced.

The homeopathic potency is all sufficient to cope with and neutralize the malignant action of viruses because it meets them on the same plane of infinitesmal energy, and both are similiar in nature and form. Similiar energies opposed dissipate each other throughout all nature.

When we review the many advantages that homeopathic medicine can bring to the world in the establishment of a safer and surer treatment of disease as well as the greatest known preventative of sickness ever given to man, it is natural to believe that the science of homeopathic medicine should be a special branch of general medicine to be taught in every medical college in the world so that better health at a greatly reduced expense might prevail. If the people of the United States were all treated exclusively by Homeopathy, medical costs would be reduced by at least one hundred billion dollars annually, more than enough to run the United States Government for a year. Then the overburdened taxpayer could hope for a substantial relief from tax confiscation and ruin.

Better health, happier lives and greatly reduced medical costs are the certain results to come when the public becomes cognizant of the preceeding array of medical facts and insists on having a truly scientific system of medical service for its needs. Only when every qualified practician of the healing art has availed himself of the doctrines promulgated by the great Hahnemann and has a working knowledge of the philosophy and art of homeopathic prescribing will medicine become truly scientific and be accompanied with an artistry transcending that of the musician, the poet, the sculptor and the painter. Then will the sordid stains of selfish commercialism be erased from the shield of Hippocratic purity and worth. Then loving service will be the driving force of action to be rewarded by a maximum of cure. Then again the Hippocratic Oath will be the guiding force of the dedicated physician on his untiring rounds of healing mercy.

The physician of the future armed with this new and perfected system of healing will be superbly equipped to meet the ravaging onslaught of all forms of disease. His success in the restoration of the sick back to perfect health will bring him fame and wealth. Better yet for him will be a satisfaction and a joy that will flow in and mellow his life with a richness beyond the dreams of avarice. The gratitude and love of hundreds of restored human beings brings a reward more precious than glittering gold and scintillating jewels.

And what about us, the followers and votaries of Hahnemann, Hering and Kent, that trio of magnificent homeopathic teachers and physicians who gave the world so much of their lives to advance the health of all mankind? For us remains the privilege and the duty to bring the homeopathic gospel of the healing art to all mankind that the race may be cleansed of the inherited ills through future generations of men and that they may be freed of suffering and sickness and live in the light of a refined knowledge that will enable them to grow spiritually as well as mentally and physically. Thus the Law of Similars in unison with all other laws of nature under Divine Providence will achieve the ideals and blessings of a healthier and happier humanity.

HOMEOPATHY VERSUS ALLOPATHY[1]

Among the greatest mass of the laity the impression prevails that there is little, if any, difference in methods of treatment between the Old and New schools of medicine. Every real homeopath resents that idea as false and misleading. In order to better understand the homeopathic concept of disease, its nature and cure, it is well to first glance back over the history of medicine past and present and then make comparisons.

From time immemorial traditional medicine, or allopathy, has been the medicine of empiricism and its dogma has been that of materialism. Its concept of disease cause has always been based on a material entity, something falling within the range of the five senses. Such a concept must necessarily need crude remedies to meet those preconceived material conditions. And there being no basic law for the prescribing of their crude drugs, a system of empiricism or experimentation came into vogue.

From the time of the Dark ages when loathsome concoctions of the excretion of animals and other obnoxious ingredients were prescribed for the sick to the present so-called scientific era, prescribing the by-products of filth and disease, in the form of serums and vaccines, allopathic medicine presents the same crude clumsy, ignorant and superstitious methods of approach to its sick victims. They prate loudly and blatantly of being scientific and progressive, but are they? "By their works shall ye know them." They have failed to keep pace with the advance of the great science of physics. The marvels of the vibratory states of matter mean nothing to them. The realm of the electron and protron might as well have remained hidden from their view because of their inability and their stubborn refusal to apply this wonderous new knowledge to the needs of the sick. The steady progress of the physicist leaves the allopathic concepts of life, of health and of disease submerged in error and darkness from whence they sprung.

---

1. From handwritten manuscript, exact date unknown. ALLOPATHY: Term coined by Hahnemann Organon §22 Footnote 12; in this form of treatment medicines are given whose symptoms have no direct pathological relationship to the morbid state, neither similar, nor opposite, but quite heterogeneous to the symptoms of the disease. Hahnmeann distinguishes allopathic from antipathic enantiopathic or palliative method i.e. giving medicines with opposite symptoms §23. Today Allopathy encompasses both this original definition of allopathic and the antipathic, enantiopathic or palliative method - i.e. improper methods. - Editor..

If we review some of the so-called achievements of the allopathic medicine we are reminded of a marriner in a storm tossed sea, without compass or rudder to guide or control his course, drifting, a hapless victim of time and circumstance. In its fight against the great white plague where millions of dollars were raised and spent, we find that the little success there attained was not due to and medical discovery or advance but in the abandonment of everything medicinal and in reverting back to natural methods of rest, open air, sunshine and change of climate, an eloquent confession of the weakness and harmful effects of its medicinal weapons against the ravages of disease. In its battle against diabetes when the world was electrified by the announcement of the discovery of a specific drug - insulin for the cure of this so-called incurable malady we see an instance of false statements based on false concepts of disease cause. Insulin never has nor can it cure diabetes, because it effects only the end results of disease, and ignores the cause; deranged vital force. Of what avail to render the blood of the diabetic sugar free and permit the disease cause to go unchecked in the economy of the patient. The disappointment and increased suffering of millions bear witness to the false doctrine of insulin as a cure for diabetes listed by allopathic propagandists as the outstanding medical achievement of the ages.

And allopathy's futile efforts against the steady increase of cancer, of heart and kidney disease, ought to be sufficient evidence of the falsity of its doctrines and concepts of life and health. The loping away by surgery or destructive burning by radium and x-ray radiations of cancerous growths has but added misery to unbearable suffering and is further proof of allopathic inefficiency and ignorance. The introduction and use in the allopathic pharmacopeia of the numerous coal tar drug derivatives for the suppression of pain of all description regardless of the cause, and for the effects of insomnia, constitutes the most potent factor in the increase of heart and kidney disease in the world today; yet no voice among the boastful scientists of allopathy is raised in protest or warning against this unscientific and deadly procedure. More alarming still is the increase of insanity and other mental and nervous diseases, many of them direct results of allopathic treatment for some preceeding physical ailment.

Allopathy builds its materia medica on knowledge obtained from experimentation on animals and on the toxic manifestation of drugs in poison cases. It not only experiments on dumb animals where no mental or moral manifestations can be observed or noted, but on sick human beings racked by disease. Hence only the destructive action of drugs on the physical plane are noted or recorded. Allopathy reasons only in the realm of effects because causes do not operate on the physical plane, and that plane is the only one known to allopathic philosophy. Allopathy is blind to causes which only operate on the higher planes of being. Mental and moral re-actions are ignored while the physical effects of such re-actions, the pathological ultimates alone constitute the guides of her intervention in the realms of disease.

Now we will present the cardinal features of the homeopathic concepts of life, of health and disease. Homeopathy perceives man as a tri-unal being dwelling in the three planes or realms of the cosmos, namely, physical, mental and spiritual. Man is subject to, and affected by his environment on all these planes. When a state of health obtains, he vibrates in harmony with the cosmos as a whole, when disease is present his rate of vibration is disturbed. If this disturbance goes unchecked over too long a period changes take place in the man's tissues and normal histology is replaced by pathology which is accompanied with misfunction of organs and will end in death of the organism if order be not restored. Homeopathy reasons from cause to effect, from first to last, from beginnings to endings, from the spirit like in dwelling life force operating down through mental processes into the ultimate of the physical body. Homeopathy perceives that no disease changes can take place in the tissues of the body without a prior causative change of vibration in the dominating life force existing in that body.

The remedies employed by Homeopathy are proven on healthy human beings and their effects are noted throughout all the planes of man's existence. That is, the changes of state of his moral and mental re-actions as well as changes in his physical body are observed and recorded in the Homeopathic Materia Medica. When these proven remedies are applied to the sick their effects as exibited in signs and symptoms must correspond to the symptoms and conditions of sickness ascertained in the anamnesis of the patient. Thus, the proving of the individual remedy manifested in symptoms produced on healthy provers must present a likeness to the symptoms and states of sickness of the individual case to be treated. The fitting of any individual case of disease to the symptoms of any proven drug constitutes the application of the homeopathic law of cure known as the law of similiars. "Similia Similibus Curantur."

Homeopathy prepares its remedies in such a way that only the weakened diseased cells are stimulated to re-action and without in any way affecting the healthy cells of the organism that are not involved. The delicate attenuated potencies of a drug adjusted by the homeopathic law renders it in selected affinity to the sick cells of the organism, its action is sufficient to change the vibratory rate of these affected cells to the normal rate of the body organism thereby restoring a state of health and leaving no residue or consequential drug effects behind. When drugs are given in crude form not only are the sick cells overwhelmed but the weakened sick organism often finds it too difficult to resist or metabolize these drugs.

Homeopathy studies the pace and direction of symptoms in the processes of natural diseases as well as in the artificial disease set up by provings on the healthy. It also notes the destructive action of crude drugs taken over a period of time, and how the mental and moral breakdown of the man is accompanied by alarming physical changes of the body organism. Homeopathy teaches the art of changing this destructive action of drugs to a curative beneficient activity of restoration and healing under the (truly divine) law of Similiars together with its accompanying art of drug potentization.

Homeopathy has no specific drug to meet all cases suffering from a given disease but it cures individuals suffering from asthma, psoriasis, eczema, malaria, syphilis, epilepsy, diabetes, tuberculosis and even cancer. These disease conditions are mentioned because allopathic authorities have pronounced them all incurable.

In the field of acute diseases Homeopathy has scored innumerable triumphs in comparison to results obtained by allopathic methods as a few comparative statistics will show.

FLU-PNEUMONIA:

Allopathic losses 10 to 40%

Homeopathic 1 to 5%

DIPHTHERIA:

Allopathic losses 12 to 13%

Homeopathic 1 to 5%

INFANTILE PARALYSIS:

Allopathic 10 to 25%

Homeopathic 1%

Crippling cases as high as 75% under allopathic treatment, less than 5% under homeopathic treatment. With these facts before us we have every reason to insist on equal opportunities and rights to practice our art without hinderence or restriction by our rivals in power.

To summarize briefly we find Homeopathy experiments, conducts its provings on the healthy and such knowledge so obtained gives us the true likeness of the power residing in drugs to change man's state either from health to disease or from disease to health depending on the manner in which they are applied. Allopathy experiments on the sick by prescribing empirically and varying the prescription with the whim of each individual prescriber and using doses only short of toxicological. And its provings are conducted on dumb animals which are poisoned to death in order to study the tissue changes in their organs. Homeopathy cures disease by the application of a fixed law with drugs prepared to operate on cells too delicate to stand the shock of crude drugs. Allopathy suppresses disease manifestations on the surface of the body which endanger the internal and more vital centers. Homeopathy treats patients whose sicknesses are expressed in the totality of symptoms and change in the moral, mental and physical functions of the body organisms. Allopathy treats diseases whenever it can name such; many times they find it extremely difficult to label the illness of their patients, (concerning which see, Cabot on the discrepencies of diagnosis before and after post mortems). Homeopathy *cures*. Allopathy *palliates* and *suppresses*. Allopathy concerns itself only with the changes wrought in the material body ignoring (when prescribing) the higher manifestations of life, and its drugs are given in crude form empirically varying with the whim of each prescriber. Homeopathy concerns itself not only in the changes of the body and its organs, but it heeds the moral and mental changes wrought by disease and remedied by medicine properly prepared and selected in accordance with a fixed law of nature.

Is it not time for Homeopathy to announce these facts to along suffering and abused humanity? Is it not our duty to tell the world of the better way of healing? True science already confirms our claims in every detail. Why are we loathing to imitate our rivals in the one respect of spearding propaganda when the world needs our knowledge and its application so urgently?

ADVANTAGES OF HOMEOPATHIC PRESCRIBING[1]

Why homeopathic medicine is superior to other methods of treating is known by the proof established through one hundred and fifty years of practice in many lands by numerous physicians. Homeopathy is broad enough in its scope to include and cure all the diseases known both acute and chronic.

Some of the outstanding advantages of homeopathic treatment are first its certain, yet gentle action leaving no consequential side effects after the cure is made. Second; the factor of economy is a vital one in this age of constantly increasing living costs. So valuable and powerful is this medical phase that if homeopathic medicine was universally recognized and accepted by the American public our vast public debt could be liquidated in twenty-five years [2] with an infinitely improved state of public health resulting.

The American public pays from fifty to seventy-five billion dollars annually[3] to manufacturing drug concerns for the almost soulless nostrums and chemical poisons that deluge our land to undermine physical and mental health. Our insane asylums are filled beyond their capacity, and much of the increased crime and lawlessness is due to ill health induced by drugging-not all narcotic. For the numerous variety of coal tar drugs are equally dangerous to mental competency even though they are more insidious in their effects.

Homeopathic doctors have long warned against these dangers and for the most part were laughed at and ridiculed by our friends of the old school. Now at last after incalculable harm has come upon the sick, some of our friends of the old school, are seeing the light from a frightening conflagration of medical horrors resulting from the over use of penicillin and other wonder drugs.

Published in THE CHICAGO AMERICAN dated April 11, 1954 are excerpts from papers read before the International Academy of Proctology, two doctors warned against the new diseases for which there are no remedies created by the over use of penicillin and other wonder drugs. Dr. Jacob Reichert of Phoenix, Arizona spoke of the increased death rate due to fungus disorders which often occurs when intestinal bacteria are abolished by prolonged treatment with the antibiotics.[4] He said:

---

1. From handwritten manuscript, exact date unknown. - Editor..
2. probably in less time. - Editor.
3. In 1994 the figure is closer to 400 billion dollars. - Editor.

"We may create a new era with new diseases[1] which will be monstrous in character, and future generations will be afflicted with new pathological problem created by the antibiotic age. Ordinarily the bacteria and fungi normally present in the intestines, hold each other in check but when the bacteria are killed off, the stage is set for the fungi to flourish" he explained. "The fungus known as monilia (Candida albicans) has proved particularly troublesome. It causes ulceration[2] of the intestine and may spread to other parts of the body to cause multiple abcesses." "Thousands of such cases have already occurred", he said, "but doctors have been reluctant to report them. Consequently medical men are learning about them only through word of mouth or hard experience." Dr. Donald C. Collins of Hollywood, California called attention to the development, during the past year, of new and alarmingly severe diarrheas[3] caused by strains of bacteria that withstand antibiotic treatment. He added: "These disorders resulting from previous indiscriminate dosing with various antibiotic drugs are becoming more and more fatal. Too many doctors are prescribing such remedies indiscriminately" he said, and went on, "This must be stopped before we are confronted with very dangerous and epidemic diseases of the colon for which there is little or no treatment." Both men declared the threat lies in the abuse, rather than the use of the wonder drugs. Dr. Reichert said that they have saved many lives but urged that they be used only under strict medical supervision. He urged doctors to be alert for the warning signals of the new diseases which may be preceded by nausea, vomiting, diarrhea and itching around the opening of the bowel. He also advised that physicians warn patients asking for penicillin for a cold of the dangers they run into, saying: "If he does not, the outraged patient

---

4. The large increase of chronic fungal disease today is mostly secondary to various antibiotics, corticosteroid preparations and other anti-inflammatory drugs - Editor.

1. §74, 75 Organon: Among chronic diseases we must still, alas! reckon those so commonly met with, artificially produced in allopathic treatment by the prolonged use of violent heroic medicines in large and increasing doses where by the vital energy is, weakened to an unmerciful extent, sometimes, if it do not succumb, gradually abnormally deranged etc.
    These inroads of human health effected by the allopathic non-healing art are of all chronic diseases the most deplorable, the most incurable and I regret to add that it is apparently impossible to discover or to hit upon any remedies for their cure when they have reached any considerable height. Samuel Hahnmeann. - Editor.

2. This increased use of antibiotics may be an explanation for the increased frequency of Crohn's disease and ulcerative colitis. - Editor.

3. NIT-AC. in potency (say the 200th) is a wonderful remedy for diarrheas after abuse of penicillin. This was first suggested by Elizabeth Wright Hubbard, M.D. one of our ablest homeopathic prescribers. - Editor.

may blame the doctor for having caused more discomfort than the original ailment, particularly when he ends up having to pay up to $1,000. (One thousand) or more in laboratory and doctor bills to get rid of the new disease."

These warnings to the public are commendable for it takes courage to tell of such dangers after all the propaganda pumped into the people concerning the miraculous action of the so-called wonder drugs in the past few years. Fortunately, homeopathic patrons may be consoled with the knowledge that their medical system has effective antidotes to cope with the evils feared by the servants of the old school. Within the portals of the vast Homeopathic Materia Medica we have remedies to meet every type of illness be it new or old. The homeopathic physician guided by the unfailing law of cure has no fear of new or little known diseases, because his knowledge is the shield that is impervious to the deadly darts of fear which spread panic in the hearts of those healers not equipped with the law and the philosophy of Homeopathy.

Another advantage that must commend the homeopathic system to every intelligent and thinking person is the inherent power of disease prevention it brings. This is especially true regarding all the chronic forms of disease which in the early or incipient stages is strikingly amenable to the homeopathic remedy. When under homeopathic care, the growing developing child escapes many of the serious ills and weaknesses that come by way of inheritance.

The accumulated taints of succeeding generations will only yield to the skilled application of the homeopathic potency, because the vibrating energy of such force alone can be attuned to that mysterious subtle and infinitely tiny group of molecules that make up the genes, those containers of the immortal traits and characteristics of individuals and races of men, animals, and plants. This picture of related facts presents a view of the beauty and unity prevailing throughout all animated nature.

It is not hard to conceive a vastly superior race of beings born and reared under three generations of homeopathic care. And because of these logical possibilities, so much needed in a world of stress and strain, it becomes a duty with those of us having this knowledge to spread the true doctrine of health for the individual and the race. Homeopathy replaces chaos with harmony, selfishness with service, and hate with love to bring forth a new order in the societies of men.

One more important advantage to the sick, only to be had in homeopathic medication, is that of palliation and comfort for those chronic incurables who have delayed too long before availing themselves of the proper treatment to effect a cure. Namely, those whose vital organs have been too greatly damaged by the prolonged action of disease, leaving the end results of disease (pathology) dominate, to impair vital function and inhibit repair in the organism. Such unfortunates are found among the victims of the painful and deforming forms of arthritis and neuritis, where pain killing drugs relieve but a short time, if at all, and their side effects are often more deadly than the disease for which they were given. Late stages of tubercular disease finds its greatest comfort in Homeopathy. Chronic forms of asthma that have been made incurable by drastic drugging can still find relief and comfort in Homeopathy. Cancer in its many forms with its awful nightmare of horrible suffering finds its most comforting friend in the homeopathic remedy.

The homeopathic physician called to treat chronic incurables,[1] most of them great sufferers, is given a heavy burden of responsibility. To be successful he must be equipped with wide and deep homeopathic knowledge that comes with much experience and constant prolonged assiduous study of the Materia Medica and the Philosophy. He must have understanding and sympathy that will spur him on with his best efforts under trying and discouraging circumstances. Above all he must have a courage born of faith in the goodness of God and all His Divine attributes including homeopathic healing. With these essential facilities he is qualified to be a veritable angel of mercy in a world of suffering.

With these rambling remarks I have tried to show you how vital and needed the homeopathic concept of healing is to the world today and for all the future. And because of that need, those of us who are aware of it, must unite our efforts and thoughts to the end, that we may devise means and ways to spread the doctrine of homeopathic truth for the good of mankind everywhere.

In the formation and development of numerous Laymen's Leagues we can evolve a mighty force for the promulgation of homeopathic knowledge which can result in homeopathic research and education for young doctors becoming interested in superior forms of healing. Many leagues when in touch and communication by co-ordinating their efforts in various ways will soon see an expanding Homeopathy in our midst.

---

1.   See article "Homeopathic Palliation in Incurables" p. 492 ff. - Editor.

Another important function of the leagues would be one of direct contact with the American Institute of Homeopathy, the parent central homeopathic organization in the U. S. That contact of the Institute and its local homeopathic organizations was lost when the Congress of States was abolished by the Institute, a most unfortunate step as local organizations and interests rapidly dissolved, cutting off growth of the Institute itself and leaving local physicians without the support or encouragement of a strong central organization. This was one of the contributing factors in homeopathic decline in recent years.

By far the greatest single factor in homeopathic decline was the loss of our colleges brought about by permitting the Old School to grade our colleges according to standards set up by them that only they could meet. Their rule was that only those medical colleges which were sufficiently endowed to pay full time professors to teach could be graded class A. Only one homeopathic college could qualify to meeting this requirement. Soon after this the state board of examiners in most states refused to permit medical graduates of class B colleges to take state board examinations for their license to practice. In this way homeopathic graduates were much restricted, and in a few years the older homeopaths in practice began to die off and there were no homeopathic doctors to replace them. Thus in the last 45 years Homeopathy has been slowly killed off at its source of supply; new and succeeding crops of young doctors to replace the departed elders.

This is a gloomy picture that now confronts us. But we, the organized homeopathic doctors of the last forty-five years are alone to blame for our present status. We have been too busy with our own individual affairs to unite our efforts along lines of endeavor that would have brought young recruits to fill our places when we no longer could carry on. When we know the causes of our misfortune and if we have faith in the righteousness and need of our cause, we need only the will directed by intelligence to rebuild our lost prestige and fortune. The pioneers of American Homeopathy began to build with but a very few men and the splendid work of the genius and unremitting toil stands out as a glorious memorial of unparalleled achievement. Their provings and writing and clinical victories against bitter opposition has left us a heritage of priceless worth to meet all ours and the future's every need. Let us not be unworthy of such a heritage built up with so much toil and sacrifice, but let us carry on united, determined, faithful and strong to emulate our worthy predecessors and leave those who follow us a fitting supplement of useful works of stored up knowledge.

WHY HOMEOPATHY?[1]

This question may be asked by those whose medical knowledge is acquired from the annals of the paid advertisements of newspapers and magazines and from the ads pushing the countless varities of antibiotics, so-called wonder drugs, pain killers, tranquilizers and mood-producing drugs which are exhibited by way of television and radio and calculated to do a most complete job of mass brain washing - all in the interest of a consciousless commercialism whose half truths and extravagant claims of cure are groundless and too often harmful to the extreme degree.

Have we not penicillin and other powerful antibiotics to wipe out pneumonia and other severe infections? Have we not specific vaccines to eradicate acute epidemic diseases? These are questions commonly asked today. Furthermore, we have numerous patented painkilling drugs to suppress every cry of pain that human flesh is heir to; and for the victims of insomnia we have a multitude of sleep-producing drugs which are guaranteed to make one sleep like a wooden Indian and wake up as refreshed as one ready for the day's work as efficient as a trained zombie obeying his master's voice. All this is the epitome of medical science as given the world today, and what a terrible price is paid for its marvels.

Then there are the mood-producing drugs advertised to give the unsophisticated victims any type of emotion or train of thought that they wish to experience. If you are depressed and sad, there is a capsule or a pill to cheer you up from the depth of gloom to the sunlight of optimism and good cheer. If you are hysterically jubilant or hilarious, they have for a price a depressant that can banish the cloudless sky of joy and hope with the chilly fog of despair.

All this does not exhaust the possibilities of modern medical science with its wonders to perform which are made known to us by a most attractive and highly priced advertisement appearing in our daily papers, current magazines and medical journals. All this is reinforced and substantiated by radio and television advertisements which are couched in semi-scientific language to give dignity and prestige, not necessarily true, for the claims made.

If you are aging too fast and your sex powers are lagging, modern medicine will help you, providing you can pay the price. If your hus-

---

1. From handwritten manuscript, exact date unknown. - Editor..

band is cross and dissatisfied and no longer interested in the warm attentions of his affectionate wife, but is prone to stray away to strange abodes, be sure modern medicine has a remedy. Or if the wife becomes cold and listless and unresponsive to the arduous attentions of her mate, yes - you guessed it - modern medicine will not let her down without giving her a panacea for her ills.

There is only one catch to modern medical science: after you have passed through all the clinics, taken all the tests of blood and body secretions, had all your organs and body parts inspected and probed, finally paid all the costs for this extensive scientific research, the happy announcement of your cure has been made, and you are sent back to work and home, you suddenly realize you need a long period of rest and special antidotal treatment to recover from the effects of your cure; for you have acquired in the course of the medical experience a serious and uncomfortable, if not a crippling drug disease as a memento of what modern medicine can do under the drive of a heartless commercialism which now dominates every phase of human society.

Many of you may think this a harsh and unfair arrangement of modern medicine, especially when you call to mind the great sacrifice and devotion of the doctor in his work, long hours, broken rest, unceasing study to keep abreast of the times, foregoing all pleasure and recreation, the dedication of his very life to the high calling of healer of the sick. This pretty picture of human virtue belongs to the earlier eras of medicine when it was indeed a dedicated calling guided by reverence and a wisdom which grew from such reverence and sacrificial devotion to the work at hand. It is because medicine has fallen from such sublime heights from the days of Hippocrates to the level of a degraded and selfish commercialism that afflicts us today that these observations are made.

Medicine must clean its own Augean stable before it can regain its lost glories and virtues. It must consider more the plight of the patient and less the urgent call of the dollar sign. It must subordinate selfish desire to the needs of true service. It must trust more in Divine guidance and place less faith in the wonders of modern science whose rainbow promises of accomplishment too often turn to ashen poison on the lips. Above all else, it must maintain an open mind to the logical truths of new concepts, principles and laws pertaining to human sickness and medicine.

Now to get back to the question "Why Homeopathy?". If we are impressed with the claims of modern medicine and accept them for their face value without question or analysis, we might well ask the same question.

If we glance through the endless array of medical vital statistics, we are appalled at the monumental increase of cancer, blood and bone disease, together with the frightful increase in mental diseases, all chronic and incurable.[1] It is even more appalling to realize that all this increase has occurred during the discovery and use of these great advances of modern medicine in the last two decades. All this makes us wonder what is wrong with the claims of modern medical science and why it has failed to stem the ever-increasing flood of human misery and sickness in the world. Yes, modern medicine has wiped out many acute and self-limiting diseases; it has stilled the cry of pain and quieted many forms of nervous tension by depressing the natural body powers of knowing or feeling. Often one realizes that the so-called cures of modern medicine are but the suppressions of symptoms to leave the patient worse than he was before he began the treatment.

One of the many reasons why Homeopathy is far superior to modern medicine in terms of cure is because the cause of the sickness is removed with all the symptoms of the patient and all the vital processes of the organisms are harmonized and strengthened to perform the manifold processes of life.

It also cures without leaving hazardous side effects. No unfortunate drug addicts are ever made by homeopathic treatment. Perhaps the greatest asset coming from homeopathic treatment lies in the field of disease prevention.

Those who have been treated consistently for five or more years with Homeopathy rarely develop cancer or other crippling chronic diseases.

When we weigh the meager successes of modern medicine (aside from surgery) against its dismal failures to cure and prevent chronic disease, especially malignancies, it should not be difficult to seek and accept new concepts and new proven knowledge for the healing of the world's ills.

For nearly two hundred years Homeopathy has met and successfully cured thousands of cases of sickness, both acute and chronic, in every climate and country of the world. Homeopathy's clientele is made up of people from all walks of life and many of the world's most intellectual people are numbered among its most ardent beneficiaries and supporters. A system of medicine that cures and leaves behind no deleterious

---

1.   §74, 75 Organon. cf. article "Advantages of Homeopathic Prescribing" p. 549 ff. - Editor.

side effects or enslaved drug addicts as a result of its treatment must be preferred by all intelligent persons everywhere.

Homeopathy with its very first tenet "The first and sole duty of the physician is to heal the sick"[1] might well be the spark to kindle and relight the fires of a new medical progress brought with deeper human sympathy and understanding of the needs of an afflicted humanity. Homeopathic concepts of sickness and healing, alone, can redeem modern medicine from the pitfalls of egotism and irrational thinking, driven by a selfish end, pityless commercialism engrossed in its own ends. Homeopathy can bring back with increased luster, past glories and crown the future with new and great achievements in the cure and prevention of disease.

While thousands of sufferers languish without hope for the cure of their ills, there will be great need for the gentle but effective power of Homeopathy.

Last and most important, Homeopathy can restore to the world its lost faith in medical science.

---

1. Hahnemann, S.: ORGANON, Article 1. - Editor.

The Status and Importance of World Homeopathy[1]

In spite of the intense propaganda of powerful drug interest against it, Homeopathy is expanding in recognition and acceptance everywhere in the world; especially among those capable of independent thinking who cannot be swayed by the extravagant claims made from the numerous so-called wonder drugs, pain killers, and nerve sedatives whose side effects are reducing the nation to a state of universal ill-health and incompetancy.

In Europe, England, France, Germany, Spain, and even Italy, Homeopathy is growing in recognition and popularity. In India, Homeopathy is wide spread, and a number of the Indian Homeopathic leaders are raising the standards of their physicians, and teaching and practicing in their Hahnemannian purity the principles and techniques of homeopathic medical science. In Mexico, Brazil and Argentina Homeopathy is gaining rapidly in prestige and power, and their schools, both graduate and post-graduate, (the latter in Argentina) are continually developing a constant new supply of good homeopathic physicians. Buenos Aires alone has four hundred practicing homeopathic physicians.

Only in the United States are we lagging and declining since our schools are gone and we no longer can replenish our ranks thinned by the death of our aging members.

Unless we replace these vacancies of declining age, the homeopathic institutions of the Unites States, built up with so much toil and sacrifice by so many inspired lives will fade away and perish from the earth. And the boon of homeopathic healing will not be available to our children's needs.

There will no longer be adequate antidotes against the dreadful abuses of unrestrained misguided drugging stimulated by the powerful soulless drug manufacturers and vendors of drastic soul destroying poisons put out in the guise of remedies. This propaganda with its extravagant and false claims goes on continually by way of television, radio, and the printed page to hypnotize the American public into a passive state of acceptance of this universal menace to the well being of our nation, because these habit-forming, pain and tension-alleviating drugs, falsely called harmless, are more deadly than bombs. Owing to their certain insidious actions on the human mind and body, they spell cer-

---

1.   From handwritten manuscript, exact date unknown. - Editor..

tain utter destruction with no hope of escape once the victim becomes enthralled in their illusive mesh. Only long tedious homeopathic treatment can restore them to a normal state of health, and ignorance of the homeopathic medicine prevents them from receiving this boon.

Allopathic medicine represented by the American Medical Association issues no note of warning against this deadly menace. A few brave and public-minded individual old-school physicians have warned against these dangers in papers read before medical conventions. Only the homeopathic profession as a body has placed itself on record against these evils and only homeopathic medication has the best antidotes against them.

Another very vital factor involving the health and welfare of millions of the citizens of Chicago and its suburbs is the question of pure water. The taxpayers of Chicago have paid out millions of dollars for the filtration plants that they might have pure clean water for drinking and cooking. Recently, a few men in places of public trust and power have, in the face of protest from representative groups of Chicago citizens and denying them the right to a referendum vote on the subject, arbitrarily begun to poison the city's water supply with the drastic health-destroying element of fluorine. In the establishment of this high-handed act of villany the precious rights of free choice of the citizens of Chicago have been abridged and nullified. Universal medication in this act is established against the will of many, if not the majority.

How easily and justly and economically this issue could have been settled with injury to none and justice to all, had the aldermen of our city voted to administer, free of charge, to those who wished flourides sufficient for their use. Then the danger of excess could have been avoided. The amounts needed for the individual could have been guided and regulated by his physician, and the more serious consequences of continuous dosing averted; and cost of buying fluorides for that part of the public wishing it would be insignificant compared to the cost of millions involved in establishing and maintaining the process of fluoridation.

Four years ago in a convention at Lookout Mountain, Tennessee, the American Institute of Homeopathy went on record against fluoridation because of its health-destroying effects.

The American Medical Association has taken no stand against the universal poisoning of the American public. Every text book on toxicology and medicine in existence attests to the toxic nature of fluorine, and thousands of industrial victims, opposed to this poison confirm these findings.

From the foregoing picture of things, it is apparent that the need for homeopathic physicians and practice is vitally needed for the welfare of the present and future. Our need is more homeopathic physicians; we could place five hundred in the Chicago area alone. But how to get them is the question. There is only one source of supply open to us. The non-medical groups of healers are all sympathetic to homeopathic principles and ideals. The osteopaths, chiropractors and physical therapy groups now can qualify to practice medicine and surgery, and it will not be long before almost all of the states will permit them to qualify for licenses to practice medicine.

These are the groups we should be sending our literature and inducements to for a better acquaintance with Homeopathy and its truly great assets to cure thus bringing fuller satisfaction for all true disciples of the healing art and conferring on humankind the great boon of homeopathic medical science for their unfailing needs.

HOMEOPATHY AND THE WORLD CRISIS[1]

Regardless of how or when the war ends, no one can be the victor, and the whole world will be the looser. The social, economic and monetary systems everywhere will undergo vast and undreamed of changes. Trade and commercial intercourse between nations will become chaotic and obliterated before a new and better order of reciprocity and universal justice will be established.

During this coming revolutionary turmoil Homeopathy may well play a most necessary and constructive role in the creation of the future new order. Economy will be the most essential watchword and force, individually and collectively, in every phase and department of government and human effort during the evolution and creation of this new and better state soon to be born into the world. The cost of war in blood and treasure together with the loss of spiritual values to the race makes it absolutely prohibitive as a means of settling disputes between the nations unless the world insists on committing universal suicide. Brute force driven on by selfishness and hatred and the lust to rule must perish and pass, as the power of justice and reason is re-instated to fashion a state built in the solid foundations of fraternity, integrity and justice.

Homeopathy spells economy and efficiency to the highest degree, even under our present disordered and antagonistic social order. Nothing in medicine has ever equaled its power in the cure of disease, and epidemic disease follows inevitably in the wake of war and famine, co-instruments of the grim reaper "Death". In the flood of mounting costs, Homeopathy will prove an undreamed of boon in medical economy, reducing medical costs a thousand-fold over those of traditional medicine while increasing the power of curing in like proportion.

Homeopaths should now begin systematic organization that they may be prepared to meet the exigencies of the near future by giving a service only they can give to this ailing time. First, let there be established, in every city and hamlet where a homeopathic physician lives, a homeopathic clinic. In the larger centers homeopathic groups can collaborate in proving the superiority of homeopathic treatment over all others in whole fields of sickness both acute and chronic. And more, Homeopathy can show the world the surest, safest of prophylactic treatment that has ever been discovered.

---

1. THE HOMEOPATHIC RECORDER, Vol. LV, No. 9, September 1940, p. 47 ff.

With such an instrumentality at our disposal and under the lash of dire necessity to society an opportunity is presented to our cause for a most transcendent and far-reaching service to harassed humanity. Homeopaths, the hour of destiny is at hand. Empires are crashing in the birth throes of a better social order. We must organize and work with unflagging faith and enthusiasm for the privilege of giving to the future the priceless boon of homeopathic healing.

ROAD TO HEALTH THROUGH HOMEOPATHY[1]

This is a time of complexities, frustrations, limitations and abnormal living. Dissipation in excess of alcohol and tobacco, together with the rapid increase of drug addictions, both within and without the medical profession proves to us that we are face to face with a condition that threatens the very existence of our social order. Institutions of science and learning as well as the many religious mentors have failed to stem the rising tide of physical decay. Mental incompetency and moral degeneracy are constantly increasing and infiltrating through every portal and ramification of society, from the humblest strata to the highest pinnacles of government. In the last forty years, the life span of one generation, we have had two world wars with a third one already starting. This has weakened the moral fiber of the race and filled the world with woe, suffering and fear.

With this has come a train of new so-called virus diseases which, so-called, scientific medicine has combatted with numerous chemical ingredients called "wonder drugs". As fast as one of these preparations fails, another takes its place. The apparent relief and cure from these substances carry in its train most serious side effects which result in serious blood changes and an ever-mounting number of degenerative diseases. Among these are cancer, kidney and heart diseases together with alarming increases of the insane and mentally incompetent.

In the presence of this gloomy picture, one may well ask: What, if any, is the remedy needed to meet it? Only the removal of fundamental causes can remove or overcome such states.

The universal acceptance and use of Homeopathy with its broad and far-reaching philosophy of life, in sickness and health, is alone sufficient to cope successfully with the complexities and dire hazards now engulfing humanity; because Homeopathy embraces and uses in its proper order and places all other proven methods of healing in the scope of its applied technique for the relief and cure of the sick. Nothing in homeopathic teaching refuses surgery where it is indicated and needed. It applies along with its therapeutic speciality physio-therapy, osteopathy, and kindred methods. Massage, dietary and sanitary procedures are used wherever and whenever needed to aid in the restoration of health.

---

1. Read before the American Association for Medico-Physical Research; September 13, 1950. From handwritten manuscript. - Editor.

Homeopathy does object emphatically to those methods and things that impair health, impoverish the blood stream, weaken the nervous system with habit-forming drugs, depressing the nerves and suppressing natural manifestations of disease such as skin eruptions of various types and catarrhal discharges from the orifices of the body, because from such depressing blood changes and suppressions of natural disease come most of the serious ailments ending in pathologic changes of the tissues and organs of the body organism.

Homeopathy scores its most effective results in the growing child and the juvenile and young adult. Herein is the formative stage of life where every impulse toward normal physiology brings about normal cell growth and development in a harmonious union of of moral, mental and physical states which enable the being to live and re-act in unison with his changing environment without friction or disturbed function - in other words, in a state of blissful health.

But even those further along in life with the piled up effects of inherited toxins of past generations together with toxic results of their own errors and mistakes of living (broken law) can be restored: This is done painfully and slowly by the benign power of the homeopathic remedy and the adherence to the wise dictums and requirements of the Homeopathic Philosophy of living.

None can be healed who do not become temperate in their desires and appetites. "He who conquers his spirit is greater than he who taketh a city." Homeopathy teaches us how to live temperately in all things. How to use and never abuse the attributes of our nature. Everything in God's creation was made for use and service. Every individual has his appointed place to fill in the broad economy of nature and in the society of his fellows.

Homeopathy is adequate to meet all acute infective causes of disease that afflicts humanity from the infant through childhood and adult life to old age. Homeopathy is sufficient to meet all painful complaints with the exception of surgical cases. These cases have come too late in the course of disease to overcome conditions of impacted stones or large tumors pressing on important organs or structures, or of obstructions which are the result of long continued inflammations and adhesions. All these conditions are mechanical and require surgical measures.

In the realm of chronic disease Homeopathy stands without a peer in its power to cure. Chronic disease is not self-limited as are acute conditions, and only the indicated remedy is sufficient to palliate, change or cure it. Without the homeopathic deterant chronic disease goes on unchecked to the end of life.

In the field of preventive medicine, Homeopathy is superior in achievement to any therapy yet discovered. It eradicates causative toxins before disease conditions can ultimate in pathologic changes in the body organism. Its prophylactic power against allergies of all kinds and acute infectious diseases such as diphtheria, scarlet fever, small pox and poliomyelitis is outstanding and certain.

With this array of superlative qualities and powers the question might be, and often is, asked: "Why is Homeopathy not more generally recognized and accepted?" It is because the agencies of publicity and purveyors of medical knowledge are monopolized by the American Medical Association who have a working agreement with the associated press that nothing pertaining to medicine, new discoveries, etc. shall go to the public without their censorship and consent. Hence only the wares of powerful manufacturing chemists and pharmacists with large financial assets can influence and convince this great worthy A.M.A. that such commercialized products are wonderful and helpful for the great American public's good. Anyone who has something better and much less expensive and every way more efficient to offer the world for the treatment of the sick is condemned as charlatans and malafactors.

Because such conditions obtain, there can be no progress in medical thought or improvement in medical technique for the cure of the sick. Wherever free competition and free thinking are shut off, there progress ceases, and ignorance with its limitless train of evils must prevail. But in spite of opposition and bitter denuncation, the homeopathic law is working its way into the consciousness of independent thinkers everywhere; and because it is part of the great universal truth, it will continue to grow and expand until the world of medicine at last is free of prejudice and ignorance. "Truth though crushed to Earth will rise again. The eternal years of God are hers. Error stung writhes in pain and dies amidst her worshipers."

Medical Research[1]

Medical research is one of the most valuable and satisfying ways of scientific investigation that the human mind can pursue. To discover the causes of human sickness and to note their effects on mind and body function as well as to find the remedies that can correct the ravages of disease are rare privileges for those who can pursue such desirable and worthwhile ends. Many millions of dollars have been spent, and many millions more will be spent for the development and extension of this valuable work.

The homeopathic branch of medicine with its concept of disease causation and its recognition of the vital life force as an important factor pertaining to disease cause and its cure can shed much light on some of the dark unsolved mysteries of life processes.

Furthermore, the homeopathic technique of reducing crude drugs to a state of electronic activity, by a special process of potentization, opens up a vast new field in the realm of physics; by the dynaminization and transformation of crude matter into dynamic energy, an energy especially adapted to act on and harmonize the activity of the vital life force, which is so important in all affairs of health and of disease and its cure.

This is an aspect of physics that has not been explored sufficiently to bring forth the many possibilities for the development of potent forces throughout the domain of nature, as yet unrecognized. These types energy, such as magnetic and electric and such as correspond to the vibrations of sound, light and color. These exist and operate in the world of cause - that unseen world out of which effects are projected into the phenomenal or physical world that is about us everywhere and of which we are a part. When these forces have been harnessed and applied, we are able to bring to the field of medicine undreamed-of powers for cure, not only in humans but throughout the whole animal and plant kingdoms as well.

There is a unity and a sympathetic relationship existing between man and both the animal and plant worlds; they are all susceptible to disease and sickness. Man depends on both animals and plants for the sustenance of his physical body. Some plants are harmful and poisonous to him; others are curative and helpful in restoring him from states

---

1. THE HOMEOPATHIC RECORDER, Vol. LXXIV, No. 10 - 12, 4th Quarter, April, May, June, 1959, p. 141.

of sickness to those of health. The homeopathic method of testing drugs on healthy human beings is the most effective way of learning the sick-making powers of individual drugs. This knowledge, when applied according to the theraputic law of similars ("Likes are cured by likes"), brings about certain and amazing results in restoring the sick to health. For over a century the homeopathic approach of treating each individual case of sickness as a law in itself (requiring its own individual remedy, whose theraputic powers must correspond in similarity of nature and symptomatology to the nature and symptoms of the sick patient) has yielded success.

Many cases generally recognized as incurable conditions, such as cancer, diabetes, epilepsy, chronic asthma and many intractable skin diseases (like psoriasis, severe types of eczema, lupus vulgaris and kel-oid) have been cured by this special aspect of medical science, namely the homeopathic approach to each individual case of sickness.

By the provings of numerous drugs on healthy human beings under scientific supervision employing safeguards and checks to insure accuracy in the provings, by eliminating the possibility of suggestive or imaginary symptoms on the part of the provers, by these careful methods the provings become established and reliable factors in the working mechanism of homeopathic prescribing.

One of the important factors in disease causation is disease suppression. This factor is too often overlooked or ignored by the practitians of general medicine, and it frequently leads into the blind alleys of disappointment and failure in the way of cure, this to the chagrin of the doctor and the loss of faith in medicine on the part of the patient. Suppressions may be brought on by either external or internal agents. When an asthma supervenes as a result of a skin disease or dermatitis, by the application of powerful salves or ointments or by drastic radiation, such as x-ray or ultra-violet light etc., we have a manifestation of external suppression. The disease condition has been driven from the skin to the mucous membranes lining the lungs. When a rheumatism has been driven from the joints to the heart by powerful pain-killing drugs, we have an example of internal suppression. Other examples of suppression are those where violently recurring headaches are constantly palliated, not cured, by coal tar types of drugs; or where severe forms of nerve tension and persistent insomnia are palliated, over recurring periods of time by sedation of various types, to finally result in a so-called nervous breakdown or in mental incompetency.

The true medical scientist must seek and find the causes of sickness and remove them at any and all costs if he would succeed in the cure of his patients. He must free himself of all prejudice and pre-conceived opinions concerning science and medicine if he would be a true exponent of the healing art. He must proceed with his work according to established laws and principles to achieve the highest standards of success in his chosen field. No sacrifice of time or effort is too great for him, whose life is dedicated to a service of such vast importance to humanity. The good physician is a teacher as well as a healer in the routine of his life's work. To instruct people in the fundamentals of proper living so as to avoid the pitfalls and ravages of disease is a work transcending even that of healing.

Enfin, the well-rounded physician and medical researcher is destined for a high place in the archives of human achievement, deserving the gratitude and acclaim of a suffering world. His reward in spiritual values exceeds material wealth or worldly station. The good his work may bring to many must be a benediction and a lasting joy to gladden his heart as long as life lasts; and finally when life passes on to the great unknown future, what a memorial and lasting heritage is left for men of succeeding generations to emulate.

HOMEOPATHIC RESEARCH[1]

At present a great wave of propaganda for medical research is on especially in the quest for the prevention and cure of cancer and polio-myelitis. It is in the realm of chronic diseases of obscure origin where the homeopathic principle and technique of drug applcation has given the world the most convincing and irrefutable proofs of curative power in sicknesses that are not self-limiting and ending either in recovery or possible death.

In the past decade a new and advanced approach to homeopathic concepts has sprung up in the regular school of medicine called psy-chosomatic medicine. This phase of medical thought emphatically stresses the great importance of the mental and emotional states in the causation of illness in even the most chronic nature such as arthritis of various forms, cancer and numerous forms of mental disease.

Since Hahnemann's time the mental and emotional symptoms have held highest rank in the treatment of the patient for the selection of his curative remedy. No drug proving is complete without a goodly number of mental and emotional symptoms, desires and aversions of the physical plane and in the sexual reactions and symptoms - on the higher planes of being, the loves and hates, the hallucinations and illu-sions, the mental abnormalities or insufficiencies, etc. Here lies one of the great differences between homeopathic and allopathic procedure in research.

Homeopathy experiments on well individuals of both sexes with the administration of a single remedial substance or drug. After its adminis-tration one takes note of all changes from the normal, in the mental and emotional spheres, changes in the secretions and excretions of the body, including changes in the blood chemistry, to form a complete picture or chart of the power residing in each proven remedial agent employed. On the basis of the well known often verified Law of Cure "Similia Similibus Curantur" such proven agents may be given to meet the conditions, symptoms and states produced by said agents to bring about normal physiological activity in the sick patient suffering similar symptoms and states produced by the curative drug on healthy humans.

In many epidemics of **poliomyelitis** during the past forty years, homeopathic methods have been notably successful in saving life in

---

1. THE HOMEOPATHIC RECORDER, Vol. LXIV, No. 4, October 1948, p. 99 ff.

most of the treated cases and securing a minimum number of crippling cases: Most of the latter being only slightly impaired. It is true that many cases are very mild and recover with little or no paralysis, but in the severe bulbar types of the disease, it is surprising how positive the curative effects of the homeopathic specific can be in the saving of life and the prevention of severe maiming.

Remedies like BELL., GELS., HELL., CUPR., CROT-H., CUR., COCC., LACH., OP., RHUS-T. and ZINC. are the leaders in serious cases of this type. In the spinal cases ALUM., CAUST., CALC-P., CALC-S., COCC., LACH., LATH., HEP., KALM., LYC., OP., PLB. RHUS-T., SULPH., ZINC. are frequently needed.

In the field of prophylaxis the epidemic remedy when it is found gives the best protection. In forty years of practice I have found LATH. one hundred percent effective. This remedy given in many thousands of individuals in many epidemics has never failed to protect, and this verifies the Law of Similars because LATH. affects the specific centers the polio virus does: namely the nerve roots of the anterior spinal column and produces a paralysis of both lower and upper extremities in its proving.

In the field of cancer research there is a much wider compass of activity to cover. It is the outgrowth of deep constitutional or inherited soil conditions. This is the homeopathic concept only partly admitted by the allopathic school of thought. Dr. Maude Sly of the University of Chicago has bred cancer both into healthy rats, individuals and families; and reversing the procedure in mate selections, she has bred cancer out of individuals and families proving convincingly the factor of inheritance as a primary causation force.

The homeopathic literature is full of reports of cured cases of cancerous tumors by such men as Cooper, Burnett, Clarke and Jones. Kent in his lesser writings developed a number of remedies that had produced cancer cures. I will mention some of them here: ALUM-SIL., CALC-SIL., AUR-S., CADM-S. and KALI-SIL. A number of physicians since his time have added many valuable remedies to the homeopathic literature CADM-MET. and some of its chemical combinations are among the most potent for the irradication of malignant conditions. The ground work is laid for many successful homeopathic research centers wherever Homeopathy is known and practiced.

Now a brief note on the procedure of allopathic research. Animal experimentation makes up most of the research in vogue today and in the past. The knowledge obtained this way is meager and completely inadequate when applied to human beings. Only the toxic effects on the tissues of animals (pathology) are found. The mental and emotional changes are unknown and undiscoverable by such means. This is the phase of medicine that marks the only real advance in traditional medicine in a hundred years and the only advance that will not be discarded for some new wonder drug in a short time.

Those of us who have had wide experience in the treatment of cancer have no delusions of finding a specific cure for cancer. There will never be any one remedy or agent to cure every case of cancer; only the specific remedy for each individual case presented will avail, and that not in every case.

It is potent to all who have worked long in this field that the prevention of cancer presents a much brighter outlook for universal success than does cure, and no one force in the world today can equal the power of the Homeopathy of Hahnemann to eradicate inherited and constitutional tendencies to chronic degenerative disease, including those of the mental and nervous spheres. This is especially true when applied to the early life of children and young adults even up to middle life. Give true Homeopathy free scope in the treatment of humanity in the early formative periods of life; and in a few generations T.B., cancer, and insanity will disappear from the earth.

Remarks on Fluoridation of Water[1]

Re: The Chicago Health Association, Distributors of medical knowledge and helpful advice regarding sanitation, dietary science and medicine.

This service is organized for the purpose of public education, bringing to the people a broad and unprejudiced view of all aspects of medical science and treatment existing today. The personnel of this organization is made up from the ranks of ten thousand experts in medicine, sanitary science and dietetics, and the service they render is free, as they serve without pay.

In times of crises and danger unusual and effective methods may be needed to meet the situation. The people of Chicago are now faced by a serious menace to their health and well being; viz. the proposal to poison their drinking water by impregnating it with fluorine, a chemical poison used to kill insects and which is deadly to all animal life.

The recognized authorities in all the medical schools, regular and homeopathic, are unanimous in their statements concerning the toxic nature of fluorine. Frank Bamford, B.Sc., State Director of the Medico Legal Laboratory of Cairo, Egypt, states that chronic fluorine poisoning manifests itself in mottled teeth, a symptom which may be produced with as little as 1 mg per litre of fluorine in drinking water. In 1932 in Denmark a much more serious symptom osteosclerosis was traced to fluorine poisoning. In one cryolite (sodium aluminum fluoride) factory fifty-seven out of sixty-eight workers suffered from the disease. Fluorides sold for the destruction of vermin have been responsible for a number of human deaths. In 1937 Roholm published an exhaustive dissertation on the subject, dealing with both acute and chronic poisoning. In a list of 34 recorded and fatal cases he mentions the following symptoms; Vomiting - 31 cases. Pain in abdomen - 17 cases. Diarrhea - 13 cases. Convulsions - 11 cases. Cattle have been poisoned when being fed on waste matter from distilleries where formerly fluorides were used to disinfect the fermentated mash. Definite thickening of the bones has been noted in sheep which have been fed on hay containing two and one half parts of fluorine to one million parts of water.

Dr. John Clarke of London, England, in his *Dictionary of Practical Materia Medica* states that fluorine in very small doses given to healthy humans for purposes of proving to ascertain its specific action on the

---

1.   From handwritten manuscript, exact date unknown. - Editor..

human organism produces abcesses, gangrene of tissue, loss of hair, liver afflictions, spinal disease, spleen and other glandular disease. It destroys the enamel of the teeth. Disturbs the nervous system and impairs the blood and the blood vessels.

Citizens of Chicago, in the name of fair play, you must prevent this great evil about to be inflicted upon a great mass of people without their consent and against their wishes. The few misinformed ones who want this drug can easily obtain it with little cost and treat their own drinking water and with the advantage of being able to discontinue its use before the adverse effects become too drastic and dangerous. Once the whole water supply is poisoned, it will be difficult and tedious to undo the harm. No project conceived by communist Russia could injure us anymore than the poisoning of the water supply of the nation; the advocates of this unreasonable scheme contemplate its establishment throughout our land; and if dupes could be made of our lawmakers and law enforcers under the guise of performing a public service, they would count it a great victory for their unholy cause.

Write or phone your Alderman and ask at least for a referendum vote of all the people on this vital issue, be safe, protect your friends and families from dangerous sickness by preventing precipitous action involving the health and happiness of millions.

Anyone doubting the truth or correctness of the statements concerning the dangers of fluorine to animal life in this leaflet can easily verify them by going to any good library and consulting any credited work on toxicology or Materia Medica.

ALUMINA STILL POISONS THE MULTITUDE[1]

Much has been said and written about the deleterious effects of aluminum poisoning chiefly caused by food prepared and cooked in alumina cooking utensils.

Some of us thought until observation taught us differently, that owing to the demand of the war needs aluminum cooking ware was mostly converted into airplanes. It is true that the manufacture of aluminum cooking utensils have ceased for the present, but for the most part all that have been produced in the past twenty years are still doing business in the same insidious and devastating way. Only a very small portion of aluminum cooking ware was turned in for the war effort.

To the homeopathic physician this subject is most vital, because while a patient is subjected to the influence of the subtle poisoning of aluminum the indicated remedy fails to act in a curative way. Many times it acts only for a few days and fails to relieve or cure the symptoms for which it was prescribed. And the antidotal remedy must be repeated too frequently to permanently relieve the patient of his natural symptoms and conditions of disease while the poison is constantly taken. Unless the supply of the poison is shut off by the patient ceasing to partake of foods prepared in aluminum it will be impossible to cure him of his chronic disease. And here is another obstacle the homeopathic physician must meet and overcome in order to effect a cure.

Old school medical authorities claim that the amount of aluminum taken in the food by way of cooking utensils of aluminum is of such small quantities as to be negligible. But our homeopathic provings by potencies given to healthy individuals prove beyond any doubt that this poisonous metal given over a period of time in even the potentized form produces a great chain of harmful and debilitating symptoms of sickness lasting for a long time and stimulating many forms of chronic diseases, such as intestinal inflammations, inertias, obstructions and even paralysis, as well as profound anemias and chronic painful neuralgias with extensive nerve and spinal inflammations and degenerations. Indeed this insidious toxin may well be one of the factors involved in the increase of cancer itself.

CADM-MET. is the most complete antidote I have found, although PLB. and OP. as well as BAR-C. have antidoted some of the special conditions produced by aluminum.

---

1. "Editorial" in THE HOMEOPATHIC RECORDER, Vol. LX, No. 5, p. 157, November 1944.

We are told that when the war ends there will be vast quantities of this metal for the manufacture of other utensils than airplanes and that the production of cooking utensils will again be resumed. If building material for houses and furniture could be manufactured instead of cooking utensils, a great menace to public health would be removed.

Impressions of the 1952 Homeopathic Conventions[1]

The National and International Homeopathic Conventions held jointly June 22 - 27 at Look Out Mountain Hotel near Chattanooga, Tennessee, were highly profitable and worthwhile to the membership and to the world of medicine in general. The papers were practical, some were outstanding in excellence and evoked valuable discussions and constructive criticism. The attendance as a whole was better than average, and the membership displayed more interest in the scientific programs than usual, perhaps because there were less outside attractions available.

However, in the delightful cool of the evening, music and dancing were at hand, under the discretely dim light of an artificial moon which looked benignly down on prowling wolves with dripping mouths and panting respirations as they whirled in the ecstatic dance to the strains of voluptuous music in the enticing arms of their would-be innocent victims. The innocent and unsophistication rendered the occasion much more attractive to the prowling dancing wolves. But this is not bad in medical conventions, especially in homeopathic conventions, where a majority of the men are either bald or grey.

The exhilarating and energizing effect of a few beautiful and youthful females was life giving to these last conventions. Feet that dragged suddenly became elastic and quickened; forms that were stooped and bent became erect and firm, and eyes dull with fatigue became luminous with expectation and pleasure in the flair and incomparable realm of youth and life at its best. Then let us have more of our youth, boys and girls, to bring back memories of less care ridden times, and the joy of living again in the warm flush of youth and romance where all is music, poetry, and high hope. Even though it be but the illusion of a Neptunian dream, we are all better, stronger and happier for the experience.

Turning back to the more serious aspect of our last meeting, one historic action was taken by the Homeopathic profession that justifies its existence and its importance for the public welfare of our country, and that is its firm stand against the poisoning of the nation's drinking water for purely experimental purposes. The courage to take this stand

---

1. From handwritten manuscript, exact date unknown. A bit of light heartedness, humour and a reminder about the dangers of fluoridation of drinking water. - Editor..

and point out the dangers of *fluoridation* of drinking water will bring the reward of public trust with an awakened interest in Homeopathy.

In closing it is well to remember and state our appreciation for the courteous and hospitable treatment rendered the membership and its guests by the management and their personnel of the Look Out Mountain Hotel. From this historic site of American greatness, brought through blood, tears, and toil, the homeopaths of 1952 will take away with them many pleasant memories, and the thought that they have contributed another mite of useful knowledge to help build a better future for our children and the children of all mankind under God, the Creator and Preserver.

Address to SHS and PAC - Fall, 1953[1]

Members and Colleagues of the Southern Homeopathic Society and the Pan American Congress, Visitors and Friends. It is a great privilege to meet you and to address you with a message from the American Institute of Homeopathy. It is a pleasant duty to extend felicitations from the Institute to the Southern Society on this memorable occasion here in the historical city of New Orleans where the Southern had its inception sixty-nine years ago. Sixtynine years of faithful homeopathic service to the world and to our country has earned the gratitude and admiration of homeopaths everywhere. A more propitious time for this eventful meeting of unified homeopathic forces could not be had than now.

From every section of our country come urgent requests for homeopathic doctors. We have not nearly enough of them to go around but we do have the potential means of making them by the establishment of a homeopathic correspondence course, which can be followed later by a post-graduate course of homeopathic therapeutics, philosophy and materia medica.

Many doctors of the regular school are not entirely satisfied with the results of modern medical practice; they are waiting for something better that is devoid of the enervating side effects attanding much of the more recent medication now used for acute ailments such as antibiotics, barbiturates, coal tar derivates, etc. all with their serious side effects. We need but show them by way of the homeopathic concept and law the superiority of homeopathic practice in terms of cure to awaken their desire for the knowledge that will enable them to obtain superior and more satisfactory results in their private practice. Once that interest is awakened and when Homeopathy is put to the test by them, more homeopathic physicians will come into being, equipped to serve humanity with the Divine law of cure, for Homeopathy is truly God-given, and Hahnemann was the gifted instrument that was privileged to bring it to his fellows the world over.

In many states of the union, osteopathic physicians are permitted to qualify for medical practice. A large portion of those graduates are already sympathetic to Homeopathy; and when they learn the great demand existing for homeopathic doctors and when they, at the same

---

1. From handwritten manuscript. Combined convention of the Southern Homeopathic Society and Pan American Congress held in New Orleans, October 1953. - Editor.

time, are informed how quickly they can acquire the necessary knowledge to enable them to do good homeopathic work, it will take but a short time for Homeopathy to expand over the length and breadth of our land, bringing a new era in our time when the Hippocratic Oath and Pledge will not be a hollow mockery dominated by selfish and insatiable code of commercialism in medicine.

The inspired healers of olden times who lived lives of purity and integrity that they might be infused with the powers emanating from the Source of All Power and thereby perform better service to the sick, whom they were privileged to comfort and restore, shall again seem to appear in our midst and multiply many fold in the near future. The better men in all schools of medical thought today are striving to correct abuses in medical practice that are the outgrowth of selfishness and greed. The true healer finds his greatest reward for the most part in the restoration of his patient to health, and any system that advances the progress of healing for the betterment of the race is certain of being accepted by steadily growing numbers of progressively informed people.

Those who have tasted the fruits of homeopathic practice and have received the benefits of such practice need not be told of its benign power for good. Our appeal must be made to the great mass of folks who obtain their knowledge of things medical from newspaper accounts and advertisements set in glowing terms and generalities of the success of the numerous experimental drugs that have deluged this generation - drugs whose certain deleterious side effects are not mentioned until after the damage is done and the truth has become apparent even to the dullest.

Undaunted by failure after failure, the manufacturing chemists and pharmacist continue to ply their trade which is eminently successful financially, but sub-zero in cure. Yes, it is the victims of commercialism in medicine that need our efforts and time to show them the true nature of disease and the means to its cure.

Besides the abuse from drastic drugs, there are many more health-destroying forces in our midst that constantly undermine public health and pave the way for the more serious forms of disease such as cancer, chronic kidney and heart disease as well as the degenerative blood diseases frequently met with and the vast number suffering from mental and emotional conditions listed under the heading of nervous breakdowns and mental incompetence. Many of today's ills are the result of processed and adulterated foods, as well as foods poisoned by chemical preservatives, meat tenderized by chemicals (sodium glycolate). The sprays used on growing fruits and vegetables are highly toxic, and small amounts ingested over aperiod of time can build up serious symptoms of illness. Foods prepared or contained in aluminum cooking utensils can cause chronic illness and even inhibit the action of curative remedies in the treatment of natural sickness.

The water supply is a constant source of illness and suffering. Water treated with chlorine, fluorine and other chemicals have caused infinitely more harm than any theoretical good they could do. These disturbing influences could be dispensed with if all who use water would have it boiled before using it. Those who doubt the power for evil that these chemicals possess need only read the provings of chlorine water and fluoric acid in Clarke's Materia Medica. The use of Aluminium chloride to soften water can prove very injurious if water treated with this chemical is used for drinking or cooking purposes.

Even the air we breathe is polluted and full of menace to health, especially in highly industrialized areas as are found in many large cities like Los Angeles, Chicago, Detroit, Pittsburgh and many others too numerous to name. Recent experiments on animals kept in the smog air that prevails in certain parts of Los Angeles indicate that definite cancer-producing properties are inherent therein. The constantly increasing amounts of carbon dioxide and monoxide gases that are poured into the atmosphere from the myriads of autos incessantly operating around us everywhere are another appreciable source of air poisoning. These gases are known to have the power of disorganizing and destroying the oxygen-carrying red blood cells; and the loss of these cells results in forms of serious anemia and death.

The sick-making power of alcohol and tobacco really needs no scientific ban to condemn them and banish them from our midst. Nevertheless, they are strong factors in the causation of certain types of serious disease affecting the heart and lungs from tobacco; and liver and kidney disease resulting from alcohol, especially when taken in excess.

We have mentioned these accessory causes of illness because the homeopathic doctor first must eliminate all causes of ill health in order to obtain successful action from the indicated remedy on the vital forces of his patient, thereby enabling him to produce a certain speedy and permanent cure.[1]

1. §77 and footnote 33 §7 Organon. - Editor.

Homeopathy has been referred to as the practice of sectarian medicine; this statement is not true because homeopathic leaders from the earliest time, including Hahnemann himself, have always endeavored to have the system incorporated into the curriculum of general medicine, and to that end homeopaths have fought only for recognition and acceptance of the principles of Homeopathy that the world might be benefitted by a better, safer and more economical means of healing.

From some quarters homeopaths have been called unscientific, but nowhere else in medical practice is a natural law invoked (the Law Similars) to find the one needed medicine to fit the requirements of each individual patient. What a contrast to the hit-and-miss method of empirical medicine with its measuring stick of trial and error. In the mechanical sciences, empiricism or trial and error may be permissible where only material things are involved and the waste and loss from error may be borne without too great a sacrifice. But in the treatment of the sick where life itself may hang in the balance, empiricism is illogical and dangerous, and human beings should not be subjected to such uncertainties and risks.

From other quarters we have heard that Homeopathy is unprogressive, stationary, fixed and unchanging in its medical methods and approach to sickness. These views are the result of prejudice and inadequate knowledge of its law and philosophy. What better way can be found to ascertain the properties and effects of drugs than to prove them on healthy human beings and to note the changes taking place in the organism while under the influence of a single drug or remedy. Changes in the emotional, mental and physical spheres of the provers, when noted and tabulated, become certain guides in the realm of cure.

When drugs are administered to animals for the purpose of learning their properties and value in the treatment of the sick, we learn very little beyond the toxic effects they produce; and even these are variable because different animals react differently to the same drug. For instance, Belladonna affects the horse profoundly in a sick-making way while the rabbit and the guinea pig can eat it and experience no harm and even seem to extract nourishment from it. The cruel methods of vivisection cannot bring us any new or useful knowledge for the purpose of cure. The pathological changes found in an animal's dead body will in no way aid in obtaining the needed curative remedy. Since the dumb animal can tell us no symptoms of his ailments, emotionally, physically or mentally, we only have the pathology found in his dead tissues as a guide to treatment; and that is of little value because in order to treat the type of pathology afflicting the patient that was produced by a certain drug, exploratory surgery would have to be resorted to in order to find the pathological processes present in the sick and employ the similar remedy against it. For several apparent reasons, this procedure would be unacceptable, but chiefly because the results in cure would be uncertain and even doubtful.

In prescribing on pathology alone, we neglect the one most essential factor of every case, viz: the totality of the symptoms. Pathology corresponds to the end results of disease. Curative medicines accomplish their astonishing effects by acting on the living organism or the vital processes of the patient. By activiating and normalizing physiological activities, normal histological units are produced in the body organism. Morbid anatomy or pathology is the result of perverted physiology.

The transition from health to disease and vice-versa is a simple one to visualize to one familiar with the known electromagnetic phenomena and laws of the Cosmos. So long as one keeps in tune with the rhythmical march of universal order, he is well; but if, for any one of numerous reasons, the silver cord of harmony is broken by adverse vibrations, ill health ensues. In the changing states of physical health a certain definite phenomena may be noted by those trained and equipped to do so. The first change noted is that of polarity in the life currents of the body, a change from the normal negative to a positive, which is a change in direction, a reversal as it were of the normal flow and flux.[1] If this adverse flux of polarity continues only a short time, there supervenes a change in the chemistry of the blood beginning in the deep unseen planes at the etheric level. If this blood chemistry persists, a change begins in the body cells and tissues which constitute the pathology of disease. It is interesting to note that the autonomic nervous system[2] and the capillary blood system are the inter changing media connecting the physical with the etheric planes of existence; any change that takes place in the physical body must come by way of the etheric plane through the medium of the capillaries and the autonomic nervous system while the polarity or direction of the life force determines the nature of that change whether of health or disease.

The homeopathic remedy is the most certain force known to control the polarity of all things throughout the realm of nature both animate

---

1. See article "Recent Concepts and New Formulas in Medicine" p. 679 ff. and article "Importance of Electronic Reactions to Future Medicine" p. 683 ff.. - Editor.
2. i.e. the ortho-sympathetic and para-sympathetic nervous systems. - Editor.

or inanimate, for matter wherever found in all its forms and states has polarity. Magnetism, electricity, gases, liquids, solids - be they animate or inanimate - all have their special rates of vibration and their own individualizing character of polarity.

In the last thirty years homeopathic physicians have employed the knowledge of this subtle form of physics to fit the homeopathic remedy to the needs of their sick patients with most gratifying results in terms of cure. The development of this relatively new concept and its application to homeopathic needs will in the near future enable homeopathic physicians to accomplish a greater number of difficult cures than ever before. Cancer and many heretofore incurable conditions will be mastered by Homeopathy with the aid of this more complete and really scientific remedy selector.

In working to extend Homeopathy, we work for ourselves, our children and the whole world throughout all the future, and what a boon that is to suffering and sick humanity. Then for this truly good and worthwhile purpose, let us unite and work with heart and mind and body as we have never worked before to bring back into full bloom the beauteous healing flower of cure, Homeopathy, for the healing of the nations.

IMPRESSIONS OF THE FALL 1953 SHS AND PAC CONVENTIONS[1]

Impressions of the Southern and Pan American Convention, held in New Orleans last October 27th to the 29th, received by those who attended, left an air of hopeful enthusiasm for the future of Homeopathy. The scientific programs both in general medicine and surgery as well as the purely homeopathic contributions were excellent and were well attended and received.

Considerable publicity was given homeopaths and their system of healing by the local press. The New Orleans city officials and representatives as well as notable medical men of the city and vicinity were generously kind and hospitable and presented a number of Homeopathy's representative men and women with certificates of citizenship and keys to the city.

Pan American delegates from Mexico and Brazil contributed greatly to a full and worth-while program, for the Pan American delegates and their presence at the meeting gave an international touch of solidarity and loyal enthusiasm for homeopathic progress throughout the Americas. These fine representatives from our sister republics came to our meeting by way of considerable sacrifice of time and money. They are ardent, tireless workers for the cause of Homeopathy everywhere. Along with their greetings, they brought urgent invitations to every homeopathic physician in the United States to attend the great planned meeting of world Homeopathy to be held in Brazil in the fall of 1954. The government of Brazil is sponsoring this elaborate program, and there can be no doubt that those who are fortunate enough to accept this invitation to attend this great meeting of world Homeopathy will experience unexpected joy to gladden the heart and stores of homeopathic knowledge to nourish and strengthen the mind.

On the evening of October 29th, the members of the joint homeopathic organizations and their visiting friends enjoyed the rare privilege of hearing Mrs. Amaro Azevedo, the beautiful and talented wife of Dr. Amaro Azevedo, render a number of charming songs in her own exquisite and inimitable way. This gracious lady lends color, charm and joy to any gathering fortunate enough to have her as a guest. Doctor Azevedo, who is one the the world's outstanding homeopathic leaders, gave the assembled members and their guests a splendid oration on the

---

1. From handwritten manuscript, probably written December 1953 and presented at the AIH Winter meeting. - Editor..

progress and needs of world Homeopathy and ended with an appeal for homeopaths everywhere, but especially those of the United States, to make preparation to accept the hospitality of Brazil for a heart-warming and soul-stirring time at their convention. In this way the bonds of friendship and understanding may be forged and sealed among the homeopathic doctors from all the continents and from all the nations of the world.

There were several meetings of the new Central Committee that was formed at Swampscott at the last Institute meeting. I have not heard the results of the meeting, but I presume a report will be made at the next Institute meeting, and it was good to see this Committee start functioning. There was also a meeting of the president and a number of the Institute's Trustees in which some unfinished business and problems of the Institute were ironed out.

Inquiries have been made as to how soon the Institute's correspondence course can be put in operation to begin the teaching of doctors. This is a matter for the board of trustees and the board of medical education to pass on and to formulate ways and means to create and maintain such a correspondence course. The Post Graduate school of the Foundation is now functioning, and it is sponsored by the American Institute of Homeopathy. By the time our correspondence course is ready to function, we should have many prospective students for the course. The rank and file of the Institute could well be at work interesting and urging prospective students who are eligible to take the course. This should be our chief objective at this time.

Our next important objective is preparing for a great meeting on July 18, 1954, at Mackinac Island, Michigan. At this meeting we can lay the goundwork for the great bi-centennial meeting of Hahnemann's birthday, 1955, at Washington, D.C.

This is the agenda that coming in an orderly sequence can assure certain homeopathic progress and expansion. Friends, let's move on, united and faithful to our principles. We cannot fail.

THE DETROIT MEETING[1]

The Homeopathic Conventions at Detroit from June 9th until June 14th, 1946, scientifically, socially and fraternally ended as a step forward for the progress of Homeopathy.

Many of the papers were intellectually illuminating and clearly demonstrated the amazing fact that science is now beginning to discover the innate principles and truths promulgated and enunciated by that incomparable homeopathic savant, Samuel Hahnemann, one hundred and fifty years ago.

So it has ever been. The gift of genius perceives the forces and laws at work in the unseeable realms of causation, and many years and much effort and experimentation are required before the materialistic and doubting scientist is able to devise instruments and equations enabling the world to visualize the truths that the illuminated flash of genius catches through an elevated consciousness.

To the doctors of Detroit and especially to Dr. W. P. Mowry and his charming wife, every member of the Institute and of the Hahnemann Association must owe a vote of thanks for the splendid entertainment and many comforts and considerations given them and their wives to make their visit at Detroit memorable and happy.

The newly elected officers of the Institute, especially Dr. Isaiah L. Moyer as president, insures loyal and efficient homeopathic leadership for the immediate future; it is up to every member to give him their best support for the good of Homeopathy.

The I.H.A. members especially and signally honored themselves by electing that matchless leader, teacher and practician of pure homeopathic practice, Dr. William B. Griggs of Philadelphia, for their next president.

The I.H.A. again is blessed in retaining the services of that indefatigable and worthy worker for the cause of Homeopathy, Dr. A. Dwight Smith, as its business manager, secretary and editor of the Recorder. No man in modern Homeopathy has given as much of himself and succeeded as well in maintaining the life and welfare of the I.H.A. as has Dr. Smith - and all without thought of recompense or emolument. As a prophet I may be wrong, but I predict that with such leaders as he, Homeopathy will come into her own and be recognized for her true worth. It is only up to rank and file of the members to emulate his

---

1. THE HOMEOPATHIC RECORDER, Vol. LXV, No.2, August, 1946, p. 61.

efforts by only a fraction of thought and effort to bring undreamed-of results.

It was a joy to again welcome our friends and colleagues from Canada. They always bring to us something refreshing and stimulating both intellectually and fraternally. They come with the freshness and sweetness of their northern summer breezes full of homeopathic ozone to quicken our lagging wits. More power to them, and may they flourish and grow in numbers and be with us always.

It was good to greet the vestor of homeopathic teaching and practice, Dr. H. A. Roberts. His presence alone stabilizes and advances all homeopathic procedure; no convention is right without him.

We missed the rich sage contribution of the presence of Dr. Royal E.S. Hayes, who always brings much of value to our deliberations and discussions, not to mention the great value of his paper full of homeopathic meat, that partaken by the wise make them wiser.

Last, but not least, we missed seeing that great, loyal and uncompromising advocate of Homeopathy, Dr. Alfred Pulford. Long may he live and thrive to bring us messages of homeopathic truth. But it was good to greet his illustrious son, Dr. Dayton Pulford, who reports that his experience with army practice has made him a more confirmed homeopath than ever. Not that Dr. Dayton was ever anything but a staunch and true practician of the homeopathic art, but his experience with old-school methods renders him glad he is privileged to practice Homeopathy.

There are so many more I would like to mention in this brief account, but space and time forbid. But I will say before closing that we were fortunate in adding some members of great promise, not gray heads full of wisdom, but young and up-coming youngsters with all the surety and enthusiasm of youth which bode well for Homeopathy's future.

Let us now begin to prepare for the next convention of 1947 to make it still greater in both the quality and quantity of its membership. As the years crowd in upon us, we look more and more forward to the friendly greeting these annual reunions bring; and if we fail to attend, we loose much that is more precious than shining gold or glittering jewels.

ADDRESS: PAN AMERICAN HOMEOPATHIC CONGRESS[1]

Friends, colleagues, and fellow members of the Pan American Homeopathic Medical Congress: It is my great pleasure and high privilege to address you on this momentous yet festive occasion. We meet here in this beauteous and historical city of fine culture and lofty aspirations, to further and advance a great humanitarian cause, Homeopathy. And no more fitting place could be selected than here, in the bosom of this Queen of Cities, which sits enthroned in regal splendor high on her loft and enduring pedestal bathed by the invigorating and purified atmosphere of the higher strata and illumined by the golden sunlight only known where the air is rare and pure. We feel uplifted and inspired in this wonderous setting and within these sweet influences. And we ferverently pray and trust that our mission of fellowship and mutual understanding and helpfullness will bring a rich harvest of homeopathic success and growth everywhere for the future. And that our children and their children may inherit the benefic boon of homeopathic healing down through the ages thereby bringing into existence a healthier, happier, nobler race of beings to adorn the earth.

No more important a subject of current scientific achievement frought with so much good to the nations can be presented for discussion than Homeopathy. It blazes forth like Bethlehem's Star of old, a heavenly messenger bringing hope and comfort to the afflicted of all lands, and it sends its beautiful rays of healing light to radiate and brighten all the dark places of the earth. Like all great truths in the march of human progress upward, Homeopathy with its founders and votaries from its inception to the present time has been beset by misunderstanding, hatred and calumny and bitter opposition both secret and open in an unsightly effort to crush and exterminate both the doctrines and teachings as well as the benefic application of its art of healing. But, Truth, though beaten down rises again and again, even rises with bleeding head and agonizing groans of pain to finally triumph in glory and recognition. Remember, the Christ was crucified and tortured by those He sought to save and help, yet Christianity abides, and expands everywhere and remains the rainbow promise of peace and justice for all the future.

I will not dilate on the achievements of the past. Such works are well known to you. A heroic band of pioneers suffered and sacrificed for a

---

1. From handwritten manuscript, exact date unknown. - Editor..

living principle of truth and human service and passed the lighted torch of knowledge to our hands for our uses and benefits. Shall we falter and fail where their glorious work ended? No! A thousand times No!, we must not fail, we cannot fail, because the fight for homeopathic truth may be likened to the perpetual battle for human freedom: and we can take heart from those immortal words of the poet Byron,

> "Freedom's battle once begun
>
> Bequethed by bleeding sire to son
>
> Though muffled oft, is ever won."

The precious heritage of truth which makes men free, vouchsafed to us, involves in its acceptance the sacred duty of the teacher and the proselyte. We, too, must be willing to suffer and make sacrifices economically and socially if need be for the perpetuation of our great medical truth, and if we wish to leave the world a little better than we found it and a little easier place to live in, and give richer dowry to our children than was ours. We who have been blessed with this light of useful knowledge and privileged to perform divine uses of healing thereby will make every effort to spread and perpetuate this beneficial and truly scientific law of healing. No labor is too irksome, no sacrifice too great to the true disciple of Hahnemann because he finds his greatest joy in the healing of the sick; and Homeopathy stands unequaled in its power to cure.

Homeopathy is the medical link between Divine Providence and His afflicted children. And the homeopathic physician is an instrument of Divine Love, dedicated to high uses and noble ends. The homeopathic physician also is an idealist, compelled to work in a world of selfish commercialism and naturally becomes a rugged individualist for the most part fighting his battles single handed. His strength and his weakness are both involved in this complexity of his life. He has developed the splendid courage and sterling character of the pioneer advancing the frontier of civilization everywhere, but unless he learns and profits from the experience of his prototype he is doomed to the same oblivion that leaves the pioneering but a fascinating memory.

The homeopathic physician must recognize the vast changes that have come to pass in the economic, social and political mechanism of organized society everywhere today where organizations and combinations of every kind work to the detriment of individual development and independence. Therefore in self defense homeopaths must organize and unite all their forces for the common good, and in fact for their very existence. They must unite their municipal units into state units and their state units into national units and their national units into an international body for the advancement and perpetuation of their science as a whole as well as for the interest of every individual member of a vast organization.

The first prerequisite of this ambitious yet necessary program is to bring into our own ranks everywhere the spirit of harmony, understanding and tolerance, thus welding our organization into a solid phalanx of opposition against our enemies. To accomplish this desirable end we must cover the shortcomings of our brothers with the broad mantle of charity and reach down the helping hand of fellowship to lift them up to the higher planes of understanding and vision. To imbue each unit of our entire organization with the stern necessity for close co-operation and fellowship for the common good, is our first and most difficult step. This accomplished, our future is assured and nothing then can stop the forward rapid march of Homeopathy to its goal of recognition and acceptance.

With a completed organization we are in a position to nullify adverse legislation aimed against us, and even to influence a more liberal legislation for all medical progress. And we can extend our activities much more universally in the form of clinics and journals both for laymen and professional subscribers.

In fact one of our most lamentable and hurtful shortcomings has been our indifference to the power of publicity and propaganda. Our opponents of the Old School have fattened and flourished on propaganda alone, for they have no real healing ability to offer outside of surgery which homeopaths can practice with much better results because of their superior methods of drug application both before and after operative procedures.

We have failed to tell the world of the great superiority of our prophylactic measures not only against acute infectious diseases but against the more stubborn chronic aspects of sickness as well. The unhygenic use of filthy serums and noxious vaccines could everywhere be profitably replaced by the certain and gentle action of the homeopathic prophylactics, removing all danger from anaphylaxis and blood poisoning or sequellae of any kind, and insuring a more certain protection as well.

I will only mention a few of the more common remedies as prophylactic medicines here in passing.

BELL. in the *smooth type of scarlet fever* is a perfect protection, a dose of the 30th potency once a week through the epidemic will protect one hundred per cent. In cases where the *coarse rash* is present the epidemic remedy at the time affords the best protection, such remedies as AIL., PHYT., RHUS-T. and SULPH. are most useful and sure for the ends desired.

In *Diphtheria* we have two remedies of great power as protective agents: MERC-CY. and DIPH. clinically have proven equally efficacious in affording perfect protection against the disease. DIPH. given in doses ranging from the 30th to the 10M centesimal potencies has removed the Klebs Leffler bacilli from the throats of carriers in from twenty-four to forty-eight hours and has rendered subjects impervious to the action of the Schick test in many test cases with no failures.

There are four valuable homeopathic prophylactics against *Smallpox*: MALAND., VARIO., VAC., and SARR. The best is the one nearest the genus of the prevailing epidemic. MALAND. is the best antidote to the terrible acute septicemias that frequently follow the act of vaccination by allopathic methods. For the chronic long lasting effects noted in weakened vitality with a train of symptoms and suffering following vaccination, (chronic vaccinosis), THUJ. stands supreme.

And now more important and astonishing than all the aforementioned things is the wonderful protection we have against that terrifying crippling malady of infantile paralysis in the remedy LATH. Nowhere in the medical world today can there be found the certain protection this medicine gives to those who know the benefic power of homeopathic science. In hundreds of cases in many epidemics in the past thirty years, I have seen no failure. Every child given a few doses of this remedy in the 200th potency proved immune though exposed to the epidemic influence of this dread malady and even when many of their school mates who were not homeopathically protected fell victims to the disease. Had homeopathy done nothing more than given the world this one remedy against this dire affliction it has earned its right for universal recognition and support.

Now a few remarks concerning chronic sickness and especially the wide spreading terrorizing plague of cancer. By many it looms large as if a menace to the existence of the human race, and in truth, humanity has no other hope of protection outside of homeopathic medication and procedure because Homeopathy meets the deep constitutional inherited soil tendencies upon which cancer, T.B., epilepsy and all other chronic manifestations of disease grow.

It also uncovers and cures the deep venereal suppressions caused by allopathic procedures all of which combined with the deleterious effects of coal tar drug derivatives such as allennol and luminal to produce sleep and suppress convulsions and paramoded, aspirin, midol and many more of a similar nature to desensitize against headache and other pains: all these combined with numerous serums and vaccines are the unholy product of a greedy consciousless commercialism that yields the answer to the alarming spread of cancer, Bright's disease and heart affections - the three leading causes of death in the world today.

Homeopathy alone recognizes these causes and has the means to nullify them. Those people, who have avoided the above mentioned things, and have been a few years under homeopathic prescribing will never develop cancer. Homeopathy affords a ninety-five percent protection against the development of cancer. It likewise cures above eighty percent of incipient cancer and in the majority of terminal or advanced cases it gives more comfort and freedom from suffering than can be found under anodynes or analgesics of all descriptions. We only need the chance of demonstrating to an anxious waiting world these indisputable claims of medical superiority in order to reach our place in the sun, whereby we may serve humanity in accordance with Divine Law and Order and obtain for it its pure birthright of blooming health with a longer life free from physical suffering and mental anguish.

A few observations concerning measures of hygiene in relation to the water supply of cities and towns everywhere. Throughout the United States and many other parts of the world there prevails the custom (which is universally sponsored by the medical men of the old school, who are in control of health departments) at attempts to purify drinking water by using deleterious chemicals of various sorts, chiefly chlorine fluorine and aluminum and copper sulphates. The provings of these substances by homeopaths have demonstrated the harmful and sick making power of these substances when taken over a period of time even in the smallest doses. So the health of the public is really harmed rather than helped by such measures. And many dangerous disease conditions such as kidney and heart complaints, asthmatic and respiratory diseases and the weakening of body resistence by these irritants have been coincident with a steady increase of cancer during the period these elements have been in use.

A few individual homeopaths have had the courage, in the face of great opposition, to oppose these harmful methods of water purification. But homeopaths as an organized whole have failed to go on record against the poisoning of drinking water. The time has come for us to act; no better time nor place than here and now can be had for us to formulate and present a resolution of protest against such unscientific and sick producing procedures.

Our esteemed colleague from Columbia, Dr. Valliante has been for many years, an outstanding and courageous battler against the wholesale poisoning under the guise of protecting health. He has been a constructive critic as well, offering a better, cheaper, simpler method of *really purifying* drinking water by an oxidation or Ozone process.

It is hard to believe that a body of educators and supposedly scientific men like those coming from the Allopathic School could be so dumb and stupid as to really think the chemical poisons they employ for water purification could be without harm. Also it is hard to think that those entrusted with the cure of the sick and the protection of public health could be so callous and indifferent to the suffering and loss resulting from their active support of, or at least their quiet acceptance of these deplorable methods. It is not a pleasing idea, but we are forced to believe it, that so august a body of real scientists, (they tell us that themselves without blushing) could be activated in their incessant practice of universal poisoning by the sordid influence of commercial interests. Great companies have been built up presenting tremendous opportunities of graft in the sale of chemicals; and when men permit themselves to be dominated by selfishness alone they are blind and insensate to all the nobler finer impulses for human service.

It is this same commercialism honeycombing medicine more than anything else that keeps up an unjust, yea, an unholy fight against Homeopathy with its certainty of curative action, its cheapness and simplicity of application. It has been stated by some of our allopathic friends that homeopaths are practicing an obsolete form of medicine, they are not scientific or educated, and that they are unprogressive and make no new discoveries or develop new techniques of value to the world. Such statements are notoriously false and spring from the pangs of envy and disappointments experienced by the physicians of traditional medicine that have been vanquished in the competitive tests of cure at the bedside of the sick. Likewise the brilliant results obtained in many epidemics of the past, such as cholera, diphtheria of malignant types, and in the war-time flu-pneumonia epidemic of more recent times still rankle deeply, and in little, unsportsmanlike minds stir up hatred and a form of fear, twin emotions of the coward's heart. Hence the calumnies and underhand attacks often delivered in the dark against Homeopathy and her practitioners.

It is known by all that homeopaths must have the same requirements, and pass the same curriculum in colleges to be permitted to be examined before the same medical boards issuing licenses to practice medicine. To this common general knowledge is added their own wonderful knowledge of homeopathic therapeutics and far more original work in laboratory and surgical techniques equating if not surpassing anything allopathy has given the world.

Simply because allopathy refuses to see the advantages of homeopathic teaching and practice does not alter the status of things. Allopaths who are prone to belittle and misrepresent Homeopathy should ponder over the fact that many of our most brilliant prescribers and champions have been converts from the old school.

No more trite or true description of what constitutes a homeopathic physician can be found than the definition given by the American Institute of Homeopathy; it is as follows: "A homeopathic physician is one who adds to his knowledge of medicine a special knowledge of homeopathic therapeutics and observes the Law of Similars. All that pertains to the great field of medical learning is his by tradition, by inheritance, by right."

It might be less in passing to give a definition of an allopathic or regular physician, as he chooses to be called. "A regular physician is a graduate of a regularly incorporated medical college. The term also applies to a person practicing the healing art in accordance with the laws of the country in which he resides."

In conclusion my friends and comrades, let me again remind you of the precious heritage given us to use and protect, and transmit in its purity and entirety to those who follow us. Well may we be proud to be called homeopath - no greater or more honorable title can be given to one who practices the healing art.

Our predecessors did their work nobly, under very difficult and trying conditions. Let us here resolve to emulate them to the utmost of our strength, that the ever brightening lighted torch of homeopathic knowledge may go on down the generations comforting and healing the afflicted ones of the Earth until the conquest of disease is wholly banished forever.

ALL PAKISTAN HOMEOPATHIC CONFERENCE 1952[1]

Brother homeopaths of the "All Pakistan Homeopathic Conference": Greetings. It is a great honor and an intense pleasure to address a group of homeopathic physicians wherever they may assemble. I am complying with the request of your honored and distingushed President Colonel A.S. Rajah M.D. to speak to you concerning the critical problems confronting Homeopathy not only in your country but everywhere in the world.

Perhaps the greatest hindrance to the spread and acceptance of Homeopathy is the selfish and commercialized propaganda put out by the manufacturing chemists of so-called wonder-drugs under numerous and varied trade names. All these agents are more or less toxic, but produce some minor superficial benefits that allow them to give a sales talk to an evanescent and uninformed public. And when the evil accumulated effects that inevitably follow their continued use are manifested, they are dropped as being disappointing, and a new and slightly different drug is put forth with extravagant claims of superiority over the preceding agents, to reap a golden harvest and sow the seeds of sickness and weakened vitality with an insiduous and enervating drug disease.

Every homeopathic physician knows that patients treated with these agents after the recovery from the disease for which they were treated, are left weak, nervously exausted, and anemic. And a considerable time under careful homeopathic prescribing is required to restore them to their normal state of health.

Homeopathic growth and expansion is inhibited by a lack of teaching or schools to educate and instruct students in sufficient numbers to keep pace with the needs of the sick public. It is true we have a number of post-graduate schools in existence. But because of prejudice and adverse propaganda on the one hand, and on the other hand lack of ability on our part to reach the students and doctors of medicine sufficiently to interest them in the worth and superiority of homeopathic healing, we find the going difficult and are faced with dwindling numbers and influence before the world.

This is not a happy picture, but we must face facts. Facts are stubborn things and will not fade away by wishful thinking and high sounding platitudes. We homeopaths have too long been rugged individualists, lone wolves as it were, doing splendid and often heroic

---

1. From handwritten manuscript. Address to The All Pakistan Homeopathic Conference March 1952 in Lahore, Pakistan. - Editor..

work under adverse conditions. But we will soon be extinguished if we do not rejoin the pack and organize to give the world not only ideal and rational healing but an educated propaganda of knowledge pertaining to sickness, its causes and the advantages accruing to the world through homeopathic medication.

Also should be stressed the dangers and afflictions inflicted on an uninformed world by empirical medicine from the earliest times to the present day. We need note, that in spite of so-called scientific medicine with its boastful claims of excellence in cures, there is an ever increasing death rate in all lands from the dreaded cancer scourge with kidney and heart diseases reaching first place as killers of humanity. While mental and nervous disorders, insanity, etc. are reaching alarming and constantly growing proportions. Palliative medication only adds fuel to the fire to increase the destruction. Homeopathy alone can cope with these terrors and over-whelming dangers to humanity.

But we must find ways and means to bring these truths to the people of the world and institute a benign propaganda and a campaign for rational medicine based on Divine Law against all selfish and irrational treatment of the sick. We must organize more homeopathic clinics everywhere that we may demonstrate the vastly more efficient results in cure. Of course we all know the Homeopathy based on truth and law cannot perish from the earth but its growth and spread depends on each individual physician and his patients.

Our predecessors, the pioneer homeopaths made great sacrifices and endured ridicule and persecution for the sake of the homeopathic healing art. And no sacrifice or toil must be too much for us to endure in the interest of this great truth which means so much for us and posterity.

As Homeopathy expands and grows the health of the race will improve and better types of humanity will develop bringing the day close to "the brotherhood of Man under the fatherhood of God". Indeed, Homeopathy is one of the forces in nature that along with its magical healing instills the lofty spirit of brotherhood. Wherever a homeopath goes in the world he will find in his brother homeopath a bond as close as that of blood brothers. For all cure is inspired by that Divine gift of healing direct from the Creator's Hand through His immortal instrument Samuel Hahnemann whose magnificent reason was only surpassed by his spiritual insight.

Let me say in closing that the homeopaths of the Americas extend the felicitations and best wishes for a most successful meeting.

President's Message for September, 1953[1]

Members of the American Institute of Homeopathy, you have made homeopathic progress of real worth at the convention of 1953 by inaugurating a correspondence course in homeopathic therapeutics and philosophy.

By this means we will be enabled to replenish the thinning ranks of homeopathic physicians, and give to our country the needed homeopathic service that has not been obtainable for many years. From a thousand desirable towns and cities in our land the call is constantly sounded for homeopathic physicians.

If we push this opportunity as we should, we can soon give to our fellow citizens this boon they need so badly. We should have not less than three or four of these teaching centers available, say one in Washington, D.C. (American Foundation), others in Chicago, Los Angeles and San Francisco. A good correspondence course followed by a term at the Foundation would quickly make homeopathic physicians who could practice homeopathic therapeutics efficiently and obtain superior results in cure.

With an infusion of young blood, guided by our veterans in teaching and practice, all our difficulties would fade away. Then let us all with all our might make effort to bring quickly into realization the vision that was brought to us by Dr. Harvey Farrington and Dr. Donald Gladish for the proposed course. And, more, let us accept with deep gratitude the generous offer made by Dr. Farrington for the unrestricted use of his valuable course, in my humble opinion one of the best ever devised. If we but bring into practical use this proposed teaching by correspondence, we shall be able to perpetuate Homoepathy for our children and their children and for all the future.

These are the things that make our annual conventions valuable to the profession as a whole and to each individual member of the organization as well; to say nothing of the added values that come from the exchange of ideas and experiences in application of the law and philosophy. Last, and most precious of all else in the renewed reunion of old, true friends made through the years - some of whom we will not see at the next convention because their work is done, but their spirits linger everlastingly with us in the work we all love. One thing more comes to mind, the meeting and greeting of new friends and converts to Homeo-

---

1. Journal of the American Institute of Homeopathy, Vol. 46, No. 9, p. 278, September 1953.

pathy who value and need our experience in the application of homeopathic practice.

Then let us all resolve to make preparations for attendance at our next convention to be held at Mackinac, July 18, 1954. This is a beautiful and most comforting spot and is easy to reach by boat, rail or airplane and even motor cars can get within a short distance of it. A magnificent golf course is available and fine fishing facilities can be had by those who wish to tarry for awhile after the convention - and the charm of the place is such that many will. Special rates will be given to members of the Institute and their friends, particulars of which you will receive later.

At this time I would like to remind you that the Southern Homeopathic Convention meets in late October in the quaint and historic city of New Orleans. These men are a loyal and progressive body of homeopaths who always have an excellent scientific homeopathic program and they entertain charmingly. We hope to meet most of the Institute's Officers and Trustees there, as many important matters concerning Homeopathy as a whole will be brought up at that time.

Though our ranks are much depleted from what they were in former years, never has there been such unity of purpose and real enthusiasm in our organizations because we have learned the value of a superior type of healing. The suffering world is in the greatest need of a truly scientific system of medicine based on unchanging law. In the face of all obstacles and organized opposition, we must, each and every one of us, go on with the good work so the future can bring a healthier, better, happier race of beings into existance.

PRESIDENTIAL ADDRESS FOR OCTOBER, 1953[1]

In retrospect:

The poet tells us to let the dead past bury its dead and to act in the living present, and that is sound philosophy in the main.[2] However, we can extract many useful lessons from past experiences when we are guided by wisdom. At least we can avoid making the same mistakes twice. Yes, we can do much more than that; we can turn the clarifying light of reason on the situation and find out the why and wherefore of the causes of unfortunate circumstances that may have dogged our steps along life's highway.

In 1906 the homeopathic profession was at the peak of its power and prestige in the United States. It had a considerable number of active small medical schools in various parts of the country. Its membership in the State of Illinois numbered around a thousand members; as many as five hundred attended some of our state conventions. Our men, in large part, were young or in the middle period of life; and there was vigor, confidence and self-satisfaction throughout our group. Our physicians attended the wealthiest and most influential clientele of the land. The Swifts, the Armours and the Rockefellers[3] were among some of the prominent people who preferred and employed homeopathic physicians to care for their health needs.

Then came the deluge. The pent-up waters of distrust and intrigue broke loose to engulf homeopathic interests into a plan of self undoing. This plan called for the classification of all medical colleges to be listed in accordance with the amount of endowment available to each. Superficially this seemed fair and just, but the barbed point of the poker struck deeply and painfully like the venomous tooth of the serpent to sap our strength and to rob us of the fruits from our laborious toil and constructive endeavors dating from our inception. We ended up with one Class A college which too soon was to pass. Class B and C students were unable to take State Board examinations in many states, and those who did qualify were handicapped and were practically medical outcasts and given inferior ratings.

---

1. JOURNAL OF THE AMERICAN INSTITUTE OF HOMEOPATHY, Vol. 46, No. 10, October 1953.
2. from Longfellow: "A Psalm of Life - What the Heart of the Young Man Said to the Psalmist". - Editor.
3. Dr.Alonzo Austin (star pupil of Dr. Kent) was the personal physician of John D. Rockefeller Sr. - Editor.

Gradually with only a little fresh blood coming into our organizations, homeopathic interests began to wane. Creeping age began to take its toll, and our members decreased with ever-increasing speed. A deadly concentrated propaganda extolling the value and advantage of a constantly increasing number of so-called wonder drugs inundated our time with its toxic flood of commercialism, and this has been and is an inhibiting factor in the path of homeopathic progress.

Yet, in spite of all obstructions, Homeopathy still lives and functions, born of the vitality and power found only in the undying germ of truth. This alone is our star of hope. We need waste no time moaning over misfortunes that were the results of our own weakness and lack of vision. We bought a gilded bauble in exchange for a false prestige tinseled with the moon light of lunacy. "We sold our birthright for a mess of pottage." Yet because of the truth that is ours, we live and carry on, knowing that the right and the good and the useful will prevail if we but remain true to the unchanging principles and tenets of our philosophy.

We have reached the crucial point in our existence. We must go forward with vigor, determination and sagacity if Homeopathy in America is to be redeemed in this generation. There is only one thing that can prevent this resurgence of new life of Homeopathy, and that is the lack of will to do so among its members. We must let first things come first, and our greatest need is more and more new homeopathic doctors.

In a day's time we could place a thousand homeopathic physicians in practice within our vast domain. The need is so great and so urgent that we must create the means to consumate this most desirable end. That is, we must begin now the training of homeopathic doctors to fill the crying need for homeopathic practice. Postgraduate training by correspondence may well be the beginning of many homeopathic physicians. Let us encourage all we can to take up this work as a life work worthy of true physicians. We should contact by every means all available physicians interested in Homeopathy and at the same time make known our need for many more homeopathic doctors that we can find places for.

That this is our first step for means of advancement and new growth to refill our thinning ranks and build a solid future must be apparent to all. We have the machinery for this work at hand, and only a little persistent effort is required to set the operation going.

"Let us then be up and doing

With a heart for any fate

Still achieving still pursuing
Learn to labor and to wait."

This is the song of the poet, and it is a beautiful and inspiring gem of thought. But already we have waited too long to start our march of victory on its inspiring way. Unless we bestir ourselves and become consecrated warriors in the great cause of a regenerated Homeopathy, our children and their children will suffer and cry in vain for the need of a homeopathic doctor to heal their hurts and cleanse their souls from inherited taints and constitutional ills. For here and now, let us not forget that the Lord in His mercy gave us through Hahnemann this devoted instrument Homeopathy for the healing of the nations.

President's Message - July 1954[1]

The question is often asked why the remarkable cures so frequently wrought by Homeopathy and reported in our medical journals are not given to the public through the medium of our numerous newspapers. The American Medical Association answers this question by stating that it has a working agreement with the Associated Press, that nothing relating to medical treatment, discovery or progress shall be published and given the public that the A.M.A. does not first censor, pass on, or endorse. Without the blessings of the A.M.A. the numerous wonder drugs and the many forms of coal tar drugs as well as vast numbers of proprietary pain killers and cold cures under various trade names would not have the wide publicity for their extravagant but false claims of pal-liation and cure that costs the American public millions of dollars annually[2] in exchange for depleted health and lessened vitality as a result of the prolonged intake of these things, often without the guide and regulation of a physician's advice.

The endorsement of Homeopathy would not find the vast profits that proprietary nostrums do, hence organized medicine as it stands today is not interested in a system that cures at a relatively reduced cost.

This does not imply that all physicians in practice today are entirely commercial in their work. We know and hereby acknowledge that in the ranks of medicine are many sincere, devoted men and women who give much of themselves to the service of helping the sick as the prime object of their lives.

The renumeration that is adequate for the support of themselves and family as sufficient; their satisfaction and happiness springs from the pure joy of comforting and healing their fellows. These are the truly born doctors whose interest might easily be awakened by the wonders of homeopathic science if only the proper medium could bring it to them.

The fact that any organization or group of individuals can control the organized news agencies of the country to throttle the free flow of thought and knowledge on a subject as vital as medical science is proof that the so-called freedom of the press is falacious and misleading. Because this situation exists, we must find ways and means to enlighten

---

1. "President's Message" in JOURNAL OF THE AMERICAN INSTITUTE OF HOMEOPATHY, Vol. 47, No. 7, July 1954.
2. Actually billions of dollars. - Editor.

the public about the superior merits of homeopathic medicine. Hence the reorganization of our state societies and the formation of more Laymen's Leagues everywhere over our country to bring direct to the public the plain and simple story of the homeopathic doctrines and achievements.

One news item of interest is the reorganization of the Maryland State Homeopathic Medical Society and State Medical Examiners for the licensing of homeopathic graduates in Maryland. Maryland has a fine group of outstanding homeopathic physicians who are a credit and an asset to the homeopathic cause.

The Institute is fortunate in having an unusually efficient Legislative Committee this year. This committee is made up of Doctors Seidel, Spalding, Swartwout and Sunnenblick; the four Ss standing for superior work. I wish to call attention to their untiring energy, their alertness and their loyal devotion to their homeopathic cause.

Our Committee on By-Laws and Amendments headed by Dr. John C. Hubbard is also very active and efficient.

The Committee on Medical Education whose chairman is Dr. Julia M. Green is busy with preparing a working program for a correspondence course in Homeopathy to be presented at the Institute meeting in July at Mackinac.

All these things give promise of enthusiastic and united effort to build Homeopathy up to the lofty heights it so richly deserves.

We in Chicago have the privilege and the honor of a visit from two of Argentine's outstanding homeopathic physicians, Dr. Pablo Taubin and Dr. Jaime Szuster, both from Buenos Aires. They plan to travel to the Pacific coast and visit the homeopathic doctors of that section. They inform us that there are four hundred doctors in Buenos Aires with a growing interest for Homeopathy among the younger members of their country.

As this is the last opportunity I will have to address the Institute before the meeting at Mackinac, I want to offer all my colleagues and friends as well as the business manager and his staff my heartfelt gratitude for the great help and support given me in the preparations for our next meeting with high hopes for a good attendance and a successful start in the expansion of all things homeopathic.

MEMORIAL SERVICE, JUNE, 1956[1]

Friends and companions of the American Institute of Homeopathy, another year has passed, and we meet again under the gracious care of Divine Providence to do honor and to commemorate the lives and services of our dearly beloved colleagues, whose passing has left a sense of grievous loss in our hearts. As we honor them with loving and fitting ceremonies, we honor and dedicate ourselves to the cause and ends they served so fully and so well, and we are uplifted and inspired by their devotion and faith in the service of human suffering. Because we are impressed and moved by the shining example of their deeds and accomplishments, we are strengthened to better perform our tasks of healing and sacrificial service if need be, for the good of that cause we love so completely.

When our departed friends selected the homeopathic method of healing for their life work, they chose a way beset with difficulties and obstacles not found in the regular realm of medicine. The propaganda and publicity of powerful drug manufacturers were not for, but against them, stirring up prejudice and false statements, constantly irritating them and inhibiting their activity and usefulness in many ways.

Furthermore, it must be remembered that the conscientious homeopathic prescriber must be prepared to work harder and longer on every case of illness which his special service demands, in quest of the individual curative remedy for each patient. His study and research in the Homeopathic Materia Medica is constant and unremitting during his whole medical life. All this must be his in common with the usual medical knowledge demanded by the State Board of Medical Examiners who issue the licenses to practice. Thus we see much more is required of the homeopathic physician than is by the physician who practices so-called regular medicine.

From these facts we know that our friends had convictions with the courage to defend them against all opposition; they often faced odium, vilification and ridicule from a prejudiced and misinformed public. In the face of these hinderances they carried on and wrought cures where some of the elite and accepted ones had failed. In the face of great odds by their service and works, they made friends for themselves and for the great system of healing they espoused and functioned in so well.

---

1. JOURNAL OF THE AMERICAN INSTITUTE OF HOMEOPATHY, Vol. 49, No. 6, June 1956.

They and their predecessors who came and went before them have left to us and the world a rich heritage of medical knowledge and accomplishment that will grow in power to cleanse humanity of its inherited racial ills and give the future a better race of humans destined to progress faster in their evolutionary growth toward a more perfected state. These dedicated votaries of homeopathic healing evinced an unusual courage and a hardihood of character that measured up to the best of our pioneer forebearers; no job was too difficult or laborious for them to take on in their constant rounds of duty. They often sacrificed comfort, health and material wealth to meet the demands of their work. They shed a glow of friendly confidence around them that made for human sympathy and mutual understanding and hopefulness everywhere they went, and that subtle aura of theirs was illuminated by the rainbow light of a sublime faith. Faith in the sure power of the Homeopathic law of cure and faith in Divine Providence and His merciful goodness to all. They lived in their service to their fellows not only in the letter, but in the vitalizing spirit of the Hippocratic oath; with pure hearts and understanding souls they toiled and gave the best they had to all those needing their ministrations.

Many times their emoluments and rewards in a material sense were few and inadequate to meet all their physical needs. But they found ample satisfaction and reward in giving comfort and hope to others in great need. They treasured the privilege of assuaging pain and dispelling the dark phantoms of fear more than they cared for the world's riches or its symbols of power. They patterned their lives after that of the Man of Sorrows who came to suffer and give His all that the weak and afflicted ones might be comforted and live. In the richness of such lives grew souls of inestimable worth who have left an indelible print on the scrolls of time and creation. Their lives were atuned to the deeper meaning and significance of a life cast into the vast eternity of living. They sensed and were aware of the deep imponderable and intangible forces operating under God for the creation and maintenance of universal order.[1]

They acquired a strange mysterious strength and fortitude to endure under constant wearing pressures. They also developed by the constant application of known laws in their demanding work a subtle wisdom not found in books or taught in the curriculum of colleges. As they worked in the unseen realm of cause to dissipate the changing effects in

---

1. Cf. article "Fifty Seven Years in the Practice of Homeopathic Medicine" p. 505 ff. - Editor.

Grimmer's Work

the material world, their consciousness was raised above the world of effects into the spiritual planes of existence from where all causes emanate. Hence their sense of values differed from those of the commonly accepted ones. But they knew the real from the unreal, the good from the evil, the worthwhile from the worthless. They knew that love and faith were more potent in the cure of the world's ills than are all the wonder drugs ever invented by puny man, because love and faith are the vivifying influxes direct from the Creator to promote rhythm and harmony and order throughout the Cosmos.

We are told that "by their works ye shall know them", and by the criterion we, their colleagues, shall know and revere them always. They not only healed and comforted bodily ills, but they were kindly and understanding consulars as well in times of stress and misfortune. From the first cry of the infant to the last wail of the aged patriarch they met all human needs through the long period of their service, and when their labors ended, they left in the hearts of those they had served so long and well a lasting memorial of gratitude and love to leave the world a better place than it was before their coming. To us, their co-workers and friends, who honor their memory and recall the beauty and worth of their lives they have bequeathed the solemn obligation to carry on in the cause of world healing with the same unflagging courage and abiding faith that was theirs for the same glorious cause - that cause fraught with so much good to all the children of the future because it represents law and order in medicine with an expanding philosophy of applied techniques that alone makes of continuous progress and advancement.

The world must not, cannot, loose the knowledge garnered and the wisdom developed by those sacrificing savants and pioneers of Homeopathy who gave all to usher in a better era of healing based on unchanging law versus evanescent theories based on empirical trials alone.

As we honor these dedicated friends today, let us all resolve to consecrate our lives and efforts to perpetuate and expand this truly benefic boon of healing vouch-safed by God through the inspired agency of Hahnemann and his true followers. To achieve in the cause of the good and the true brings its own reward of great and lasting happiness not known by those who covet the glamour of wealth and place it above the paths of duty and service. In closing, let us also resolve to work with the same untiring zeal for the good of our fellows that distinguished our friends that we honor here tonight and thereby preserve and perpetuate the better philosophy of healing which alone can bring about a freer and better world to live in for all the children of the future. In this way we can build the finest memorial to their worth that the human mind can conceive or the human heart desire.

Let us pray and invoke the supreme forces of good for strength, faith and wisdom to perform the duties presented to us in the orbit of our lives and works. Above all give us sympathetic hearts and understanding minds and sharpened sense to better meet the needs of the afflicted ones who come to us for succor and comfort. Equipped with these heavenly attributes we can better bring a share of added knowledge to the great fund built up by our predecessors whose precious memories and achievements we are privileged to gratefully receive and honor here tonight. Imbued with the same faithful spirit and desires that fashioned their glorious lives and devoted to the needs of human suffering, we cannot fail to bring an added luster to the cause of Similia.

The Doctor of the Future[1]

It has been stated that "coming events cast their shadows before". As we gaze over the field of medical accomplishment up to the present, we note much confusion, uncertainty, and disappointment in the cure of diseases afflicting humanity in their many different forms.

True, epidemics of disease have been mitigated by the use of hygiene and sanitation, including better sewerage disposal, but not by medical treatment. This observation applies especially to typhoid, malaria, and yellow fever for which sanitation and mosquito control sufficed to lessen the ravages of epidemics. Specific remedies for these and all other diseases stated by name have proved disappointing in curative power, producing only dangerous suppression and inimical side effects that have added misery to the suffering of natural sickness and complicated the road back to health with additional obstacles more difficult to contend with than the illness itself.

The wide-spread employment of serums and vaccines in the past three decades (with its three major wars[2]) for the presumed prevention of acute epidemic disease has inoculated the race from the cradle to the grave with an insidious toxemia that deprives the blood of much of its defensive power against the more deadly resistant chronic blood diseases, like the many forms of cancer, anemia, kidney and heart diseases - all of them exacting a terrible toll, not from the aged and worn out alone, bout also from multitudes of those in early middle life, the most productive period of human endeavor, who are victims. With their activities and uses aborted and lost, with forced invalidism, suffering, and material and economic loss thrust upon them and their families.

Of what avail to prevent acute diseases by doubtful means when such diseases are self-limiting in action with good chances for recovery by the unassisted power of the body defense mechanism? Then why endanger the health and well being and even the lives of multitudes with dangerous and subtle poisons that can and do bring on many destructive disease conditions that are difficult or even impossible to help when they become established in the economy? Only the manufacturers and vendors of these harmful things, who with their paid propaganda of false and extravagant claims of cures and benefits to a misinformed public, can keep such iniquities alive for profit.

---

1. From handwritten manuscript, exact date unknown. - Editor..
2. World Wars 1, 2 and the Korean War. - Editor.

In some states, laws have been passed compelling people and their children to submit to inoculations against their wishes, depriving them of the heaven-born right of free choice in medicine and preventing the free exercise of their constitutional guarantee of protection in their pursuit of happiness and liberty of action. We have now come to a place in our social order where the individual has lost all right of choice in the care of his body which is sometime called "the temple of the Lord". Yet the holy place is profaned with laboratory filth, in poisonous form, against all protest of logic and experience so that the coffers of the powerful drug interests may be constantly replenished.

Not only is our blood polluted with sick-making agents, but the air we breathe is loaded with disease-producing elements from the marts of industry. While our water supply is poisoned with dangerous, life-destroying chemicals by our so-called guardians of health, our food is processed and adulterated, thus greatly impairing its nutritional value which also tends to impair health. Adding to all these things the fallout or radiations resulting from the testing of atomic weapons is another threat to racial health and well being, especially to the new incoming generations of humans because of the effects on the genes. We are indeed beset by a multitude of health hazards that present a gloomy picture for the health of the race in the near future, unless these hazards are recognized and means taken for their elimination and control.

These pressing and vital aspects of medical facts are being voiced by upstanding medical men from many quarters, and soon new and more rational concepts of sickness and cure will evolve in the practice of the healing art.

Now is the time and the place to demonstrate to a distraught and confused medical world the certain efficacy of homeopathic medication. We have a certain safe and easily applied protection against the ravages of polio in our often tested remedy, Lath., which has been one hundred percent effective in the hands of many homeopathic physicians during the past fifty years. Homeopathy holds the key that will unlock the door of that sanctuary of knowledge, the use of which will free mankind of the race-born inheritances that stem behind all chronic manifestations of sickness, including cancer in all of its dread aspects.

It is in the realm of prevention that we can do our most effective work against kidney and heart disease, cancer, arthritis and the numerous forms of baffling mental diseases existing everywhere around us today. That does not imply that we cannot cure them with our methods when they are presented, but it is so much easier to prevent these things than to cure them because much time and labor are involved in the processes of cure and because some of these cases have advanced too far and built up extensive pathologic changes in vital organs making a cure impossible. But even in such cases, Homeopathy can give longer life and more comfort than any other means known to medicine.

In the lives of children and young adults, it is a God-sent blessing rounding out a fuller, more competent and healthier life for the best performance of its uses. Even in declining age, it is a great comforter and helps prolong life, strength and ambition far beyond the average time alloted today.

Because of these things, the doctor of the future will put aside preconceived prejudices concerning the treatment of the sick and seek knowledge and help wherever it may be had and use it for the good of his patients and the glory of himself. He will be a teacher as well as a healer and provide his charges with the necessary knowledge of both mental and physical hygiene, scientifically proven diets, sanitation, directed physical exercise, and all the other assets for the attainment of normal living. He will improve his own growth and ability to cure by the study and the investigation of all established and generally recognized means and methods of healing outside of his own accustomed and narrow groove of medical practice. He will cease to be bound and restricted by the static limitations of custom and tradition. He will break the shackles of so-called medical authority and become a free soul responding to the light of reason wherein his every step forward and upward will be guided by the sure compass of principle and law. He will seek the causes of sickness, find and remove them as the first step in the realm of cure.

When he has advanced this far on the road of progress, his eyes will be opened to new and beautiful vistas reflecting Divine Goodness; and undreamed truths of Cosmic unity will be revealed that will help him become a fit and valuable instrument of healing for the benefit of his fellows and the achievement of his own happiness. When he has traveled this far in his search for the crowning diadem of healing and can rejoice in its attainment, he will have acquired the clarity of vision and the wisdom essential for the evolution of a homeopathic physician.

Let us not forget that Homeopathy in all its detailed ramifications and purity rightly belongs in the broad field of medicine to be used by all for the good of all. Hahnemann made every effort to have it accepted and incorporated as a progressive part of medical science, and many of his most enthusiastic followers have endeavored to bring about the same ends. Today every homeopath should ask nothing more than the recognition of the law and the philosophy that has evolved throughout one hundred and sixty years of practice and clinical experience. We feel that these things are priceless to the race and must not be lost and that they should be preserved and developed for the use and well being of all the future.

Through the circumstances of necessity, the physician of the future will be both a teacher and healer and get back to the ideals conveyed in the Hippocratic oath to live a life of purity and service, free of the urges of avarice and content with an emolument sufficient for his needs and rewarded by an enduring love and reverence from all those he is privileged to serve.

THE POWER OF PROPAGANDA[1]

In the world of the past and the present as well as that of the future, the mighty force of propaganda shapes the destinies of men, all organized institutions and things.

We need but recall the spectacular rise of men like Adolph Hitler and Benito Mussolini to an undreamed zenith of power by means of intensive propaganda. And because it was evil and selfish in character, they fell and perished in shame and humiliation. Wrought with their ruin came suffering and impoverishment for all mankind.

On the other hand, we may note that the rise and spread of all religious philosophies, including our own Christian doctrines, are born, nurtured and grown by the power of a benign propaganda to bring hope and righteousness into the lives of the multitude. Because it is based on unselfishness and is compatible with Cosmic law, they shall continue to grow and function for "good and truth" through the everlasting realm of eternity.

In the sphere of things related to healing and medicine, we can see this same potent force of propaganda at work around us today. Some of it is good and true, but much of it is false and evil. A factor of interest to all is the steady growth that the nonmedical cults of healing such as the naturopaths, sanipractors, chiropractors, osteopaths are achieving. Because these practicioners have much that is good and useful (although not enough to meet all the needs of the deeply sick), they will grow, prosper, and abide in the place where their special uses are required. On the other hand, traditional or old-school medicine in spite of constant intensive propaganda is slowly sinking and dying of a corroding dry rot that will soon spell its doom as a system of medicine. This comes as a result of false propaganda based on superficial empirical knowledge apart from law and order.

Behold the disappointing and even baneful effects of the so-called "wonder drugs" now too numerous to mention, but all launched under false claims and producing destructive reactions on the human economy often of a more serious nature than the illness for which they were given.

With these observations before us, we wonder why Homeopathy based on eternal law and with a highly developed philosophy of practice does not grow but is fast declining in numbers and patronage. The

---

1. "Editorial" in THE HOMEOPATHIC RECORDER, Vol. LXV, No. 1, July 1949, p. 18 f.

answer is as clear as the shining stars of heaven. We failed to employ the mighty force of a good propaganda to which the homeopathic concept of healing lends itself most forcefully and appropriately.

To summarize: *The Homeopathic Law of Similars* is but one of nature's unchanging laws. The knowledge of homeopathic principles is obtained by experimenting on well human beings, proving of individual drugs given to produce an image of illness with all its signs and symptoms. Hence the empirical practice of trial and error on the sick has no place in the homeopathic field of practice or experimentation. No dumb helpless animals are tortured or done to death, nor are sick humans made sicker in the search for healing knowledge.

Homeopathy heals gently, safely, surely and permanently. Homeopathy heals without leaving in its wake any consequential drug disease. It is a boon in cases of burns, cuts and bruises, broken bones. Also, bones that will not knit because of disease or weakness heal with alacrity under the chosen remedy.

In the fields of acute and chronic disease, Homeopathy stands at the head without equal. Even in incurable disease it has proven the most efficient and comforting palliative known. Degenerative diseases like heart and kidney affections occurring so often in early middle life (the time of greatest use and productivity mentally and spiritually if not physically), will obtain greater comfort and longer life under homeopathic care.

In the realms of preventative medicine, Homeopathy is most effective because its use builds the human being into a state of harmony with his ever-changing environment, as well as increasing his resistance against acute infectious disease by removing susceptibilities to allergies of all kinds.

Homeopathy is the only force in nature that can antidote and irradicate inherited toxins and soil conditions that spring from tuberculosis, syphillis, sycosis and even cancer. Hence, an intelligent application of the homeopathic law can and does prevent cancer and all other degenerative diseases afflicting the race today.

Homeopathic prophylaxis in severe acute disease is the most efficient and safe method at humanity's disposal ever discovered. Epidemic diseases such as small pox, diphtheria, scarlet fever, whooping cough and poliomeylitis may find the most unfailing protection ever known by the gently yet forceful and certain action of the homeopathic epidemic remedy.

In the dark hopeless realm of mental sickness of all kinds, Homeopathy is the only force that can cope successfully with the threatened destruction of the human mind. The fearful increase of mental sickness demands Homeopathy's balm of healing where nothing else in the world of medicine can help.

The world is in dire need of these facts pertaining to the healing power involved in the homeopathic law, an attribute of Divine Goodness for sick humanity languishing in hopelessness and suffering. What will organized Homeopathy do about giving the world this much-needed propaganda of medical education of the true concept of sickness, its causes and cure?

Organized Homeopathy will do what each individual homeopathic physician wills and does in this vital and stupendous project. If we are to survive as an organized society of healing, we must act at once and in unison. Ways and means should be discussed and planned at the coming convention at Cincinatti, and the plans that are made executed with thoroughness and dispatch.

It is necessary that every homeopathic doctor give this matter deep and concentrated thought for the consummation of this work. The time is ripe now, for the world senses the need for a more effective art and science of healing without the deleterious effects resulting from empirical or the regular school of medicinal practice.

Homeopathy's Contribution to the World of Medicine[1]

Most of the real advances and progress of modern medicine have come as a result of applying the cardinal principles of Homeopathy, too often in a crude and materialistic sort of way. To mention a few instances: the application of vaccines and serums against small pox, polio, rabies, diphtheria, typhus fever and tuberculosis. While the side effects of these agents have been severe in many cases and with some fatalities, enough success has been obtained to verify the efficacy and accuracy of the law of Similars.

Had our friends of the old school followed the Hahnemannian technique into the wonderful realm of infinitesimals and potentizations, they could have obtained infinitely better results with no deleterious side effects resulting, thereby proving the law of Similars and the incomparable advantage accruing from the use and application of Hahnemann's method of attenuating remedies used for the cure of human sickness.

For the past one hundred and fifty years, Homeopathy has successfully antidoted the ill effects of vaccines and serums and also has supplied successful antidotes in attenuated form against the diseases aforementioned with no sudden deaths from anaphylactic shock or no long, lingering suffering so often the results of vaccines and serums administered for protective purposes. In the past fifty years poliomyelitis has been highly amenable to the homeopathic remedy both curatively and as a highly successful prophylaxis. In ninety percent of the cases for which it was employed, it was successful; and many thousands were, without a single exception, immunized against polio.

Homeopathy has given the medical profession an unsurpassed method of case history taking with few variations as it was introduced by Hahnemann himself. This method is now employed in every hospital and clinic in the world today.

The influence of Homeopathy on medical practice has been tremendous and most outstanding as seen in the prescribing of the single dose and in the abandonment of polypharmacy. Another notable and ever-growing procedure in medical practice is the gradual reduction of medicinal doses, approaching in some instances the infinitesimal. Thus we see some of the progressive steps toward homeopathic concepts taken by general medicine in recent years. The tendency to study the

---

1. From handwritten manuscript, March 9, 1957. Read before Bureau of Homeopathy, American Institute of Homeopathy, June 12, 1957.

individual patient and to strive to find a remedy suited to each patient, rather than the disease, is strictly homeopathic.

The recognition of the importance of allergies as causative agents in many forms of sickness, together with the susceptibility of certain patients to certain drugs, foods, pollens and many other disease-producing substances, is a cardinal homeopathic tenet now accepted as true by modern medical science.

Since the days of Hahnemann, the drug THUJ. has not only proven a curative and prophylactic agent against smallpox, but it is also one of the most reliable and effective antidotes against the evil effects of smallpox vaccination which has produced more chronic sickness and suffering than has smallpox itself. Only the unprejudiced homeopathic physician is able to recognize the widespread and far-reaching mischief that universal vaccination has brought upon the race, mischief which Homeopathy alone can eradicate.

The world now knows that the sanitary engineers have done more in preventing the spread of infectious and epidemic disease than any other factor in the world. We need but cite yellow fever, malaria, typhoid and typhus fevers to prove this statement. Where good sanitary conditions obtain, epidemics of diphtheria and scarlet fever are less virulent and more easily brought under control. The serum shooter claims credit for the decreased virulence or incidence of these diseases; but the credit really belongs to better sanitation and hygiene.

One of the logical objections to all serums and vaccines is the fact that they are disease-producing proteins to which many individuals are allergic. A physiologic reason against this form of protection is the fact that the vaccines and serums are foreign proteins and, when introduced into the blood stream, can be a source of great danger to health and life itself. The great wonder is how one familiar with these facts and one trained in hygiene and taught to avoid all forms of sepsis and contagion could bring himself to the position of deliberately polluting the human blood stream, fresh from the Creator, with laboratory filth. Is it because some half-baked[1] savant has labeled such an act scientific? Or is the desire for sordid gain, regardless of result, the motive for the practice of this unholy traffic in human misery?

The ugly force of commercialism now dominates the activities and practice of modern medicine; powerful organizations made up of the pharmaceutical houses and manufacturers and dispensers of proprietary drugs are reaping huge sums of money annually from the sale of many

---

1. i.e. inexperinced or stupid - Webster's Dictionary. - Editor.

varieties of antibiotics and pain-killing and mood producing drugs. These organizations dig deeply into the lives of millions in such an adverse way as to threaten the moral, mental and physical stability of the nation.[1] From the vast profits these organizations amass, they are able to control the policy of organized medicine and to employ the vast facilities of the press, radio and television for publicity and propaganda purposes. These vicious nostrums that are undermining the strength and competency of the nation could not long exist but for the endorsement and blessing of organized medicine.

Claims have been made that there exists an understanding that nothing medical in the way of new discoveries or cures or that any medical subject can be printed for the public's consumption without the sanction and censuring of the American Medical Association. One thing is sure: any medical article written for the enlightenment of the public by a physician not recognized or endorsed by the A.M.A. would not be published by any member of the Associated Press. Because such conditions exist, it is not possible to enlighten the public concerning medical abuses and false claims and statements concerning the efficacy and use of manufactured or proprietary drugs.

So many Americans have gloried in the freedom and independence of our so-called "free press"; but if things medical that are of interest to all can be controlled and obliterated from the public by a biased group, even though that group be the majority, it is obviously a most unhealthy and deplorable state of affairs where not only individual liberty but all liberty is endangered.

Many physicians of all schools of medical thought deplore the present low and unscientific status of medicine as it is today but they are afraid to attack the evil because of the organized power and wealth behind it. Unless some effort is made by the real physicians to correct the conscienceless cupidity of commercialism in medicine where progress is throttled by organized selfishness, we will decline to the level of the dark ages in things medical.

From these aforementioned facts, we can see why the wonderful achievements in cure by Homeopathy can never reach the public for its enlightenment and benefit. Only our adversities and loss of schools and prestige are stressed by them; and these were brought about largely from the corrupting machinations of the powerful drug syndicates whose deathly influence controls state legislators, organized medical

---

1. See for example: Coulter, Harris: Vaccination, Social Violence and Criminality: The Medical Assault on the American Brain, North Atlantic Books, 1990. - Editor.

societies and a venal press, who are willing to further a false, misleading propaganda clothed in scientific language to mislead and confuse an unsuspecting and gullible public for the sole purpose of amassing more wealth and power extracted from the millions suffering from the many hazards to health and life from poisoned food, poisoned water, and poisoned air - all impregnated with the destructive forces of radiation from the continued explosions of the atomic and hydrogen bombs and all these hazards aggravated by blood-corrupting, mind-destroying drugs manufactured only for profit.

Not only our atmosphere is saturated with these deadly forces; but every ocean and all the creatures in them, every lake and river and likely every drop of water anywhere on earth is polluted with radioactive poison. And all animal and plant life is already imperiled by this destructive force. In the face of the widespread menace, some of our so-called scientists have the brazen audacity to tell us there is no more radiant energy around us than a watch with a radium dial would give off. How can we accept such men as authorities and guides when instruments of precision inform us that all animated nature is now already reeking with radioactive poison?

Even now it may be too late to stop experimenting with these deadly playthings that man in his egotism created for his own destruction. If the folly of these drastic experimentations can be stopped in the next few months, homeopathic science can furnish humanity with an adequate antidote to this universal poison and in time restore a sick world back to a normal level. PHOS. and a number of the STRONTIUM COMPOUNDS, namely the carbonate, phosphate, iodide, bromide, and nitrate compounds properly prepared and given in potentized forms and given on individual indications, in ascending potencies with properly spaced doses, will prove to be the only effective antidotes sufficient to cope with the deadly radioactive poison that now threatens to exterminate man and all his fellow creatures from the earth. It might well be that this is the test needed to convince an unbelieving world of the truth of homeopathic claims of its superior efficacy in the realm of healing.

Recently many cases of sickness of a baffling and insidious nature have appeared. They are difficult and resistant to medical treatment. Such illness has been ascribed to viruses for which no remedies are known outside the tenets of Homeopathy. The medical world has not yet awakened to the awful danger now already upon us of universal radioactive poisoning with its more remote effects on future generations because of its drastic action on the genes.

Homeopaths, get ready for the battle. Put on your armor and sharpen your best weapons, for the needs of humanity will be multiplied a hundredfold, and your strength and courage will be tested as never before in the great battle for survival that now faces us. All other hazards that have beset us in the past are trivial compared to the one you soon will be called upon to face. Let our watchword and our faith be God and Homeopathy.

In closing, it is fitting to note that Homeopathy's contribution to the world of medicine has brought more than new discoveries and advanced concepts; it has brought higher ideals that come from better understanding and closer bonds of sympathy with sick humanity. These ideals can have no traffic with the selfish aims of commercialism, which places profit above duty and selfish gain before service.

The ideals of Homeopathy, like those of the early votaries of the healing art, have ever embraced the principles of faith and reverence and unselfish service in the broad realm of cure. We believe the physician of the future will come back to the saving grace of unselfish service which distinguished the physicians of ancient Greece which gave to the world Hippocrates, truly the "Father of Medicine".

Postscript

The occurrence of radioactive rains in various parts of the world at various times recently should be sufficient evidence to convince everyone of the wide prevalence of the subtle poison polluting even the upper stratas of our atmosphere. These radioactive rains, falling on the grass and herbs growing in the earth, have carried sufficient toxicity to produce radioactive milk in cattle that ate the grass which was made radioactive by the rains precipitated from the clouds formed in the upper layers of the atmosphere.

Our criticism against the trend of modern medicine for its descent into the mire of commercialism is offered for the constructive purpose of helping to restore medicine back to the high ideals and uses it once treasured and lived by in the glorious past.

If the Russian's proposition to discontinue the experimental testing of hydrogen and atomic bombs is sincere, it is hoped for the good of all the world that the United States and Great Britain will speedily join in that resolve and bind themselves together in a pact to interdict the practice of exploding both the atomic and hydrogen bombs and thus save the peoples of the earth further suffering from the deadly fallout which follows the exploding of these bombs.

To Members of the House of Representatives Washington, D.C.[1]

We, the undersigned citizens of the State of Illinois, respectfully petition that the medical regulations governing the personnel of the United States army and navy be so amended to grant soldiers and sailors in the service the option of refusing the various so-called immunizing inoculations now imposed on every recruit regardless of his own rights and beliefs in such medical procedure.

The appalling recent casualty list of 28,000 cases of sickness with 63 deaths from the yellow fever inoculations alone, in spite of the supervision of what was considered the best medical minds of the service, is convincing proof of the dangers of such purely experimental methods. Medical science has safer and more efficient means at its disposal in the use of certain specific drugs for protection against all the tropical and epidemic diseases to which the armed forces may be exposed.

The evil lasting effects on the health of great numbers of the nation's defenders both in World War I and II have created a sense of fear against the drastic procedure of injecting foreign proteins directly into the blood stream because such procedures are contrary to the laws of physiology and hygiene. Some soldier and sailors have preferred imprisonment and disgrace to the pollution of their blood by laboratory products of disease.

"Freedom from fear" is one of the freedoms we are fighting to maintain, and this war's outcome shall determine whether or not it will remain with us. And it is highly essential and vital to our cause that our defenders, their dependents and loved ones be assured that such freedom shall be no longer denied them.

The right of choice in medical matters where the issue is purely speculative and empirical should be given to the individual in the interest of this great cause of human freedom now engaging the efforts of the whole world. Such an assurance of individual right and peace will add greatly to the country's war efficiency and render our deeds consistent with our claims that the fight is one for human liberty in all its ramifications throughout the social order.

---

1. From handwritten manuscript, about 1950. Letter written to the Members of the House of Representatives. - Editor..

Homeopathy's Friendly Enemies[1]

Since its inception, Homeopathy has had to contend with secret enemies masquerading as friends within its ranks as well as its avowed antagonists without. Men advocating the combination of a number of remedies in a single prescription (combination tablets) and the use of drugs only in low potencies or in crude form exclusively was the first almost mortal wound that split the homeopathic ranks wide apart and left scars remaining after sixty years.

The second blow came after a fair degree of recovery and harmony had made Homeopathy a respected and growing institution with a large number of flourishing colleges in all parts of the country and an increasing number of students and physicians annually produced and patronized by many of the wealthiest and most influential families of the nation. Then a few homeopathic leaders were persuaded to permit their colleges to be accredited and classified by old-school medical authorities as a friendly gesture. It was claimed this action would bring peace and harmony in the whole ranks of medicine and make for progress.

Every homeopath now knows the sequence of that treacherous deal. From many flourishing colleges we now have two; one of them only recently dropped the name "Homeopathic" from its title; hence no real homeopathic physician can hold anything but contempt and disgust for a faculty that could so betray the great trust reposed in it by converting the funds raised and designed to teach Homeopathy to the coffers of the old school for the purpose of teaching only so-called regular medicine. Really only one of all our colleges of the past remains. However, the new Hahnemann College of the Pacific is the most recent additon to our cause where the names Hahnemann and Homeopathy are cherished and used proudly and defiantly.

For the past twenty years the oligarchy of the American Medical Association has sought membership in the ranks of homeopathic graduates, requiring them not to practice medicine, as they term it. In other words, they (the Homeopaths) could wear the collar of bondage by foregoing the precious birthright of free thought and free expression of principle and action. Thus, by a process of benevolent assimilation, they sought to swallow and digest all homeopathic organization, but they have only succeeded in acquiring a case of severe indigestion. For

1. "Editorial" in THE HOMEOPATHIC RECORDER, Vol. LVII, No. 2, August, 1941, p. 102.

somehow, those who once bask under the benign light of the homeopathic sun find it impossible to forget its warmth and truth.

The latest proposition from one in our own ranks is to drop the name "Institute of Homeopathy" and substitute for it the "Institute of Therapeutics", thereby appeasing the old school and making ourselves acceptable for membership in the A.M.A. Those who attended the recent convention of the American Institute of Homeopathy know how completely that proposition was repudiated by the great majority of its members. Not only that, but the Institute and the whole homeopathic fraternity found itself cleansed and regenerated and infused with new life by the sloughing off of the many decadent barnacles from the body politic. Much credit is due for that herculean job to Dr. McKenzie and the forward-looking men and women supporting him throughout that ordeal. That we have some in our ranks who sincerely believe that a union of the homeopathic school with that of the traditional school of medicine would be beneficial for all, as well as make for general progress, is true without a doubt.

But a slight review of the recent past in medicine should convince all that such a union would be most disastrous to homeopathy and detrimental to the progress of the old school itself. Whatever progress that has been made by old-school therapeutics is due to the direct influence of the homeopathic concept of sickness and drug application to the same. Beir of Germany and McDonald of England are two noted instances of the complete acceptance of the homeopathic dogma in its entirety by acknowledged leaders in old-school medicine. All progress in the world of thought, philosophy, science, medicine, politics must come by the clash of opposing concepts even though one side to the controversy constitutes a minority.

We homeopaths need but remember that the truth for which we stand and strive for is the greatest unifying and most progressive force in the world today. Homeopathy ministers to all God's children regardless of race, creed or station. It rests on the solid foundations of philosophic truth, and its key word is service.

It came to us by sacrifice, courage and faith of the founders. It is our privilege to carry that shining torch even through dark and rugged ways and to transmit it undimmed to those of the future for use in the development and fruition of the great new race of beings soon to appear on earth.

We cannot, we will not fail to carry the enlightened banner of Homeopathy unsullied and victorious over grinding greed and blind prejudice.

HOMEOPATHY, A BOON TO CHILDREN[1]

Children are the special wards of our Saviour as babes who come into a harsh, rugged world from an abode of heavenly innocence to grow and learn through earth experience the lessons that love and truth can bring them. Though born in innocence and purity of Spirit, they carry the seeds and forces of inherited evils, sin and disease in their physical bodies. Verily, the sins of the fathers do visit and afflict through many generations.

But the mercy of the Lord is ever present and never failing. His love passeth all understanding; only in the Word can we grasp the significance of the power of love. Love is patient and kind; love is not emulous of others. Love is not insolent and rash, is not puffed up, does not behave in an unseemly manner, does not seek its own, is not quickly provoked, does not impute evil, does not rejoice at iniquity but rejoices with the truth, bears all things, believes all things, hopes all things, endures all things. Love never fails. (Corinthians 13)

From its first breath, the child has the unflagging protecting love of its parents to nurture and guide its life through infancy and early childhood to the time of maturity when it becomes an independent being equipped to face the exigencies of life. Parental love under God also supplies the love of teachers, religious instructors, medical care, friends, companionship and all the spiritual and educational needs of the normal human being. All this and more are supplied by influx from Divine goodness.

Medicines produce natural cures by their action on the wondrous autonomic nervous system, that complex defense mechanism of the body organism, a replica of Divine Order and perfection, used in the protective and regenerative processes of life.

As life progresses in infancy with growth and body development, mental and emotional changes manifest themselves; and traits of character begin forming. This is the time and stage of most vital importance in the life of every human being born into the world. It is a time where every constructive agency available must be employed to establish a character that is benign and harmonious to grow in a physically healthy and normal body.

A cursory glance at the aspects of early life, fresh and innocent and so recent from the heaven world, might lead one to infer that the sched-

---

1. From handwritten manuscript, exact date unknown. - Editor..

ule for a good and useful life is easy to establish. But intermingled with all the innocent beauty of childish life and happiness, like weeds springing up and growing in a bed of flowers, come thoughts of selfish desires to dominate, to hate, to commit cruelties and even to kill insects and small animals, to tease and torment their playmates and to fight and contend for selfish ends.

Many physicians and psychiatrists have rejected the claims of that great leader in psychiatry, Freud, that most mental and moral irregularities and abnormalities of character have their causative origin in the sexual sphere, but multitudinous observations from numerous and various scientific sources have confirmed these claims. The sexual nature and urge (so closely allied to the creative fiat) insure the purposeful ultimate in the scheme of all created nature. As long as that urge flows in normal channels and is satisfied in reciprocal union with its counterpart, nature's end is obtained, and health and happiness result.

When physical irritants and inherited constitutional miasmatic toxins supervene, vicious harmful habits develop to undermine the whole moral and physical being. Sex symptoms and urges begin to manifest very early in child life; and under the impact of the forces mentioned above, the habit of masturbation in members of both sexes may be formed to later lead to more ruinous states and weaknesses. The earlier in child life preventive and constructive measures are instituted, the better chance there is for the development of a healthy normal child amenable to all the influences wrought by the sciences superimposed by the all-powerful spiritual laws of God.

In the light of the conditions that exist common to child life, the use and value of circumcision come up for consideration. The ancient rites of the Jewish holy men mentioned so forcefully and extensively throughout the Old Testament and also in many books of the New Testament, suggest a spiritual significance, figuratively spiritual purification; physically, an aid to fecundity. Mohamedans also practice this rite. Aside from the religious aspects, circumcision does remove the possibilities of local irritations intimately associated with the autonomic nervous system by way of the terminal nerve endings. Irritations occurring at this vital place can disturb the function of the whole economy, which, if not corrected, may end in organic disease or in severe types of mental and moral disturbances. These irritations are not confined to males only. Female children often suffer from a hooded clitoris with binding and restricting adhesions which can be the source of severe irritation, sufficient to produce convulsive states even to an alarming degree. Epileptic states have also stemmed from this source. Before leaving this subject, it is well to stress the need of unusual care and skill in correcting these conditions. If the operative measures are poorly done, a worse condition can result with more adhesions and scar tissue present than existed before the attempted corrective means were made. When physical causes have been corrected and habits of hygiene and cleanliness have been established, the homeopathic physician is able to do his best work for these little ones launched on the rough seas of life and buffeted by the winds of adversity and suffering.

Very recently we have been appalled by the accounts of rape and murder perpetrated by very young adults. These tragedies with the wide circle of suffering involved make all this a subject for serious thought concerning causation and the possible prevention of recurrences of these evils.[1] We believe the solution for this problem is largely medical and that homeopathic medicine carefully and skillfully applied along with the measures suggested, together with very early religious training, can prevent such horrors. The child must be taught the sacredness and the use and purpose of his organs of generation. He must be made to realize as soon as possible that he is the custodian, under God, of a wonderful power which, if conserved and preserved for its intended use, can be the source of physical, mental and moral power giving him strength and courage with a sense of well being and sheer joy in life. But if wasted and perverted, will lead to weakness and degeneration physically and spiritually.

To get back to the medical aspects of our subject. Only remedies capable of removing or antidoting the inherited miasmatic toxins common to the race can harmonize the life force of these little ones to build healthy lovable minds to dominate and control strong, healthy bodies to serve and bless the future.

SULPH., being the king remedy of the anti-psorics, is the first remedy to be given in a series of potencies, preferably from the thirtieth to the ten thousandth only to be interrupted by acute remedies in case of some severe acute condition arising. The first dose should be given very soon after birth.

I would choose MED. as the best anti-sycotic remedy to follow. Many good prescribers might prefer THUJ., which could well be better indi-

---

1. The work of Harris L. Coulter shows a clear connection of criminality with vaccinations. See his book: Vaccination, Social Violence and Criminality: The Medical Assault on the American Brain; North Atlantic Books, 1990. - Editor.

cated in some cases. The reason my choice is MED. is because one of its prominent symptoms is the marked tendency to masturbation, especially in children, in which condition it has produced curative results many times. Suppressed sycosis is all too wide spread in the race; and when it is complicated with psora, we get the most intractable types of sicknesses which often require a series of complimentary remedies to unravel them and cure them. Sometimes a series of potencies may be required of each of the remedies given. Only as the case evolves under the action of the remedies can we act with precision and certainty.

Homeopathic medicines are especially adapted to the needs of the growing child in the formative stages of his life where the impetus in the right direction can mean so much in terms of character as well as in his physical well being. The type of character formed in the child determines greatly the kind of destiny under which he will develop. It is apparent that homeopathic medicine is essentially a medicine of prevention. With the eradication or even the modification of the deep inherited miasms, the vital force is left free to perform its important life functions to the fullest bringing health and happiness to the being that can be blessed by the highest type of homeopathic prescribing.

The Father in Heaven has given His children not only life and love but, under the inspired instrumentality of Hahnemann, the priceless boon of homeopathic healing for world-wide use. Let us perfect ourselves in that use and pass it on for the good of the children of the future.

HOMEOPATHY AND MEDICAL PROGRESS[1]

Every little while the world is the recipient of a new and wonderful medical discovery. Recently the newspapers were full of praise for what was said to be a new discovery in the form of the curative properties found by medical scientist in the African plant STROPHANTHUS HISPIDUS, which contains the substance found in the pituitary glands of pigs: Cortisone, the new and wonderful specific for rheumatic and arthritic diseases of severe types.

Homeopathy discovered STROPHANTHUS, proved it and found its action specific in rheumatic and cardiac conditions. These facts were published and given to the world by Dr. John Clarke of London in his *Dictionary of Practical Materia Medica*, 1902, vol. III, pgs. 1286 - 1289.

About five years ago several old-school physicians by way of newspapers came out in glowing terms about the efficacy of RHUS TOXICODENDRON for the cure of poison ivy. Over a hundred years ago Hahnemann proved RHUS-T. and gave us an extensive account of the curative power of the remedy in a wide variety of illnesses including severe skin afflictions besides that of rhus poisoning.

Another discovery made by allopathic scientists a few years ago was that of the venom of the Moccasin snake *(Toxicophis)*. This venom was found specific for persistent chronic nose bleed and acclaimed one hundred percent efficient.[2] Again if we refer to Clarke's *Dictionary of Practical Materia Medica*. We will find the effects of the bite recorded which brought out an annual periodicity of the symptoms of pain and toxicity at exactly the same repeated time for many years. In common with all the snake poisons, hemorrhage is a marked condition because of the profound effect that is produced on the blood elements and constituents by the venoms.

Before Pasteur introduced his rabbit serum for hydrophobia, Dr. Constantine Hering had potentized and proven the salavia of the rabid dog and made cures of hydrophobia - that remedy is called HYDROPHOBINUM or LYSSINUM.

None of these discoverers of new medical wonders ever mention Homeopathy, although in every instance it preceeded their announced discovery from fifty to a hundred years. We would suggest to our brethern of the old school that, before any more announcements of new mir-

---

1. "Editorial" in THE HOMEOPATHIC RECORDER, Vol. LVII, No. 7, January 1942, p. 360.
2. See article "Homeopathy's Future" p. 524 ff. - Editor.

acle drugs are made by them, they avail themselves of the medical wealth only to be found in the archives of the *Homeopathic Materia Medica*. In this way, they may avoid the odious status of plagiarism in the future and at the same time find much material to expand their medical knowledge for the benefit of themselves and their patients.

MEDICAL PLAGIARISTS [1]

Every little while the American public is given a shot in the arm via the daily press in the form of a so-called new scientific medical discovery of unusual value as a more or less specific cure for some stated condition of illness given a diagnostic handle.

Not long ago, some New York doctors, members of the old school, claimed to have discovered that the venom of the Moccasin snake (TOXICOPHIS) was of great value for the condition epistaxis in severe forms actually curing the majority of the cases treated.[2] A little before that time, other old-school scientists announced they had discovered wonderful curative powers in cases of epilepsy from the application of the rattle snake venom and of Lachesis, venom of the South American snake. It is only a record of history of Hering's heroic proving and introduction of LACHESIS in the year 1828, and the first published cases that were given the world in 1835. So one gets a fair idea of the pace of progress made by traditional medicine one hundred years after Hering had published his researches on this venom. Old-school scientists give to the world a fragment of Hering's incomparable knowledge and appropriate it as their contribution to the world of medicine.

A couple of years ago another plagiarizing scientist of the old school gave the world by way of the daily press a discovery of the marvelous curative powers against angina pectoris contained in the venom of the black widow spider (LACTRODECTUS MACTANS). If one will refer to the *Homeopathic Recorder* of July, 1889, he will find the account of this wonderful remedy introduced by Dr. S.A. Jones and Dr. A.J. Tafel, purely homeopathic sources.

And so it was even with the great Louis Pasteur with his semi-homeopathic ideas of administering the virus of rabies by attenuating it through the media of rabbits' spines and giving it hypodermetically to patients bitten by a rabid animal to prevent the development of the disease. Pasteur's work was antedated by the homeopathist Hering many years in applying the virus of the dog in potentized form (LYSSIN or HYDROPHOBINUM) by mouth for the prevention and cure of rabies. Hering's work along these lines was first given the word in 1833.

Very recently an old-school doctor proudly announced to the world that he had made the discovery that RHUS TOXICODENDRON poisoning

---

1. THE HOMEOPATHIC RECORDER, Vol. LIV, No. 1, January, 1939, p. 47.
2. See article "Homeopathy and Medical Progress" p. 627 ff.

could be cured by small amounts of the RHUS TOXICODENDRON extract. Samuel Hahnemann made the first proving of this drug early in his homeopathic work, and from that source comes our most complete knowledge of the drug's curative values.

In the light of these facts pertaining to medical discoveries, one wonders at the amazing egotism as well as the stupid duplicity of such members of a moth-worn, weather-beaten system of medicine and ethics. Also one must be impressed with the startling contrast existing between an antiquated and chaotic conglomeration of empirical procedure and a system of medicine based on law and order.

HOMEOPATHY AND PROGRESS[1]

Prior to the advent of Homeopathy, the world of medicine was in a state of chaos and confusion made up of illogical and conflicting theories concerning life and the cause and cure of disease. Dietary science and sanitation were non-existent. Anatomy and physiology were only beginning to emerge from the foggy realms of ignorance and superstition. Pharmacology still reeked with the damp musty air of the dark ages. Surgery was largely performed by barbers and rated little above the menial tasks of society. Psychology and psychiatry were yet undreamed of. Only a rampant and irresponsible and conscienceless empiricism made up the practice of medicine.

Hahnemann was among the first to distinguish between what he termed indispositions[2] caused by faulty diet and unsanitary living conditions, poor ventilation in the sleeping rooms, etc., and true disease - either acquired or inherited. The former needed only the correction of living habits and environment to restore health; while the latter required the careful selection of the homeopathic remedy to restore harmony in the flow of the life force to produce a healthful state of the whole body. Thus from the practice of Hahnemann and his followers was born dietary science and later a program of sanitation where clean and purified living conditions would obtain to eventually bring into being a system of sanitary science which now exists in every well regulated community throughout the civilized world. So that now pure air, proper food, measured and tempered sunshine, together with correct sanitation constitute a generally recognized medical procedure essential for the insurance of health.

Hahnemann was a pioneer in the humane treatment of the insane and in recognizing the physical conditions associated with mental failure. The numerous cures of so-called incurable mental disease made today by the homeopathic law all vindicate the existence of the great law of similars. These beginnings have markedly changed the attitude of dominant medicine regarding treatment for the insane. Today every hospital in the world follows the Hahnemann scheme of case taking and record keeping. Hahnemann stressed the importance of mental and emotional symptoms in the taking of each case of sickness, and for the selection of the indicated remedy gave them the highest value.[3] Today

---

1. "Editorial" in THE HOMEOPATHIC RECORDER, Vol. LIX, No. 12, June, p. 493.
2. §150 Organon. - Editor.

the new sciences of psychology and psychiatry are coming much to the front, and we hear a great deal about the baneful effects of frustrations and fixations on health states. We are told how fear, anger, hate and greed all change the chemistry of the body fluids and thus impair health. More and more the materialistic-minded scientists and doctors are beginning to see and acknowledge the power of intangibles on health.

The studies of Crile with his concept of the electrical man and the reactions of Abrams, now just beginning to be accepted at Yale, although called by another name - viz. bio-electric phenomena - are only approaches to the Hahnemannian doctrine of the vital force so long the butt of ridicule by the uninformed.[1] Perhaps after another hundred years of growth and progress, modern science will discover for itself the great truth and fundamental principle of the homeopathic law.

In the meantime, the humble and unselfish homeopathic physician must carry on with his prescribing and teaching and give the succeeding generation of young doctors, any of whom may evince interest in the law of healing versus empirical and uncertain medical procedure, the certain knowledge that Homeopathy alone bestows.

Verily we are but torch carriers to light the way along the path of medical progress for the physical salvation of the future. Though the way be beset with strain and stress, the reward is great if we but succeed to pass on to the future the accumulated medical knowledge from Hahnemann until now. Our children and their children's children will crown our efforts with gratitude as they receive the incomparable blessings and happiness of radiant health. In that sweet time warfare will give way to peace and good will among all men under the common Fatherhood of God.

---

3. Organon, §210 - §213 - Editor.
1. See article "Recent Concepts and New Formulas in Medicine" p. 679 ff. and article "Importance of Electronic Reactions to Future Medicine" p. 683 ff.. - Editor.

Homeopathy in Chronic Disease[1]

Old-school doctors have a trite saying that "a large percentage of sufferers from acute disease will recover without the aid, and often in spite of, the physician's treatment through the mystic life forces of the body organism".

We hear much about antibodies' inherent powers of resistance that confer natural immunity against acute infectious disease and induce curative results in many cases of acute sickness.

But in the realm of chronic disease, we hear another story: only palliative measures of doubtful value are urged here. Neither the natural forces of the body organism nor the artificial powers and methods of scientific medicine can avail against the resistless and inevitable march of chronic disease.

That which cannot be surgically helped nor palliated must take the ever downward descent into the abyss of suffering and death; and surgery at best is useful in removing piled up pathology too far advanced for medicine to remove or help. Such surgical palliation, however, can in no way be regarded as a cure.

Such in brief are the aspects of modern scientific medicine which bring to a suffering world a minimum degree of help and a maximum amount of laboratory technic and consequential expense.

In spite of the so-called progress of medical science, degenerate diseases of the heart and kidneys, cancer, T.B., and mental and nervous disasters all are constantly increasing in virulence and numbers. Epidemic disease alone has been stemmed, not by any medical process but by the application of hygiene and sanitary science.

On the other hand, the homeopathic speciality in the field of medicine, both acute and chronic, presents a picture of amazing success both as a cure and a prophylactic all through the whole realm of epidemic disease. Flu, pneumonia, rheumatic fever, diphtheria, yellow fever, and typhoid and typhus fever of the past have yielded to the certain power of the homeopathic law. But it is in the sphere of chronic disease that the "Law of Similars" takes its most definite place as a cure for disease, and because of this high place in the service of suffering and sickness the world must soon be compelled to recognize and accept it because of its high use and worth in the treatment of disease.

---

1. The Homeopathic Recorder, Vol. LXII, No. 8, March, 1947, p. 285.

Commercialized interests in medicine are the chief reasons that prevent its spread. But an awakened intelligence among true physicians of all schools of healing as well as a better informed public will soon bring an upheavel in homeopathic education and practice that will mean a real and lasting triumph in the whole realm of medicine responding to the benefit of sick humanity everywhere.

Medical Mistakes[1]

Among the numerous demands for money from a public already over burdened with taxes and ever-increasing numbers of charities is the insistent drive for funds by the medical profession to be used especially in research for cancer and heart disease.[2] These medical groups work subtly and under the dark cover of a fear propaganda to achieve their ends, employing sub-groups from women's clubs, fraternal and church organizations; and even the theaters and moving picture shows are invaded with pleas for money to be used chiefly by laboratory specialists and technicians to seek the cause and cure of cancer and heart disease.

For the past twenty-five years or more "intensive research", as it is called, has been operating in the hands of ultra scientific medicine for those objectives. Millions of dumb animals have been tortured and killed in animal experimentation; numerous serums and vaccines, filthy products of disease, have been produced and used experimentally in the vague hope of a cure; but only polluted blood streams and worse sicknesses resulted. Countless numbers of hapless victims of cancerous disease have been subjected to deep x-ray and radium burning only to have agony added to misery and hopelessness piled upon fear and despair to end in impoverishment and utter ruin. The cost of these twenty-five years of fatuous and fruitless research has run into billions of dollars because modern medical thought and procedure lack philosophic law to direct their efforts into rational channels, hence the resulting chaos and confusion of their work.

Pathological end results of perverted life processes have been mistaken for and accepted as disease causes. So long as medical effort is directed to the effects of disease and not its cause, that long must their efforts be in vain. Only by the sane approach of working from cause to effect can success in the cure of any or all sickness be obtained. Only by a philosophic grasp of living processes related to environment can we know anything about the realm of causes and their effects. Only by the orderly force of biologic laws can morbid processes be arrested and restored to a harmonious action of health processes. Before the implacable scourge of cancer is subdued, medical efforts must get back to the

---

1. THE HOMEOPATHIC RECORDER, Vol. LXIV, No. 1, July 1948, p. 19.
2. And today there are drives for many other chronic diseases. - Editor.

simpler but well known laws of sanitation and individual hygiene, together with the rational science of diet and nutrition.

To make a beginning advance in the age-long battle of man against his most relentless and unconquered foe, medical mistakes and short-comings of the past must be cast aside as wreckage and debris and be destroyed so that the way may be cleared for the better and stronger forces of knowledge and achievement to follow. The polluting of the human blood stream with the by-products of disease, serums, vaccines and animal extractives must cease to be given before health can abide in the human body. For at least a generation, the universal administration of these inimical products from the cradle to the grave has been lit-erally forced on a patient long-suffering public with the result of a steadily increasing volume of degenerative diseases such as Bright's dis-ease, cardiac disease, cancer and an alarming increase in mental and nervous disease, all of a chronic and incurable nature.

The unbridled advertisement and sale of pain-killing, sleep produc-ing drugs, all coal tar derivatives, depressants and blood destroyers such as the barbitol, anacin, midal, phenacetin and numerous others must be stopped, or more jails and insane institutions must be steadily provided to care for the ever-increasing flow of mental incompetents these things produce. Physicians of all schools of medical thought must forego any pecuniary benefits from the use of these things and organize to make a united effort to halt these appalling evils that threaten to destroy civili-zation if not the race itself. This threat is far more real than the threat of atomic warfare with its dire consequences because it is less patent to the lay public and more subtle in its approach. Another generation of these evil forces operating unchecked in the race will leave little that is worth-while for even the atomic war fare to destroy. Outraged nature will exact the supreme penalty death - for the orgy of sin and broken law indulged in through ignorance and indifference.

Physicians will do well to get back to the fundamentals of life and wisdom taught them in their infancy at their mother's knee: Truth and power emanating from faith first vouchsafed by a mother's love to her young, fresh from God's eternal fount of mercy and goodness. Let them dig deeply into their reasoning minds and recall the God-given attributes inherent in every human being for growth development and repair after injury, shock or disease and behold a true reflection and likeness of their Creator. Let them trust more to the mysterious and ever-active and alert life force with its power to restore and harmonize rather than pervert or subdue its action by injecting foreign and poisonious materials into the crimson tide of life to carry morbidity instead of the materials for health to cells and tissues of the organism. Let them be teachers to teach the power of right thinking and right living and the harm that comes from wrong thinking and living. Teach of the evils that come to those who live by the impulse of unholy desires and blind passions. Teach of the dangers to health that ungrounded fears and untrammeled anger may bring upon the body. But above all, teach them, the children of man, of the power of faith in God over the ravages of disease; tell them of the healing and regenerating force of unselfish love. Do these things, and never again will they profane the temple of the Lord, the human body, and blood stream with impure disease-laden material bringing suffering and sickness by its presence. When these things are done, they are then fit to become a true knight in the army of healers.

Then will their hearts and minds be open and prepared to receive the sublime teaching of homeopathic philosophy with its practical application of the only known law of cure. *Similia, Similibus Curantur* with its vast armamentarium of proven remedies to meet the numerous causes of each individual sickness the physician is called on to treat. This way the physician of the future will not only excel in the cure of disease but be supremely superior in the field of prevention both in acute and chronic manifestations of sickness. Homeopathy is eminently potent in the prevention of cancer and all other forms of degenerative disease.

To attain his greatest success in healing, the physician of tomorrow will make use of every force available in nature, and he will operate in accordance with all law on every plane - spiritually, mentally, emotionally and physically. For these laws are co-relative and function in unison to maintain the harmony and unity of the Cosmos.

HOMEOPATHY AND NATIONALIZED MEDICINE[1]

The recently elected administration is pledged to a program of nationalized medicine involving an outlay of billions more of the already overburdened tax payers' wealth to meet it. But the thing that concers every homeopathic physician most is what will be the status of Homeopathy itself within the frame of such a program?

Will he be permitted to practice his special brand of medicine under the nationalized program of medicine? Or will he be compelled by law to practice allopathic medicine under the supervision of political office holders appointed by the government? These are but a few of the vital questions we should consider individually and collectively and seek with all diligence the answer - if there be such.

Our institutions of instruction are gone, but our organized societies remain; and through them we may find the means of obtaining recognition to the God-given right to practice the medicine of our choice, even in a socialized medical order. Our leaders should already be consulting with astute legal minds to pave the way by law to give those citizens desiring homeopathic medicine that privilege, and also to grant homeopathic doctors the right to serve those desiring such service.

It would be well to inquire from our homeopathic colleagues in Britain just what has happened to Homeopathy and to homeopathic physicians under their nationalized system of medicine. We already know what has happened to the general practitioner; he is reduced to such straits that he cannot support his family.

Homeopaths, let us unite and work together as we never have before for the preservation of the greatest and most scientific concept of medical approach the world has ever known.

Humanity must not be deprived of this benign and precious force of healing balm. All the effort, sacrifice and toil of those fearless sublime men and women who went before us, our teachers and leaders, who founded the science and perfected the art of prescribing for the sick everywhere in all lands must not, cannot be in vain. The matchless outstanding works of Materia Medica and homeopathic philosophy cannot perish or be destroyed. For these priceless things we all should give our all, if necessity demands it. Let everyone of us begin to work and organize to discuss ways and means to protect the great privilege of being a homeopathic healer.

---

1. THE HOMEOPATHIC RECORDER, Vol. LXIV, No. 8, February, 1949, p. 223.

One very important move is for each one of us to get the names of our patients on a petition expressing preference for homeopathic medicine and treatment. We should be able to obtain at least one million names which will impress the legislators sufficiently to entertain the proposition of having homeopathic practice incorporated and recognized in any law enacted.

Come on, brothers and sisters, let us hear from you. Put on your thinking caps and send letters and ideas to the Recorder Editorial staff for our common use.

THE CALL OF DUTY[1]

We still get calls for homeopathic doctors from far and near. Too may of the old boys and girls who have been the bulwark of homeopathic practice and teaching the past thirty years are leaving us at that inevitable summons none can evade; and there are no substitutes to take up their work. They did a wonderful job with their lives dedicated to the service of their fellows. They brought hope and comfort and good fortune to hundreds and in that way procured for themselves much happiness.

But they were remiss in one very important thing: they failed to provide healers for their faith to take up their work when they no longer could respond to that sacred call of duty, whose clarion note had been the moving force of their lives over the years. They were so busy meeting the problems of their busy lives they did not make the effort or give the time to train young, eager students in the art and science of homeopathic healing.

We cannot recover the lost opportunities that were ours when the homeopathic sun was shining high in the heavens and success attended all our efforts. Like the improvident grasshopper we lived in the golden present and gave no heed to the needs of the future. But vain regrets for lost changes and misspent time will not mend our fortunes. If similar conditions and circumstances for success no longer exist, we must devise ways and means to create them, because the cause is precious and the need for that cause is urgent and great.

Let the world know by every means possible how great the demand is for homeopathic physicians. Then start the processes of training and perfecting them in the art and science of homeopathic practice and finally placing them in contact with the clientele that is eagerly waiting for their services. There is no other way left to us to preserve Homeopathy for the future. Let us all give thought and effort to this vital subject.

---

1. "The President's Message", JOURNAL OF THE AMERICAN INSTITUTE OF HOMEOPATHY, Vol. 46, No. 11, November, 1953, p. 344.

Homeopaths Can and Will Do Their Bit[1]

Our world is now divided into two definitely antagonistic groups. One is the aggressor and predatory group made up of purblind[2] slaves driven by mad unscrupulous blood-lusting dictators, the perpetuators of ruin and utter desolation of not only the material riches but also the spiritual and intellectual values that have been built up during five thousand years of slow painful evolutionary effort of man in his journey from the primitive state to the present time.

The other group comprise those who love the principles of freedom of thought and speech for each individual and for each nation without unjust hinderance from any source. Those who live by a tolerant and free interchange of thought with all their fellows everywhere. Those who believe in orderly government based on the consent of the governed. Those who select their rulers not as unbridled dictators with the power of life and death, but as equals and servitors in the commonwealth of equal rights. Those who stand one for all and all for one, a banded brotherhood under the Fatherhood of God. Those who, though they loathe the horror and devastation and filth of massed murder called war, hear the clarion call of human rights sounded now and for all the future, and for all races of men to unite them in a solid phalanx of righteous resistance against the slavish tools of would-be universal tyranny.

The United States is now a member of the free nations and peoples striving against the agressor group and has dedicated its powerful resources materially and spiritually for the eradication of tyranny and brute force from the earth and for the establishment of all those precious things summed up in Liberty, Equality, and Fraternity. Our country is the melting pot of the nations where men of every clime and race and shade of devotion and philosophy have gathered from the four corners of the earth to live in peace and in tolerant regard and mutual respect. All are imbued with gratitude for these privileges they enjoy, and today stand as one in loyalty and strength and courage for service in defense of those inalienable rights that millions died to create and maintain in a warring world.

As homeopathic physicians whose lives have been dedicated to the high mission of conserving human life, the beastiality and destructive-

---

1. The Homeopathic Recorder, Vol. LVII. No. 7, January, 1942, p. 360.
2. Purblind = slow in perceiving or understanding - Webster's Dictionary. - Editor.

ness of total war is abhorrent beyond words to describe. But duty to the God-given cause of human freedom will enable us to see above and beyond the thunder clouds and the consuming flames of war to the shinning rainbow of a just peace. With such a goal enshrined in our hearts and souls, we stand ready for any service and any sacrifice needed for the great work at hand.

Because of special training and equipment in the realm of internal medicine, it is regretable that our homeopathic doctors could not be assigned to strictly medical cases, especially those of epidemic disease such as flu and pneumonia wherein homeopathic prescribing has scored such notable successes in past epidemics. And were it possible to have a homeopathic medical unit or base hospital for strictly medical cases where the great advantage of specific homeopathic prescribing could be obtained, it would prove a fortunate asset in the saving of many soldiers' lives.

But even if these things are not realized, we all stand ready to serve in any way or assignment required of us. Even those of us who cannot serve at the active front will be doubly needed in civil centers because of the shortage of doctors sent to the front with the fighting forces. And it would be well for us to organize our efforts for the emergency that now is here. Soon we will have to meet a more subtle and devastating force (epidemic disease) than the legions of war.

Let us instruct our public first against the certain dangers of self-medication which is so constantly and blatantly advertised by radio and other means. The warning against the coal tar drugs such as aspirin, the barbitals, the salicylates and many of the other so-called miracle drugs - all of which can be obtained without a doctor's prescription in most places - cannot be too strongly or too often mentioned because such drugging is one of the underlying factors in a highly increased death rate in flu and pneumonia.

Those homeopaths left in the home centers must keep in communication in order to develop quickly the epidemic remedies in the different sections of the country if our best results are to be obtained. One of the little things that nevertheless is highly important is the homeopathic antidotes against the evils of serums and vaccines. The experience from the last war and of this one up to the present has enabled us to relieve much suffering with the use of Bry. This remedy is especially efficacious against the typhoid inoculations.

Lastly, we homeopaths can provide each and all of our soldier and sailor friends with a small case of a half dozen remedies with a few cardinal indications for the use of each remedy. A nice and very frequently needed brief list of remedies to which others may be added is made up or ARN., ARS., BRY., CARB-V., GELS., EUP-PER. and SULPH., all in the 30th potency. These remedies will cover not less than eighty percent of the flu colds. When the epidemic remedies are known, it will be very easy to provide protection for any number of people even without seeing them.

Let every homeopathic doctor get in line, resolved to do his bit for the duration of the emergency; and results will justify the need of preserving homeopathic methods and concepts.

HOMEOPATHIC OUTLOOK FOR THE FUTURE[1]

Members of the Illinois State Homeopathic Society, colleagues and friends, it is both a privilege and a pleasure to address you on this happy occassion.

Our subject concerning the status of Homeopathy is especially interesting and vital to us all. Most of us here today can look back some thirty years and recall Homeopathy as an independent, militant, expanding minority group in medicine, well organized with numerous active colleges, efficiently run and turning out an annual supply of young doctors more than sufficient to replace the older adherents that may have dropped out. We were also supplied with many high-class medical journals to meet all our needs, and better still our clientele were the wealthiest and most influential among the country's citizens.

Today we stand the remanent of the Old Guard of that grand army of homeopathic physicians that sprang up in America from a small group of homeopathic physicians of unusual ability and tireless energy and irrepressible enthusiams. By the sheer power of their incomparable healing, they built colleges and hospitals, established periodicals and medical societies that spread over the length and breadth of our nation. They added new remedies and new provings and built up new techniques in homeopathic research to expand and perfect the homeopathic Materia Medica and philosophy. Their myriads of papers on clinical medicine and confirmed cures make up many volumes of medical lore of priceless worth which must be preserved for the future. That is one reason why our state societies must be maintained by however few of us that may be left to carry on. This picture of slow, steady decline in our fortunes can in no sense be encouraging.

But there is another side for us to note and ponder on. Traditional and empirical medicine is today in a most chaotic state. The ballyhoo and extravagant claims made for the so-called healing power of the wonder drugs and antibiotics have not only fallen down as flat failures of cure, but they also have become the number one health menace according to some of the leading physicians of the old school, producing conditions of disease (especially intestinal) for which they have no remedy.

---

1. Held at the meeting of the Illinois State Homeopathic society, probable date June 1954. JOURNAL OF THE AMERICAN INSTITUTE OF HOMEOPATHY, Vol. 47, No. 8, August, 1954, p. 239.

The too-frequent application of the antibiotics renders them inert against the bacteria that the initial doses of the drug at first contolled. We are told certain bacteria are needed to control and inhibit some of the more deadly fungi and viruses that invade the organism at times; when the balance between the bacteria and viruses is disturbed by the antibiotics, new and terrible disease conditions obtain as a result of this imbalance between germs and viruses.

With the so-called progress of medical science with its numerous massed inoculations constantly taking place from the cradle to the grave, together with the deadly sulpha drugs and ever-increasing varities of antibiotics, the race is fast becoming cancerous - that is, that part of it not afflicted with heart and kidney disease or mental incompetency.

All these maladies have increased to an alarming percentage of the population in the past thirty years, since 1917 when the United States went into World War One. From this, we plainly see that medical progress is impotent against cancer, heart and kidney disease and mental deterioration. These killers and destroyers move on with increasing deadliness, unchecked and untouched by anything empirical medicine has to offer as an agent of help or restraint against the implacable onslought of disease everywhere about us.

Homeopathic medicine is the only agent in the world today adequate to cope with the disease conditions that beset us on all sides. Homeopathy in conjunction with proper hygiene and sanitation together with correct dietary measures alone can save the world from its massed, suicidal tendencies imposed by many forms of state medicine.

Polluted air in highly industrialized areas, poisoned water supplies from the compulsory use of harmful chemicals put into the water by edict of law and municipal regulations. Inoculations which are blood poisoners (the product of disease itself) for the vast array of every acute disease known and tabulated constitute some of the disease-making causes afflicting us today. Because Homeopathy removes causes - constitutional and environmental - is the reason for its success where other methods have failed. From these cited facts, we can see why Homeopathy can survive through adverse times and circumstances; it is nurtured by the fountains of eternal truth, and it will rise again and again to face the tyranny of error.

Because Homeopathy and homeopathic physicians are needed so badly today to meet the dread scourge of disease in its hydraheaded forms is reason enough for us all to put forth our best efforts to restore this boon of the healing art, not only to its recent past glory but to the sunlit heights of supreme medical achievement in terms of cure. From our predecessors we have inherited a mass of precious knowledge built up for us with infinite toil and great sacrifice. Shall we, the custodians of that knowledge, permit it to lie dormant and useless while so many sufferers languish and perish for the need of it? Or shall we go forward in the face of obstacles and opposition as the brave pioneers of Homeopathy did in the early years of its inception?

Here in this land of ours, a few dauntless souls imbued with the love of truth in a few decades built up a wonderous and complete new system of healing, founded colleges and hospitals, launched periodicals, formed state and local societies that covered our nation from ocean to ocean and spread beyond our borders to our Canadian neighbors on the North and our Mexican neighbors on the South.

What a few men accomplished with nothing but their own indomitable will and courage, we, their privileged successors and benefactors, surely can do, armed as we are today with the means and instrumentalities they created for us to use in the great cause of a truly natural healing art. Already organized Homeopathy is at work planning to educate more physicians in the homeopathic way and to enlighten an anxiously waiting laity of the superiority of homeopathic medicine that cures without leaving consequential injurious side effects and at a cost that is within the means of the humbler members of society. In fact, the mounting costs of medical service are fast becoming a serious economical factor of our time. The reduced financial aspects involved in homeopathic medicine may well be one of the impelling forces compelling universal acceptance by the public and governmental agencies as well.

In Europe, in India, in Mexico, Brazil and Argentina, Homeopathy is spreading fast with well equipped colleges and agencies to educate and license a constant stream of new, young physicians to expand and enrich the ranks of Homeopathy in all these respective countries.

Now is the time for us to move on the wave of homeopathic upsurge that is occurring everywhere in the world today. We cannot fail because we are strong in the knowledge that our cause is implemented by the force of the unchanging natural law of Similars. The complete picture of Homeopathy's past and present status presents an aspect the nature of which depends on what we homeopaths do now. If we begin building and organizing our forces constructively, we can start an upsurge in our fortunes that will place us on the highest pinnacle of success to attain wide public recognition.

We need to widely publicize Homeopathy as a superior method of cure minus any side effects. Laymen's leagues, magazines and bulletins regularly and discriminately sent out to the proper and most susceptible places and people can accomplish much useful help to aid us in our aims. We must educate and obtain many more homeopathic doctors and help place them in strategic places all over our country. To do these things, we must organize and build up all our homeopathic medical societies - municipal, state and national into enthusiastic, militant groups who are willing to work and make sacrifices in time and money for the consummation of these ends.

With the accomplishment of these desirable ends, viz. the recognition and establishment of homeopathic medicine as an important asset to general medicine for the good of all. Such recognition will insure the future welfare of all posterity and lay the groundwork for a healthier and better race. The realization of this desirable boon will be ample reward for all the effort and sacrifice we may make to obtain it.

Resume[1]

Resume of the tentative program for the Congress of States Meeting at the Hotel William Penn, Pittsburgh, Pennsylvania, February 2, 1947, from membership, with ways and means to maintain and increase the same and with a streamlined constitution with omissions and inconsistencies corrected; thereby to govern our organization and its individual members along truly democratic and representative lines and to guarantee and safeguard the rights and privileges of all as well as to inculcate a sense of duty and loyalty in an awakened and united body of enthusiastic homeopaths who will then proceed successfully to the goals set by our worthy and ambitious president, Dr. I.S. Moyer.

With membership secured and enlarged, especially with a sizeable transfusion of young blood in that membership to add strength, vigor and enthusiasm to the councils and activities of the veterans who have carried on long and well in the great cause of homeopathic medicine in America in the past one hundred years.

With such a start, we may pass on to hospitals, interns, resident physician, etc.; but such will hardly be available before the subject of Homeopathic Post Graduate education is met and successfully established. The well known and highly competent doctors selected as essayists on this most important subject will leave nothing unsaid or undone to bring forth a complete program for the establishment and maintenance of Homeopathic Post Graduate education which is the very keystone of all future homeopathic development and growth in the United States.

"Protection of the Homeopathic Practitioner in His Rights as a Physician" by Dr. Seaver Smith[2] is timely and most vital to our very existance; for without equal rights and privileges with all other schools of healing, Homeopathy as a school would soon cease to exist. Any infringement of the right of any individual homeopath should immediately bring forth the influence and power of our several homeopathic organizations to the front in a determined legal fight to right such wrongs and ensure justice and fair play for all homeopathic practitioners. By maintaining our own selfrespect and fighting for our rights, we will gain the respect of even those who cannot agree with our principles.

---

1. JOURNAL OF THE AMERICAN INSTITUTE OF HOMEOPATHY, Vol. 40, No. 8, August, 1947, p. 274.
2. From the JOURNAL OF THE AMERICAN INSTITUTE OF HOMEOPATHY, exact date unknown. - Editor.

Grimmer's Work

Homeopathic education must be second to none; a broadly educated physician develops into a better homeopathic physician. The doctors selected for essays on this subject are all renowned teachers of broad experience which insures an excellent program for homeopathic education.

"Research Work to Develop and Prove the Fundamentals of Our Homeopathic Law" by Dr. Charles Bryant and Dr. Harry W. Eberhard is a stupendous job and one that is rich in possibilities beyond the dreams of an Edison.

The consummation of this task will place Homeopathy on its rightful throne of dominance in the world and vouchsafe to suffering humanity the benign boom of homeopathic healing.

MEDICAL LIBERTY[1]

We are told that the war now devastating the world is being waged in the cause of universal human liberty, enlightment and happiness; versus slavery, degradation and despair.

We have also been told that we have four freedoms or legal rights bought by the blood and tears of our country's founders. These fundamental freedoms have been specifically names as "the right of free speech, including a free press; the right of public assembly, the right to vote and choose our public servants or rulers, and the right to worship God according to the dictates of our own conscience."

Unfortunately the founders of our great and beloved Republic failed to give another freedom equally important to the common citizen and more essential to the public welfare than all the others combined for reasons mentioned later on. This fifth freedom would give every citizen the right of choice in the selection of his own medical treatment and the right to accept or reject any experimental medical cult or system of treatment for human ills that his intelligence and reason might dictate. With this added freedom operating throughout our land, greater efficiency and contentment would prevail in the ranks of all industrial and social life, and greater progress in the successful treatment of all disease conditions would obtain because of a free and unrestrained competition among the various systems and advocates of the healing arts.

Such free competition would soon prove to the world the best system of cure for ailing and sick humanity, and society could then more accurately place each system and method of healing where it could accomplish the most good.

Under the present social set-up, a small minority of organized medical men dominate all medical thought and treatment. This is especially true in the army and navy where a medical political machine appoints only those of its choice and prevents the representation of all other systems of treatment from participating in the care of the sick. And more pernicious still, this same clique at the suggestions and behests of various manufacturing pharmacists and chemists are polluting the blood stream of the nation and its defenders with the various products of disease, serums and vaccines under the guise of prophylaxis against certain specific diseases.

---

1. "Editorial" in The Homeopathic Recorder, Vol. LVII, No. 10, April, 1942, p. 518.

To this is added the baneful effects produced on the body politic by the numerous coal tar drug derivatives, barbitals, etc. with various sulfanilamide types of drugs for the suppression of pain and fever. All these drugs are acknowledged to be blood destroying agents by those who use them; yet the public is encouraged in the persistent and universal application of these poisons through the propaganda via radio and the daily newspapers instigated by commercialized manufacturers and vendors of these pernicious things.

Thinking men of the United States are asking why, in a country professing equal rights for all its citizens, is a minority permitted to deprive the majority of having the privilege and the right to choose their own doctor and kind of treatment suited to their needs. Christian Scientists and many non-medical cults, such as osteopaths, chiropractors, naturopaths as well as minority medical groups such as the homeopaths and eclectis, all are compelled to submit to high-handed medical dictatorship that is repugnant to their reason and principles of life and ruinous to their health and well being.

Another question asked by these thinking and investigating men relating to public health is especially important at this time. Why, in the light of so much organized and scientific medicine, is heart and kidney disease together with cancer and insanity increasing so rapidly?

Surely empirical medicine with all its boastful science has proven a weak reed for ailing humanity to lean on. Its greatest blessings have been a golden shower to the manufacturers of chemical nostrums and laboratory products of disease that poison and pollute the blood stream of the infant, the growing child and the young adult and end in premature old age and sudden death.

While we are engaged in the glorious struggle of free men and free women against the tyrant and the oppressor, we will do well to secure our all-important rights vouchsafed us by the founders and preservers of the Republic. And still better, if all the disfranchised groups in medicine would unite as a voting unit, we could then secure just and equal rights for all that would make for better public health and increased security, happiness, and prosperity.

We believe these criticisms are just and constructive in nature. For what avail is the lavish expenditure of money and time, consumed in acquiring a scientific education that is designed to equip one with the essential knowledge and training to treat the sick, when those so prepared turn dispensers and peddlers of proprietary rubbage produced solely for commercialized purposes and profit?

And this evil fearfully aggravates the situation by adding to the natural diseases of man the frequently more dangerous calamity of drug and serum-born diseases throughout the whole body politic.

Even the old-school doctor stands rigidly for his right to treat his patient as his conscience and his reason dictate without interference from any source.

THE MENACE[1]

One hundred and sixty-three years ago, a dark and slave laden world was electrified with hope by a proclamation stating that "all men are created equal, that they are endowed by their Creator with certain inalienable rights, that among these are life, liberty and the pursuit of happiness. That to secure these rights, governments are instituted among men, deriving their just powers from the consent of the governed, that whenever any form of government becomes destructive of these ends, it is the right of the people to alter or to abolish it and to instate new government, laying its foundation on such principles and organizing its powers in such form as to them shall seem most likely to affect their safety and happiness".

Within the beginning paragraphs of that immortal document of human rights, the American Declaration of Independence, there is contained philosophic truths that have not only enlightened and inspired our beloved country from its inception but has fired the whole Western continent by that flaming message of human liberty. The whole world, even into its remotest corners and darkest places, has vibrated these clarion-like reverberating words of truth and justice that echoed back to heaven over that never-to-be-forgotten 4th of July, 1776.

Following the tenets of that document, a great nation dedicated to those principles and consecrated to those truths was founded. A nation whose shores have been a haven and refuge for the oppressed of all lands. A nation unequaled in progress and spiritual power whose very name carries the magic import of peace, security and happiness, where men of all beliefs exercise freely their God-given rights and dwell together in mutual respect and without anxiety.

Today we are confronted with another document, a proposal to change the letter and the spirit of the first, which has been our guiding star these one hundred and sixty-three epoch-making years of the world's progress. On July 28, 1937, Senator Lewis, Democratic Senator of Illinois, introduced Senate Joint Resolution 188 providing for the following: It shall be compulsory for physicians to render any medical aid requested of them by the indigent Bills for such services shall be paid by the Social Security Board. Jail sentences of three months and fines of not over $1000.00 or both for doctors who decline their services, make excessive charges or try to collect from the patient.

---

1. "Editorial" in THE HOMEOPATHIC RECORDER, Vol. LIV, No. 5, May, 1939, p. 45.

Senator Lewis says we are to have not State medicine but Federal medicine, that every doctor must take out a federal license in addition to his present qualifications, that the profession is to be placed in the position of complete obedience to Federal law, that doctors must serve the citizen, that their compensation is to be fixed by some board - which he piously hopes will not be political - that this board shall also have power to pass on the quantity and quality of professional services and the number of patients that the doctor shall care for daily.

When the medical profession is reduced to a state of servile obedience to the whims of politicians, how long will other professions and occupations escape a like predicament? And where will the vested rights and individual liberties paid for with so much blood, suffering and sacrifice be? These will be relegated to oblivion, sweet memories of a better age, given place to brutal and callous commands of the Dictator's unjust might and merciless ambition.

Men and women of America, not homeopathy, not doctors, but patients of all shades of religious and medical beliefs, rise up in united strength and demand in the name of American liberty and progress that these hateful dogmas of red Russia, of Nazi Germany and Fashist Italy conceived in inequity, born in ignorance and nurtured in dictatorship and tyranny, shall not be placed on the fair pages of American jurisprudence. Now is the time to act. Flood Congress with millions of protests against this noxious foreign poisons that would undermine all that is sacred of our glorious past and would blight our present and future with loathsome forms of slavery and degradation. Remember the sage statement of Patrick Henry, "Eternal vigilence is the price of liberty".

Already taxation and waste have become so burdensome that the sources of wealth are being undermined, and the threat of utter ruin and complete destruction of our social structure is a certain result if the same forces and tendencies of the past eight years are allowed to remain to complete their program of enslavement and ruin.

It is within our power to choose and to have either a blind unscrupulous dictatorship or the blessings of the free institutions established by our fathers that have made the American Union the symbol of freedom and progress in the past and the haven of safety for the present and the rainbow of hope in a storm-blasted world for a future free-born race to live in.

Arise, friends. Let no past political ties bind us to the dead carcass of a past glorious political organization that once stood for freedom and equal rights but now symbolizes tyranny and serfdom in their worst and most subtle forms.

Under a benign form of patriotism the present administration has championed the cause of the unfortunate who are without support or means of earning a livelihood because of unforseen economic failures. This laudable action has been used as a smoke screen to undermine the independence and stamina of our free institutions as well as to deprive the individual citizen of his vested rights and equal opportunities before the law.

In other words, the unfortunate are given enough crumbs to maintain life for the surrender of their birthright. Of what avail is life spent in serfdom away from the sunlight of freedom and advancement? What chance remains for noble incentive and achievement in the service of a free people under the malign reign of a political dictatorship with all its unscrupulous graft and unfair indifference to the rights of the individual.

The shades of Washington, Jefferson, Lincoln amid the millions of free men who died to create and maintain this glorious land of opportunity and justice mutely implore us to shake off the cobwebs of indifference that have blinded us to the dangers that threaten to overwhelm and destroy us and our children after us.

The Hour of Decision[1]

The hour of decision is at hand and the choice is ours, homeopaths of America, to survive and carry on with the great crusade, to perpetuate the only truly scientific system of medicine based on natural laws existing today, or to objectively surrender all our prerogatives and privileges gained with so much sacrifices and labor by our predecessors.

If we choose or accept the terms of defeat and apathy we will soon cease to exist as an independent medical system of incalculable value for the need of the world today and for all the future. If we decide to fight for the great privilege of establishing and securing the stability of the benign system of homeopathic medicine which alone can meet the medical needs of the world we will have to unite and strive and sacrifice time, labor and substance as we have never done before. All our efforts must be directed by intelligent planning and organization. Our steps must be timed, synchronized and correlated to meet each and all of the numerous problems that will confront us in our march to our goal. I believe the rank and file of the American Institute of Homeopathy together with their elected officers stand as a unit for the preservation and development of homeopathic medical principles. Because of that belief and faith in the integrity and generous courage of my colleagues I know our cause is secure.

The culminating circumstances resulting from activities of certain non-medical groups and individuals in various states of the union, wherein, the attempt to destroy or take over homeopathic state societies by political chicanery and other means, has become a serious threat to our existence as a medical body. The object of these activities is not to teach or further the interests of Homeopathy; but to establish diploma mills that will turn loose on an unsuspecting public a flood of incompetent medical practitioners. It becomes our duty for our safety and our honor to prevent the consumation of these unworthy objectives. The best way to achieve our desired results is to reorganize our homeopathic state societies wherever we can and teach homeopathic principles by way of correspondence and post graduate courses sanctioned by the Institute.

To do this the Institute must provide and man the machinery to inaugurate these procedures. By request of several of the Institute's

---

1. President's address No. 13 in Jounal of the American Institute of Homeopathy, vol. and date unknown. - Editor.

members your president has appointed a competent committee to take up this work at once and proceed with it until our July meeting when the Institute and its officials may take over for further development.

At this time it is well to remember our need for intelligent publicity, not a paid publicity, but one that we can create for our use along many lines. I refer to the formation of as many Lay Societies as we can organize everywhere there exists a group of homeopaths. Such groups are useful nuclei which can awake public interest and bring help and influence to further the spread and acceptance of homeopathic principles and ideals.

Because of the importance and vital significance of these things it becomes a moral duty for every member of the Institute to be present at the July meeting at Mackinac and aid in the solving of our numerous problems for the good of ourselves, our families, friends, patients, our country and the world.

Necrology No. 1. Presidential Address No. 8[1]

Homeopaths, friends and colleagues, Again we meet to renew and strengthen the bonds of affection and faith that has made the American Institute of Homeopathy an outstanding medical organization for over a hundred years. Also on this occasion we set aside a period for meditation and dedication, that we may honor the memory of those dearly loved and highly respected colleagues who finished their earthly labors in the Divine realm of healing and passed to their reward, where rest and peace abide with them. We love them because they were faithful to a great cause, whose work must be carried on in the face of opposition and ridicule from powerfully organized and entrenched forces of selfish interests. They carried on often far behind the line of duty through changing seasons and times, day and night, unremittingly with sacrifice of personal pleasures and too many times a neglect of family duties, applying the benign law of cure to the utmost of their ability to ease pain, assuage grief, allay anxiety and save life.

Our gratitude and respect goes out to them because of their courage to practice in the cause of truth and in the face of harmful opposition and unjust criticism. Truly, they have shown us how to live and extract happiness in the service of others as well as how to die unafraid and content with a full life well spent for the good of all. Indeed the span of their existence could be likened to "a glorious day in time and space, a day with a beautiful sunrise touching all nature with its light and warmth, momentarily broken by cloud and storm to be followed by more and greater light, and finally to end in the beauty of a gorgeous sunset with its inimitable display of changing color merging into the purpling twilight of evening the worlds of which precedes the night of well earned sleep - the blood red poppy of enchanting rest".

Words are idle and meaningless to our beloved departed friends; in honoring their memory we honor ourselves, and our acts of dedication must be the dedication of ourselves and our talents to the great good cause they loved and struggled for, and for which they gave the full measure of their devotion.

It is for us, the survivors of the storms and battle, to close ranks and carry on with the same faith and courage displayed by those of our predecessors who laid the foundation and built the superb superstructure of homeopathic truth for the good of all mankind in all the future.

---

1. From handwritten manuscript, exact date unknown. - Editor..

It is for us to maintain and strengthen our organizations and build them into citadels and repositories for the perpetuation and the preservation of all homeopathic writings, essays and papers, magazines, etc. that American Homeopathy has contributed to the common cause in the hundred years of its existence.

The world must not and will not loose this precious heritage of healing knowledge needed now more than ever before, because of the sorry failure of empirical medicine in spite of extravagant claims of success made by it.

In closing let each and all of us resolve to give the best we have in thought and effort for the building up and perpetuation of homeopathic principles that our children and their children can live and grow under the cleansing protective power of homeopathic law.

NECROLOGY NO. 2[1]

Friends and colleagues of the American Institute of Homeopathy, the passing of another year again brings us the privilege and the sacred duty of honoring the memory of our comrades and co-workers who have earned the reward and rest that follows a life consecrated to the healing service of his fellows.

Words of praise from us to them are now futile, but our affectionate recognition for the valuable contribution to the cause of homeopathic healing that they made in the practice of the art and science of homeopathic medicine is altogether right and appropriate. And as we honor the memory of the departed members, we honor ourselves and rededicate our lives to this same cause that they gave so much for.

Since the time of Hippocrates, the great Greek physician, known as the Father of medicine, the healing art has occupied a high and enviable position in the minds of men and in the social order, and justly so, as inspired by word and precept of the great Greek physician and his ever living Hippocratic Oath which is given to every graduate of medicine since his day to the present time.[2]

That we may again know and feel the impact of that oath, I will quote it now: "I swear by Apollo the Physician and Aesculapius[3] and health and all heal and all the Gods and Goddesses, that according to my ability and judgment I will keep this oath and this stipulation to reckon him who taught me this art equally dear to me as my parents, to share my substance with him and relieve his necessities if required, to look upon his offspring in the same footing as my own brothers and to teach them this art if they shall wish to learn it without fee or stipulation and that by precept, lecture and every other mode of instruction I will impart a knowledge of the art to my own sons and those of my teachers and to disciples bound by stipulation and oath according to the law of medicine but to none others. I will follow that system of regimen which according to my ability and judgment I consider for the benefit of my patients and abstain from whatever is deleterious or mischievous. I will give no deadly medicine to anyone if asked, nor suggest any such consul, and in like manner I will not give to a woman a pes-

---

1. JOURNAL OF THE AMERICAN INSTITUTE OF HOMEOPATHY, Vol. 50, No. 6, June 1957, p. no. unknown. - Editor.
2. The present day doctor of medicine no longer takes the Hippocratic oath. - Editor.
3. Roman mythology: The god of medicine; the son of Apollo by the nymph Coronis. - Editor.

sary to produce abortion. With purity and with holiness I will pass my life and practice my art, I will not cut persons laboring under the stone but will leave this to be done by men who are practitioners of this work. Into whatever house I enter I will go into them for the benefit of the sick and will abstain from every voluntary act of mischief and corruption, and further, from the seduction of females or males of freemen and slaves. Whatever in connection with my professional practice or not in connection with it I see or hear in the life of men which ought not to be spoken abroad I will not divulge as reckoning that all such should be kept secret. While I continue to keep this oath unviolated may it be granted to me to enjoy life and the practice of the art respected by all men in all times, but should I trespass and violate this oath may the reverse be my lot."

Those practitioners of the healing art who mold their lives and practice in accordance with these ideals are indeed fortunate for themselves and for their patients as well, and they lend a luster to the lofty traditions of past greatness and goodness.

Sick man as envisioned through the homeopathic concept of health and disease is something more than a group of chemicals miraculously fused together to make blood, nerves, flesh and bone needed to construct the animal body. He is life, love and intelligence - all priceless gifts of God. His possibilities, like the Divine source from which he came, are limitless when his life is directed by love. When his life is not guided by love, he becomes the author of his own misfortunes and in his uncontrolled egotism and desire for power may even destroy himself. But the achievements of these mental powers and intelligence in the natural world have expanded his ego and dimmed his spiritual vision as well as dulled his sense and love of the beautiful nature, which make up the real though apparently intangible values in the cosmos.

Since the inception of Homeopathy from Hahnemann down, the modern homeopathic physicians of today desire to give to general medicine the benefit of homeopathic discoveries confirmed by more than a hundred of years of successful practice. We believe the day is not too far away when Homeopathy will be accepted as a specialized branch of therapeutics and incorporated as a part of general medicine to be taught in all medical colleges as a necessary part of their medical education.

Homeopathy treats the sick man as a unit: spiritually, mentally, emotionally and physically to make the whole. Homeopathy recognizes the cause of sickness as a racial, constitutional inherited miasm that must be eradicated before health can be established throughout the organism. Because of individual susceptibility to their own peculiar sick-making forces, illustrated by allergies, only the one appropriate remedy can remove the susceptibility and restore order.

Another cardinal feature of Homeopathy is that the sick individual's blood chemistry must correspond to the nature of the remedy needed to restore harmony in the play of the vital processes of the patient. The sick patient is the one treated, not the name of his disease.

Homeopathic remedies are prepared in such a way, a process called potentization, that brings curative results without any deleterious side effects which follow the action of crude drugs, especially when these latter are administered hypodermically.

Homeopathy has demonstrated the powers of infinitesimal forces which arm us with the awareness of grave hazards to health and life in the form of attenuated toxins in the air we breathe and in our food and water supplies. Specifically these hazards are the adulterations and preservatives in our food, the chemicals in our water supplies, the sprays used on our vegetables, the sulphur and carbon dioxide in the air we breathe and the radio-active poison permeating the air and waters and all growing things of the earth. Because these things are ingested in such a small amounts, many so-called scientists believe them harmless. They forget that these things taken in the infinitesimal dose continuously can build up a destructive force in the body organism that can end in its death. Plant life, including large trees, will die if long exposed to sulphur dioxide with as little as one part to a million floating through the air (this corresponds the 6x homeopathic potency).

While different opinions are expressed by recognized authorities concerning the radio-active fallout now permeating the air and waters of the earth with its effect on life and health because of its relatively attenuated amount, it is reassuring to know that its harmful effects are being investigated. Geneticists and men of noted medical standing such as Dr Bentley Glass of John Hopkins University, Dr. James Crow of the University of Wisconsin and Dr. Herman Muller of Indiana University all expressed definite conclusions about the threatened harm to health and life both now and in the future. In all, two thousand scientists have expressed grave fears concerning the far-reaching ill effects or radioactivity now and for future generations.

Homeopathy has the most effective remedies to antidote these subtle poisons which is one reason why more physicians schooled in the philosophy and techniques of homeopathic medicine are needed. The homeopathic physician of the future has knowledge and prescribing ability built on the vast labors of those who have gone before us. They have left a heritage of priceless knowledge that will help bring into being a better race living in a better world.

Slowly but surely thinkers of the dominate school of medicine are discovering homeopathic facts and the ravages of proprietary drugs, most of them habit forming, mind and soul destroying agents whose repercussions are beginning to be noted. More and more physicians of all schools of medicine are becoming aware of these destructive evils which are pushed on the public by organized selfish interests operating for huge profits which enable them to maintain an unceasing propaganda of false claims and half truths. With the great wealth amassed by these powerful drug interests, they are enabled to dominate medical thought, to direct and control legislation and influence the press, to mold public thought, to further their selfish ends. To combat these evil influences, we need men and women who fashion their lives based on laws and principles of living, who develop character to give them integrity and courage that they might successfully combat and expose the unhealthy conditions that the selfishness and rapacity of men have brought upon every segment of the social order.

In medicine more than anywhere else we need such workers to restore the high ideals that once directed medical thought and practice for the great good of the sick and afflicted.

The men whose memory we here honor tonight were of that nature. They devoted their lives to and with a minority group, beset by difficulties that arose from lack of understanding and unreasoning prejudice, but they chose to work in this group because it brought to the world a superior type of service based on the unerring truth of natural law that cannot be found anywhere else. These men were unassuming and unselfish in their devotion to their chosen work of healing the sick. They amassed no great wealth, nor did they attain world fame; but they achieved more than riches or passing fame could give; the friendly living regard of so many simple folk, who found happiness and well being from their kindly ministrations were satisfaction surpassing the understanding of those engrossed in pure selfish interests. They shaped and lived their lives much like the simple but beautiful philosopher expressed so clearly by the poet Longfellow in "A Psalm of Life":[1]

Tell me not, in mournful numbers,

---

1. Longfellow: "A Psalm of Life - What the Heart of the Young Man Said to the Psalmist". - Editor.

"Life is but an empty dream!"
For the soul is dead that slumbers,
And things are not what they seem.

Life is real! Life is earnest!
And the grave is not its goal:
"Dust thou art, to dust returnest,"
Was not spoken of the soul.

Not enjoyment, and not sorrow,
Is our destined end or way:
But to act, that each to-morrow
Finds us further than to-day.

Art is long, and time is fleeting,
And our hearts, though stout and brave,
Still, like muffled drums, are beating
Funeral marches to the grave.

In the world's broad field of battle,
In the bivouac of life,
Be not like dumb, driven cattle!
Be a hero in the strife!

Trust no Future, howe'er pleasant!
Let the dead Past, bury its dead!
Act, - act in the living Present!
Heart within, and God o'erhead!

Lives of great men all remind us
We can make our lives sublime,
And, departing, leave behind us
Footprints on the sands of time; -

Footprints, that perhaps another,
Sailing o'er life's solemn main,
A forlorn and ship wrecked brother,
Seeing, shall take heart again,

Let us, then, be up and doing,
With a heart for any fate;
Still achieving, still pursuing,
Learn to labour and to wait.

Longfellow

THE SYPHILIS CRUSADE[1]

The loathsome clinical aspects and the far-reaching constitutional effects of syphilis through succeeding generations readily supply a reason to organize for the control and eradication of such a scourge. But the methods adopted by the Public Health Service, which is entirely dominated by one school of medical thought (allopathic), will in the end do more harm than good.

The foolish and misleading results that must follow from universally testing everyone, children and adults alike, with the Wasserman blood test for diagnostic purposes, is nothing short of a most revolting crime against the individual and the public weal.

We are warned by the leading allopathic authorities on the subject that a diagnosis of syphilis should never be based on a positive Wasserman alone, because the blood of a large percentage of people not having syphilis will give a positive Wasserman reaction. The negro race is especially prone to give a Wasserman positive; tuberculosis, chronic malaria, jaundice, visceral cancer, yes, and even a pregnant woman may give a positive Wasserman reaction.

On the other hand a negative Wasserman is not a guarantee that an individual is syphilis-free; for many known cases of nerve, spinal and brain syphilis will give a negative Wasserman blood reaction.

In the light of these facts, why brand hundreds of innocent and syphilis-free individuals as social outcasts and pestilential units of infection as well as subject them to a false, inappropriate and harmful treatment for a disease they do not have? All of this will add tremendously to the increase of illness instead of its curtailment and mitigation.

It is hard to believe that the real leaders of scientific medicine could endorse such a loose and indiscriminate procedure as is now being pursued in Chicago, viz. the insistence on a Wasserman blood test for all. If the disease has reached the high percentage claimed, 15 to 20% of the population, we can find no comfort from the methods and ministrations of empirical medicine since such methods have dominated the field of control and treatment in the past, and present conditions with the whole gloomy picture are but the result and sequence of such empiricism.

Not long ago the world was intrigued by the experiments with the drug 606 (Ehrlich). These experiments were repeated with the drug 909

---

1. "Editorial" in THE HOMEOPATHIC RECORDER, Vol. LI, No. 9, September, 1937, p. 430 - 431.

and finally faded away into thin nothingness to be followed by many experiments in other hands with the various PREPARATIONS OF BISMUTH.

Prior to these experiements of Ehrlich were those made with massive and poisonous doses of mercury in numerous forms, all of which took a heavy toll of the hapless victims suffering from a horrible disease made doubly destructive by ignorant and unscientific treatments. Judged by the facts, the only benefit derived from this hysterical and brazen crusade will accrue to the manufacturing medical chemists, laboratories and empirical doctors, for which the public must pay in greatly increased sickness and consequent expense.

The world is ready to receive a program of education and instruction for the disbursement of useful knowledge treating of the habitasis, origin and causes of the disease with the object of prevention rather than of doubtful cures.

If the public could be impressed with the certainty of venereal infection and with the uncertainty of its cure, together with the attendant sufferings and far-reaching effects resulting from promiscuous and illicit sexual intercourse, far more good could be accomplished for the eradication of all venereal infections than has been done by all the so-called treatments of empirical medicine.

Things Homeopathy Does Not Do[1]

Our brothers of the dominate school doubtless have heard of many wonderful things in the way of cure accomplished by the homeopathic Law of Similia. Said law is applicable in every field of and branch of illness the race is heir to; and it is fitting that we homeopaths in our enthusiasm and perennial faith in the efficacy of this law, should pause and remind both ourselves and our brothers of the traditional school of medicine of some of the things homeopathy does not and cannot do.

First in the field of prophylactics against smallpox, diphtheria, scarlet fever, malaria, poliomyelitis, etc., the results obtained in successful immunication against these diseases have been startling, at least 95% good. But that which homeopathy does not do in these cases is still more interesting and revealing.

There are no sudden deaths from anaphylactic shock. There are no consequential septicemias and no long train of systemic diseases resulting from homeopathic immunication as the long painful history of vaccination shows.

No unfortunate victim of so-called neurasthenia, neurosis, insomnia and numerous other nerve conditions ever was consigned to the ward of an insane institution as a result of homeopathic treatment; homeopathy has remedies highly efficacious in power to cure with none of the disappointments and dangers that follow the administration of allonal, luminol and many other depressant drugs developed from the coal-tar derivatives.

No case of destroyed white blood cells could follow the administration of a homeopathic remedy as frequently follows the prolonged use of the barbital preparations. Homeopathy cures pain by removing its cause; the agents above mentioned temporarily alleviate pain by lessening the reactive forces of the body to the sensation of pain at tremendous cost in vitality and health.

No new agent of cure introduced by homeopathy could produce the horror of wholesale death of nationwide extent as we have recently witnessed in the new drug sulfanilamide so blatantly and extensively heralded as a cure for septicemia and other virulent types of infection because homeopathy experiments on healthy beings, not on the sick, not on guinea pigs and rats. All this illustrates the difference of working according to a definitely proved law and working from the haphazard empiricism.

---

1. "Editorial" in The Homeopathic Recorder, Vol. LI, No. 12, December, 1937, p. 575 - 576.

MEDICAL ASTROLOGY[1]

From most ancient times and civilizations down through the middle ages and as late as the eighteenth century Astrology and medicine have been closely associated and used in the treatment of the sick.

Hippocrates, the father of medicine, was an ardent advocate and practician of the starry art as well as a most successful physician, not only of his time but of all time since. His observations relative to the course of fevers and their remissions are recognized as still true and accurate today. The course of fevers correspond closely to the motion and phases of the moon. In fact all sickness, acute and chronic, stem in some way from the inharmonious play of planetary law in the life of the individual victim of ill health.

This fact was almost universally accepted as proven truth down until the eighteenth century when material science usurped first place as a guide for the thinking of the multitudes of the so-called progressive nations of the world. But material science with all its advances is far from an unmixed benefit and often leaves in its wake a train of evils to eclipse the benefits gained by its use.

The highly advertized achievements of modern medicine and its wonder drugs with so-called benefits are often followed by far more disastrous side effects to the afflicted than the natural diseases for which they were given. For the most part these create in the hapless victims an artificial sickness more deadly and difficult to cure than natural sickness operating under natural law.

The envisioned benefits that may come from the application of atomic energy to our daily life are certain to bring a host of unfortunate ills to humanity in the form of radiation sickness and pernicious genetic changes in the race which will be difficult if not impossible to eradicate. All of this together with the great danger of widespread atomic warfare over the world could spell universal destruction, incurable sickness and unmitigated misery ending in the annihilation of the human race, and the entire structure of civilisation with its host of material and spiritual advances.

It could well be that only through the medium and a sane application of Astrologic Law to the needs of these changing and fateful times that the world will be able to advert and mitigate the many hazards that

---

1. Dr. Grimmer was an accomplished astrologer. This article was taken from his handwritten manuscript (written in 1956) and was probably never published. - Editor.

now threaten the race from many sides. As a prelude and significant sign of great impending changes in the history and affairs of men and the world that is now at hand, astrologers are noting an Astrological phenomenon probably never occurring in all past recorded history and never again to happen for eons of time to come. We refer to the almost simultaneous change of all the major planets of the Solar system into new signs in this year of 1956.

June 9th of this year, Uranus entered the sign of Leo to remain there for the next 7 years. Oct. 10, 1956 Saturn entered the sign of Sagittarius to remain there for about two and one half years. Oct. 26, 1956 Neptune entered Scorpio where she remains until June 26, 1957 then retrogrades back into Libra and remains there until August, 1957 when she goes back into Scorpio to remain there fourteen years. Nov. 1, 1956 Pluto enters the sign of Virgo conjoining the great fixed star, Regulus remaining in Virgo until about Feb. 1, 1957, when it retrogrades back into Leo remaining there until Sept. 1, 1957 after which he goes back into Virgo where he will remain for the next twenty years. Dec. 18, 1956 Jupiter enters Libra to stay there until February when he returns back to Virgo where he remains until August 7, 1957, then again entering Libra to remain for about a year. Added to all of this Mars, who has remained for many months in the sign Pices, will on Dec. 4, 1956 enter the sign Aries and remain there until Jan. 29, 1957.

These mutual planetary aspects and changes among these heavy slow moving bodies add tremendous force to this unusual and notable astral phenomena. Saturn and Pluto in square aspect from common signs, Virgo and Sagittarius (Water and Fire) Leo.

Pluto and Neptune will remain in sextile aspect over a relatively long period from water and earth signs. Also Saturn and Uranus behold each other by trine from the fire sign of Leo and Sagittarius. Jupiter from Libra throws a benefic sextile to Uranus in Leo and Saturn in Sagittarius, this is a harmonizing and benefic influence that could neutralize much mischief. The fast moving Mars during December, 1956 and January, 1957 contacts by aspect all the heavier planets. Jupiter by opposition from fire and air, Uranus by trine from fire, and Saturn by trine from fire. Pluto by inconjunct 150° aspect (fire and earth). Neptune by 150° aspect from Aries and Scorpio (fire and water).

Within the scope of these unprecedented planetary forces and involved two of the eminent fixed stars, Regulus in Virgo with Pluto, and Antares in Sagittarius with Saturn and more yet, Pluto, Saturn and Uranus are all parallel of declination with each other at the same time with the sun also in declination with these three heavy planets from fire and earth.

Who is wise enough to interpret these world shattering portents of near and stupendous change in world affairs? Not only economically and politically but mundane changes of great import in the crust and structures of the earth itself may be expected.

Pluto and Saturn from earth and fire fore shadow intense volcanic activity and earthquake action of deep and widespread proportions. Some parts of the Earth's surface will sink and be submerged in the ocean depths and new Islands and lands long submerged will rise again and reappear to the earth's surface. Fritz Brumhubner's interesting book on the planet Pluto and his aspects and effects on mundane affairs. Dec. 11, 1956 when the moon joins Mars in Aries and Mercury square both from Capricorn may well be a day long remembered and most eventfully.

What does all this have to do with Medicine? From the position of Pluto in Virgo, the natural sixth house of Health and Saturn in the natural ninth house of science, philosophy, etc. both these planets beholding Jupiter in Libra in the natural seventh house of enemies and partners, Saturn sextile and Pluto semisextile at the same time, Uranus in Leo, the natural fifth house of children, education, sports and speculation and games, etc. and Neptune being involved in this tremendous array of planetary forces, we have presented a rare astrological picture potentious of strange unexpected events and changes now at hand.

From this complexity of mutual astral aspects among the heavy planets especially the position of Pluto in Virgo, the natural sixth house of health and disease, and Saturn in Sagittarius, the natural ninth house of science and philosophy we may well see an advance in the science of medicine with outstanding discoveries bringing an entirely new concept in the treatment of the sick wherein the finer forces of nature are brought into play to achieve outstanding cures in chronic and intractable forms of illness heretofore impervious to the action of remedial measures.

More important and notable still, the science of disease prevention or prophylaxis will be developed and employed with the attainment of far reaching, beneficial results to the future of the whole race.

Mental and spiritual attributes of the human being will be harnessed and used as most potent, curative agents for the healing of mind and body.

The starry science that flourished in the ancient civilizations of the past will again come into use as a certain guide for the diagnosis of disease and an efficient and reliable aid for its prevention and cure. The transit of Neptune through Scorpio, the natural eighth house will deluge the world with epidemics of loathsome and devasting debility of the blood and nervous systems with worldwide sickness as a frightful harvest of serum poisons that have polluted man's blood stream for the past fifty years together with the suppressed general poisons, signs of the antibiotics, and these things will be difficult to cure because the antibiotics of modern science are useless against the subtle viruses that even now prevail.

William Lily, a notable Astrologer and Physician who lived in England in the Sixteenth century has left a valuable and notable work on questions of the hour, or Horary Astrology. The section devoted to sickness is replete in uncanny knowledge that may be obtained from erecting a chart of the heavens at the moment the patient is stricken, or when he first seeks to aid of the astrologer physician concerning his case. All the old time astrologers gave their medicine under the most favorable stellar forces obtainable at that time.

Paracelsus compounded his remedies and administered them only under favorable heavenly auspices and acquired a fame and recognition as a superior healer of his time.

Coming down to our present time, Max Heindel of Rosicrucian fame, has given the world a remarkable and valuable work on the diagnosis and cure of diseases with the aid of astral law entitled "Astro Diagnosis". This work will reward any medical man or the votary of any branch of healing with added power for good in the broad field of healing.

By far the most lucid and informative writer of modern times on Medical Astrology is the great English Astrologer, Allen Leo. His observations and aphorisms concerning stellar forces in their relation to human sickness are most accurate and can be verified with very little labor and effort by anyone at all familiar with Astrologic technique.

Allen Leo mentions three vital centers in the horoscope that effects the life and health of every individual born. First the sun is ruler of the vital, or life force. The solar orb, as it rules and sustains the solar system being its center and life, rules the body organism giving it life and vital force by its rule over the vital centers viz. the brain and spinal cord from which all nerve impulses both efferent and afferent come and go; the heart and blood circulation that supplies oxygen and nutrition to every part of the organism from center to circumference is under solar rule in the horoscope. Also the eyes and the vision come under the joint rule of sun and moon, afflictions of the lights impairs, and sometimes destroys the sight. Serious affliction of the malific to sun and birth bring about various forms of heart disease and brain and spinal cord conditions. Depending on the place of the planets in the signs and houses of the nativity hence the ascending sign together with its ruler and the planets that occupy it are deciding factors in the state of vitality and health.

The acending signs rule the physical body and its appearance and individual peculiarities as well as its power of resistance against the forces of environment. The power and importance of the sun's place in the horoscope and its relationship to the other heavenly bodies especially with that of the moon determines the state of health as well as the character and destiny of each individual born into the world.

The moon is next in importance to the sun in the horoscope. Quoting Allen Leo further: "The moon is the medium of relationship, the conveyor and distributor, and because of its brisk passage through the circle of the zodiac it rapidly takes up magnetic force from the other bodies as aspects are formed and dissolved, and as quickly lets go thus producing change and acting as an expulsive alternative and cleansing agency." It is the minima evestrum of Paracelsus. The lunar person is ever a rover, restless, variable, mobile, inconstant. Our satellite then becomes chemically convertive, integrative, secreting, metamorphic and assimilative in action. It is the receiver and preparer and is therefore intimately allied to the stomach, uterus and breasts and so of a peculiarly powerful import in a woman's nativity. As Leo and the sun are identified with the masculine, electric positive active, so cancer and the moon are with the femine magnetic, negative passive. The one is vital heat, the other radical moisture. The one is the sperm the other the matrix of nature. Serous and mucous surfaces are dominated by Luna, as also the lymphatics and lacteals. Taken in the abstract, the luminaries together are sun spirit and moon matter; one is the reality essential eternally existent, the other illusion may be transitory experience, organic decay. From them result two series of planetary expression, a solar and a lunar, the former always clamoring for deliverance from the latter, which implies bondage to matter, thralldom of the flesh fate. The moon then may figuratively be regarded as a sort of alembic in which the processes of fermentation and decomposition are carried on. Those substances under lunar sway are extremely liable to fermentation and decomposition, and putrefaction, cabbage fungi, etc. for example, these grow with astonishing celerity mostly by night have much consistency but little vitality or staminia and ferment and putrify with most rapidity. They may be accounted for by the lymphatic temperment of the vegetable world. Luna has special rule over the stomach and alimentary canal, the brain substance, the breast lymphatic and lacteal systems and the lachrymal apparatus, also a general one over the fluids of the body.

Mercury, the spiritus of Paracellsus is somewhat of a protean artist, taking various forms according to the manner in which it is aspected. This body is a connector, mediator, translater and reflector, distributor and co-ordinator. The specialized mercurian function is in common with the nerves. Gemini, whose lord is Mercury indicates this trait. For since this sign and the associated house (3rd) hold sway in the world over means of transit and communication, railroad, telegraph, correspondence etc., so in the physical body these are represented by the ramifications of nerve tissue. Insignificant as the body of the planet appears yet its influence is of the most important character from a physiological standpoint. And although movement and muscular force are denoted by muscle, the excitement is evidently due to nerve forces. Hence the motor nerves depend not only on nutrition of muscle, but also on actual control; the intensified form of muscular contraction, termed spasm, is directly the result of and dominated by the octave of Mercury. Under Mercury we find the nervous system, mental faculities, breath, hands and tongue. Together Moon and Mercury govern the brain substance and function and their affliction in any scheme of nativity is a powerful argument of unbalanced mentality amounting to actual madness if the malefics are dominate.

However intimately we may be acquainted with the intrinsic virtues of members of the solar system, the knowledge will only avail us to a limited extent. We have now to draw the threads so as to finally adjust and lighten up the whole scheme. It remains for us to consider in order what increase or surcease of virific and morbific energy is induced by the aspects and the actual planetary location in points of the natal chart.

The points of great value to the physician are first the nature and power of the disease to harm of endanger the life of the patient. Second the time element, and third, the possibility to cure.

Pluto is said to strongly influence the rule over the pineal gland as well as the very subtle and fine complex of the central nervous system and the automaticity which produce the amazing involuntary reflexes to external stimuli according to Fritz Brumhubner. It is iminently connected by a fluid the center or starting point of which is the vital center of respiration the lengthened spinal narrow in the nape. He says, "I place the seat of the ego center of life center here because all nerve ganglia meet in the nape of the neck". It may be mentioned by way of illustration, that immediate death will take place if one sustains a blow on this center and if the minute nerve is hit in such cases the ganglia of nerves which maintains the connection with the whole organism is severed. Here we see why the so-called rabbit punch of professional boxers is ruled illegal and interdicted; breaking the neck causes immediate death because the vital nerves are involved. Where Pluto is prominent in horoscope the native is endowed with a more refined sensitivity and awarness to impressions even to the point of clairvoyance. Pluto produced warped over-sized personalities as well as geniuses and individuals of unusual power and talents occult powers and gifts. The diseases involving the nervous system deeply, produce epilepsy, catalepsy, drastic blood changes, abnormal growth, and abnormal development of organs and body parts. Congenital defects, etc. are found under severe Pluto afflictions. Severe blood disorders and infections are ruled by Pluto. Psychic afflictions of the most stubborn nature are also prominent.

In Memory of My Grandfather[1]

As he has lived in the sight of God so do I long to follow.

As he has loved God the Father and Christ the Son so do I seek to love the Almighty.

As he had faith in the light of the Redeemer so do I pray for such faith.

As he was blessed with the gift of wisdom so was I blessed with his teachings.

And as he was blessed with a love for mankind so was I blessed in receiving his and giving my love.

Lord, I pray, rest his soul in the peace of Heaven, for truly he has served Thee well on earth.

---

1. Written in 1976 or 1977 by Karen Bayler, granddaughter of Dr. Grimmer.

Electronic Reactions of Abrams

Grimmer's Work

RECENT CONCEPTS AND NEW FORMULAS IN MEDICINE[1]

Among progressive thinkers today, the ETIOLOGICAL concept of disease is vastly different than it was even a decade ago. Materialistic causation factors are largely replaced by a knowledge of the subtle forces producing distunement in the vital and physiologic processes of the organism, *disturbed life force* and changed polarity in the electro-magnetic currents of the body which renders the being out of harmony with the rhythm of the Cosmos.

Hence the patient's inability to react in a normal way to his environment and the bringing about all the so-called infections and allergies that medical science has cleverly enumerated and classified, and more recently has devised for each new virus or germ (designated as a causative entity) a specific new *wonder drug* to destroy it. But alas, soon the germs and viruses become immune to their would be destroyer and new brain throbs conjure forth new wonder drugs to go the way of their predecessors leaving poor suffering humanity with an added load of toxemia to harass it and endanger life and comfort because of the so-called side effects which engraft on the hapless victims (or patients if you wish) a lingering debilitating drug disease not easy to cure.

One of the more logical medical concepts of recent years known as psychosomatic medicine states that sickness of all kinds for the most part has its origin in unrestrained and imbalanced emotions. Fear, anger, envy, hate, avarice, lust etc. are said to be the causative factors in such chronic diseases as arthritis and cancer and innumerable mental disorders. This line of thought is similar to the teaching of Hahnemann and is largely accepted by homeopaths everywhere.

For the removal of these causations *wonder drugs* would not only be useless but extremely detrimental. Mental and spiritual guidance, and adjustment together with the homeopathic remedy and an improved environment are the only procedures to help or cure such conditions. The body of man and animal are made up of and contain the chemical ingredients of the earth. This mass of chemistry however is activated, balanced and controlled by the same subtle force that illuminates and vivifys the sun and stars throughout the realms of space; keeps the planets in their ordered orbits without clash or friction; and gives us the changing seasons and all the natural phenomena about us. In generous profusion plants, shrubs, trees and flowers all evolve and grow because

---

1. THE HOMEOPATHIC RECORDER, Vol. LXVI., No. 6, Dec. 1950, p. 167.

of this God-given life power. The chemical body of man is formed in the pattern of a huge storage battery comprised of twenty six trillion bipolar electric cells. Each cell is a separate unit yet all are *wired* together to perform work for the whole organism. Through oxidation processes electricity is manufactured and distributed from the deepest centers to the remotest extremities to maintain growth and all the activities of life and to repair injury or the ravages of disease in the body.[1]

So much for the physical body of man, animal and plant corresponding to the crust of the earth of which they are a part existing in the phenomenal and seen aspect of nature. In the unseen and causative realm of nature there exists an etheric bond linking the physical body of man and nature with the creative and animating forces of life which proceed through the medium of the sun, stars, and innumerable other suns, from the fountainhead of all power: God, the Creator and Governor of the universe - mysterious, orderly, ever changing, yet eternal in cycles of perfection and beauty. *The Lord God formed man of the dust of the ground, and breathed into his nostrils the breath of life. And man became a living soul.* (Gen. II. 7)

From the above observations it is logical to conclude that causes exist in and proceed from the unseen realms of nature and manifest their effects in the phenomenal world of matter.

All chemical, all disease changes in the body of man manifest first in his etheric body by means of the life principle emanating from the fountainhead or source of life. Any disturbance or impairment of the etheric body which hinders the free and harmonious flow of the life force immediately renders the material body or its parts inert and lifeless and soon subjects it to the process of decay and disintegration. All remedial action must be directed to the causative plane in the etheric body to effect a cure.

In recent years we have heard much of vibrations and vibratory rates and how the science of physics is contributing useful advances in medical technique of diagnosis and treatment for the sick. The phenomena of color, the speed of sound, the changing physical nature of water from ice to steam are all governed by the rate of the vibrating particles of these substances. Yet the phenomena of color and sound would be nil if the retina of the eye or the tympanic membrane of the ear did not exist to receive these vibrations. The changes in the state of water exists

---

1. Crile, George W.: A BIPOLAR THEORY OF LIVING PROCESSES; The MacMillan Co., New York 1926.

entirely on the physical plane and require no special medium to register its change in vibration. These things are mentioned in order to introduce the Hahnemannian discovery of the potentization of remedies - one of the outstanding advances in the annals of medicine and only faintly recognized by some medical investigators at the present time.

Science has proven that not only light and sound vibrate but every solid substance and element in nature vibrates at a rate consistent with its own form and existence. Also that temperature, friction, division and chemical action may all change the rate of vibration as well as the form and nature of the substance acted on. Hahnemann's process of potentization reduced the crude drug to a state of ionization rendering it highly active and expansive and deeply penetrative which enables it to act on the deeper etheric planes of nature. The Law of Similars operates by a strong natural affinity to bring the delicate force of the ionized or potentized drug to the affected part of the etheric body to produce equalization, balance and cure from within out, from center to circumference; by releasing the vital force, harmony and health prevails throughout the whole organism.

Professor Einstein is said to have formulated a theory where all natural phenomena including gravitation and magnetism may be solved and measured in mathematical formulas and symbols. The progressive medicine of the near future will be based on and operated by proven mathematical equations in conjunction with the homeopathic Law of Similars within the broad scope of Homeopathic Philosophy, for that has been built on the solid rock of one hundred and fifty years of untiring work and effort from many minds, hearts, and hands of votaries from many lands.

Already the vibratory rates and polarities of remedies and diseases are known and used in the successful treatment of disease in its worst forms. For our present use in medicine there are four polarities always present throughout nature including man, animal and plant and even all inanimate things and substances.

When a patient's blood registers a positive polarity he will require a remedy in the negative class. Not any or all negative remedies will restore the balance of health but only that negative remedy whose vibratory rate is similar to the sick patient's; and that is found by placing the remedy in the circuit with the patient's blood and noting the ensuing action. This action is measured by a rheostat or resistance box which records the findings in ohms of electrical resistance; in this case the blood is changed when the remedy is in the circuit with it, from positive which measures +.12 of an ohm resistance to negative -.12 ohms resistance.

When a sick patient is found over negative (less than -.12 ohms) he requires a positive remedy found in the same way as stated before. A patient whose blood is neutral, that is balanced neither negative nor positive requires a neutral remedy with a similar vibratory rate to the patient and this remedy is found by trying each individual neutral remedy in the circuit with the blood until the rheostat changes the readings of the blood from neutral to -.12 ohms of resistance. For all persons whose blood registers -.12 ohms are in approximate health, at least his life force is flowing in harmony with the rhythm of the Cosmos.

A patient registering a bi-polar reaction is recorded on the rheostat as -.04 +.12 (or 1/25 ohm negative resistance and 3/25 positive resistance). For this patient a bipolar remedy in the circuit that restores the blood polarity to negative .12 exactly, no more no less, will prove curative.

This vibratory and electro magnetic method of remedy finding is a boon to the hard working homeopathic prescriber because it combines accuracy with much time saving, providing the prescriber is well grounded in Homeopathic Philosophy and the Homeopathic Materia Medica. First he must take his case history carefully and completely as outlined in the Organon. Then the personal and family history together with the high grade generals with rare and peculiar symptoms by repertory study will reduce the vast Materia Medica to a dozen or so remedies. When the patient's blood polarity is obtained or known three fourths of the remedies may be put aside as the similium will be found in the proper polarity group only. The few remedies needed for further study can yield the one most appropriate when placed in the circuit with the blood. It is a mistake to infer that one can successfully employ this method without a good knowledge of the Homeopathic Philosophy and an assiduous study of the Materia Medica. Without the coordination of these elements success will be infrequent and failure a common experience.

This work is only in its incipiency. There is a great deal more research needed together with more delicate instruments than those we now have. The vibratory rates of remedies are far from complete. When these factors are completed a much higher percentage of good prescriptions will obtain and the advance in Homeopathy will be marked and world recognition will be attained.

IMPORTANCE OF ELECTRONIC REACTIONS TO FUTURE MEDICINE[1]

The discovery and development of the Electronic concept of disease and its cure, is destined to place the whole field of medicine on a really scientific basis in the near future. The kaleidoscopic aspects of empirical medicine with its so-called discoveries of new wonderful remedies (*wonder drugs*) for specific diseases will no longer be able to deceive and afflict suffering humanity. Many chronic disease conditions are caused from the abuse of coal-tar and other toxic drugs. Heartless commercialism in medicine will then be replaced by a sure benign service with an undreamed of economy and efficiency in cure.

Since each disease has an individual rate of vibration and a polarity or patron strictly its own, it follows that the remedical measures must have a similar vibratory and polarity energy to the disease conditions for which they are suited in order to effect a cure. Hence the various remedies present their electronic and polarity patrons which may be fitted to corresponding disease conditions. It need not surprise us if in the very near future the whole process cure may be reduced to a simple process of arithmetic; subtraction of the remedy vibrations to the disease vibrations.

Traditional medicine has been slow to advance with the pace of the physicist, and as a result it is still floundering in the mire of empiricism, wherin the process of trial and error is the measuring rod and the end product has been up to the present chiefly error.

All substances in nature have rates of vibration and polarity. There is a persistent feature concerning polarity when determined and measured in the Abram's circuit that is basic. If the rate for magnetism is set and either end of the bar magnet is placed above the dynamizer the energy will measure $\frac{3}{25}$ (.12) of a unit, no less, no more.

An approximately healthy blood specimen in the dynamizer will measure when rate 35 is set just $\frac{3}{25}$ of a unit on the negative side. Anything less than $-\frac{3}{25}$ is abnormal (negative) and requires a positive remedy. Most positive bloods measure $\frac{3}{25}$ positive, no more.

The bi-polars are irregular generally $\frac{1}{25}$ negative and $\frac{3}{25}$ positive.

When no polarity reaction is found on either side it is a neutral case.

---

1. From handwritten manuscript, exact date unknown. - Editor..

Neutral and bi-polar cases require respectively neutral and bi-polar remedies to effect cures. The positive cases require negative remedies and over negative cases need positive remedies with similar vibratory rates to the disease to cure.

To ascertain the best remedy for a given case three requirements must be met: First, the polarity of the patient's blood must be normalized - it must register negative $\frac{3}{25}$ exactly. Second, all disease reactions must be eradicated. Third, the vital wave must be raised to the maximum. When these three requirements are met by placing the remedy in the circuit with the blood specimen the physician may be certain of obtaining certain curative action.

Sometimes due to drug, food and other toxins such as serums and vaccines one remedy is insufficient to take off all the toxins together and a complimentary remedy must soon follow - this remedy is obtained in the same manner as stated before.

Through this great concept of Abram's, life and all nature unfolds before our vision in a beauteous and orderly process of universal law where vibrations, wave lengths, polarity and potentials are common terms expressing life's complex phenomena.

One object we have in bringing this subject to you is to show the harmony and confirmatory relationship existing between Homeopathy and other very subtle forces in nature. If we pause and view the scientific world today as a whole we will be struck at the tremendous advance made by the physicist over that of modern medicine in general.

From the mighty globes of fiery light circling in the never ending vastness of interstellar space down to the most infinitesmal electron vibrating even beyond the ken of the ultra-microscope, the physicists have captured, measured, classified and discovered the underlying harmony of immutable law linking the greatest with the least where each and every particle acts and reacts on each other in unending cycles of activity and perfect balance. Each unit from the mightiest sun to the smallest point of light, keeps its appointed place in its orbit without clash or hindrance, obedient to the one universal self perpetrating eternal first cause or Law.

Man has been called an epitome of the universe within whose body all substances and forces in nature meet and blend to build an organism endowed with creative intelligence and with inherent powers of adaptability to changing environment as well as the capacity for growth and repair. And because of this creative intelligence man may modify and control his environment to a large degree by avoiding the destructive forces in nature or utilizing them to his purpose and his will, by means of inventive talents. As long as man works and operates in accordance with law there is almost no limit to what he may accomplish in the upbuilding and perpetration of his life and his happiness. By orderly processes of organization where by the inventive wonders of this age and what is yet to come can be marshalled into use for the common good, man can and will replace the present chaotic fog of economic gloom (with all its health destroying powers) by the benefic sunlight of unselfish and intelligent cooperative service each for all, and all for each.

In that new day health will flow through natural processes and be tapped at the source of vital energy with all the ease and facility that we now receive from the boundless ether waves, our selective strains of music by the simple tuning apparatus we are all so familiar with. Nothing the imagination conceives is impossible of realization if patience and persistent intelligence be applied.

For the perfect utilization of these finer forces we must develop more subtle instruments than we even now possess. Those we now have are sufficient however to indicate tremendous and far reaching possibilities for the future in the realm of cure.

Homeopaths and physiotherapeuts are not alone, engaged in the investigation of these subjects. Experimentors at Yale University employing a vacuum tube microvolt meter for the measurement of what they term, *bio-electric phenomena* have discovered many interesting facts relating to the state of health in cells, tissues, organs and organisms. Ultra microscopic organisms are now known to carry electric charges of definite polarities which enable the investigator to identify and differentiate toxemia of infinitesimal quantities with the recognition that this bioelectric phenomenon involved in the processes of all living and even non living things is the modus operandi pervading and animating all nature. Confirmatory of the Hahnemannian Law of Similars this bioelectric phenomenon reveals the subtle powers residing in drugs whose vibratory rate and polarities are similar to those found in disease toxemias which invade the blood and tissue of men and animals to bring on disease by disturbing the bioelectric balance in the body organism. Thus each drug presents a patron of bioelectric activity peculiar to itself.

In presenting this paper I am aware that a great deal of prejudice and misconception relating to this subject exists not only outside our ranks but within as well. But fear of criticism will not deter the true scientist from expressing his conclusions and his reasons for holding them. Had Hahnemann been afraid of the storm of opposition and even hatred that his discoveries brought forth from the bigoted and the ignorant, we would not today be privileged to heal the sick under the certain and gentle process of a beneficent law of cure.

POLARITIES OF REMEDIES IN RELATION TO THE POLARITIES OF DISEASES[1]

Many electronists ignore the polarity of diseases, in spite of the fact, that the founder of Electronic Medicine spent much time and labor in working out the polarity of the various diseases, as a glance through the Atlas will prove.

The sciences of physics and chemistry are especially interested in polarity. Even the astronomers are beginning to recognize that polarity and gravitation, are one and the same; and lastly the great Einstein has reduced electro-magnetism to terms of mathematical formulas.

As our vision expands and we become aware of new and increasing varieties of cosmic forces we are impressed with the great importance of POLARITY in the scheme of all creation. Every particle of matter, every shade of energy in the universe is moved, controlled and directed by this mysterious and ubiquitous agent.

POLARITY: From the infinitely small to the infinitely great, organic and inorganic substances alike, are moved, attracted, or repelled by this unseen but ever potent eternal power.

Whence it comes or whither it goes we know not, only its ever dominating presence and manifestation, co-existing with eternity and boundless space, is sensed, the "*Alpha And The Omega*" encompassed in the enchanted circles of life and knowledge, where the interchange of matter and energy is ever going on in unending cycles, evolving new forms and species, in uncountable myriads. Vivifying forms, or reducing them to ultimates, thus changing or sustaining established orders throughout the universe this amazing imponderable force reigns as the supreme attribute of Diety. Constellations and solar systems and their whirling retinues of planets, with all the fiery cometary wanderers of the unfathomed heavens, move in orderly procession under the certain sway of this Divine emanation. Matter from its most gross forms to its finest divisions and forms - molecules, atoms, electrons, elemental substances, light, electricity, radiant energy and the cosmic rays generated beyond the realm of the fixed stars - are obedient to the UNIVERSAL LAW OF POLARITY.

Reflecting on these facts makes it easy to visualize the relation existing between disease energy and the substances or energies called remedies, when these forces meet and manifest in the economy of man.

---

1.   From handwritten manuscript, exact date unknown. - Editor..

Man has been truly called an epitome of the universe. Every substance of Earth and sky is found in the body of man, and every energy of the Cosmos vivifys and sustains him through his predestined cycle of life. In his evolutionary march from birth to death he is subjected to many conflicting forces and disturbances resulting in a certain peculiar, individual development and growth and form, and in the crystalization of certain personal characteristics. This individual form and character with its inherited proclivities and acquired susceptibilies resulting from environment, habits of living and etc., constitutes a miniature replica of the universe.

While the life energy of this wonderous organism of man is flowing harmoniously, that is, polarized correctly, for the maintainance of the electro-chemical processes of metabolism, health is present. Anything interferring with this life force, i.e. reversing its normal polarity, results in disease. And order can only be restored by recovering the normal polarity of the vital force. If a reversed polarity exists for too long a time changes begin in the chemistry of metabolism which are soon followed throughout the cellular elements of the body by a change in structure ultimating in some pathologic process. After all disease is only a change of the electro-magnetic state of the body organism and health is the harmonious flow and play of vital processes.

A review of Dr. Abrams polarity findings relating to diseases reveals the cause of sickness in the animal organism. To illustrate we will recall only a few of the disease condition listed: Carcinoma is listed as a positive electro-magnetic energy and every step forward in the march of scientific advancement confirms these observations. Photography now is able to capture the energy emanating from a malignant tumor on a photographic plate, and no such energy comes from a benign growth.

The experiments of Crile so ably set forth in his *Bi-polar Theory of Living Processes*[1] prove that the carcinoma cell has changed from the bipolar energy of the normal cell to a positively charged cell (has lost its negative end).

Our observations have gone a little farther, by using Abrams technique, vibratory rate 35 for magnetism, and stroking over the positive area, in every case of developed and active carcinoma, we have found the blood of such patients, registering a positive reaction with all negative reactions absent.

---

1. Crile, George W.: A BIPOLAR THEORY OF LIVING PROCESSES; The MacMillan Co., New York 1926.

In every case of developed and active tuberculosis the bloods of such patients are neutral; Abrams also found tuberculosis neutral. Abrams observed that syphilis and sarcoma gave out a bipolar energy and when either of these diseases predominate in a patient his blood will register bipolar.

Streptotoxemia in the early and inflammatory stages gives a negative reaction to the blood, this is also consistant with Abrams findings of a negative polarity in the streptococcus.

As every particle of matter or energy in the universe contains some form of polarity it follows that remedies for the cure of sickness must also have a specific polarity. And they fall into four classes of polarity energy as follows: positive, negative, neutral and bi-polar, corresponding to the four classes of energy found in disease producing causes, infections and toxines of all kinds.

Clinical experience and observation has taught us the proper remedial energy to employ against every case of disease energy to effect an equilibrium and obtain the processes of health. Against disease polarity of a positive nature only negative energy can neutralize or cure. The negative diseases require positive remedies, while the neutral and bipolar diseases will only yield to the neutral agents for the neutral diseases, and the bipolar forces for the bipolar sicknesses.

We have been taught that in order to annihilate disease cause, we must employ an energy of a similar rate of vibration or wave length; but we must have added to the similar vibratory rate the correct polarity energy as well. Polarity is the direction taken by the lines of force, vibratory rate the wave frequency.

We only partly cure or even suppress disease conditions, unless both these forces, polarity and vibratory rate, are used in the treatment of the sick. Remedies not consistent with the required laws of both polarity and vibratory rate can never be ideal or produce the best results in sickness.

These hastily gathered facts and observations are presented to you with the object of aiding in the construction a more proficient treating machine than any now existing. The perfected treating machine will deliver energy of both the required vibratory rate and the necessary polarity to produce results that will prove amazing in terms of cure.

E.R.A. Changes the Prescribing of Drugs from an Art to a Science[1]

The history of medicine is one long nightmare of disappointment. The empirical application of repulsive substances given mainly on superstitious grounds were the earliest attempts of man to combat disease.

A little later followed the giving of drugs all more or less toxic based on the whims and theories, and entirely bereft of anything savoring of law or logic; in fact, this still obtains down to the present time.

The regular practitioner of medicine who is so proud of his learning and his science has no definite guide for the administration of drugs; he is long on diagnosis that at best is 50% right, and short on cure that is 90% wrong. Hence, a large majority have turned medical nihilists having no faith in the efficacy of drugs to heal, and who depend entirely on the reactive powers of the sick organism to elaborate the necessary antibodies, antitoxins, etc. to overcome disease. With the aid of general care, nursing, rest, diet, etc. a higher degree of success has been obtained than the regular application of drugs has brought.

Through all this dark night of the mind with its groping and stumbling there shone forth one bright star of hope in the medical sky. The *Law of Similars* was discovered and announced by *Samuel Hahnemann*. He was the first to prove drugs on as near healthy human beings as could be obtained and to record those *provings* and compile them into a *Materia Medica*. Having found the way drugs derange or change from normal the thoughts and bodily functions of man, it was then ascertained that a very light or attenuated application of a drug would mitigate pain, reduce fever, and restore to normal function in a very short time, providing the disease for which it was given contained a symptom image of the drug in its provings made on the healthy. Here at last was something definite and guiding and capable of being proved by all whose minds were free of prejudice and who were seeking the truth. One of the requisites of a scientific proposition is the ability of any one or more experiments (using a given technique) being able to obtain the same results repeatedly and whenever tried under the same conditions and circumstances. This has been accomplished by those who were willing to work hard and long and unremittingly.

---

1. E.R.A. = Electronic Reactions of Abrams

The percentage of cures alone is the variable factor and depends upon a complimentary law. It remained for *Dr. Albert Abrams* to lay the foundation for its discovery and elaboration contained within the reactions of disease and the corresponding vibratory rates he discovered and gave the world. This is the *Law of Polarity.* Dr. Abrams taught and proved that every substance has polarity and he likewise gave us the vibratory rate of magnetism which may be used to obtain the polarity of any blood specimen (or the vital energy of any patient) or any drug or substance in nature.

All things in nature below man contain all the elements that destroy him. From the animal world down through the vegetable kingdom, down into the mineral realm we find vibratory rates corresponding to the disease vibration found in the blood of sick humanity.

Even corresponding pathologic states obtain at least down to the plant life. Many plants and many animals show cancer growths and tubercular changes, and the Abram's reactions demonstrate syphilis in the blood of the lower animals and even in plants and minerals. And it is because of these facts that plants and minerals and animal products when properly attenuated and given in susceptible doses attuned to the disease vibrations and polarity of the sick, are able to eradicate disease and restore order and equilibrium in the plane of the life forces.

The life force maintains function, repairs and eliminates waste when in harmonious play.[1] When distunement obtains in the life force, the electronic elements first, and then the cells of the body break down and undergo change. Most blood specimens, (about 90%), and human energy show a negative polarity. This is the natural waste of negative electrons thrown off in excess in the process of normal functions and obtains in approximate health, or at worst in functional disease with no serious change in tissue. About 5% show a positive polarity. This condition has been noted in those who have tissue changes in cells or organs and occurs in those who are breaking down from disease and who are wasting an excess of positive electrons. The other 5% show no polarity, this has been noted in those whose processes of repair and waste are about on a par; frequently early tuberculosis conditions show this polarity. Of course many of the 90% of those of negative polarity are sick but their sickness is more capable of reacting to remedial agents and has not progressed to serious tissue changes.

Now the protein molecule given by Dr. Abrams as a probable index to the life duration is a most interesting factor taken in conjunction

---

1. §9 Organon - Editor.

with its reacting to the polarity of various remedies. Vibratory rates do not affect the protein molecule. Polarity has a most decided effect.

If a patient whose blood polarity is negative be given a remedy of the positive polarity his protein molecule will be increased from $\frac{3}{25}$ to $\frac{7}{25}$ of a unit measured on the reflexaphones. If the same patients be treated with a negative remedy his protein molecule will fall from $\frac{3}{25}$ to $\frac{7}{25}$ of a unit. Not only that but all the endocrine activities of the patient may be stimulated, retarded, or balanced with the substance suited to the polarity of the patient. Vibratory rates of remedies only destroy disease reactions in the blood and in no way affect the protein molecule or the endocrine functions of the patient which after all is the fountainhead of health. The dangers of drugs wrongly applied as well as the advantages of drugs suitably applied is shown from the above law. Of course, of the 90% of human beings, not too sick drugs empirically given may not kill (even though they do harm if not given in harmony with the laws above mentioned: of *Similars, Vibratory rates,* and *Apropriate Polarity).* Of the 10% seriously sick drugs wrongly given will prove rapidly fatal.

The phenomena of the two fundamental laws relating to sickness and cure (viz, Vibratory Rate and Polarity) will easily explain the findings of some of the early electronists victimized by so-called scientists (investigators) who sent in animal blood specimens and got findings of cancer and tuberculosis and syphilis in return. These self-constituted scientists (investigators) ridiculed the findings as absurd but can they prove the contrary? Most emphatically, No. Even ultra-conservative doctors admit that animals and plants both may be cancerous and tubercular. Paint and chemicals were also sent in, but the bunglers contaminated the specimens with their own body energy and, of course, syphilis and other disease reactions were recorded all of which only substantiates the correctness and delicacy of the Abram's reaction and in no way disprove the claims made for E.R.A.

No real electronist should fail to get animal blood reactions when present, but he may get also human blood reactions from contamination of those who handled the specimens and sent them in for tests. E.R.A. practitioners have a technique that must be observed closely in taking and handling blood specimens to avoid contamation. Those not familiar with that technique or who ignore it necessarily render the specimen to be tested useless as an index of disease reactions of a given case.

Electronic Patterns of New and Old Remedies[1]

In presenting this paper I am aware that a great deal of prejudice and misconception relating to this subject exists not only outside our ranks but within as well. But fear of criticism will not deter the true scientist from expressing his conclusions and his reasons for holding them. Had Hahnemann been afraid of the storm of opposition and even hatred that his discoveries brought forth from the bigotted and the ignorant, we would not today be privileged to heal the sick under the certain and gentle process of a beneficant law of cure.

One object we have in bringing this subject to you is to show the harmony and confirmatory relationship existing between Homeopathy and other very subtle forces in nature. If we pause and view the scientific world today as a whole, we will be struck at the tremendous advance made by the physicist over that of modern medicine in general. Vibrations, wave lengths, polarity, and potentials are the common terms expressing life's complex phenomena.

From the mighty globes of fiery light circling in the never-ending vastness of interstellar space down to the most infinitesimal electron vibrating even beyond the ken of the ultra-microscope,[2] the physicists have captured, measured, classified, and discovered the underlying harmony of immutable law linking the greatest with the least where each and every particle in the universe acts and reacts with every other particle in unending cycles of activity and perfect balance. Each unit from the mightiest sun to the smallest point of light, keeps its appointed place in its orbit without clash or hindrance, obedient to the one universal self perpetrating eternal first cause or law.

And man has been called an epitome of the universe within whose body all substances and forces in nature meet and blend to build an organism endowed with creative intelligence and with inherent powers of adaptability to changing environment as well as the capacity for growth and repair. And because of this creative intelligence man may modify and control his environment to a large degree by avoiding the destructive forces in nature or utilizing them to his purpose and his will, by means of inventive talents.

As long as man works and operates in accordance with law there is almost no limit to what he may accomplish in the upbuilding and per-

---

1. From handwritten manuscript, written in 1938. - Editor.
2. Today it would be the electron microscope. - Editor.

petration of his life and his happiness. By orderly processes of organization whereby the inventive wonders of this age and what is yet to come can be marshalled into use for the common good, man can and will replace the present chaotic fog of economic gloom (with all its health destroying powers) with the beneficial sunlight of unselfish and intelligent cooperative service each for all, and all for each.

In that new day health will flow through natural processes and be tapped at the source of vital energy with all the ease and facility that we now receive from the boundless ether waves, our selective strains of music by the simple tuning apparatus we are all so familiar with. Nothing the imagination conceives is impossible of realization if patience and persistent intelligence be applied.

For the perfect utilization of these finer forces we must develop more subtle instruments than we even now possess. Those we now have are sufficient however to indicate tremendous and far reaching possibilities for the future in the realm of cure.

Homeopaths and physiotherapeuts are not alone engaged in the investigation of these subjects. Experimentors at Yale University employing a vacuum tube microvolt meter for the measurement of what they term, "bio electric phenomena" have discovered many interesting facts relating to the state of health in cells, tissues, organs and organisms.

Ultra-microscopic organisms are now known to carry electric charges of definite polarities which enable the investigator to identify and differentiate toxemias of infinitesimal quantities with the recognition that this bioelectric phenomena involved in the processes of all living and even non-living things is the modus operandi prevading and animating all nature.

Confirmatory of the Hahnemanniam Law of Similars this bioelectric phenomena reveals the subtle powers residing in drugs whose vibratory rates and polarities are similar to those found in disease toxemias which invade the blood and tissue of men and animals to bring on disease by disturbing the bioelectric balance in the body organism. Thus each drug presents a pattern of bioelectric activity peculiar to itself.

THE POLARITY OF REMEDIES IN RELATION TO THE POLARITY OF DISEASE[1]

The law of polarity is universal, its ramifications are everywhere, it permeates every substance, and animates every force.

The phenomena of chemical affinity and gravitation are the result of this law.

The various color vibrations are only a varying degree of polarity, a changing rate in the speed and direction of the electronic units of the light particles. Medicines either crude or potentized are grouped into four distinct classes as to polarity - positive, negative, neutral and bi-polar. Every food is also similarly classified. Specific diseases have the same grouping. Human beings show in their blood the same classification. Even the lights of heaven are embraced in this same law. The sun's rays (ultra violet) are positive; the moon's rays vary with her phases, that is, her aspects to the sun, when at full or in conjunction she is positive. When at trine or sextile her light is negative unless conjoined with the positive Jupiter or Mars - then her light is neutral. When in square aspect, her light is neutral.

Those individuals whose blood shows negative reactions, that is where an excess of negative electrons are thrown off, chemically appear nearer to normal states of health than those of the other groups.

Those whose polarity is neutral are in a balance, either coming up from a lowered state of vital weakness, or descending down to a serious state of sickness preceeding or accompanying tissue changes.

Those of a positive reaction are always sick whether they know it by their symptoms or not, they are breaking down positive electrons in excess and serious tissue changes are taking place.

The Streptococcus infection is the most prominent of the negative diseases. Influenza, tuberculosis, diabetes, and typhoid are neutral diseases.

Carcinoma, sarcoma, the venereal infections, diphtheria, scarlet fever, epilepsy, and malaria all give a positive reaction and cause destruction of the positive electronic elements in the tissues. All this does not necessarily mean that the patient's blood as a whole will register positive, the majority of cases will be neutral, and some in the early stages of positive disease may even be negative.

---

1. From handwritten manuscript, exact date unknown. - Editor..

It is the advanced cases that will show positive as a whole and these must be met with negative energy both as to their medicines and to their foods in order to reverse their polarity and establish health and blot out disease energy and raise positive energy activity and balance and establish harmony.

The negative cases require positive energy to establish health and blot out disease energy; whereas the neutral cases require neutral energy to blot out the same reactions, and the bipolar cases require bipolar energy to achieve harmony.

The various endocrine chains: pituitary anterior lobe is positive; posterior lobe is negative and extract from the whole gland is neutral; supra-renal, spleen, brain, and spinal substances are all positive. The liver, kidneys, pancreas, thyroid, and thymus glands all neutral. Gonads and ovary are positive.

The heavy metals are mostly negative (ex. plumbum, radium). Most animal poisons such as the snakes and spiders would produce are bipolar. Two spider poisons so far tested ARANEA DIADEMA and TARENTULA are the exceptional negative remedies. APIS is positive. About a third of the vegetable kingdom is positive. Most of the acids are bipolar. The halogens are bipolar. All the earth salts and earth metals are positive. At least a third of the vegetable remedies are negative. All the silaecea, most of the nosodes, the pure carbons and silicates, and all salts made of positive and negative substance such as the union of an acid and an alkali or those produced by the union of a heavy metal with a halogen as in the case of FERRUM IODATUM and AURUM IODATUM are all neutral. The only exception so far noted in the nosodes have been in the case of ANTHRAC. being bipolar and MALAND. being positive. The housefly TROMB.(According to Clarke TROMB. is a parasite found singly or in groups on the common house fly) and the grass hopper, are two exceptions among the insects as they are neutral.

The question will be asked how do we know when to use one energy and not another. Also, how do we determine from a proven scientific basis that their is a definite unchanging law underlying the giving of medicines according to the relative polarity of patient and remedy.

It has been noted that workers, independent of electronic practitioners have noticed changes in the polarity of the cell in cases especially of malignant disease. This change also includes one of relationship between the centrasome and the nucleus, being histologic in nature; but it nevertheless is preceeded and accompanied by an electromagnetic change in the electronic elements. These always change prior to any morophological change of the cell.

And on the subsidence of pathologic states with a clinical picture of health the changes in the cell mentioned above have assumed their normal histological form and appearance.

And most important of all other proofs are those of clinical evidence observed in hundreds of cases. The restoration of the sick to health with the remedy of the indicated polarity and the evidence of symptoms and illness produced on healthy subjects by remedies of the highest potencies given in the inimical polarity. Laboratory proofs of this law has been confirmed by other electronic physicians and may be so confirmed by anyone desirous of so doing.

Take a bar magnet over a known specimen of blood, the polarity of which has been determined by the Abrams method setting the reostat at rate 35 and bringing the action through the proper area on the subject. The polarity of the bar magnet is a known element and serves as a check for all other substances, for if that registers correctly it follows; others will do likewise. Other known elements are the positive acids and negative alkalis together with their neutral salts. All these known substances comes through unvarying and certain. And these known things always coming through according to their known polarity it justifies our confidence that the reactions of unknown substances conform to the same law and are correct in the indications shown.

There are several reactions found in the human blood and known to electronic physicians that indicate a patient's vitality or life force. One of these points comes through the sex area on the subject at rate 22 on the reostat. This is known as the protein molecule and in a negative blood specimen it will raise appreciably in value if the opposite pole of the magnet be placed above the blood and it will decrease a proportionate degree if the negative or same pole of the magnet is used. Both poles of a horseshoe magnet (neutral energy) has no influence on either negative or positive bloods, but it raises a neutral blood's vitality in the same way as the others do when indicated.

The above is the basis for the clinical procedures that followed, and while a remedy of the indicated polarity may not always be the most effective one in a given case, it will require at least another remedy of the same polarity to effect the cure. For the remedy must not only be of the indicated polarity, but must contain all the vibratory rates corresponding to those in the blood of the patient. If cancer is present only those remedies of correct polarity that also have the similar vibratory rates to cancer and all the other vibratory rates such as subtoxemia, gallstones, etc. that may be present in a given case if it will cure. Never will a known cancer remedy take off the reaction from the blood or cure the patient if the polarity of patient and remedy is inimical.

A knowledge of the polarity of remedy, diseases, and the blood of patients is of great value to the homeopathic physician, as it aids him greatly in the selection of the similium. The similimum is always found in the polarity group indicated by the polarity of the patient's blood. This important knowledge is only valuable when used in conjunction with the homeopathic symptomatology together with the homeopathic philosophy as taught by Hahnemann and Kent. Often failure and disappointment will come if the attempt be made to prescribe with this method apart from the symptomatology and philosophy of homeopathy. The knowledge and application of polarity added to the proven and accepted methods of prescribing conceived of and taught by the master prescriber such as Hahnemann, Hering, and Kent, will simplify and insure greater accuracy in homeopathic prescribing.

Because of these facts, every homeopathic physician should be equipped with these facilities in order to do their best work with a minimum amount of time and labor. When the polarity of a patient's blood is found and known, approximately three-fourths of the remedies in the materia medica can be eliminated from the study of any case in the search for the similar remedy because the best similar will be found in the polarity group indicated by the polarity of the patient's blood.

FOLLOWING ARE THE POLARITIES OF THE:

ANTI-PSORIC REMEDIES

Agaricus-mus.	0	Argent -cyan	3
Ailanthus	-1+3	Arg- met	-3
Allium cepa	0	Ars-alb	-1+3
Alumen	0	Ars-sulph-flav.	-1+3
Alum-phos	0	Ars- sulph-rub	-1+3
Alumina	-3	Asterias-rub	-3
Alum-sil	-3	Aur-met	+3
Anacardium	-1+3	Aur-.mur	0
Ananthereum	-3	Aur. -iod	-1+3
Ant-crud	+3	Aur. -sulph	+3
Ant-sulph-aur	-3	Bar-carb	-3
Ant-tart	0	Bar-mur	-1+3
Aralia-rac	-3	Blatta-orient	-3

Anti-psoric Remedies ...

Bromine	-1+3	Condurango	-1+3
Bryonia	-3	Corallium-rub.	-1+3
Bufo.	-1+3	Crot-casc.	-1+3
Cactus-grand.	-3	Crot-hor.	-1+3
Cad-met	-3	Curare	-1+3
Cad-phos	0	Elaps-cor.	-1+3
Cad-sulph.	-1+3	Equisetum	0
Calc-ars	0	Ferrum-met	+3
Calc-carb.	-3	Ferr -iod	-1+3
Calc-caust.	-3	Ferr. Phos.	+3
Calc-fl.	-3	Fluor Acid	-1+3
Calc-iod.	-3	Formica	0
Calc-phos.	0	Graph.	+3
Calc-sil.	-3	Guaiacum	0
Calc-sulph	0	Heloderma-hor.	-1+3
Carb-an.	-1+3	Hepar-sulph	-0
Carb-ac.	-1+3	Hippozeninum	-3
Carb-ox.	-1+3	Hydrangea	-3
Carb-sulph.	+3	Hydrastis	-3
Carb-veg.	0	Hydrocyanic acid	-1+3
Card-marianus	-1+3	Hyoscyamus	-3
Caust.	-3	Hypericum	-3
Ceanothus-am	-3	Iberis	-3
Cedron	0	Ignatia	-3
Cench.	-1+3	Iodine	-1+3
Chimaphila-umb	-3	Ipecac	+3
China	-3	Iris	0
China-ars.	0	Jaborandi	-3
China-sulph.	0	Kali-ars.	0
Chionanthus	-3	Kali-bi	0
Cina	-3	Kali-brom	-3
Cinnabaris	+3	Kali-carb	-3
Cobalt-met.	0	Kali-cyan	0
Cobalt-mur.	-3	Kali-iod	-3
Cocc-ind.	-3	Kali-mur	-3

ANTI-PSORIC REMEDIES ...

Kali-nit	-1+3	Ranunculus-scel	-1+3
Kali-phos	0	Raphanus	0
Kali-sulph	0	Ratanhia	-1+3
Kalmia	0	Rhod	-1+3
Lachesis	-1+3	Rhus-arom	-1+3
Lactrodectus-mac	0	Rhus-rad	-1+3
Lapis-alb.	-3	Rhus-tox	+3
Lyssin	0	Rhus-ven	0
Mag-carb.	-3	Rumex	-3
Mag-mur.	-3	Ruta	+3
Mag-phos	0	Sabadilla	-1+3
Mag-sulph.	0	Sabal-ser	-1+3
Mag-pol-amb	-1+3	Sabina	-1+3
Mag-pol-arct	+3	Sambucus-nig.	0
Mag-pol-aust.	-3	Sanguinaria	+3
Manganum-met.	+3	Sanic	-3
Manganum-mur.	-3	Sarracenia	-3
Med.	0	Sars	-3
Merc-sulph.	+3	Scutellaria	-3
Nat-ars.	0	Secale	-1+3
Nat-carb.	+3	Selenium	-1+3(?+3)
Nat-hypochlor	0	Senecio	-1+3
Nat-mur.	0	Senega	-1+3
Nat-phos	0	Sepia	-1+3
Nat-sulph	-1+3	Silica	0
Nit-acid	-1+3	Solanum-olec	-1+3
Opium	0	Solanum-nig.	0
Phos-acid	-1+3	Spigelia	0
Phos.	-1+3	Spongia	-1+3
Physostigma	-3	Stannum	+3
Phytolacca	-3	Staphisagria	-3
Plumb-met	-3	Stramonium	-3
Psor.	0	Strontium-carb	-3
Radium-met	-3	Sulph	+3(?-1+3)
Ranunculus-bulb.	+3	Sulph-iod	0

ANTI-PSORIC REMEDIES ...

Sulph-acid	-1+3	Uran-nit	0
Sumbul	0(?-1+3)	Urtica-urens	0
Syph	-1+3(?0,?-3)	Ustilago	-1+3
Tabac	+3	Valeriana	-1+3
Tarent	-3	Variliolinum	-1+3
Tell	+3	Viburnum	0
Terebenth	-1+3	Verat-alb	-1+3
Thallium	-3	Viscum alb	0
Thuja	-1+3	Verat-viride	0
Tub-bov	0	Zinc	+3

ANTI-SYCOTIC REMEDIES

Agar	0	Ferrum-met	+3
Alumina	-3	Fluoric-acid	-1+3
Alumen	0	Graph	+3
Ant-tart	0	Hepar	0
Apis	+3	Iodum	-1+3
Arg-met	-3	Kali-c	-3
Arg-nit.	+3	Kali-sulph	0
Aster	-3	Lachesis	-1+3
Aurum-mur	0	Lyc	-1+3
Bar-carb	-3	Manganum-met	+3
Bry	-3	Medorrhinum	0
Calc-carb	-3	Merc-sol-H	-1+3
Calc phos	0	Mez	-3
Calc sil	-3	Nat-sulph	-1+3
Calc sulph	0	Nit-ac	-1+3
Carb-an	-1+3	Petr	0
Carb Sulph	+3	Phyt	-3
Carb Veg	0	Puls	0
Caust	-3	Sabadilla	-1+3
Cham	-1+3	Sabin	-1+3
Cinnabar	+3	Sars	-3
Con	-3	Sec	-1+3
Dulc	-3	Selen	+3
Euphrasia	0	Sepia	-1+3

Anti-sycotic Remedies ...

Sil	0	Sulph	+3
Staph	-3	Thuja	-1+3

Anti-syphilitic Remedies

Arg-met	-3	Hepar	0
Ars	-1+3	Iodum	-1+3
Ars-iod	0	Kali-ars	0
Ars-sulph-flav.	-1+3	Kali-chl	-3
Ars-sulph-rub.	-1+3	Kali-iod	-3
Asaf	-3	Kali-sulph	0
Aur-iod	-1+3	Lachesis	-1+3
Aur-met	+3	Ledum	+3
Aur-mur	0	Merc	+3
Badiaga	0	Merc-cor	0
Benz-ac	0	Merc-i-fl	-3
Calc-iod	-3	Merc-i-rub	-3
Calc-phos	0	Mez	-3
Calc-sil	-3	Nit-ac	-1+3
Calc-sulph	0	Petr.	0
Carb-an	-1+3	Phos-ac	-1+3
Carb-veg	0	Phos	-1+3
Cina	-3	Phytolacca	-3
Cinnabaris	+3	Sabadilla	-1+3
Clematis	0	Sars	-3
Conium	-3	Sil	0
Cor-rub	-1+3	Staph	-3
Crot-hor	-1+3	Still	0
Dulcamara	-3	Sulph	+3
Elaps-cor	-1+3	Sulph-iod	0
Fluoric-ac	-1+3	Syphil	-1+3
Guaj	0	Thuja	-1+3

Tuberculosis and most of the viruses are neutral - 0. Most of the nosodes are neutral. Tuberculosis, polio, flu, and other virus diseases are related and neutral. Diabetes is mostly 0 (neutral). Purely scycotic disease is 0 (neutral). Syphillis is mostly -1+3 (bi-polar); the exceptions are due to a fusion of the miasms, especially if psora is dominant. It will be noted that the anti-psoric remedies are made up various polarities. This is likely due to a combination of the several miasms occuring in the pathogenisis of these remedies in cases of sickness. Many of our remedies are anti-psoric, anti-syphilitic, and anti-sycotic in their scope of cure. The following group are those remedies and are as follows:

Psoro-sycotico-syphilitic Remedies

(All Three Miasms)

Alumen	0	Fluoric-acid	-1+3
Alumina	-3	Graph	+3
Alumina-phos	0	Hepar	0
Alumina-sil	-3	Iodum	-1+3
Ant tart	0	Kali-bic	0
Apis	+3	Kali-carb	-3
Arg-met	-3	Kali iod	-3
Arg-nit	+3	Kali mur	-3
Aur-iod	-1+3	Kali nit	-1+3
Aur-met	+3	Kali-phos	0
Aur-mur	0	Kali-sulph	0
Bar-carb	-3	Lachesis	-1+3
Bry	-3	Lyc	-1+3
Calc	-3	Manganum-met	+3
Calc-phos	0	Medorrrhinum	0
Calc-sulph	0	Merc-cor	0
Carb-an	-1+3	Mezer	-3
Carb-sulph	+3	Nat-sulph	-1+3
Carb-veg	0	Nit-ac	-1+3
Caust	-3	Phyt	-3
Cham	-1+3	Puls	0
China-off	-3	Sabadilla	-1+3
Cina	-3	Sabal	-1+3
Cinabaris	+3	Sabina	-1+3
Con	-3	Sars	-3
Dulc	-3	Secale	-1+3
Euphrasia	0	Selen	+3
Ferr-met	-3	Sepia	-1+3

Psoro-sycotico-syphilitic Remedies ...

(All Three Miasms) ...

Sil	0	Thuja	-1+3
Staph	-3	Zinc-met	+3
Sulph	+3		

Within this group of sixty-one remedies will be found to be the curative remedy for seventy-five percent of the cases coming to the average doctor in general practice. Hence, this group is of great value for study, especially in chronic cases of disease. A close study of the symptomatology of this group of remedies will be very rewarding and helpful in finding the simillium in a majority of the cases coming to the average physician.

The question may be asked why the need of the many remedies of our vast Materia Medica. The obscure, difficult, and one-sided and unusual cases may require a search through the whole Materia Medica at times to find the one needed curative remedy for a given case. However it is readily seen that a relatively small group of remedies containing the nature and pathogenisis of the three miasms must be a valuable starting point for study in quest of the simillium. The SNAKE POISONS with few exceptions belong to the bi-polar group. NAJA and VIP. are neutral exceptions. The acids are mostly bi-polar. Lactic, Salyiclic, Benzoic and Butyric acids are neutral exceptions. The metals are found in positive and negative groups about equally divided. The royal metals gold, platinum, mercurius, copper, and zinc are positive. Alumina, thalium, selenium, plumbum and silver are negative. The compounds of these metals are for the most part either bi-polar, negative or neutral; only a few are positive. The carbons and silica are neutral. The halogenes are bi-polar. The spider poisons are either neutral or bi-polar, only a few are negative - Theridion, Tarentula, and Aranea diadema are the negative exceptions. Later a complete list of all the remedies of our Materia Medica will be submitted to enable the physician to find the exceptions occuring in the groups aforementioned.

Diabetic disease is largely neutral although some cases are cured with bi-polar and negative remedies very few in the positive group.

Following is a group of remedies with a polarity and nature corresponding to malignancy in its several forms. Most cases of malignant disease that is established in the economy occur in patients whose blood is positive; therefore they require negative remedies to relieve or cure their troubles. The following group of mostly negative remedies which have been proven electronically to be homeopathic to various forms of malignant disease, with confirmation of their curative action in numerous cases:

MALIGNANCY REMEDIES

Alumen	0	
Alumina	-3	
Alumina-sil	-3	
Am-mur	-3	arthritis
Anantherium	-3	
Ant-ars	-3	
Ant-iod	-3	
Ant-mur	-3	especially useful in skin cancer
Ant-sulph-aureum	-3	
Aranea-diad	-3	
Arg-cyn	-3	
Arg met	-3	
Aster-rub	-3	
Asaf	-3	bone disease
Bellis-p.	0	tubercular ulcers of breast
Blatta-orent	-3	affections of lungs, bladder
Bomhenia	-3	uterine hemorrhages and cancer
Bufo	-3	
Bryonia	-3	lung cancer
Cactus-grand	-3	heart disease
Cad-met and oxide	-3	
Cad-bichromate	-3	lung cancer
Cad-calc-fl	-3	bone disease antidotes fluoridated water
Calc-caust	-3	epilepsy
Calc-iod	-3	
Calc-phos	0	
Calc-sil	-3	
Calc-sulph	0	

Caust	-3	
Ceanothus-amer	-3	
Chenopod-anthel	-3	
Chimaphila-umb	-3	bladder and prostate
China-off	-3	
Chionanthus-virg.	-3	
Cina	-3	
Cobalt-mur	-3	lung cancer
Cocculus-ind	-3	
Colchicum	-3	
Condurango	-1+3	lip cancer
Con	-3	breast cancer
Cypripedium	-3	
Dulcamara	-3	
Equisetum	0	uterus and bladder cancer
Eryngium-aquat.	-3	
Eucalyptus	-3	
Euphorbium	-3	
Gnaphalium	-3	
Graph	+3	cancer in surgical scars
Guaj.	0	lungs and arthritis (chronic)
Hell-foet	-3	
Hippozaeninum	-3	malignant ulcerations
Hydrastis	-3	liver cancer
Hyos	-3	
Hypericum	-3	
Jaborandi	-3	
Kali-brom	-3	
Kali-iod	-3	
Kali-mur	-3	
Lapis-alb	-3	
Mag-mur	-3	
Mag-carb	-3	
Merc-cyan	-1+3	
Mez	-3	
Millefolium	-3	hemorrhage in cancer
Mygale-lasiodora	-3	

Myristica	-3	
Naja	0	
Nux mosch	-3	
Nux-vom	-3	
Origanum	-3	
Paeonia	0	rectal cancer
Plantago	-3	
Plumb-met	-3	
Radium-met	-3	
Ratanhia	-1+3	rectal cancer
Sabadilla	-1+3	
Sanicula	-3	
Sarsaparilla	-3	
Sarracemia	-3	
Scutellaria	-3	
Selenium	-3	
Solanum-tub		
Sol. aegrotans	-1+3	rectal cancer
Staphisagria	-3	bladder cancer
Stellaria-media	-3	
Stramonium	-3	
Stront-carb	-3	bone cancer, antidote radio-active vibrations
Tarentula	-3	
Theridion	-3	liver cancer cured

In the cancer group there are 88 remedies which are cancer potentials for any patient where the polarity and symptoms and family history may indicate it. The specific remedy needed may be found from this group.

A small group of remedies that correspond in their pathogenesis to the three miasms and at the same time contain the electronic elements relating to malignancy with clinical confirmations of their curative action in such cases is the following group of 68 remedies which can be viewed and studied with profit in the search for a helpful remedy in cancer cases:

MALIGNANCY & ALL THREE MIASMS

Alumina	-3	gastrointestinal cancers and ulcers
Aranea-diad	-3	cancer of blood, lungs, and glands
Antimon-mur	-3	skin cancer
Ant-sulph-aureum	-3	gastric cancer
Arg-met	-3	cancer of glands and lungs
Arg-cyan	-3	cancer of tongue
Asaf	-3	cancer of the bones
Asteria-rub	-3	cancer of breast
Bellis-per	0	cancer of the breast and blood vessels
Blatta-orien	-3	cancer of the bladder
Bomhenia	-3	uterine cancer with hemorrhage
Bufo	-3	cancer vibrations
Bryonia	-3	lungs
Cactus-grand	-3	heart cancer
Cad-met and oxide	-3	cancer of stomach, antidotes alumina poison...
Cad-calc-fl	-3	antidotes aluminium fluoride found in the drinking water
Ceanothus	-3	cancer of spleen, liver and pancreas
Chenopodium	-3	
Chimaphila	-3	cancer of bladder and prostate
Chionathus	-3	liver and gall bladder cancer
Cobalt-mur	-3	cancer of lungs
Condurango	-1+3	cancer of lips
Conium	-3	breast cancer
Cypripedium	-3	
Dulcamara	-3	cancer vibrations
Equisetum	0	uterine cancer
Eryngium	-3	
Eucalyptus	-3	mucous membranes, sinuses

Euphorbium	-3	
Gnaphalium	-3	
Graphites	+3	cancer in scar tissue
Guaj	0	lungs and joints (chronic arthritis)
Hell-foet	-3	
Hippozaeninum	-3	malignant ulcers
Hydrastis-can	-3	liver cancer
Hypericum	-3	
Jaborandi	-3	
Kali brom	-3	
Kali-iod	-3	
Kali-mur	-3	
Lapis-alb	-3	cancer of bones and glands
Mag-carb	-3	
Mag-mur	-3	
Merc-cyan	-1+3	
Mezer	-3	
Millefolium	-3	hemorrhagic cancer
Mygale-las	-3	
Myristica	-3	lungs, glands
Naja	0	cancer of breast cured
Nux-mosch	-3	
Nux-vom	-3	
Origanum	-3	
Peonia	0	rectal cancer
Plumb-met	-3	
Rad-met	-3	
Ratanhia	-1+3	rectal cancer, fissures
Sanicula	-3	
Sarracenia	-3	
Sarsaparilla	-3	cancer of kidney, irritation from stones
Scutellaria	-3	
Selenium	-3	
Solan-tub-aegrot	-1+3	
Staph	-3	

Stellaria-med	-3	
Stram	-3	
Stront-carb	-3	bone cancer, antidotes radio-active poisons; compare Phos.
Tarent	-3	
Theridion	-3	liver cancer cured

After many years of cancer study and treating thousands of cancer cases with strictly homeopathic remedies used in various potencies, I am convinced that there can never be a one individual specific remedy for cancer disease occurring in many different patients. First, because the many etiologic factors that enter the field of causes such as irritations from blows (trauma), burns, intense heat and cold, drugs, processed and adultered foods, made noxious by poisoned metal containers like aluminum, and poisoned water supplies from aluminum fluorides; poisoned air from carbon and sulphur dioxides and lately radio-active fallout - all are hazards to health in our modern environment and these are all cacinogenic agents.

Second, the known and proven constitutional cause that runs through many families, this factor may not be universally recognized because a generation of tuberculosis may be followed by one of cancer, and even individual patients may develop cancer on advancing tubercular disease.

Third, each individual case of sickness has a body chemistry peculiar to itself and only reacts to the curative remedy called for by the polarity and blood chemistry of the individual victim of sickness. In the hands of many homeopathic prescribers for several generations of doctors, the homeopathic approach in medicine has its worth in the cure and palliation of cancer.

Since homeopathic methods attack the basic constitutional cause of all chronic and degenerative disease and removes all harmful irritations common to the environment at the same time, it occupies a superior place in the treatment of chronic disease including malignancies in the vast realm of healing. And because individual patients can only react to the curative remedy called for by their own peculiar symptoms and constitution, it becomes apparent that no one single remedy or drug can possibly cure every case of cancer occurring in the human race. From these facts we are justified in concluding that the homeopathic method of cure is more logical and effective, although it makes no claim for specific remedy for cancer or any other disease. It is effective only when it is indicated in the individual cases of sickness regardless of the diagnostic name. It is in the field of cancer prevention that homeopathy is destined to achieve its greatest triumph and use.

In a practice of over 50 years where many thousands of cases were seen and treated for numerous forms of sickness, mostly chronic in nature, some of these cases come for treatment now, mostly for acute minor conditions, their chronic states having long ago cleared up. But the important fact relating to this long medical service is the relatively few cases of cancer that developed in the numerous patients over the space of 50 years (excepting those came in with the cancer already developed). Only three in a hundred who had five or more years of treatment developed cancer in any form.

In questioning many of my homeopathic colleagues I found they could report about the same results from two to four cases to the hundred that had received five or more years of homeopathic treatment. Vital statistics inform us that one in every eight human beings past forty years will die of cancer. These facts afford convincing proof of the evident value of homeopathic treatment for the prevention of cancer. This same condition obtains regarding other forms of degenerative disease also. It is difficult to estimate the percentage of cancer cures under homeopathic treatment as they vary with the stage of the disease when treatment starts, early cases being more amenable to the curative power of the homeopathic remedy. And cases organically sound and vital respond more readily and completely.

A conservative estimate that 25% of all cancer cases can be cured with homeopathy. And the 75% not cured will live longer, from five to ten years, and be enabled to carry on with the affairs of life and enjoy more freedom from pain rarely with a need for narcotics to the end, often with a painless death. Because of these encouraging factors, homeopathic research should be encouraged and sponsored by every adequate means we can obtain. Indeed this presents a great privilege and opportunity for an individual or an organized group interested in human welfare to perform a most worthy and outstanding service of lasting benefit to sick and afflicted humanity.

We need to reprove those remedies that have clinically been effective in cancer cures and relief. We must develop many new remedies by provings and clinical application that show electronic possibilities for cancer cure. This approach gives us the key to the inherent nature and power residing in all medicines. Homeopathy with its extension and incomparable storehouse of curative remedies atuned to meet all human ailments, has the golden opportunity of giving to the world of medicine an elevated position in the realm of healing by bringing solace and well being to millions of suffering humanity.

Some years ago Dr. Guy Buckley Stearns wrote a most enlightening paper entitled, "An Approach to Reality"[1] which stressed the value and use of the vibratory concept for the selection of the homeopathic remedy. I am sure this paper can be found either in the archives of the Journal of the American Institute or The Homeopathic Recorder. The late Dr. Boyd of Glascow, Scotland used this method extensively for the selection of the curative remedy for many years in his extensive practice. I cite these eminent and recognized homeopathic practicioners and scientists to vindicate my faith in the accuracy and value of this work as yet little understood by many of our fine homeopathic doctors. This work is presented to the homeopathic profession for their unprejudiced attention and investigation.

Notes On V. R.

While working with this method of remedy finding and diagnosis, we must realize that it is a phenomenon of the superphysical operating beyond the realm of the physical world. It might be more accurate to say the material world because we are dealing entirely with energies vibratory in character. The vibrations traveling by way of the ether wave require no wires to transmit them. Wiring devices were formerly thought necessary to establish a circuit, but a circuit exists between the blood specimen, the operator, and the reagent, viz. the chamois covered jug.

When the right remedy is placed in the circuit with the blood specimen, a sympathetic state of resonance is established between the blood of the patient and the remedy needed for it to cure. There is another phase of this work that may increase its effectiveness and accuracy and that is to employ the vibratory rate of the patient and match it with a remedy having the same vibratory rate, such a remedy will prove to be the true similium not just a similar. We are now experimenting with this aspect of the work and will have more to say about it later. The late Dr. Guy Buckley Stearns of New York City made some very interesting observations of the effect of homeopathic potencies on the autonomic

---

1. The Homeopathic Recorder, Vol. LV, No. 11, Nov. 1940, p. 3; Vol. LVI, No. 3, March 1941, p. 99 and no. 5, May 1941, p. 195.

nervous system. The percussion sounds in the chest were changed by the similar remedy as much as 50 feet away.

The pulse, its rate and character were altered or normalized by holding certain remedies in the hand. Also the pupilary reflexes were markedly effected in the same way. Also, Dr. Boyd of Glascow, Scotland made a number of scientific tests that were accepted as accurate by a prominent group of medical scientists of London, England. Every homeopathic physician knows that if the correct homeopathic remedy is found, any curable state of sickness can be cured with it, however drastic the case may be.

Because of that fact, it is well to avail ourselves with any proven method or means of obtaining the best remedy in any given case of illness. The homeopathic remedy is the great harmonizer, restoring normal activity to the central and cerebral spinal nervous systems, the cardiac and circulatory system, the respiratory system, the endocrine chain, and glandular system, these are all normalized by the homeopathic remedy. All this is followed more or less gradually and slowly by improved mental and emotional states. It must be born in mind that this method cannot possibly dispense with the symptomatology of the Materia Medica and the homeopathic philosophy in the search for the similium, but it is a valuable aid in confirming the accuracy of the prescription and is often a great time saver in the finding of the remedy. Perhaps the most important factor in obtaining the best prescription is in the taking of the history both family and personal. To get the high grade therapeutic symptoms of the patient by the Hahnemanian method of questioning is an art well worth cultivating as it will pay off abundantly in terms of success.

To obtain the vibratory rate of the patient, set the reostate at 49 and stroke over the sex areas on the right side for a female, on the left side for a male, then measure the intensity of the life wave (rate 49) one ohm at a time until the reaction is spent, the number of ohms of the life wave is the V. R. of the patient. To find the V. R. of remedies, the remedy that neutralizes or blots out the V. R. of the patient has the same vibratory rate as that of that patient. I am now testing all remedies for their V. R. It will take some time before the V. R. of all our remedies are found but we will soon have a list of our more frequently used remedies with their V. Rates.

LETTER FROM E. GARCIA-TREVINO, M.S., M.D. TO DR. GRIMMER

Dated November 17, 1961

Dear Dr. Grimmer:

I must apologize for having delayed this letter so much, but I wanted to write after sending you the grafts of the 50 Milesimal Potencies that I prepared for you, and the excerpts from the Organon and from my paper, that will tell you something about the use of them. But last month I had to take another unexpected trip to Mexico and was away most of the month.

We have just received a letter from Mr. & Mrs. Murdock, from Florida, and were sorry to know through them that you had a set back in your condition; but then they tell us that by the time they were visiting you there you were much better. We hope and pray that you have remained well. We are also glad to know that Mrs. Grimmer was feeling better and stronger.

It is possible that you have received by now the box of these remedies prepared in the 50 Milesimal scale. I know that you are going to be delighted to experiment with them, according to Hahnemann's last instructions. I am also sending back to you the copy of the Instructions for the Polarimeter. This copy was intended for you when I gave it to you. I have taken notice of your additions. Thanks. I have also typed your notes on Vibratory Rates, of which I am keeping a copy. I have been able to check on the selected remedy the way you advise in those notes, and have found it correct in getting the similimum. We had been using another method, also suggested by you before you went to Florida, and have found that both methods confirm each other. You will recall that you had suggested to test the selected remedy on the area of Blood Vitality with the rate set at 49 - 48 (91 in our machine) and that the remedy that comes through that rate is the best. But we had found that often there would be two or more remedies coming through that rate, but we have been selecting the one that gives the highest reaction in that rate, as measured in hundred of Ohms; that is, the one that will go over 0.12 hundreds is the best. Checking this procedure with your new method, they both give the same result.

With kindest regards to all of you. Cordially yours,

Signed *E. Garcia Trevino*

Abram's Work[1]

Abram's rate for magnetism 35 (+) positive and (-) negative. See diagram for areas where reactions come in. See Figure 1.

Figure 1

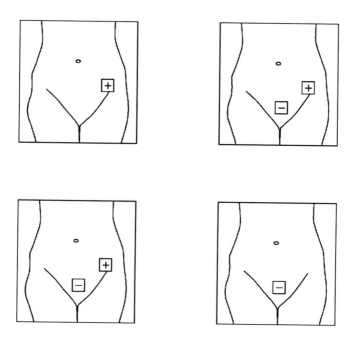

BI-POLAR: Reaction found at both areas but measuring in different intensities. The negative side measures -.04 intensity and the positive .12 intensity (-1 and +3 twenty-fifths ohm).

Some basic things to remember. Take a bar magnet over the blood-box or dynamizer with rate 35 on and each end of the magnet will measure but .12 intensity. A blood sample in the dynamizer or blood-box with rate 35 on, if it be from one in approximate health, will measure .12 intensity in the negative area (i.e. -.12).

---

1. See the Electronic Atlas by Albert Abrams, a reference book showing the polarities of diseases. - Editor.

All blood specimens fall into one of four polarity groups as do remedies, or in fact any substance in nature they are negative, positive, bi-polar, and neutral.

A glance will show how, by the law of polarity alone, three-fourths of our remedies can be discarded by selecting that group required for the given specimen or case. Negative bloods that measure less than -0.12 intensity require a remedy from the positive group. Bloods that are positive require a negative remedy. Bloods that are bi-polar require bi-polar remedies. Bloods that are neutral require neutral remedies.

The most homeopathic remedy when placed in the circuit with the blood specimen will render that blood just exactly -0.12 (negative), no more, no less, regardless of what that blood polarity is. The remedy must come from the group required by the particular blood specimen's polarity as noted above. Positive remedies for negative cases. Bi-polar remedies for bi-polar cases. Neutral remedies for neutral cases. Negative remedies for positive cases.

The blood changes polarity from the effects of disease. (See Atlas.) Cancer is positive; tuberculosis is neutral; streptococus highly negative less than -0.12 intensity; sarcoma generally bi-polar. The correct remedy changes the abnormal blood polarity to the normal polarity that always accompanies approximate health, namely -0.12 (negative).

I use a mechanical reagent that sits in the Abram's circuit in the same place occupied by the human subject. It is made up of a glass or light crock jar of about a gallon capacity covered entirely over with chamois skin. Below is a crude illustration with circle for areas marked as those occurring on the human subject's abdomen. In this jar is suspended a photo-electric cell connected with the reflexophones (see Figure 2).

Reactions obtained by using a non-metallic glass or hard rubber rod over the surface areas of mechanical subject. A distinct sticking of the rod is felt when reactions come in.

Use same areas shown by atlas as on human reagent.

FIGURE 2

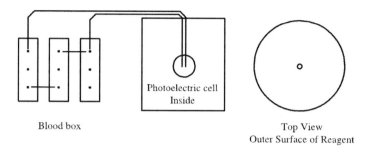

Blood box

Photoelectric cell
Inside

Top View
Outer Surface of Reagent

LIST OF REMEDIES ACCORDING TO THEIR POLARITY (MAGNETIC)[1]

This list is far from complete and quite a few revisions and corrections have been made as well as many additions. After extensive clinical trials in the application of polarity of remedies to the indicated polarity of patients which is summed up as follows: Patients with positive blood require negative remedies. Patients with over negative blood require positive remedies (magnetic polarity measures .12 of an ohm of electrical resistance). Patients with neutral blood require neutral remedies.

From observation of many thousands of cases tested we have proven that the best remedies for patients regardless of symptoms, or better stated, including symptoms present, will be found in that list of remedies called for by the indicated blood polarity of the patient.

From the facts just cited, it is seen that roughly three-fourths of our remedies can be eliminated in the study of any case in the search for the indicated remedy by obtaining the patient's blood polarity.

Out of the special group needed we have a lesser number of remedies to study for the finding of the individual similimum. A few general and high grade mental symptoms can narrow the search to a few remedies after which a little reference to the Materia Medica will bring in the one indicated remedy needed, and lastly this is confirmed by placing the single remedy found over the patient's blood which is immediately restored to the normal, negative polarity measuring .12 ohms negative.

In the study of cancer from a homeopathic view we must not loose sight of the constitutional and miasmatic cause residing in every human born. To this basic cause are added the numerous irritations of environment such as processed and adulterated foods, poisoned water supplies, polluted air, together with all the psychosomatic forces inherited and acquired that beset the race. Included in the environment is the excessive intake of drugs, alcohol, tobacco, coffee and tea all of which debilitates the organism and lessens resistance to disease that they help to create.

The early stage of disease is manifested as a disturbed vital process or morbid physiology. If this morbid physiology is not arrested to eliminated morbid histologic cell growth or pathologic change of tissue result. During the stage of functional disease and especially in childhood and early adult life, the homeopathic remedy is the most potent solvent yet found to eradicate cause by restoring order in the flow of the

---

1. From handwritten manuscript, exact date unknown. - Editor..

life force. This brings a normal state throughout the whole organism from center to circumference because the polarity of the blood and its chemical reactions are rendered normal instantly after the remedy is administered. If functional disease is not checked in time a change of cells and tissues take place ultimating in pathology. These changes embrace the various and numerous organic diseases of the brain, the nervous system, lungs, liver, spleen, kidneys, heart, glands, gastro-intestinal tract, and the blood.

It is this later developed type of disease that test the ingenuity and skill of the physician especially the homeopathic prescriber seeking the one single remedy that can arrest the process of disease toward death and dissolution and reverse the process toward life and regeneration.

In the progress of this change we see old symptoms and conditions return to be superceded by radiant health.

In functional disease a remedy from any polarity group that is indicted may be the similinum, but in the chronic cancer states only those remedies in the negative group will prove sufficient except where the tubercular constitution is dominate and then neutral remedies like NAJA, SYMPH. and TUB. will be needed, sometimes to be followed by deep chronic remedies from the negative group.

Today we are beset by the universal and insidious toxine of aluminum which not only acts as a causative irritant in many cancer constitutions but prevents the smooth action of the indicated remedy while it remains a factor in the case. It behaves like one of the miasms inhibiting the process of cure until it is antidoted and removed. CADM-O. has proven the most efficacious antidote to this poison and at the same time it is one of the most potent remedies we know against cancerous conditions of all kinds. The oxide is the most active of the cadmium group.

Cancer cases may be divided into two groups viz. the pre-cancer functional states and the ultimated pathologic states. In the first group any homeopathic remedy from any of the polarity groups may be the one needed for the case to be treated. Hence, those treated homeopathically while disease is functional have little or any chance of developing cancer. Exceptions occur in those who come from cancerous parents from both family lines. Here we see why a clear and complete family history is so important for both patient and physician. Knowing the family lines enables the physician to apply his most potent weapons for his patients welfare with good chances of preventing cancer even in those individuals with inherited tendencies to the disease. Here indeed is homeopathy's greatest field, prevention. Cures are most desirable but they are difficult and uncertain. Prevention eliminates the necessity of tedious cure.

Homeopathy has both the complete knowledge of the many causative factors in cancer and adequate means to successfully combat it in our wonderful Materia Medica guided by the law of cure and a matchless philosophy.

While any remedy in the negative polarity group may be useful and needed in any given cancer case as they are all anti-cancerous in vibration and magnetically, but clinically out of this group of over a hundred remedies and in over thirty years of practical application to cancer patients we only have thirty-five that have shown consistent curative power against the disease. There are ten or fifteen others still in the process of trial that need further confirmation before they can be included in that magic list. Here for your ready reference is that list:

Acalypha-indica	Lung cancer; hemorrhage
Alumina	Rectal cancer
Alumina-fl.	
Alumina-mur.	
Alum-sil	Breast cancer, ulcers on whole breast, periodic pain
Ant-mur	Skin cancer
Aranea-diad.	Lung cancer, hemorrhage
Arg-cyan.	Larynx cancer
Arg-met.	Larynx cancer
Benzoquinone	
Bomhenia	Uterine cancer with hemorrhage
Cad-cyan.	
Cad-fl.	
Cad-met.	Breast cancer
Cad-ox.	
Cancer Astoc.	
China	Weakness from hemorrhage
Conium	Breast cancer
Euph.	Bone cancer, pains of cancer
Glyorolide (?)	
Hippoz.	Brain, breast, glands cancer
Hydrastis-can.	Liver cancer

Kali-cyan	Prostate cancer with mets
Koch (Cancer)	
Lapis-alb.	Bone cancer and glands
Millefolium	Hemorrhage of cancer
Phytolacca	Breast cancer
Plumb-met.	
Rock and shell	Not in Materia Medica
Scolopendra	Hard palate cancer cured
Scrophularia-nodosa	Breast and glands
Symphytum	Sarcoma especially of jaw
Theridion	Lung and liver

NEUTRAL GROUP

A
Abies-can.
Abies-nigra
Acetanlidium
Acetic-acid
Actaea-spic.
Adonis-vernalis
Adrenalin
Aesculus-hipp.
Aetusa-cynap.
Agaricus-muscarius
Agnus-cast
Agrostemma
Aletris
Allium-cepa
Allium-sativa
Alloxan
Alnus-rubra
Aloe
Alumen
Alumina-mur
Alumina-phos.
Ambra-gris.
Ambrosia

Amyl-nitrosum
Anagallis-arv.
Angustura
Antimonium-mur
Antimonium-tart.
Antipyrinum
Apocynum-andros.
Apocynum-cann.
Aquilegia
Arbutus-andr.
Argentum-chl.
Argentum-iod.
Arsenicum-brom.
Arsenicum-iod.
Artemisia abs.(Absin.)
Arum-triphyllum
Asclepias-syr.
Asclepias tuberosa
Aspirin
Aurantium
Aurum-calc-carb-fl.
Aurum-kali-fl.
Aurum-kali-mur.
Aurum-mur.

Aurum-natrum-fl.
Aurum-natrum-mur
Avena-sativa
Aviare

B
Bacillinum
Badiaga
Balsam of Peru
Baptisia
Barium-sulph
Bed Bug Lig
Bellis-perennis
Benzoic-acid
Berberis-aquif.
Beryllium-nitr.
Beryllium-phos.
Bismuth-iod.
Blue Electricity
Bolen
Boletus
Bombyx
Bothrops-lanc.
Bovista

NEUTRAL GROUP ...

Brachyg-repens
Brassica-nap.
Bromquin
Bromo-seltzer
Buboine
Butyric-acid

C
Cadmium-ars
Cadmium-phos.
Cahinca
Calcarea-ars
Calcarea-oxal
Calcarea-phos.
Calcarea-pic.
Calcarea-ren-phos
Calcarea-sulph.
Cannabis-indica
Cannabis-sativa
Carbo-veg.
Carboneum-hydrog.
Carcinoma-breast
Carcinoma-k
Carica-papoya
Cass-chrom.
Cauloph-thal.
Ceanothus
Cedron
Cerabonium
Cereus-bonplandii
Cereus-serpent.
Chaulmugra-oil
Chimaphila-umb.
Chininum-ars.
Chininum-bisulph

Chininum-sulph.
Chocolate
Chrysophanic-acid
Cimex
Cimex
Cimicifuga-rac
Cineraria
Citric-acid
Citric-acid
Citrus-lim.
Clematis
Cobalt-met.
Cobalt-nitr
Coccinella
Cocc. septempunctata
Coccus Cacti
Codeinum
Comocladia
Convallaria-majalis
Copaiva
Cornus-circ.
Coto-cortex
Coyotillo
Crataegus-oxy
Cresol
Crocus-sativa
Croton-chloral
Cuprum-iod.
Cuprum-met
Cuprum-mur
Cyclamen

D
Daphne-ind.
Datura-arb.

Digitalis
Dioon Edule(?)
Dirca-palust.
Dolichos
Drosera
Duboisinum

E
Egg Plant
Ephedra-vulg.
Epigea-repens
Epilobium-pal.
Equisetum-robust.
Erigeron
Erodium
Eucalyptus (?negative,
    ?neutral)
Eugenia-jamb
Eupatorium-per.
Euphor-heter
Euphrasia
Eupionum

F
Fagopyrum-escul
Feldspar
Felix-cap.
Felsal(?Fel-sui)
Ferrum-iod.
Ferrum-cyn
Filix-mas.
Formica-rufa
Fragaria

NEUTRAL GROUP ...

G
Gallic-acid
Gambogia
Gaultheria
Ginseng
Gladiola
Glonoin(?Glanderine)
Glycerinum
Granatum
Green Tomato
Grindelia-root
Grossularite
Guaiacum
Gun-powder

H
Hamamelis
Hedeoma-puleg.
Hedera-helix
Heliant-ann.
Helix Tosta.
Helonias-dio
Hepar-sulph-calc.
Hepar-sulph-kali
Heracleum
Hydrophyllum-virg.

I
Ichtodes
Influenza
Insulin
Iodoformum
Iris-tenax
Iris-vers

J
Juniperus
   Communis

K
Kali-ars.
Kali-bichromicum
Kali-cyn.
Kali-fer-cyn
Kali-fl
Kali-nitr.
Kali-perman
Kali-phos
Kali-sulph.
Kalmia
Kamala

L
Lactic-acid
Lanth. (?Lachn.)
Lactrodectus-kat
Latrodectus-mactans
Larynx-tuberculosis
Lathyrus-sativa
Lecithin
Lemna-minor
Lepedium-bon.
Leptandra
Lilium-tigrinum
Limulus
Lipps
Lobelia-erinus
Lobelia-inflat.
Lobelia-syph.
Lonicera-tart.

Lycopus-virg.
Lyssin
   (Hydrophobinum)

M
Magnesia-mur.
Magnesia-phos.
Magnesia-sulph
Magnet-pol-ambo
Magnolia-glauca
Mancinella
Manganum-mur
Mangifera-ind.
Maple Sap
Marenalin
Medorrhinium
Mentha-pip.
Menyanthes.
Mephites
Mercurius-cor.
Mercurius-praecipt-alb.
Metastatic-melanoma
Methylene-blue
Methalum (?)
Metrazol
Minucent
Mock-orange
Morgan
Morphinum
Moschus

N
Nabalus
Naja
Naphthalinum

NEUTRAL GROUP ...

Narcissus
Natrum-ars.
Natrum-cacodyl
Natrum-chlor
Natrum-dilantin
Natrum-fl.
Natrum-hypochl.
Natrum-hyposulph.
Natrum-iod.
Natrum-mur.
Natrum-nitr.
Natrum-per.
Natrum-phos.
Natrum-salic
Natrum-sil.
Natrum-sil-fl.
Nembutal
Neo-silver (silvol?)
Nitro-muriatic-acid
Nitr-spirit-dulc
Nuphar-luteum
Nyctanthes-arb.

O
Odoroform
  (Iodoform?)
Oleum-animale
Oleum-jecoris-as
Oleum-santali
Ornithogalum-umb.
Opium
Osmium
Oxalic-acid
Oxytropis-lam
Oxydendron-arb.

Ovarian (Ovinum?)

P
Paenoia
Papain
Paraffin
Parotidinum
Parthenium
Pecten-jacob.
Penicilin-Sodium
Petroleum
Petroselinum
Phaseolus-nana
Phos-mur.
Phenacetin
Phellandrium
Physostigma
Pinus-sylvestris
Piperazinum
Pituitary
Platinum-mur.
Plumbum-ars.
Plumbum-iod
Plumbum-mur
Poconeol
Polygon-sag.
Psorinum
Ptelea-trif
Pulsatilla
Pyrus-amer.

R
Radium-brom.
Radium-iod.
Raphanus

Ratanhia
Rhus-ven.
Russula-foet

S
Salicylic-acid
Salix-nig.
Saly Theop.
Saccharum-off.
Sambucus-nigra
Sanguinaria-nitr.
Sanguinaria-tart
Senna
Serum-Ang.
  Ichthyotoxin
Serum-Leg.
Seuic Uson
Silicea
Silica gels.
Sodium-cacodyl
Solanum-nigrum
Solidago
Spartein-sulph.
Sphingurus
Spigelia
Spiraea-ulm.
Squilla
Stannum-iod.
Stearic-acid.
Sticta-pul
Stillingia
Strophans Gaiggs
Strych-ars.
Strych. Bi-sed
Strych-phos.

Neutral Group ...

Strych-sulph.
Strych-valer.
Succinic-acid
Sufonal
Sulph. Fachion(?)
Sulph-iod.
Sumbul
　　(?bipolar,?neutral)
Syco-syphlinum
Sycotic Co.
Symphoricarpus-Rac.
Symphytum
Syphilinum
　　(?bipolar, ?neutral,
　　?positive)

T

Tartaric-acid
Taxus-bac.
Tedral
Tela-aranea
Terminalia-arjuna.

Teucr-marum
Teucr-scor.
Thymus
Thyroidinum
Trodis
Tuberculinum-bov
Tuberculinum-Heath
Tuberculinum-Koch
Tuggin

U

Umckaloala
Upas
Uranium-nit
　　(?bipolar,?neutral)
Uric-acid
Urtica-urens
　　(?bipolar,?neutral)

V

Vanadium-met.
Vanadium-ars.

Variolinum
Vat. Saly
Veratrum-vir.
Verbascum
Veronal
Viburnum-opulus
Vinca-min
Vipera
Vipera-aqua
Viscum-alb.
Vitamin D.
Vitamin K.

X

Xanthoxylum

Z

Zacum (?)
Zinc-iod.
Zinc-mur.
Zinc-valer.

Negative Group

A

Acorus-calamus
　(Calamus aromaticus)
Aethiops-mineralis
Alfalfa
Alumina
Aluminium-met (?)
Alumina-silicata
Alumina-sulph.
Alum-sulph-sil-calc
Amino-acetic-acid
　　(Glycocollum)

Ammonium-mur.
Amygdalus-persica
Anantherum
Anhalonium
Anilinum
Anthrakokali
　(Anthracokali)
Antimonium-ars.
Antimonium-iod.
Antimonium-mur.
Antim-sulph-aureum
Aralia-racemosa

Aranea-diadema
Arctium-lappa
　　(Lappa-arctium)
Areca-catechu
Argentum-chlor
　　(muriaticum?)
Argentum-cyan.
Argentum-metallicum
Arlome
Asafoetida
Asparagus-officinalis

NEGATIVE GROUP ...

Aspidosperma-
  quebracho
Asterias-rubens
Asvagandra (?)
Aureomycin
Avocado Skin.

B
Baryta-acetica
Baryta-carb
Basalt Scori
Benzoquinone
Beryllium
Bismuth-natrum-tart.
Black Radish
Blatta-amer.
Blatta-orient
Bomhenia
Bryonia
Bufo (?bipolar,
  ?negative)

C
Cactus-grandiflourus
Cadmium-barium
  -iodatum
Cadmium-bichromate
Cadmium-calcarea
  -carb.
Cadmium-calcarea
  -fluorica
Cadmium-calcarea
  -iodatum
Cadmium-calcarea
  -silicata

Cadmium-caust.
Cadmium-chrom.
Cadmium-fl.
Cadmium-kali-brom
Cadmium-kali-cyanide
Cadmium-kali-iodatum
Cadmium-kali-mur.
Cadmium-mag-carb
Cadmium-mag-mur.
Cadmium-mal
Cadmium-met.
Cadmium-natr-mur.
Cadmium-oxide
Cadmium-phos
Calcarea-carb.
Calcarea-caust
Calcarea-fluor
Calcarea-fluor
Calcarea-iod
Calcarea-lac.
Calcarea-mur
Calcarea-ox.
Calcarea-pent.
Calcarea Silicata
Calcarea & Salt
California Redwood
Calotropis-gigantea
Carcinosinum
Carduus-benedictus
Carious-tooth
Cascara-sagrada
Causticum
Ceanothus-amer.
Cheiranthus-cheiri
Chelone-glab.

Chenopodium-anth
Chimaphila
  -umbellata
China-off.
Chionanthus-virg
Chloral-hyd.
Cina
Cistus-canadensis
Citrus-sinensis
  (orange sucker)
Cobalt-muriaticum
Cobalt-phos.
Coca (Erythroxylon)
Cocculus-indicus
Colchicum
Conchiolinum
Conium
Corpus
Corpus-luteum
  (?Folliculinum)
Corydalis-formosa
Cotyledon
Culex
Cypripedium
  (?bipolar, ?negative)

D
Darthronol
Dicalc-phos & Calc
  -gluco-with Vit. D
Diubut
Doern Ser.
Dulcamara

Negative Group ...

E
Earth salts
   (Sales terrestres)
Eggause Energy
Elaeis-guin
Eosinum
Epiphegus-virg.
Eriodictyon-calif.
Erodium
Eryngium-aqua.
Eucalyptus
   (?neutral, ?negative)
Euonymus Atrop.
Euphorbia-lathyris
Euphorbium

F
Fagus-sylvatica
Ferrum-met.
   (?positive, ?negative)
Ficus-benghalens
Ficus-religiosa
Formalin
Franciscea-uniflora

G
Gaertner
Gallium
Gnaphalium
Granite
Guarana
Guland (?)

H
Haematoxylon

Helleborus-Foet
Heptuna & Folic Acid
Hippomanes
Hippozaeninum
Hoang-nan
   (Strychnos
   gaultheriana)
Homarus
Hura-brasiliensis
Hydrangea
Hydrastis-can.
Hydrastis-mur.
Hydrocotyle-asiatica
Hyoscyamus
Hypericum

I
Iberaman
Iberis
Ice Plant
Ignatia
Ilex-aquif.
Inula-helenium.
Isene

J
Jaborandi
Jacaranda-caroba
Jalapa
Jatropha-cur
Jequirity

K
Kali-brom.
Kali-carb.

Kali-chlor.
Kali-iod.
Kali-mur.
Kali-sil.
Kali-thio-cyn.
Kalmect (?)
Kaolin
Khanpap (?)

L
Lapis-alb
   (?negative, ?bipolar)
Linum-catharticum
Lithium-benz.
Lithium-brom.
Lithium-carb.
Lithium-lact.
Lithium-tart
Lycopersicum

M
Magnesia-carbonica
Magnesia-mur
Mag-pole-aust
Malic Acid
Manganum-mur
Mannitol-hexa
   -phenobarbital
Medusa
Melilotus-alba
Merc-iod-flav
Merc-iod-rub.
Mexican-root
Mezereum

Negative Group ...

Millefolium
  (?positive, ?negative)
Mono-sodium
  -glutamate
Morbillinum
Mullo (cholorphyl)
Mustard-gas
Mygale-lasid.
Myristica
Myrtus-com.

N
Nabalus-alb
  (serpentarius)
Nakamo
Natrum-hexa
  -meta-phos.
Natrum-pentholate
Natrum-thio-cyn.
Nicconexine
Nux-mosch.
Nux-vomica
Nylon

O
Oreodaphne-calif.
Origanum-marj.
Ovi-gall-pell.
Oxygen
Oxy-clori. (?)

P
Parthenium-hyster
Paris-quad.
Pertussinum

Physalia-pelagic
Physostigmine
  (?bipolar, ?negative)
Phytolacca
Plantago-major
Plumbum metallicum
Podophyllum
Potassium
Prontosel
Prostigmin
Punaranum

R
Radium
Red Vulc.
Resorcin
Rhodium
Rhodium-met
Rumex
Rutin

S
Samarsakite
Sanicula
Sarracenia
Sarsparilla
Scorr. Equi.
Scirrhinum
Scolopendra
  (centipede)
Scopolamine
Scorpio
Scrophularia-nodosa
Scutellaria

Selenium (?positive,
  ?negative, ?bipolar)
Sempervivum
  -tectorum
Silecea-calc-kali-carb.
Silver-maple-seed
Skookum-chuck
Sodium-cyn.
Sodium-pent.
Solanum-integri
Spiranthes
Spiritus-gland-quer.
Staphysagria
Stellaria-media
Strammonium
Streptomycin
Strontium-carb.
Strophanthus-hispidus
Strychinum
Sycotic Co.
Syzygium

T
Tanacetum-vulg.
Tannic-acid
Tarentula
Thallium-iod.
Thallium-met.
Thallium-oxid.
Thallium-sulph.
Theridion
Thiosinaminum
Tilia
Tillandsia-usneoid
  (Spanish Moss)

NEGATIVE GROUP ...

Titanium-met.
Triona
Tungsten-met.
Turnera-aphro
　(Damiana)
Twigs & Moss

U
Unicaps
Uranium-met.
Usnea-barbta

V
Verbena-hast.
Viburnum

Viscum-album
Vitamin B-12
Vitamin C

Z
Zema Cap.
Zirconium-met.
Zizia-aur.

BI-POLAR GROUP

A
Ailanthus
Aletris-far.
Alon-flour
Alum-mur
Amalgum
Ammonium-carb.
Ammonium-caust.
Ammonium-iod.
Ammonium-phos.
Ammonium-valer.
Anacardium
Anthrax
Arctium-lappa
Arnica
Arsenicum-alb.
Arsenicum-sulph-flav.
Arsenicum-sulph-rub.
Arsenicum-ter-sul.
Aurum-iod
Aurum-kali-brom.
Avocado-seed.

B
Baby-sea-mussel
Barium-iod.

Barium-mur.
Benzedrine-sulph.
Bismuth-natrum-tart.
Black-rock
Blister-bug.
Borax
Bothrox Atrox
Botulinum
Bromium
Brucella
Bufo
　(?negative, ?bipolar)

C
Cadmium-brom
Cadmium-cyn.
Cadmium-ferr.
Cadmium-ferr-iod
Cadmium-iod.
Cadmium-lac.
Cadmium-merc.
Cadmium-merc-chrom
Cadmium-mur
Cadmium-natr-sil-fl.
Cadmium-nitricum
Cadmium-sulph

Caltha-pal.
Camphora
Camphora-mono-brom.
Cancer-ast.
　(Astacus-fluviatilis)
Cantharis
Carbolic-acid
Carbo-animalis
Carboneum
　-hydrogenisatum
Carboneum
　-oxygenisatum
Carduus-marianus
Castor-equi
Cenizo
Cench-contortrix
Chamomilla
Chaparro-amarg
Chininum-phos
Chininum-salicylate
Chloroformum
Cholesterinum
Chromic-acid
Chromium-oxydatum
Cicuta-virosa
Cistus-can

Bi-polar Group ...

Colostrum
Condurango
Congo-red.
Coral-rub.
Crotalus-cas.
Crotalus-hor.
Cuprum-calc-iod
Curare
Cypress-law
Cypripedium
  (?negative, ?bipolar)

D
Datura-arb.
Diamond
Diptherinum

E
Echinacea-ang
Elapps-cor.
Emerald
Eryngium

F
Ferrum-brom
Ferrum-iod
Ferrum-oxid
Ferrum-pic
Fluoric-acid.
Frax-amer
Fucus-ves.

G
Gratiola
Gymnocladus

H
Heckla-lava
Heloderma-hor.
Hemiloln
Hydrocyanic-acid

I
Illicium
  (Anisum stellatum)
Indigo
Iodum

K
Kali-nit
Koch-Cancer
Kreosotum

L
Lac-caninum
Lac-defloratum
Lac-humanum
Lachesis
Lapis-alb.
  (?negative, ?bipolar)
Latrodectus-mactans
  (?neutral, ?bipolar)
Laurocerasus
Lycopodium

M
Magnetis-poli-ambo
Malandrinum
Mastuerzo
Menigoccinum
Meningoccus-antitoxin

Merc-ars
Merc-cyn.
Merc-iod-Kali-iod.
Merc-prec-alb.
Merc-sol-H.
Murex
Muriatic-acid
Myrica-cerifera

N
Natrum-sulph.
Niccolum-met.
Nitric-acid.
Nosodes

O
Ocimum-can

P
Panthro
Pariera-brava
Parotidinum
Phlorizinum
Phosphoric-acid.
Phosphorus
Physostigma
  (?negative, ?bipolar)
Picric-acid
Piper-methysticum
Piperazine
Pituitary
Placental-substance
Pyrogen

Bi-polar Group ...

R
Radium
Radium-brom.
Radium-cad.
Radium-Chlor.
Radium Clor.
  & Spongia(?)
Ranunculus-scel
Ratanhia
Rhamnus-cath.
Rheum
Rhododendron
Rhus-aromatica
Rhus-rad.

S
Sabadilla
Sabal-serrulata
Sabina
Saccharum-lactis
Secale-cornutum
Senecio
Senega
Sepia
Sililcea-atlantis
Sisyrinchium
  -galaxoides
Solanum-oleraceum

Solanum-tuber-aegrot.
Spiritus-glandi-quercus
Spongia
Sulfo-Kreosol
Sulphur
  (?positive, ?bipolar)
Sulphuric-acid
Sumbul
  (?neutral, ?bipolar)
Syphilinum (?neutral
  ?positive, ?bipolar)
Syzygium

T
Tallium Sta.
Taraxacum
Terebinthinum-oleum
  (?positive, ?bipolar)
Thiosinamine
Thlaspi-bursa-pastoris
Thuja
Thyroidinum
Tissue Salts
Toxicophis.
Tuberculinum-test.

U
Uranium-aceticum

Uranium-nitricum
  (?neutral, ?bipolar)
Urtica-urens
  (?neutral, ?bipolar)
Ustilago
Uva-ursi

V
Valeriana-off.
Variolinum
Veratrum-alb
Viola-odorata
Viola-tri
Vitamin-A

X
X-Ray

Y
Yohimbinum

Z
Zinc-arsen.
Zinc-nitricum
Zinc-phos.

Positive Group

A
Aconite
Agave-amer
Antimonium crudum
Apis-mellifica
Areca-nut (catechu)

Argentum-cyn.
Argentum-nitricum
Argentum-phos.
Argentum-pitur. (?)
Argentum-sulph.
Aristolochia mihomens

Artemisia absinth.
  (Absinthium)
Atribine(?)
Atropinum
Aurum-ars.
Aurum-cyn.

Positive Group ...

Aurum-met.
Aurum-sulph.
Avocado-pulp

B
Belladonna
Berberis-vulg.
Bismuth-met.
Brassica-nap-oleifera

C
Caffein-citr.(?)
Calendula-off.
Cajuputum
Carbo-fl.(?)
Carboneum-sulph.
Cayoid(?)
Chelidonium
Cherry-pit
Cinnabaris
Cinnamomum
Coffea
Colocynthis
Conchiolinum
   (?negative,?positive)
Cotyledon
   (?negative, ?positive)
Croton-Tig
Cuprum-ars.
Cuprum-Ferr.(?)
Cuprum-met.
Cuprum-met
   -Mang-Phos.
Cuprum-phos.
Cuprum-sulph.

D
Dental-rubber(?)
Derris-pinnata
Digitalis
Digitoxinum

E
Ephedrin
Ether
Euphorbium

F
Ferrum-cuprum (?)
Ferrum-met.
   (?negative,?positive)
Ferrum-phos
Ficus-relig.

G
Gallstones
Gelsemium
Glat-amer. (?)
Graphites
Gros.
   (?neutral, ?positive)
Guarea-trich.

H
Hippozarina (?)

I
Indium-met.
Ipecacuanha
Iridium-met

K
Kali-ferro-cyn.
Kurchi.

L
Lac-humanum
Leburnum
Ledum

M
Mag-pol-arc.
Malandrinum
Manganum-phos.
Manganum-sil.
Mathicola
Mathicola Groc.(?)
Mercurius-vivus
Merc-chrom
Merc-iod-fl.
Merc-sulph.
Millefollium
   (?negative,?positive)

N
Natrum-carb.
Natrum-nitricum
   (?neutral,?positive)
Natrum-phos.
   (?neutral,?positive)

O
Ogymun
Oleander
Onosmodium
Orchitinum

POSITIVE GROUP ...

Oxalic-acid

P
Palladium
Pineal-gland
Piper-nigr.
Platina
Primula (?veris, ?vulg)
Primula-obconica

R
Radium-sulph.
Ranunculus-bulb.
Rhamnus-calif.
Rhus-tox.
Robina-pseud.
Ruta

S
Salvia-son.
Sanguinaria
Sauerkraut
Schth (?)

Selenium(?negative,
    ?bipolar,?positive)
Silphium-lacinatum
Solanum-carolinense
Solidago
Stannum
Sulfanilamide
Sulphur
    (?bipolar,?positive)
Sulphuric-acid
    (?bipolar,?positive)
Sulph-terebinthinum
Supra
Symphytum (?)
Syphilinum (?neutral,
    ?bipolar, ?positive)

T
Tabacum
Tellurium
Terebinthiniae-oleum
    (?bipolar,?positive)
Thlaspi-burs.

U
Urea
Uric-acid

W
Wyethia-hel.

Y
Yohimbinum
    (?bipolar ?spelling)
Yohimbinum-mur.(?)

Z
Zinc-met.
Zinc-oxide
Zinc-perman
Zinc-pic
Zinc-sulph.
Zingiber-off

Cancer

Cancer and Chronic Disease

The Homeopathic Research for Cancer and Other Chronic Diseases

Homeopathic Cancer Research

Remedial Measures: Homeopathic and Dietic - Developed in the Homeopathic Cancer Laboratory of Chicago

New Concepts of the Cancer Question

Cancer - It's Cause, Prevention and Cure

The Homeopathic Philosophy of Cancer Cause

Homeopathic Treatment of Cancer

Homeopathic Science Will Conquer Cancer

The Conquest of Cancer by Homeopathy

The Homeopathic Concept of the Etiology and Cure of Cancer

Cancer and Specifics

Diet for Cancer Patients

The Application of Homeopathic Remedies to Cancer Cases

Cadmium Cures of Cancer

Further Results in the Homeopathic Treatment of Cancer

Some Cancer Remedies and Their Indications

Homeopathic Remedies that have Cured Patients Suffering from Cancer

Remarks on Breast and Prostate Cancer

Cancer and Chronic Disease[1]

The homeopathic approach to chronic disease and cancer differs from the approach of traditional medicine. Homeopathy takes cognizance of the intangible forces operating in and around us; these forces are related to causes and work on the unseen planes of nature.

Force, though material is imponderable, and without form and unseeable, yet knowable by and through its effects in the material forms of matter. The life force in man, that maintains function, growth and repair in his body, is the primary factor in health and disease as it is the source of animation and all life activity. This force cannot be seen, contacted or analyzed; it can only be influenced, retarded or stimulated by other agents or forces as subtle in nature as itself, viz. morbific agents (like viruses or other infections; mental, emotional, physical traumas or inherited traits etc.) and intangible changes in environment may produce sickness which will require a suitable remedial force (or dynamic) to restore equilibrium (or harmony) in the life force with ensuing health.

Before any change takes place in the cells or tissues of the body there is a change in the life force and chemistry of the body; these changes are first observed in the blood stream which carries all nourishment to the remotest parts of the organism. The result of a continuous normal flow of the life force is normal cell growth and development or histology. The result of an interrupted or retarded life force is morbid anatomy or pathology. Hence the homeopathic scientist concerns himself less with the presence of pathology and attacks it by seeking to correct its cause, which is faulty physiology or impaired life force. When the life force is restored to normality the chemistry and tissues of the organism take on normal function and repair to attain a normal cell growth.

Our allopathic friends and colleagues approach this problem of disease from an opposite view point. They believe they are attacking the cause by removing the pathology with surgery, x-ray or radium and other caustic forces. It is true old school scientists are doing commendable and progressive work in the study of blood chemistry, but their attempts to normalize it with highly toxic drugs must end in failure because of the certain side effects produced which are often as harmful to the patient as the disease for which they were given to dispell.

---

1. The Homeopathic Recorder, Vol. LXVI, No. 6, December 1950, p. 357.

From these facts just mentioned it is patent why homeopathic research stresses the necessity of discovering and developing more and more remedies similar in nature to the numerous disease conditions and manifestations afflicting humanity today, for only by the proven law of similia can disease be prevented and irradicated. Homeopathy also stresses the value and importance of prophylaxis for the prevention of sickness both acute and chronic. In this field of preventive medicine it is superlative over all other known methods of therapy because when the life force is normal and unencumbered, resistance is at par and health is present.

The Homeopathic Research for Cancer and other Chronic Diseases[1]

Under the auspices of the Homeopathic Foundation a clinical laboratory is now established to treat patients suffering from cancer, tuberculosis, arthritis in its many forms, heart and kidney diseases, polio myelitis, diabetes and all other chronic forms of chronic illness.

The homeopathic concepts of sickness and its treatment stresses the importance of the individual symptoms and blood chemistry of the patient apart from the disease. Also homeopaths realize that all sickness regardless of name stems from a weakened or obstructed vital force of the sick individual, and that must be treated and normalized in order to obtain a cure.

Not all patients suffering from the same disease can be cured with the same remedy. Each individual requires his own specific homeopathic remedy for his cure. Hence the fallacy of a specific drug for a specific disease as an entity apart from the patient. The homeopathic approach of normalizing the patient's vital physiological processes is a potent factor in the prevention of any or all sicknesses, providing the treatment is instituted before the disease has ultimated in the pathological changes in the tissues and organs of the body. After the pathologic changes have come the treatment requires more time to bring about a state of health and well-being.

The Homeopathic Laboratory will seek out causes of illness, such as heredity and the effects of environment, diet, habits, work, meteorological factors, etc., on individual health; it will also take cognition of the mental and emotional states, frustrations, worries, fears, hates, etc., that are powerful factors in the production of disease. But most of all the Homeopathic Laboratory will concern itself in the discovery and perfection of remedies to meet the appalling increase and variations of sickness afflicting humanity today. Many more remedies than we now have to meet the needs against the cancer scourge will be discovered and developed, enabling the physician to obtain a greater degree of efficiency in the relief and cure of this intractable disease. The Foundation will start with centers in seven of our large cities and gradually spread to many of our smaller cities all over the country. In that way Homeopathy will gain recognition and patronage, and attract physicians who

---

1. THE HOMEOPATHIC RECORDER, Vol. LXVI, No. 3, September, 1950, p. 88.

really want to be proficient healers from the dominant school of medical thought as well as from many of the other schools of healing.

This is homeopathy's golden chance to convince the world, by the wonder of its works, of its superiority over all other methods of healing. Thus it behoves every homeopathic physician and every patient and friend of homeopathy, who have known and felt its benign power, to rally and unite with purpose and determination of making the Foundation's wonderful plan a certain, far-reaching, and ever-growing success.

From time to time the readers of the *Recorder* will have reports of the progress and accomplishments of this wonderful project.

Homeopathic Cancer Research[1]

Homeopathic Cancer Research is far more comprehensive in its scope than is that of the Old School. This comes as a startling statement to the misinformed, but a brief survey of the following facts is conclusive evidence of its truth.

Old School research confines itself to the study of the pathologic processes of cancer chiefly hoping thereby to find its cause. Such procedure has led them constantly in circles and they are, by their own admissions, utterly lost regarding the causative factors involved in the growth and development of cancer in its many forms.

Homeopathic philosophy treating of the nature of illness takes up the study of sickness from its beginnings and even surveys and studies conditions and circumstances prior to such beginnings.

Taking up the pathologic changes of the cell ultimating in cancer and going back a step we find that a chemical change has preceded the cellular change, and that chemical change is admirably illustrated in the splendid work performed by that learned and able worker in THE BEHAVIOR OF THE BLOOD COLLOIDS IN HEALTH AND IN DISEASE, by Dr. Archie Jones, whose achievement in this valuable field has won the admiration of the homeopathic profession and must soon compel recognition from the scientists of the dominate school as well.

Preceding the chemical change in the cells one finds an electro-magnetic change in the currents and life forces of the body, and even the diseased cells take on a change in the polarity.[2] These electro-magnetic changes in the body in health and in disease are now captured and shown on specially treated and super sensitive photographic plates; not only the magnetic waves or emanations of the body are photographed, studied, and classified, but the emanations from malignant tumors are also caught, while no such waves (called mitogenetic) can be obtained from benign growths. This photographic work has been accomplished by German and Italian scientists. Gurwitch, the German, and Cremonese, the Italian, have developed this photographic study to such a state of perfection that an accurate diagnosis can now be made of many obscure and baffling conditions that formerly was not possible by the older methods and techniques. These scientists now look upon the ani-

---

1. From handwritten manuscript. - Editor.
2. See "Recent Concepts and New Formulas in Medicine" on p. 679 ff. and "Importance of Electronic Reactions to Future Medicine" on p. 683 ff.. - Editor.

mal economy of man as being but an electro-magnetic unit in the universal cosmos, with health and disease resulting only from a change of state in the flow of the universal electro-magnetic force dominating everything, organic and inorganic, from the smallest to the greatest in the universe.

For over a hundred and fifty years homeopaths have recognized these things and have gone even farther, for they are able to go back to the fundamental causes of the electro-magnetic changes out into the mental sphere, all of which is now confirmed by the leading physicists of the day. Compton, of the University of Chicago, has been quoted as saying that all evolutionary changes in nature may have been or may be influenced by the power of thought.

Prolonged emotional stress and strain are often leading factors in the change of the electro-magnetic currents of the body, reversing them from a state of health to the opposite direction of a state of disease. Irritants of various kinds, such as the prolonged use of chlorinated water for drinking and cooking, various metalic poisons, such as alumina, copper, lead, zinc, etc., brought about by preparing foods in containers made of these various metals, the abuse of serums and vaccines, and the use of foods deficient in normal mineral content or lacking in vitamins, are proven factors in changing first the electro-magnetic balance of health and later the chemistry of metabolism that finally ultimates in histologic changes in the cells of the body organism itself.

The most basic and fundamental factor in the growth of cancer, that of heredity, was first discovered and announced by homeopathic scientists. Only recently confirmed by the work in animal experimentation very ably conducted by Dr. Maude Sly of the University of Chicago. Because of this basic fact now generally accepted by all as true, homeopaths are better able to successfully cope with the cancer cause.

By eradicating these constitutional or inherited soil causes with the carefully prescribed homeopathic remedy or remedies, (for it often takes a series of complementary remedies, to bring an individual to such developing cancer) we can thus attack this problem at its root.

From the nature and origin of cancer as observed by many able clinicians we know it is an insidious creeping monster slowly undermining the vital processes, starting only as a slight sore or patch, or an enlarged gland or cyst generating toxins as it expands and grows defying all the orderly processes of the body organism, until it becomes a dominating force of destruction ending in death.

Because of this deadly devastating nature, the pre-cancer stage presents the best time for a successful cure to be effected. As the disease advances it becomes increasingly more difficult to control or inhibit it in its deadly march of anarchistic reign. Late stages can only be deferred and the attendant sufferings mitigated by the homeopathic remedy; a cure is out of the question.

From the above mentioned facts it is easy to see the necessity for early treatment if calamity and tragedy is to be avoided. Starting with the child, and instead of depriving him of valuable defense organs or glands like the tonsils, we as homeopaths can, by careful prescribing, successfully restore the so-called infected tonsils to normal appearance and function, leaving the child in a more normal and efficient state to combat other infections and toxins to which he is subjected in his early life environment. (If vital organs, like the heart and lungs, when infected are amenable to homeopathic remedies, and clinical experience proves they are, then how much easier it is to cure a small gland near the surface of the body like the tonsil.)

Instead of an artificial immunity against certain specific infections brought about by injecting directly into the blood stream the toxic by-products of disease we must establish a natural immunity (brought about in the organism by stimulating its automatic defense mechanism with the application of the homeopathic specific) and thereby avoid a host of evils and dangers involving vital organs such as the heart and kidneys. Indeed the blood serum of one animal is inimical to the organism of another (as physiologists have proven) and who can say or measure what great harm or disturbance may result from the injection of so many foreign proteins into the blood of innocent and defenseless children. What abnormal changes may be set up in the endocrine chain of these innocent victims of commercialism and ignorance to mature into moral, mental and physical derelicts. Add to the above mentioned outrages against the bodies of children the abuse of coal tar and other depressing drugs, consumed by those of all ages, without and in spite of medical advice, and we have a host of evil forces perverting and destroying health on an appalling scale.

Still another factor in cancer cause that homeopathic observers have proven beyond any semblance of doubt is the one of suppression. Old School practice consists largely in suppression of disease manifestation in its attempts at cure. Skin eruptions of a chronic nature are suppressed with powerful salves and ointments, headaches and various nerve pains and coughs are suppressed with narcotic and coal tar drugs all of which prevents the normal expression of disease surfaceward by the action of the vital force against disease of toxemia.

If cancer is successfuly treated all the aforesaid irritating and suppressive causes must be removed and careful homeopathic prescribing instituted instead. The fearful and startling increase in cancer, kidney disease, together with insanity and mental diseases under the regime of Old School medicine which deals in and depends largely on surgery and suppressive measures for curative results makes it the duty of every homeopath to spread the gospel of medical light. Both to the brother practicians of the Old School, many of whom are ready for better things, and to the laity who are the victims of a vicious system of commercialism and medical fallacy.

The highly beneficial results obtained in cure under homeopathic treatment in a large percentage (60 to 80 percent) of proven cancer cases is very heartening. This showing excells any and all other methods together thus demonstrated. And for that reason on the broad grounds of humanity and sympathy for the tragic suffering that is the common lot of the cancer victims, I will close with an appeal to every homeopathic doctor to go back to the first principles of homeopathic doctrines and perfect himself in this glorious heaven-sent work for the physical salvation of the sick.

REMEDIAL MEASURES: HOMEOPATHIC AND DIETIC

DEVELOPED IN THE HOMEOPATHIC CANCER RESEARCH LABORATORY OF CHICAGO[1]

This cancer center is only in its formative stage and the work to date has been accomplished by a few men. The number of our workers recently have increased and we have promise of encouraging financial support in the near future from a number of our interested lay friends.

We have recently acquired a home wherein we may conduct our clinics and better pursue our laboratory studies. Our results are mostly of a clinical nature; but so largely beneficial as to open up very hopeful possibilities for the prevention and alleviation of the ever increasing number of cancer sufferers. No research in cancer can hope to accomplish much unless the treatment facilities are associated with the research laboratory.

We are stressing the importance of cancer prevention over any specific cure that may be developed in this work, since the studies of the subject have brought abundant proofs of the advantage of preventive measures over the possibility of cure in the strictest sense (at least in the advanced stages of the disease).

The most important factor in any case as well as in the sub-total of all cases is a complete and detailed personal and family history including all essential laboratory tests used by all investigators. To the homeopathist such a history has a dual significance involving both causative elements and therapeutic means. The constitutional and inherited soil tendency of cancers as fundamentally causative was first advanced by the homeopaths. This fundamental fact is now accepted by all cancer authorities and all schools of medical thought.

The animal experimentation of Dr. Maude Sly of Chicago University has established the inheritability of cancer in families beyond all doubt. The investigations of Crile and others show that the cancer cells have lost their normal bipolar electrical state and taken on a positive electric state with a resulting change in the position and size of the cell nucleus. More recent investigation in the behavior of the colloids in the blood of healthy and cancerous subjects show a marked electromagnetic and chemical change in the blood preceding the pathology of the

---

1. THE HOMEOPATHIC RECORDER, Vol. XLVI, No. 3, March 1931, p. 172.

cells ultimating as cancer. Many secondary or subcauses enter the field as multiple factors in the growth of cancer.

Recent discoveries by means of an improved technique in photography has enabled an Italian scientist of repute, Prof. Cremonese, to photograph the "vital rays or emanations of the human body". This achievement may well be regarded as one of the most important discoveries of all time fully confirming the hypothesis that life is an oscillatory electromagnetic phenomen. The Italian savant is quoted as saying: "This discovery is the missing link without which it was hitherto impossible to fully understand and explain the mystery of life."

"Its effects will be of incalculable value especially, because having once ascertained that the nature of life is purely physical, the treatment of disease will have to be conducted on different lines, starting from the idea that disease is nothing but an alteration of the oscillatory state of equilibrium of the organism, both in the physical and psychic field".

"The photograph of vital radiations had already been attempted, but with unsatisfactory results. In 1922 Gurwitch said that the rays emanating from the roots of onions were capable of inducing an increased cellular growth in other roots. Hence the name of Gurwitch's mitogentic radiations."

"Numerous scientists have devoted themselves to the mysterious problem. Among the pioneers must be mentioned two Germans, Reiter and Gabor, who were able to confirm the existence of mitogenetic radiations which are ultraviolet rays of a wave length of 2,000 to 34,000 angstroms (the angstrom is equivalent to the ten millionth part of a milimeter i.e. 10^{-7} mm)."

"They discovered that malignant tumors emit mitogenetic radiations and benign tumors do not. After several vain attempts they came to the conclusion that it was impossible to photograph the vital rays."

"It is very probable that in the near future, with an improved technique, we shall be able to diagnose special pathological or heriditary conditions by means of the photography of vital rays."

"My discovery proves in a most conclusive manner that life is a purely physical phenomenon to be placed in the field of electromagnetism. This is of the greatest importance because it opens up new possibilities in physioloy and pathology."

"If we admit that the real cause of disease is a lack of equilibrium between the internal rays of the body and the external ones, and that disease is not the result of pathogenous agent but of the state of the individual, it is obvious that the alterations of this wonderful oscillatory circuit, namely disease, can only be cured by opportunely modifying the oscillatory rhythm, thus restoring equilibrium, which means health."

"As Science progresses", concluded Prof. Cremonese, "it is more evident that we are electromagnetic atoms vibrating in unison with the great throb of the universe."

How marvellously similar is all this to the formerly ridiculed "vital force" of Hahnemann.

The work of Tharaldsen exhibiting the effect of shock: electrical, chemical or physical on normal cells is another evidence of how the currents of the body organism are the primary forces that either break down or repair it in accordance with the direction they may be forced to take.

Among the sub-causes is the one of irritation, chemical or physical, commonly produced by the abuse of crude drugs, especially those of the coal tar group. Also the extensive use of serums and vaccines employed for prophylaxis and in the cure of infections of various kinds. These agents affect the cells of the body by inhibiting or reversing the electromagnetic currents of the organism, thus changing the blood chemistry and later instituting actual changes in the histological elements of the body.

The effects of abuse of curde drugs on the body organism as it develops the toxemias and chronic changes called cancer might well suggest curative possibilities to the homeopathist employed in potentized form and in accordance with our well proven law of therapeutics. It might also provide an answer to the observed fact that cancer is continuously occurring in younger individuals in each succeeding generation. Also may not the almost universal practise of tonsilectomy in children have some bearing on that phenomenon as well.

Another place where remedies of a certain type and form may be successfully employed is to restore an unbalanced mineral content in the blood stream; these are brought about either by a diet of processed foods such as white flour and refined sugar or by foods lacking the sufficient amounts of the primary elements commonly known as the tissue salts (such foods having been grown on exhausted soils or soils deficient in these essential mineral elements). In this way are produced blood, cell and nerve changes in the body; resistance to infections is thereby lowered and irritations of various kinds result. A blood replenished by low potencies of these necessary mineral elements will often restore many incipient cases and even some advanced cases of cancer, provided a consistent diet rich in the necessary mineral ingredients and free of the irritating ones is persistently and consistently taken by the patient. Dr. Kaust of Chicago claims he has authentic records of over 200 cases of cancer in various stages cured by the application of the tissue salts.

Some of our remedies given in high potencies act as catalysts to restore the mineral balance in the blood providing such mineral defeciency has not been too far reduced by waste and disease. Another observation first noted by Hahnemann and only recently mentioned by several investigators of note are the pre-cancer symptoms and states occuring in cancer victims together with the interchangability of several systemic chronic disease conditions such as tuberculosis in one generation alternating with epilepsy and cancer in a succeeding one; or in members of the same family some having one and some another of these complaints. Diabetes and cancer frequently alternate. Asthma and chronic skin diseases also many times alternate in the same individual and in succeeding generations of the same families. All this is consistent with Hahnemann's conception of the basis of chronic diseases having a common cause viz. in the inherited soil condition of the family setting and secondly in an altered or perverted flow of the individual's life processes or Vital Force. This may be reduced to more modern terms viz. that normal physiology produces and sustains normal cell growth, normal histology and anatomy while abnormal or perverted physiology produces abnormal histology and pathology and these changes are preceded by a changed activity in the colloidal electricity and chemistry of the blood. And this chemistry of the organism with its specialized groups of cells, endocrine glands, etc., and its multitudeneous functions and activities are controlled by the nervous systems voluntary and involuntary, conscious and sympathetic moving in harmonious unity in all the complex and automatic processes that ultimate in and perpetuate the wonderful manifestations of life. The electro-magnetic currents of the organism (produced by the continuous exchange of gases in the lungs wherein the oxidation of the blood is consumated), produce the recurring cycles of physical life.

This picture of the changing and perishable body of the material world, wonderful and beautiful, is only the visible part presented by scientists and physiologists whose work we all admire. Back of all this marvelous mechanism of the material or sense world is the inner or internal man which exists and operates and constitutes the life force of Hahnemann. Scientists are only now contacting this force that he perceived 150 years ago.

The physicists who lead the world of science have probed and analyzed the nature and behavior of the finest particles of the atom so far known - the electron, the proton and the neutron - and have arrived at the point where matter and energy are interchangeable; and still the baffling mystery of life remains unsolved. The intricate science, involving the new mathematics[1], as evolved by the genius of Einstein, can do no more than trace the relative nature of time and space and the interchange and relationship of matter and energy.[2]

Compton is said to have announced that thought may be the dominating influence in the material process of nature. These mighty savants now bow down to the sovereign power of thought as something immortal and dominating in the domain of nature, a force defying their analysing scrutiny yet vibrant with possibilities as the key to unlock the vault holding the riddle of life enshrouded in the immortal circle of eternal truth.

In medicine, if not in physics and science, homeopaths have been pioneer observers in the boundless and pregnant archives of thought. They are the Einsteins of medicine who interpreted and correlated thought forces with the changing processes of health and disease. The mental symptoms of our proven remedies have always held first rank as guiding symptoms in the selection of the curative remedy to the specific case. More recently the vanguard of the old school have begun the study of thought processes and the emotions in relation to disease. Psychoanalysis and psychology are now quite common and useful in the study and technique of every recognized nerve specialist.

These things are mentioned to impress upon your minds the value of the homeopathic philosophic concepts of health and disease. We need no longer apologize for such tenets. (Some homeopaths have, in the not so distant past, done more - they have denounced such doctrines as visionary and foolish). Before now the leaders of scientific thought had

---

1. Actually Dr. Grimmer was referring to Einstein's Theory of Special Relativity which actually involved well known mathematics (at least to scientists) but new to the layman. - Editor.

2. The equation of Einstein, $E=mc^2$, states that when 1 g of matter is converted into energy, the energy liberated is 900,000,000,000,000,000,000 ergs or 3,770,000,000 kilocalories; to express it differently: enough heat to boil 37,000 tons of ice water.
   It has been suggested that this equation $E=mc^2$, that governs the relation between matter (mass m) and energy E explains the great power of our homeopathic remedies as they are prepared by trituration and succussion. - Editor.

been led by slow and tortuous byways to the threshhold of our abode where light and sustenance await to aid them in the tedious climb up the mountain heights of knowledge.

But the homeopathic cancer clinic will endeavor to correlate and use all the knowledge so far gathered by the workers in the vast field. All will contribute in the upbuilding of our edifice dedicated to the alleviation of suffering and the upbuilding of better health. The study of the chemistry of foods in health and in disease will be assiduously followed. And led by our wonderous therapeutic law we will develop remedies of great power for the prevention and cure of this heretofore baffling but not unconquered monster. For our records are replete with numerous cures and therein lies the hope for humanity.

And this brings us to the most important phase of the whole subject: the mental or psychological feature, both individually and collectively. The mental attitude or psychology of the dominant school of medicine is fatally prohibitive of progress or success in the fight against the cancer scourge. They are whipped before they start to fight; to them it is useless to try to cure and palliation is the most they strive for. Such an atmosphere can not hearten physician or patient; hence it has come to pass that a diagnosis of cancer be it right or wrong is equivalent to the sentence of death. The terror, the suffering, the childish helplessness and the utter hopelessness of modern scientific medicine in its application to cancer is a universal tragedy.

The alarming increase in cancer victims of the last two decades must be a concern for all physicians and lay people alike. Remembering that every one individual in eight past forty years of age will die of cancer, we cannot treat this thing lightly. We know not where the blow will fall: some loved member of one household or some devoted and valued friend may be the next victim or even anyone of us assembled here may be called upon to tread the path down to the dark shadows of the grave; no flesh is immune to the inroads of this hideous terror.

Only the God given truth of Homeopathy offers any hope of the successful conquest of this devastating woe. A surprisingly few patients who have had the advantage of real homeopathic constitutional prescribing (over an adequate period of time, say from two to five years), will suffer from any form of cancer. And if a preventive diet, one that is meat free, is followed at the same time their chances for health will be still more improved and cancer even less likely.

Contrast the homeopathic psychology with the dismal weakness presented by the old school leaders and investigators of cancer today. They say: "we do not know its cause we have no remedy to cure, only surgery and radium might ameliorate suffering and prolong life. We have nothing more to offer."

But a suffering world has come to know how futile and inadequate these measures are when weighed by their clinical results. Only a heavy financial burden has been saddled on the back of misery to plunge the hapless victims down to the depths of despair.

In Homeopathy's law of cure may be found the arsenal of healing power; that they who wear her shining armor and wield her flashy sword are sustained by a faith born of knowledge, and heartened by a courage begotten of oft repeated victory in the grim battle against disease. They radiate hope and bring strength to the despairing and the afflicted. They are messengers and instruments of the Inscrutable all pervading, all merciful, eternal architect of the universe because they labor with love and move and work with the immutable currents of the irrevocable law.

New Concepts of the Cancer Question[1]

Every advance in the investigation of cancer leads more and more to the conclusion that the cancer cause exists in an inherited susceptibility or soil condition which only requires some exciting irritation to start the morbid processes that ultimates in cancer. Cancer has been likened to an anarchistic group of cells refusing to be governed by the body organism and gradually encroaching on and destroying the surrounding adjacent cells until finally the organism is overwhelmed and killed. While this likeness is a good one, it does not convey all the truth of the nature and relationship of cancer to the body organism as a whole. Because such a rebellious group of cells never could exist if the dominating vital force (physiologic functions) of the body were not first, disturbed and weakened by some inharmonious element (inherited toxine).

This concept is consistent with the Hahnemannian doctrines of sickness and health. We know now that no chemical change takes place in the organism until after an electro-magnetic change has occurred, and further, no pathologic process occurs until a change in the chemistry of the blood and other vital secretions (endocrines, etc.) have transpired. These processes are reversed under the action of the exact homeopathy remedy, first, the electro-magnetic currents of the organism are restored to a harmonious state and then instantly the chemical reactions in the blood and glands assume normal conditions starting repair and the removal of waste (pathology). While these processes are instantaneous, it may require some time before waste products are removed and normal tissue cells are restored. The time element is governed by the amount of pathology present while functional changes take place much faster.

Old school methods in the treatment of cancer are entirely material in concept. The allopaths attack the morbid growth and pay little if any attention to the patient or his physical and mental requirements during the course of that treatment. Surgery, x-ray and radium[2] are the main agents of "scientific" medicine and in spite of the fact that the results obtained in cure by these agents have been dismally disappointing. In the past two decades these methods have failed and left the medical world dark and helpless in the face of the cancer scourge. We are told

---

1. From handwritten manuscript. - Editor.
2. And today chemotherapy. - Editor.

there is nothing else to do outside of surgery x-ray and radium. And any one differing with them or attacking the problem from another angle is branded as a charleton and becomes a medical outcast.

But why pursue methods and follow leaders whose failures to cure or even mitigate are acknowledged even by themselves? Why burn, torture and mutilate to a purposeless end, and add financial burdens many times impossible to bear upon these unfortunate victims of a dire malady? Why do all these things, when we have at our hand a better, surer means of combating this implacable foe of mankind. Our old school friends have been searching since the early dawn of medical history for a specific serum, vaccine, or what not, for cancer, and today in the light of all their boasted scientific knowledge they are as far or farther than ever from their goal.

No specific will ever be found outside of the homeopathic specific for each individual case of cancer, because each patient, with his individual susceptibilities and reactions to stimuli and irritants, requires the specific that meets the sum total of symptoms plus the blood chemistry of each individual. Our homeopathic materia medica abounds in authentic cures of cancer conditions from its inception to the present day.

Burnett, Cooper, Clarke, Kent and a host of others whose ability to diagnose such conditions cannot be questioned, because of the facts just cited, make it our sacred duty to give this knowledge to a suffering world. Homeopathy is the only force in the world today equipped to meet successfully this terrible menace to humanity's very existence.

But we need better organization and more team work, and we must know the limitations of our weapons in order to obtain a maximum in results. It need not be stressed that the more advanced the case the less the chance for a cure. And cases complicated with damaged vital organs, such as heart, kidneys or lungs, are less able to respond to a curative remedy; only severe aggravation of symptoms follow the administration of the curative remedy in these cases[1]. Palliative remedies instead of curative ones must be used in these conditions, and the potencies must be low instead of high. Most of the early cases under the exact remedy, if no vital complications exist, will get well.

But our greatest field is that of prevention. And the earlier we see and administer to our patients the better results can be obtained. Homeo-

---

1. Sometimes the curative remedy (similimum) in low potency may be a palliative. For these and other remarks see references at the end of this article. - Editor.

pathic prescribing through early and middle life will reduce the possibility of cancer affliction a thousand fold in the first generation. If true and exact homeopathic prescribing be followed through the second generation the chances against cancer will be million to one. And if pursued to the third generation there will be no cancer tendency left.

Think of the possibilities in health and well-being, that homeopathy offers to the world now deluged with uncertainties and fear; think of the burdens lifted, of hopes revived, of happiness assured in the light of this God-given knowledge sent through the illumined mind of the faithful servant Hahnemann.

Hahnemann suffered poverty, calumny and banishment because of his unswerving faith in the power of his enlightened doctrines of healing. We have inherited the blessings of these truths hardly without effort. Shall we let them perish from the earth when they are needed so sorely. Shall we not proudly and fearlessly be the standard bearers, and true disciples and workers in the glorious cause, which means the physical salvation of the race.

I would like to give you a full treatise of remedies and their indications for this dreadful plague but time and space prohibits. I can mention only a comparative few remedies that are frequently needed. Cadm-ar., Cadm-i., Cadm-met., Cadm-s., are powerful curatives and frequently are helpful even in advanced cases, their indications from the symptomatic angle are still very meager with the exception of Cadm-s., which is given in The Guiding Symptoms by Hering; Kent has also given a splendid picture of this remedy's possibilities in his materia medica. These stand as representative of the group. In the early stages of the disease any well indicated remedy of our materia medica will prove useful. For the preventive measures the broad constitutional lines of prescribing will bring the best results.

I will close by presenting a list of useful remedies taken from Kent's repertory listed under cancerous affections in Generalities page 1346. This group will serve as a valuable study group for those engaging in cancer work.

Acet-ac., alum., alumn., *apis, ambr.,* **Ars.,** *ars-i., aster., aur., aur-m.,* bism., **Brom.,** *Bufo, cadm-s., calc., calc-s., carb-ac.,* **Carb-an.,** *carb-v., carbn-s.,* caust., *cist.,* clem., **Con.,** cupr., dulc., *graph.,* hep., *hydr., kali-ar., kali-bi., kali-s., kreos., lach., lap-a.,* **Lyc.,** *merc., merc-i-f.,* nat-m., **Nit-ac.,** ph-ac., **Phos., Phyt.,** sep., **Sil.,** *sulph.,* sul-ac., *thuj.,* zinc.

Two very valuable remedies for study in cancer of the tongue are Kali-cy. and Rad-br.

What we need in this country is a homeopathic cancer center in every big city or even in every city where a half dozen or more homeopaths can work together for homeopathic research. Besides the great amount of good that would occur to many unfortunates, the knowledge that cancer can be cured and prevented through homeopathic methods would become more quickly and widely circulated, thus increasing our usefulness to the world a thousand fold.

References (by the Editor)

1. Kent, J. T. Lectures on Homeopathic Materia Medica, Fourth Edition. Philadelphia: Boericke & Tafel, 1956. KALI-C., p. 599. PHOS. p. 786. HEP. p. 543.
2. Kent, J. T. Lectures on Homeopathic Philosophy; Lecture XXXV Prognosis After Observing the Action of the Remedy. Calcutta: Sett Dey & Co., 1961, p 227 ff.
3. Kent, J. T. New Remedies, Clinical Cases, Lesser Writings, Aphorisms & Precepts. Calcutta: Sett Dey & Co., 1963. What is Homeopathy? p. 375 - 380.
4. Kent, J. T. Repertory of the Homeopathic Materia Medica. Fourth Edition.

Cancer - its Cause, Prevention and Cure[1]

Millions in wealth for research have been spent, and millions of lives have been sacrificed in a vain search for the cause and cure of the cancer scourge. When we think of the worse than useless mutilations by surgery alone, we must be appalled at the sum total of increased suffering such procedure brings. Still more disappointing in beneficial results obtained, and heart rending and discouraging to the deepest degree, have been the application of radium and x-ray radiation to the cancer problem. Only unreasonable extortion in expense, and increased agony have been added to the suffering and depletion common to the cancer victims.

But not wholly vain the sacrifice and suffering of these unfortunates, because during their travails a collection of basic facts have been gathered which will help materially in the prevention and eradication of cancer from the race.

Until recently there existed two distinct and opposing views concerning the fundamental nature of cancer:

One school of medical thought maintained that cancer was but a local manifestation of a local irritation and not in any way related to the organism as a whole, except that as it developed and infused more of its toxines into the blood stream it then affected the organism adversely and gradually overwhelmed and destroyed it. The cure was said to be found entirely in surgical or mechanical means, in short, extirpation of the growth at its first incipiency; but alas, how inadequate such treatment proved, for in from two to three years most cases were dead. Many moles and warts that had lain dormant and harmless for years were suddenly turned to malignant growths of a rapidly destructive nature by the irritating effects of cauterization, radium and x-ray radiations. This is one fact that disproves the purely local nature of cancer - the destruction of the growth only served to increase suffering and hasten death.

The other concept, mostly, though not entirely sponsored by the homeopathic school is that cancer is a constitutional disease, whose soil tendencies are inherited, and the result of a disturbed or morbid physiology. Hence the treatment must be directed to the removal of soil conditions, and to the restoration of normal physiologic processes. And

1. From handwritten manuscript. - Editor.

when a healthy physiologic state is obtained the gradual disappearance is inevitable, leaving the patient in every way well and normal.

A few observed facts gathered from numerous and various sources will serve to shed a great light upon the dark background of superstition and error that envelopes and obscures the cancer cause and its proper treatment.

As all homeopaths know, Hahnemann and his followers were the first to observe, and announce, that constitutional and inherited causes were fundamental as cancer cause; and that it was a systemic affliction, even before the first faint manifestation of cancer ultimates appeared.[1] This concept was denied and ridiculed by the dominate school of medicine, until recently one of their own members, Dr. Maude Sly of the University of Chicago, by observations made in the breeding of many thousands of families of mice, has proven beyond question the truth of the claims made so long ago by Hahnemann:: first, the constitutional or inherited soil condition as a basis; second, the systemic rather than the local nature of cancer.

It follows that if the above is true, that any effort directed to the cancer growth apart from the attack on the fundamental internal cause, is worse than futile, because increased suffering and harm can only come by dealing with effects instead of causes.

Dr. Field Buckley observed by actual statistics compiled over a long period of time and from many thousands of cases, that ninety percent of the cancer patients operated on were dead after a lapse of two years. An eminent surgeon of Boston of many years experience recently told me while discussing the cancer question, that he would not operate on any more cancer cases under any circumstances as suffering was increased and the span of life shortened by surgery, x-ray and radium applications as these things could in no way remove the underlying systemic cause of cancer.

Dr. Buckley was one of the first to recognize the importance and advantage of a carefully selected diet, mostly of fruits and vegetables for the cancer sufferer; and wonderful results in a large number of cases were obtained by such a diet. The diet phase of treatment is complimentary to the medicinal side, as both are related to the blood chemistry of the patient which is the all important factor that must be changed before pathologic processes can be arrested and curative action instituted in any given case. Elimination of accumulated cancer toxines is

---

1. §185-203 Organon - Editor.

also favored, by the proper diet, which is of importance in the early treatment stage of the disease.

By far the most valuable contribution to the early diagnosis of cancer and the pre-cancer state is that given the world by the late lamented, but much unjustly villified Dr. Albert Abrams.[1] The application of his discoveries linked up with the selection of homeopathic remedies for the individual patient by electronic methods is destined to be the chief force that shall drive that heretofore resistless destroyer and agony producing scourge from the earth.

I know this statement will be challenged by the unthinking and the misinformed, and by a third class, the venal commercialists in medicine who fatten on the suffering and anguish of the cancer victims and their relatives. I know also there are many of my colleagues here in this society who will doubt the wisdom and use of that statement. But duty to the high calling of a physician, compels me to speak of what I have proven to be true. The anguished cries of crucified millions, the stench of slowly dying and decaying body cells, the uncounted mutilated deformities, and the bloody shambles every modern hospital presents, answered by the disconsolate wail of despair from present-day scientific medicine, makes it incumbent on every man with any knowledge however meager it may be, to give it to the world, regardless of consequences to himself. And we homeopaths have found something that can help change this dismal picture. In the language of the great Hahnemann, the ideal physician is without prejudice and is tolerant of others views and stands ready to receive truth where ever found and in any guise.

The work of Dr. Crile, of Cleveland,[2] is unique for originality and utility. His experiments show a conception deeper in scope than the average research worker, he has found that an electro-magnetic change takes place in the cancer cell, from the normal bi-polar state of healthy cells; the cancerous cell becomes positively charged with a resulting change in the cell nucleus. Strange that these findings confirm the claims that Abrams made ten years or more ago; viz. that the cancer cell is electro-magnetically positive. And right here is the crux of our whole problem; the restoration of the normal electro-magnetic polarity

1. See "Recent Concepts and New Formulas in Medicine" on p. 679 ff. and "Importance of Electronic Reactions to Future Medicine" on p. 683 ff.. - Editor.
2. Crile, George W.: A Bipolar Theory of Living Processes, The Macmillan Co., New York, 1926. - Editor.

to the affected cells. The causes of this changed polarity are found in an inherited weakness, plus certain toxines engendered in bad habits of living, eating, serumization, drugging, etc., and in many other irritations related to environment.

The cure is in removing environmental subcauses, by normal living and in changing inherited weakness and the actual polarity of the diseased cells with the properly selected homeopathic remedy. Experiments over the blood of many hundreds of cancer patients give us a comparatively narrow group of remedies out of our vast materia medica, that are really curative in cancer conditions. Among the most efficient for carcinomatous conditions are the various preparations of CADMIUM. Sarcoma demands another group of remedies for its cure. In the past four years a number of apparently complete cures have been made with cadmium preparations, I say apparent because sufficient time has not yet elapsed to state positively that there may not be a return of this disease in at least one of the cases.

Enough good reports are coming in from many parts of the country concerning the cure of cancer with homeopathic remedies selected by some modification of the electronic method, to encourage our efforts along this line, with every promise of far greater success in the near future. Every cured case is a great victory that inspires hope and courage throughout the profession; and even our failures are teaching us new means of attack, and the avoiding of possible mistakes a second time.

The blundering procedures of surgery and radiation of various kinds because of poor results obtained, will serve to warn us away from all attacks on the end results of the disease, because it is never local but always systemic and must be met on broad systemic lines of treatment.[1]

The microscope and the test tube have taught as much as can be learned by such methods. Millions of dumb animals have been tortured and slaughtered and the lavish expenditures of millions of dollars by an army of trained technicians have all failed to stem the rising toll of cancer deaths.

The wise ones are more mystified and helpless than ever before. They say we do not know the cause and have found no cure for this immedicable woe.

From the failures of the past we may learn much by avoiding their methods of technic and their many subsequent mistakes in treatment. We are approaching the problem from a different angle and with differ-

---

1. §185-203 Organon - Editor.

ent equipment and with a vastly different strategy. We are convinced that any research laboratory apart from clinical treatment must end as it always has in the past, by disappointment and failure.

Our first and greatest need is proper hospital facilities, where our methods of diet and remedy treatment can be carried on without interference and where we can have complete and sympathetic cooperation, in the treatment of our cases.

The great possibilities for the prevention of this dread scourge that exists in the homeopathic therapy and methods is only one of the reasons for the great drive for homeopathic institutions now being launched in Chicago. We want a place to take our suffering cases, we want above all other things a place to train our young men and women in methods that have proven successful in the prevention and cure of this awful malady.

We cannot let preconceived ideas of medicine nor prejudice deter us from supporting such institutions, where so much good for suffering humanity may be consummated. Those of us who have seen the miracle of cure wrought by the homeopathic remedy will not falter in the great work that soon shall unfold for us to do.

No greater heritage can be left to the future than the perpetuation of the homeopathic healing art, it has stood the test of corroding time; its votaries had to meet hatred, calumy and ridicule at the hands of organized power. Shall we the recipients and guardians of this great fund of useful knowledge, obtained by so much sacrifice and suffering, not find joy in sustaining and perpetuating these great truths until the future be free from weakness and disease?

Can we remain deaf to the evergrowing wail of anguish and despair of victims languishing without hope or help except what the starlit truths of homeopathy offers?

Too long we have stood with the balm of healing in our hands mute and dumb before this Saturnalia of agony and black despair that mocks our gaze wherever we turn.

The hour has struck for action and for united homeopathic effort in the conquest of man's most implacable foe, The Dread Dragon, Cancer.

The Homeopathic Philosophy of Cancer Cause[1]

Though cancer has been known from the most ancient times for its devastating and implacable ravages, Hahnemann was the first observer to perceive its true nature and etiology. A vital force weakened by a blending of inherited miasms, the chief of which is psora, constitutes the fundamental underlying cause. Irritations, mostly those resulting from drugs, serums, vaccines, processed and demineralized foods are secondary and exciting causes, but these latter will not produce cancer in a constitution free of the fundamental inherited miasmatic causes. These facts announced by Hahnemann are now being proved to the world by Allopathic scientists.

Dr. Maude Sly of University of Chicago, by her extensive and comprehensive experiments on rats, having bred thousands of families and many generations of rodents, has succeeded in establishing beyond all doubt the factor of inheritability as the fundamental cause of cancer. By selecting cancer free parents all their children, even if wounded or subjected to various forms of irritation, were free of cancer. One cancer parent produced cancer in a high percentage of the children. Both parents cancerous transmitted to most of their offspring the cancer disease. By the process of selecting cancer free parents cancer can be bred out of the race.

Crile, of Cleveland,[2] has shown that before any chemical or pathologic change takes place in the body cells, there is a preceding change in the electrical polarity of such cells destined to become cancerous. Hahnemann observed that cancer, tuberculosis, eczema, epilepsy and many other so-called chronic diseases were all only manifestations of the one underlying chronic miasm, psora. These various forms of illness may not only alternate in the same individual, but they may also change their manifestations in children suffering from cancer or epilepsy. For years homeopaths were laughed at because they spoke of the evil effects of the suppression of chronic skin disease by the topical application of metallic salves. How many times asthma, of an alarming type, has supervened upon such suppression, and the action of the homeopathic remedy has relieved the asthma and restored the skin dis-

---

1. The Homeopathic Recorder, Vol. XLVII, No. 2, February 1932, page 134.
2. Crile, George W.: A Bipolar Theory of Living Processes, The Macmillan Co., New York, 1926. - Editor.

ease to the body surface, where it no longer could menace the vital centers.

Hahnemann speaks in the Organon of the great power of drugs over natural disease, saying that the reason of their ability to cure, comes from their innate power to effect the vital force of man and make him sick.[1] Drugs, given in material dosage over a long period, may so disturb the economy of even robust individuals that an artificial disease is produced, sometimes ultimating in pathological end results. Thus with the advent and abuse of the numerous coal-tar drugs, has come the marked and alarming increase in kidney and heart disease. Cancer has increased in the last decade more rapidly than ever before, very possibly due to the irritating effects of aluminum poisoning, from the almost universal custom of cooking and preparing foods in utensils made of aluminum.

Formerly cancer was a disease peculiar to the period of middle and advanced age, now it frequently occurs in early adult life.[2] How much the wholesale sacrifice of the tonsils of children, together with the various so-called immunizing vaccines and serums given to prevent acute infectious diseases, have to do with this phenomenon, is hard to know. It is certain that these things all shock the nervous system and pollute the blood stream thereby weakening the defense mechanism of the body to all forms of disease producing causes. With the vital force weakened by these things it might easily be made more susceptible to the effects of metallic and other poisons.

Today there is a wide difference of opinion expressed by medical men concerning the baneful effects of aluminum. But homeopaths who study the provings of the various aluminum salts and preparations must acknowledge the chronic far-reaching, though very subtle, insidious effects of this poison on the race. It is true, that those weakened by other causes, are more liable to the influence, but even the robust after a sufficient time will feel the enervating force of this potent destructive element. With these facts before us, how solicitous we must be for those consigned to hospitals and sanitariums by force of circumstances, because, perhaps without exception, this universal poison of aluminum is even there in evidence as they all employ aluminum ware in the preparation of the foods for their sick. How much more tedious must be

---

1. §25 - §32 Organon - Editor.
2. And today 1996 more and more so in children as evident in the large increase in hospitals devoted to treating children with cancer. - Editor.

recovery under such conditions. Why is the medical world so stupid and bigoted as not heed these patent things when homeopathy, chemistry, and even common sense and observation, all teach the truth about this subtle ubiquitous poison. Or, is it the greedy hand of commercialism, red with the blood of its uncountable victims, that holds back the march of progress with its corrupting, selfish power?

Hahnemann laid stress on the importance of the mental symptoms in sickness and in the provings of remedies, and modern physiological research proves the wisdom of his claims. Tests of the body secretions in health and under the influence of thought emotions, show a great change, the normal, alkaline secretions becoming acid. Therefore in cancer cause, the mental and emotional stresses and disturbances from normal must play an important part. Who can say how much hatred, envy, fear or selfish greed may enter into the formation of every cancerous growth? We do know that remedies can produce great emotional changes in healthy individuals and by that same law can cure them in the sick, if they are suitably prepared and selected. When the moral and mental states are normalized in the individual he can build up a better defense against the destructive agents that are constant concomitants of his environment.

Occult students tell us that mental and emotional symptoms are the result of disturbances in the astral and mental bodies which function respectively on the astral and mental planes of existence.[1] All this brings us to realize that as physicians, we must treat something prior to and beyond the physical body alone. Failure to grasp these fundamental facts, and failure to realize exact definitions of health and disease in all the forms and aspects, spells failure in the realm of cure.

Next in importance in the treatment of cancer, as well as any other chronic disease, is the subject of nutrition or food. Foods should contain all the necessary elements for growth and body repair, and they should, at the same time, be free of irritating and unwholesome ingredients. Also foods must be studied from the homeopathic angle, that is, the susceptibility of the individual (regardless of the disease afflicting him) must be first considered. Even some diabetics may tolerate, not only without harm but with benefit, certain forms of sugar. So throughout the realm of disease, we may extend the homeopathic philosophy individualizing both the food and remedy of the patient.[2]

---

1.   See the articles "Occult Causes and Material Effects" on p. 238 ff. and "The Occult Side of Homeopathic Philosophy" on p. 231 ff. in the section Philosophy. - Editor.

To summarize then, we must first grasp Hahnemann's conception of all disease cause, or vital force disturbed and weakened by the miasms of the three chronic diseases plus all drug and irritational food disturbances. Next, with Hahnemann, we must recognize the tremendous importance of mental states in the cause and cure of all sickness. Then we must select foods containing all the essential elements of nutrition, purged of all irritants and compatible with the individual patient's needs. Finally, we must establish orderly habits of thinking and acting, living in accordance with the natural laws of health, thereby making the acquisition of health, mentally and physically, the most important business in existence. When these things are accomplished then will the prescribing and administering of all homeopathically indicated remedy truly perform miracles of cure.

---

2.   See Kent's Lecture on Bryonia paragraph 20 in Kent Lectures on Homeopathic Materia Medica. - Editor.

HOMEOPATHIC TREATMENT OF CANCER[1]

Cancer cases fall into three groups: viz. those in the pre-cancer stage, those in the early or incipient stage and those in the late or advanced stage.

Those in the first group are far more numerous than are those of the other groups and obviously the probability of cure at this stage is more likely, and hence presents an especially fertile field for homeopathic treatment. At least ninety-five per cent of these cases will end in cure.

Cases of the second group are less numerous and their chances for recovery and cure are much less certain. About seventy-five per cent can hope to get well. In the advanced group only about 10 % can hope to get well. Yet in these advanced and incurable cases the majority are helped under the properly selected remedies. One remedy is rarely sufficient, but a series of complimentary remedies are required to cope with these conditions and bring the necessary comfort to these sufferers without the use of narcotics or pain killing drugs.

To ILLUSTRATE: Twenty years ago while lecturing at the Post Graduate School in Boston, Dr. Woodbury introduced me to one of his patients, a lady about forty-five years of age whose right breast was half necrosed away with carcinoma. A biopsy had been made. This patient's breast healed entirely and she carried on socially and in her home in a most active way for eighteen years, without pain or inconvenience. Then a cancerous condition of her bony structure supervened and she had to remain in bed to prevent the breaking of her brittle bones. Shortly after she died without pain.

Many late cases will respond to treatment and live in apparent health and comfort for ten or fifteen years, and then die of cancer but without suffering.

Some seven years ago Dr. Farrington[2] and myself saw a boy about nine years of age with a bone sarcoma in the upper arm. Doctors who saw the boy before we did after taking x-ray pictures and blood findings diagnosed sarcoma and advised immediate amputation of the arm at the shoulder, which the parents refused to have done. Thanks to CADM-MET. given in repeated doses in a succession of ascending potencies from the thirtieth up to the fifty thousandth this boy is now a vigorous

---

1. JOURNAL OF AMERICAN INSTITUTE OF HOMEOPATHY, Vol. 43, No. 6, June 1950, p. 121 - 123.
2. Dr. Harvey Farrington (son of E. A. Farrington). - Editor.

young man with a normally functioning arm and only a slight enlargement of the bone remains.[1]

Another case seen with Dr. Farrington June 27, 1938. A man then
aged fifty developed a round celled sarcoma of the jaw after tooth
extraction. Biopsy was made. He experienced pain and swelling involving the jaw and face, taking on the so-called frog faced appearance. The
man had always been in good health and gave no therapeutic symptoms to prescribe on. His family history was equally vague: his father
died in an accident at sixty years of age and his mother died of a stroke
at eighty-one. The prognosis was grave, with six months to a year to
live, but SYMPH. in a succession of potencies from the 10M to the CM
left this man well in about eighteen months time. He is still well and
vigorous now, twelve and one half years after the sudden development
of his trouble.[1]

A woman age fifty years has sarcoma of the bones of the skull with a
swelling as large as a half grapefruit in the right temporal region, diagnosis made from x-ray and blood pictures. Surgery. and radium treatment was refused. Under homeopathic remedies the woman remains
well without pain and no further increase in size of skull bone after
seven years CADM-MET. and CALC-F. in potency were the chief remedies
used in this case.

October 2, 1947 a woman of about forty-six years of age was brought
into my office by a trained nurse. She was suffering intense pain, was
extremely weak and cachectic and had lost forty pounds of her body
weight, weighing at this time 100 lbs. In spite of pain-killing and sleep-
producing remedies the patient was a constant sufferer and obtained
only a little broken sleep. Following is the case history of the family
physician, the doctor preceding me on the case. The history sheet is not
dated but it must have been in March or April of 1947. Mrs. G. R. D.
age forty-five. Seven years ago patient noted pink staining from uterus.
Six years ago gave birth to a male child. Nothing abnormal was
observed by attending physician. After delivery there was an increase in
volume of discharge and staining was more deeply colored. From the
spring of 1945 until the fall of 1946 patient had sunlight lamp treatment
for what was diagnosed uterine ulcer. As healing did not take place the
physician giving treatment recommended seeking further medical
advice.

---

1.   See article "Some Clinical Cases" on p. 406 ff. in the section Clinical Cases. - Editor.

Fall of 1946 an examination was made by a surgeon who sent a specimen to be analyzed. The report came back "positive malignancy in early stages". After consultation the surgeon turned the case over to a cancer specialist who during October administered twenty x-ray treatments of one hour duration. The following month the patient was hospitalized and given radium treatment for four days, after which she was returned to her home for ten days then back to the hospital for three more days of radium treatment.

She gained weight and felt well until May, 1947. Then she began to have pain in her legs, then the buttocks, then the rectum and thereafter pains all over. Constipation set in, appetite vanished, blood count was low and there was loss of weight.

June, 1947 a cancer specialist examined patient at the hospital and said it looked like a recurrence. July, 1947: "no cause for alarm". August, 1947: "definite recurrence". The patient was turned over to the family physician by the specialist. Sept. 4, 1947 the family physician examined patient and saw no evidence of recurrence. Intense pain and suffering especially extreme intestinal discomfort was attributed to reaction caused by x-ray and radium treatment. Sept. 18, 1947 superficial examination, all O.K.

Sept. 20 the patient had intense pain (sciatica) lasting three hours. Liver injections were given and an effort was made to control pain by use of Frosts 292. The tablets helped to control pain but were very constipating. Mineral oil was prescribed but constipation persisted. Patient took enema every four or five days which was followed by two days of diarrhea, then extreme weakness.

A normal, average diet was prescribed plus one and one half quarts of raw vegetable juices, mostly carrot, since Sept. 10, 1947. After ten days of vegetable juices patient had intestinal hemorrhage which family physician said was a sloughing off of scar tissue caused by radium burns.

This case presents several important lessons to the thoughtful physician, mainly that x-ray and radium do not cure cancer, but they shorten life and intensify suffering and inhibit the action of curative remedies and processes.

As noted in the beginning of this report this woman was sinking rapidly deathward on October 3, 1947. On March 7, 1948 this patient returned to my Chicago office from Canada on her own power without an attendant or nurse. She had regained her normal weight and presented the picture of radiant health and was a most happy and grateful being. Up to this writing, October 3, 1949 she remains well and happy only reporting by mail to tell me all goes well with her. She is restored to health and to her loved ones from the brink of an open grave.

This seeming miracle of cure was wrought by a few potencies of Cadm-met. 30 to the 10M at in-frequent intervals of from thirty to fifty days apart. A second remedy, Benzoquinone was given in the 200 and 10M potencies after the Cadm-met. had antidoted the evil effects of radium and x-ray. All this was consummated in the short space of five months.

I will mention briefly one more most interesting case of mylogenous leukemia, a patient of Dr. Guild of Chicago. It was my privilege to be a consultant with Dr. Guild in prescribing homeopathic remedies. This case first came to my notice in the later part of 1942. At this time the patient was at a very low ebb in the tide of life, having but a few months to live at best. It is now seven years past and Dr. Guild's last report was the patient is well and performing her functions in all affairs of life. In this period of seven years this patient required sixteen different homeopathic remedies given on the blood indications of the patient. Two nosodes were among the most effective, viz. Metastatic melanoma and Tub. Dr. Guild has the laboratory reports and findings of the blood.

From the preceding reports the victims of this dread disease need not despair entirely, several encouraging factors appear and they are very much in favor of homeopathic procedures.

However the fact remains that only ten in a hundred of the late cases recovered, all too gloomy a picture from the point of cure, yet on the other hand there is a degree of encouragement from the fact that cancer well advanced in its worst aspects has been conquered and cured.

We need much more homeopathic research because at present we have only about twenty-two remedies that really correspond to the likeness of cancer in its various manifestations and in its ultimate destructive stage.

The remedies with power to cope with cancer in advanced stages are as follows: Alum-sil., Anan., Ant-ar., Ant-i., Arg-met., Bell-p., Benzoquinone, Cadm-chr., Cadm-met., Cadm-s., Calc-f., Con., Hydr., Kali-thio-cy., Lap-a., Metastatic melanoma, Nat-hexa-meta-phos., Phos., Phyt., Scir., Scroph-n., and Symph. If the Cadmium combinations are added we might increase the number to thirty.

As time and experience guides us along we are finding and proving new possible cancer remedies. Every new remedy enlarges the scope of usefulness in the treatment of the disease.

If the doctor gets the case in the incipient stage the number of useful and possibly indicated remedies are greatly enlarged, in fact any one of the deep, broad remedies of the Materia Medica might be found useful. As was stated earlier, seventy-five per cent of these cases can be absolutely cured.

From these facts we see the importance of early diagnosis and discovery of the malady. Also the importance and use of accurate blood tests to detect the cancer virus at the earliest possible time. These things plus a carefully taken homeopathic history of the patient and his family will reveal to the intelligent physician much useful knowledge concerning the patient's tendencies and susceptibilities.

When we view the cancer question from a broader sense, that is if we add the combined cures of the true cancer group made up of the incipient and developed cases with a recovery record of eighty-five per cent the situation presents a far brighter aspect and stamps the homeopathic methods of cure as not only the most scientific but also the most successful practice against the cancer scourge ever given the world.

Add to this picture the matchless power of the homeopathic treatment in the pre-cancer stage. That stage embraces all the countless manifestations of chronic disease such as diabetes, epilepsy, psoriasis, eczema, arthritis in its many forms, asthma, hay fever and numerous tubercular affections as well as the venereal diseases together with the numerous abnormal mental and emotional afflictions which harass the race today.

All this further aggravated by the suppressive and drastic effects of serums, vaccines and coal tar derivatives, "goof pills" and what not that literally deluge humanity.

Is it any wonder that heart and kidney disease, cancer and mental incompetency are increasing at most alarming rates. Traditional medicine stands helpless and palsied before these death dealing forces. Only the homeopathic law courageously and intelligently administered is equal to cope with this alarming situation.

To summarize: those who practice homeopathy to the utmost of their ability especially in the field of chronic disease can but arrive at a most apparent conclusion, that our usefullness and success in the treatment of cancer finds its greatest scope in cancer prevention.

It is a fact that those receiving true scientific homeopathic treatment over a course of a few years even though they come of cancer families and with bad inherited tendencies rarely develop cancer. Homeopathic physicians know that cancer can be arrested and cured. Homeopathic literature abounds with accounts of notable cures from the early times.

But homeopathic physicians and their patients have been slow to tell the world about these things, while so-called science stimulated by commercial zest and profit have been loud, far reaching and rampant in their praise of one wonder drug failure after another. Yet unabashed they carry on without hindrance or cessation to fill the world with woe and error and increased suffering, piling evil upon evil in their insatiable greed.

In the face of these errors and iniquities why should homeopathy hide its light from the dark places and habitats of men who need light and truth so sorely. Homeopaths, if you wish to help yourselves, your friends, your families, your country and the world you must cooperate, organize and go forth to spread the one true science and doctrine of the healing art.

Give these truths to the lowly and the mighty alike, but above all give them to the high and mighty, to the teachers teaching only what, not how to think; to the scientists whose chief energies are centered on the atom bomb and kindred instruments of destruction, and last to the empirical doctors whose methods of treatment change faster than the shifting winds around them because they have no fixed principle or law to guide them in their work dedicated to the cause of mercy.

An organized benign propaganda taken to the multitudes may well change the world's chaotic state not only in medicine but in economic and spiritual values to one of health and stability bringing in its wake happiness and security to all.

Homeopathic Science Will Conquer Cancer[1]

I am honored and happy to comply with the request for an article on cancer to meet especially the requirements of the laity for this valuable publication, "The Messenger of Health".

Those in the profession who are still able to observe phenomena and reason independently and who have the courage of free men and dare express what to them is true, know that much of the so-called cancer knowledge given the lay public by the so-called experts and specialists is erroneous, because such knowledge is based on a false premise. The said premise being, that cancer in its beginning is only a local manifestation and can be easily irradicated either by surgery, x-ray or radium. Of the results of such treatment more will be said shortly.

Let us touch briefly on the known causes which may be designated first as constitutional or inherited and second as exciting or irritational.[2] Until recently the preponderance of medical opinion held that no systemic cause existed, but the experimentation on animals, mice, rats, guinea-pigs, chickens, fish, etc., have forced an acknowledgment that the inherited factor is the underlying fundamental cause of cancer. If we study the irritational or exciting side of causation we find it lacking and inadequate to explain cancer phenomena in its entirety. Every woman suffering traumatic injuries to the breast does not develop cancer, every man exposed to excessive ultraviolet rays of the sun does not develop a skin cancer. Only those individuals who have an inherited predisposition to cancer are affected by irritations of all kinds.

The concept of the Homeopathic school of medical thought has always held heridity to be the underlying causative factor in all chronic forms of disease. More important still homeopathy teaches that cancer, tuberculosis, epilepsy and most forms of insanity are but different manifestations or outgrowths from a common soil and that they often alternate in individuals and in families. Thus it follows that if the constitutional cause of cancer be proven true, and clinical observations covering great periods of time, experimentation on hundreds of thousands of animals all furnish indisputable evidence of that truth, it becomes obvious that any treatment neglecting this underlying consti-

---

1. The journal THE MESSENGER OF HEALTH where this article was published could not be located, therefore the article was taken from the handwritten manuscript. Judging from the previous articles on cancer, this artickle must have been written around February 1950. - Editor.
2. See also the "The Homeopathic Concept of the Etiology and Cure of Cancer" on p. 781 ff. - Editor.

tutional cause of cancer must be wrong and doomed to failure, and success can only be obtained by treating the constitution or fundamental cause through the blood stream with remedies selected by the only known and proven law of cure.

All criticisms made in this article are in no way personal, we are attacking false principles and systems with the force of proven facts and the logic of correct deductions. In the past twenty five years we have seen tremendous expenditures for cancer research and animal experimentation. Surgery, x-ray and radium therapy have been universally praised and practiced and all to no purpose. Cancer victims continue to increase and recognized medical measures remain dismal failures while suffering and impoverishment make up the resulting harvest. Why continue to exploit a system of disappointment, misery and failure? Why persist in torturing, burning, mutilating and impoverishing the great multitude of sufferers for the benefit and satisfaction of an antiquated system of medicine that has failed to find either cause or cure and which in spite of its own short-comings, condemns all other methods, and dogmatically refuses to investigate or use remedies or systems that do not subscribe to the decadent and dying propaganda of Regular Medicine whose foundations rest on the quicksands of publicity obtained through the medium of a venal press.

No knowledge of cancer or any other medical subject can be presented to the public in the daily press that the heads of the Regular school of medicine do not sanction. The American Medical Association has boasted that no medical article of a cure or method of treatment or medical discovery will be published by any member publication of the associated press without the consent and censorship of this medical trust: the A.M.A.

While the field of medical knowledge is dominated and restricted to one school of thought there can be no progress or advance over that now existing. The treatment of cancer has not materially changed in the past twenty-five years because it is based on the theory that cancer in its early manifestations is purely a local affair and if this early symptom is eradicated by surgery or by radium or x-ray or cautery a cure is obtained. A quarter century of such treatment has not only failed to cure the majority of cases, but has proven harmful and added increase of suffering and tremendous expense to the cancer victims. This group of self-respecting medical scientists have spent much time and effort in warning the public of the dangers and injuries that may come from unscrupulous advertising medical men whom they are pleased to call quacks and charlatans profiting on the misfortunes of the cancer afflicted. All of which reminds one of the story of the pot calling the kettle black.

As scientists, medical men should be ready to abandon any theory or system of procedure that fails to produce resultant cures after twenty-five years of trial; think of the thousands of sufferers who perished under the false hope held out by medical science. As scientists, medical men should be open minded, free of prejudice and ready to try any feasible method to save life or help human suffering, even though such methods run counter to their own preconceived opinions. Only by trial and error can science finally arrive at the goal of truth.

Much more might be said concerning the shortcomings of traditional medicine but it is of little use to tear down an old structure unless we can replace it with a better and more serviceable one. The science of homeopathic medicine is such a structure of use with simplicity and beauty. Promulgated and given to the world one hundred fifty years ago, by that flaming genius Samuel Hahnemann of Germany, it has stood the test of time and emerged victorious against prejudice, persecution and misrepresentation. Its methods of approach, inquiry and experimentation have never been surpassed or even equaled but its methods of history, case taking have been imitated by the very ones who have ridiculed it. The homeopathic materia medica is built on the pure experimentation of the action of a single medical substances on healthy human beings; although the effects, especially the chronic effects of poisonings, have also contributed to its completion. These drug substances when given to the healthy produce changes in the state of the nervous system. Alternations of sensation and the reactions to stimuli and to environment are changed; mental and moral reactions are noted, appetites, desires and aversions are set up, changes in the blood and secretions may be found, and finally, disfunction of organs and a general state of inharmony shows forth, as an artificially produced disease or sickness. After a period of time, these drug effects pass off, leaving the healthy person in his normal state. These artificially produced sicknesses are known as provings. Every medicine given by a homeopathic physician has been tested on healthy humans. No experiments are made on the sick. When the patient presents a sum total of symptoms or a symptom picture that simulates one of our proven remedies it has been found that that particular remedy will cure that particular case of disease, restoring a sick individual to health in the safest, gentlest, and speediest manner. This comparison of the symptoms of the patient with the symptoms of a proven drug is known as the *Law of Similars*, the only definitely known law of cure that the field of medicine presents. Hence homeopaths work in accordance with a proven law of nature when administering their remedies to the sick.

Hahnemann not only discovered the *Law of Similars*, but he developed the art of preparing remedies or drugs suitable to be received by oversensitive sick organisms. In sickness, the system is much more sensitive to stimuli of all sorts, the forces of environment, light, temperature changes, electro-magnetic changes, foods, drugs and infective causes produce their effects much more certainly and profoundly. So it follows that even the correctly indicated remedy will often produce a severe aggravation of the symptoms if it be given in the crude form that it was given to the healthy prover to produce its effects and symptoms. To avoid such aggravations, Hahnemann was impressed with the need of attenuating the drug substances to a degree where the aggravation was very slight if at all, thereby effecting the cure in a gentle, rapid and certain manner. The process of attenuation and sucussion of drug substances eventually became known as potentization because it was soon found their power for cure was greatly enhanced and that even almost inert substances such as sand and charcoal, took on wonderful power as curative agents under this process of potentization.

No longer does this fact, wherein the potentizing of a substance increasing its activity, seem absurd or impossible. The wonderful discoveries and advance of the physicist explain the phenomenon by showing the interchangeability of matter and energy. Matter reduced to its electronic units confers tremendous energy to those ultra microscopic changes of electricity that are the building blocks in the construction or ultimation of all substances. The scientific world is no longer impressed by ridicule concerning the infinitesimal dose, for all forces and substances in nature have their origin in these ultra microscopic units of energy, electrons, protons, etc. Even old school medicine is impressed profoundly by the infinitesimal organisms, called bacteria and filtrates, some of the latter so infinitely small they cannot even be seen by the most powerful lens. Then what is better suited to meet and overcome the infinitely small causes of disease operating on infinitely small nerve cells at the centers of life, than the specific medicine, selected by a definite law, administered in an infinitely fine and suitable form to meet and operate against a like force on the occult plane of the organism where the invisible life forces have their origin and action. Perhaps the efficacy of those substances, known as vitamins, on repair and growth obtains because of their similarity to a homeopathic potency in the infinitesimal quanity they present; in fact the vitamins are rather a quality of energy than a quantity of substance. All this shows us that science is slowly but surely discovering in its own way some of the underlying truths of homeopathy. Such is a brief resume of homeopathic law applied to oppose the natural manifestations of human sicknesses.

Now let us present some of the clinical observations concerning the working of this law especially such as relate to cancer. Over a period of thirty years I have treated many hundred cases of cancer in various forms and different degrees of development and in all stages from incipiency to finality. Case histories were taken and records kept and the prescriptions were given in accordance with strictly homeopathic principles. Cures resulted in sixty percent of the cases and in those cases that failed to be cured, there was almost entire freedom of suffering and a prolonging of life in comparative comfort and use without the employment of narcotics or anodynes of any kind. This record is in no way exceptional for many other homeopathic doctors are doing as well or better in the percentage of cures made. It is the common reward of real students of homeopathic methods. Our literature is rich in reports of cures from the hands of many doctors from its beginning to the present time. And it is available to any medical man willing to have it in exchange for the work and study required to obtain it.

But magnificient as is this record in the cure of malignancy through the medium of the homeopathic law, there is a still greater work to be accomplished by its use and that is in the field of prevention and immunization. Forty percent of failures leave a heavy load of depression and regret in the heart of the true physician and he cannot rest until a greater work is consummated. In the thirty years of my practice not less than thirty thousand cases of chronic disease have been treated by the exclusive and strictly homeopathic procedure and of that vast number less than one hundred have developed cancer, tuberculosis, epilepsy or insanity - all forms of an inherited racial tendency to disease, all outgrowths of a common soil condition. And this again is a very common experience in the lives of a great many homeopathic doctors where it is rare and exceptional for a case of cancer in any form to develop in a patient that has had several years of constitutional homeopathic treatment. The aspects and possibilities of this phase of homeopathic prophylaxis against the development of cancer in the individual and the race must be the goal and ambition of every true practitioner of our glorious law. If we review the figures of vital statistics issued by the U.S. Public Health Service and those of the various state health departments together with those of a number of the leading life insurance companies we will be shocked to learn that about one in ten of every individual past forty years of age will die of cancer. In the light of these comparative figures, we are justified in our claims of the conquest of cancer by the application of the homeopathic law. And we are glad to be able to preach a new doctrine of hope for the afflicted now doomed to suffering, mutilation, impoverishment and death. And better still, this promise and hope is based on the solid foundation of a natural law, proven and confirmed in many hands in many lands over a period of one hundred fifty years and by the testimony of thousands of cures.

THE CONQUEST OF CANCER BY HOMEOPATHY

The last two decades have witnessed the most intensive study and scientific investigation of cancer in all its multitudinous manifestations together with the search for the underlying etiological factors involved.

Strange that after all this expenditure of time and money no definite change of treatment has been instituted. Surgery, and the topical applications of x-ray and radium are still the chief reliance of the large majority of medical men and in spite of the fact that curative results have been on a low average. In fact they have been nil if we exclude the skin cancer from the lists. Many of the so-called cures of skin cancer if followed up, will be found to be but suppressed conditions induced by the massive doses of the rays. Many of these patients die of cancer of the liver or uterus or other vital organs in later years.

After twenty years of intensive research in animal experimentations, it has been quite generally accepted that cancer is a hereditary disease with only a local manifestation at first. Dr. Maude Sly of the Chicago University has bred cancer out of mice families and in the immune families has bred cancer in them, and clinical observations by myriads of clinicians of the human victims of the disease have confirmed these findings.

Homeopathic physicians who follow Homeopathic doctrines closely have always claimed cancer to be a constitutional and inherited manifestation of disease, that must be attacked by systemic remedies acting in the blood stream, thereby changing and harmonizing the chemistry of the organism. Crile in his work "A Bipolar Theory of Living Processes"[1] states that the cancer cell has lost its normal bi-polar polarity and has changed to a positive state. With the change of cellular polarity there comes a corresponding change in chemistry, unless this change is soon normalized by the proper remedy or reagent.

Ten years of experimental work with blood radiations (electromagnetic) emanations with a radio hook up has proven the specific action and power of homeopathic medicines to alter and normalize these reactions that are basic in all changes in the organism from health to disease and vice versa from disease back to health. Before any chemical change comes in the tissues of the body there must be a change in the electro-magnetic currents that dominate all physiologic activities.

---

1. Crile, George W.: A BIPOLAR THEORY OF LIVING PROCESSES, The Macmillan Co., New York, 1926. - Editor.

Hence the life force of Hahnemann in the light of science's more recent discoveries takes on a greater significance than ever before.

Slowly but surely the men of the sciences are proving the Homeopathic theory of disease to be sound and based on the foundations of discovered and proven truth. The Homeopathic similium acts as a catalyst to harmonize the chemistry of the living organisms and this maintains balance and a state of health. It is likewise the best antidote to the cancer toxines which soon become such dominant factors in the control of body repair, developing what has been so aptly termed the anarchistic cell growth known as cancer. The hope engendered by so many leaders of the dominant school of medical thought for a specific remedy for the disease is doomed to disappointment.

For individual peculiarities and idiosyncrasies call for remedies similar to their individual symptoms and types. Although the remedies in the cancer group are comparatively small in number, still there is no one remedy for cancer to fit every case. We must individualize family histories and symptoms to find the best remedy out of the comparatively small group whose provings and clinical confirmations are related in similarity to the cancer disease in all its manifestations.

Remedies that influence growth and body repair are all more or less related to cancer because they are basic and alone are capable of removing constitutional or inherited tendencies. These same remedies readily take on blood changes and correspond to the cachexia that is so typical of malignancy. The more one studies and observes the nature and action of cancer the more convinced he becomes that the best time to cure cancer is before its first symptoms appear. In other words the best cure is to be found in preventive treatment, the earlier it is started the better. For the farther cancer advances the less chances there are for recovery. And right here is where our homeopathic therapeutics can do more than is offered any other treatment.

A cancer history in the family, yes we will go a little further than that and include T. B. and epilepsy and even many of the chronic skin diseases with diabetes are related and spring from a common soil cause. Hence these diseases are related and interchangeable to some degree. T. B. is especially closely affiliated with cancer. Tuberculosis parents frequently have offspring of strong cancer tendencies and vice versa cancer parents beget T. B. offsprings. Clinical observation has noted the interchangeability of these diseases and the homeopathic remedy irradiacates them both effectively. It is necessary to cover all the chronic manifestations of sickness when treating a patient with the best constitutional remedy. Such a remedy given in time to the child and the young adult will almost certainly immunize against the inroads of cancer. Of course the removal and avoidance of all irritations, the proper diet and general good hygiene all are helpful factors in the escape from the cancer scourge.

In the list of *irritations* I would be remiss if I failed to mention the deleterious effects that the universal use of drugs more especially those derivitives of the coal tar products. Such drugs depress the vital resistance to all disease producing cause, and weaken vital organs like the kidneys and heart, likewise they unbalance endocrine harmony. Another harmful and predisposing cancer cause is produced by the almost universal and frequently repeated use of scrums and vaccines. These products of disease injected directly into the blood stream give the organism no chance to provide antidotal reagents to them and the system must eliminate them in a slow and imperfect manner. In many cases the baneful effects are never eliminated and the patient retains a life time of sufferings if he survives the first shock of the poison.

Only a commercialized system of medicine would retain such harmful products in its pharmacopoeia, because the world has witnessed myriads of tragic effects from these things. And, this same commercialized medicine is seeking to compel by law the universal and forceful acceptance of these toxic materials, all in the face of the recent fatal results in the use of a poliomyelitis serum that was so destructive in the results it produced that the U. S. Health Service was compelled to take notice and warn the profession and the laity of the dangers attached to its use. It is true that all serums are not as deadly and quick in their action as this one proved to be but they are nevertheless deeply innervating and health disturbing even if more insidious in their action as innumerable proofs have shown from the fatal results that have been recorded from time to time, but a few instances will suffice. The tuberculosis vaccine of the French killed a large number of babies at one time. The early use of the Dick serum against scarlet fever produced a number of sudden deaths immediately following its injection. Even the much lauded vaccine of small-pox has produced death and long painful lingering sickness, from tetanus, streptococcus toxemia, and mouth and hoof disease leaving in its harmful wake myriads of human wrecks along life's highway, mute yet eloquent witnesses of a commercialized medical procedure, built on superstition and ignorance, a kick back and a relic of the dark ages, and on a par with other filthy and abhorrent prescriptions employed by medical men of that period. In the light of modern hygiene and physiologic teaching how can medical men square such procedures?

Why expect health to ensue from the direct injection into the blood stream of a foreign material and the direct product of disease? I am aware that these criticisms must expose me to bitter attacks from those who are unconsciously or otherwise the tools of avarice. A physician's duty includes the protection of both his individual patient and the public as well against all dangers from disease. It is more than the simple giving of a remedy; if he is a scientist, he notes the things that threaten and impair health.[1] And he must have the courage to speak and to act without fear or favor for that which he knows to be best and right in the interest of all. The menace from this cancer problem has become so overpowering and terrible that we must attack it from every angle and from all fundamental factors if we are to succeed in stemming the deadly and almost irrevocable tide that is sweeping myriads of our fellows, some of them loved ones, into a painful and early death. If the above statement of facts will start a few more conscientious and unfearing physicians thinking and investigating it will be well worth while. We need team work, we need knowledge much more than we now have, we need courage and self-sacrifice and we must cast aside all prejudice and preconceived theories and face the solid unyielding blocks of facts as we find them and build our plans and lives of effort accordingly if we are to be victorious in this unrelenting battle.

On the prevention side of cancer is the development and recognition of a recent blood test that is said to show pre-cancer states; such an asset would prove of incalculable value.

However, we homeopaths need not await such a development for our work. Our knowledge of the fundamental cause and evolution of disease as outlined in our philosophy enables us to predict with unerring certainty the trend toward cancer or tuberculosis. This knowledge combined with our inimitable therapeutics will enable us to prevent innumerable potential cancers ever developing. In the past thirty years of my practice I have treated not less than 50,000 cases of chronic diseases who were not cancerous and out of that vast number I can record less than a dozen cases who subsequent to a course of treatment lasting two or more years developed cancer or T. B. *in any form.*

A recent bulletin of U. S. Vital Statistics stated that one person out of every eight past forty years of age would die of cancer. Compare these two statements and you have an idea of the wonderful power within the scope of homeopathic therapeutics in the positive and certain prevention in the spread of cancer and T. B.

---

1. §4 Organon. - Editor.

THE HOMEOPATHIC CONCEPT OF THE ETIOLOGY AND CURE OF CANCER[1]

There are two distinct etiological aspects[2] of cancer generally recognized by the majority of medical researchers.

FIRST: The basic constitutional inherited susceptibility of a tendency to the disease that is inherent in every cancer victim.

SECOND: The exciting or irritational causes operating on both the physical and psychic planes of existence.

Listed among the physical causes are injuries, wounds, burns, (chemical, thermal, electrical, radiation - either internal or external), excesses of alcohol or tobacco, poisons, drugs, etc. They are potent irritants and are carcinogenic in nature. Some irritational factors may come by way of improper food and water supply. The latter treated with aluminum flouride is spreading the seeds of disease in ever widening circles; this insidious poison is cumulative and builds up in the animal economy serious tendencies to destructive diseases of various forms affecting the blood, glands, bones, nerves and ligaments ultimating in progressive crippling types of arthritis as well as in many forms of malignant disease, including the anemias and leukemias. Another source of carcinogenic irritation more recently on the scene, but universal in scope, is radio-active fall out resulting from the testing of the atom and hydrogen bombs by the U.S., Russia, Great Britain and France. The realm of the psychic, mental and emotional side of life, with the fears, frustrations, resentments, hatreds, compunctions and compulsive drives afflicting the race today is another source of cancer producing forces. This statement is substantiated by the psychosomatic group of medical research whose observations have proven the close relationship which exists between physical disease and mental and emotional states and conditions.

A careful review of cancer research by many investigators and medical scientists over the past two hundred years has established a number of cardinal and valuable facts related to the etiology and cure of cancer. Perhaps the most significant and verifiable fact is this, that many isolated cases of cancer have been cured by different methods, remedies and physicians, but there has been no one specific remedy that can cure

---

1. From handwritten manuscript. - Editor.
2. See also the "Homeopathic Science Will Conquer Cancer" on p. 771 ff. - Editor.

or even help all cases of cancer. In other words, there has not been found a single specific remedy for the cancer disease.

Within the broad scope of the Homeopathic Materia Medica there are a great many remedies for the relief and cure of patients who suffer from the ravages of cancer, as attested by many clinical cases over the past one hundred and fifty years by physicians applying the homeopathic approach. This evidence should teach the medical world that the most successful approach to the cancer problem must come by the individual study of each case of cancer presented for treatment. Before presenting the philosophic portion of this paper it will be instructive and interesting to call attention to the various claims of a few physicians and surgeons whose wide experience in the treatment of cancer is well known. Dr. John Abernethy, renowned English surgeon, claimed that cancer is a constitutional disease not confined to local growth. Dr. Abernethy with other eminent surgeons, Dr. Charles Mayo, Dr. George W. Crile, Sr., and Dr. Isidor Ravdin, stressed the futility of surgery as a cure for cancer.

The dietary treatment of cancer has proven efficacious and curable in a large number of cancer patients in the hands of a number of prominent physicians of the past. One of the earliest advocates of a fruit and vegetable diet, Dr. William Lamb of London, England, was successful in curing cancer cases and he received favorable attention from Dr. Abernethy. Dr. Forbes Ross, of London, England, was another advocate of a properly selected diet for cancer sufferers and he obtained considerable recognized success as a cancer doctor. Dr. Lucius Duncan Bulkley and Dr. Max Gerson, of New York City, strongly advocated the constitutional and dietary treatment of cancer. Dr. Bulkley's methods were highly successful in a large percentage of cases, mainly in prolonging life with its continued uses and in rendering his patients more comfortable and less susceptible to pain and body weakness. His treatment was not only palliative but was credited with a number of definite cures. Dr. Gerson believes the liver holds the key to the cure of cancer; he accomplished a number of astonishing cures in the most serious types of cancer. Other physicians who were successful in the treatment of cancer were Dr. Emanuel Revici of New York City, and Dr. William Koch of Detroit, Michigan. There are many other physicians who treated cancer with varying degrees of success but the list is too great in number to mention in this paper. This information can be found in the book entitled THE CANCER BLACKOUT by Maurice Natenberg.[1] This book contains a most complete fund of useful knowledge related to cancer research during the past two hundred years, with the names and methods of many prominent doctors and scientists, along with a number of lay researchers empirically seeking a specific cancer cure. It also reports graphically on the attitude of organized medicine toward these men and their work. This valuable work of Maurice Natenberg should be read by every medical practitioner in the world, as well as by all the non-medical healers practicing their art. It imparts a comprehensive account of all that has been attempted and done, the results obtained and the repeated failures and bitter disappointments suffered by both patients and doctors in their long hard march along the road of empiricism in the search for the holy grail of medicine, a specific remedy for the cure of cancer. Every layman who wants to be fully informed on this vital subject could find no better source for a broad, unbiased and enlightened knowledge of this subject than that contained in this book.

Among the great contributors of useful and truly scientific knowledge in cancer research is Dr. George W. Crile, Sr., of Cleveland, Ohio. He is an experienced and well-known surgeon, but the world is even more indebted to him for his stupendous work envisioned in the book entitled, A BIPOLAR THEORY OF LIVING PROCESSES.[1] It is difficult to describe the value of this extensive work and its vital importance to the world of medical science and to the needs of mankind in a brief treatise such as this. I will quote some basic principles and facts which coincide with the tenets and concepts of the homeopathic philosophy regarding the phenomenon of life in its many forms and expressions, especially those changes which occur in normal cell growth and differentiation and the chemical changes which supervene and the type of energy involved during the transition of the normal cell in health to that of the pathologic cell in malignancy.

For a better understanding of this vast subject a brief view of Dr. Crile's Bipolar theory of life is helpful, scientific and logical. "Any theory of the nature of life must account not only for the common fundamental phenomena of life in all forms of living beings from the simplest to the most complex, but it also must identify the fundamental form of energy to which the reactions or life can ultimately be traced. It must identify a uniform pattern or plan for the transformation and utilization of energy. It must account for the necessity for such everpresent characteristics as the acid-alkali balance, the lipoid films, the

---

1. The Cancer Blackout, Maurice Natenberg, Regent House, Chicago, 1959.
1. Crile, George W.: A Bipolar Theory of Living Processes, The Macmillan Co., New York, 1926.

omnipresent electrolytes. It must show why a continuous supply of oxygen and continuous oxidation are necessary. It must show the mechanism of stimulation and specific response to stimulation. It must account for the phenomenon of memory. It must account not only for reproduction but also for the transmission of acquired characteristics. It must identify the operation of the unicellular and of the multicellular organism with the operation of protoplasm itself. It must show the mechanism of the creation of living matter-protoplasm from the energy and matter of the environment. It is obviously beyond the present scope of human knowledge to meet all these requirements. It is feasible, however, to present a theory which appears at least to point to a reasonable explanation of the essential characteristics of living organisms and of the phenomena of life itself." Mathews has stated that the difference between the living and the lifeless is a difference in the energy content of the molecules. "The difference between the reactive molecules of protoplasm and the same unreactive molecules outside of protoplasm is a difference in energy content. The various chemical and physical powers of protoplasm which so strikingly differentiate it from the lifeless are due to the increase in the energy content of the molecules. Living matter contains molecules having a high content of energy and capable of passing to a more stable dead form in which they contain less energy."

"The central fact regarding living organisms then is that they are transformers of energy and that they must be operated by means of one or more of the following six forms of energy: (1) heat, (2) light, (3) gravitation, (4) intermolecular forces, (5) chemical energy, and (6) electromagnetic energy. It is obvious that the organism of a rabbit, for example, is not operated by heat energy; nor by light energy; nor by gravitational forces; nor by surface energy. It follows that the probable driving force of living organisms must be either electrical or chemical energy or a combination of both."

"We therefore propose the theory that living organisms are bipolar electric mechanisms. If this theory is tenable it must meet the following requirements:

1. That electricity is a constant phenomenon of living processes. This has long been known.

2. That the application of electricity to the muscles or glands, or to their nerve supply will cause them to perform their natural functions. This is a basic fact which is universally accepted by physiologists.

3. That the materials of which animals are constructed are specifically adapted to electrical processes. Certain generally known facts regarding the principal constituents of the body will be cited and new evidence submitted.

4. That in structure and function the unit cells which drive the organism not only are adapted to fabricate, to store and to discharge electricity, but that this is true also of the protoplasm itself. Certain generally accepted facts and certain new evidence which tend to establish this requirement will be cited.

5. That the organism as a whole is a bipolar electric mechanism bearing the pattern of the unit cells and that the unit cells are constructed on the pattern of the atom. Experimental data which tend to support this requirement will be offered.

6. That the normal and the pathological phenomena of man and animals can be interpreted in electrical terms. Summaries of experimental researches undertaken to establish this point will be given."[1]

Sir Arthur Thompson tells us that "the human organism is made up of twenty-eight trillion cells. These are bipolar electrical units each performing its own special function while co-ordinating with the organism as a whole."

"The unit of structure and of function of the animal organism is the cell. An animal may in fact be regarded as a disperse system of cell suspensions. It is primarily essential therefore to consider the operation of the cell as a bipolar unit."

"The nucleus of the cell is comparatively acid, the cytoplasm is comparatively alkaline; the nucleus and the cytoplasm are separated by a semipermeable film of very low conductivity. These characteristics of the cell indicate a difference in electric potential between the nucleus and the cytoplasm."

"We may therefore consider the cell as a bipolar mechanism, the nucleus being the positive element, the cytoplasm the negative element. The oxidation in the nucleus appears to be on a higher scale than the oxidation in the cytoplasm; and therefore as the electric tension increases in the nucleus, the current breaks through; the potential in the nucleus falls and in consequence the current is interrupted. Since the potential is again immediately restored by oxidation, we conceive that

---

1. Crile, George W. - Ibid, p. 11.

an interrupted current passes continually from the positive nucleus to the negative cytoplasm and in consequence a charge is accumulated on the surface films. These films of infinite thinness and of high dielectric capacity are peculiarly adapted to the storage and adaptive discharge of electric energy."

"Why is the extreme thinness of these films of advantage? The work of the cell depends on its capacity for oxidation; oxidation, as we believe, in turn depends on the electric energy seated between the nucleus and cytoplasm; this energy depends on the voltage in the cell and on the electric charge the lipoid films will hold; the electric charge the lipoid film will hold is dependent on the thinness of the film - the thinner the film the greater the charge. Dr. Fricke has found that the film which surrounds the cells is of the order of 4/10,000,000 of a centimeter thick; and that this lipoid film has electric capacity of a high order, viz. 0.8 microfarads per square centimeter."

"We may consider then that electricity keeps the "flame of life" burning in the cell; and that the flame (oxidation) supplies the electricity which is the "vital force" of the animal. In accordance with this conception, therefore, the cell is an automatic mechanism; life as we view it is the expression of the activity of this automatic mechanism."

"In accordance with this conception, it is of infinite advantage to have the organism made up of trillions of units called cells instead of an equal mass in a single unit.[1] Also the body organism as a whole, is a bipolar mechanism, the positive pole is the brain, the negative pole is the liver with many lesser circuits between the various organs and the endocrine chain all centered in the brain, the governing center."

Such is the ultra scientific conception of life and its processes operating through its physical natural forms. It is interesting to note how close the homeopathic conception of life's processes seem to coincide, with slight variations, with the tenets and accepted facts of the more recent discoveries of science. Before proceeding with our homeopathic philosophy it will be helpful to present a few observations taken from the various sources discussed in this paper, related to human life in health and in disease, especially as related to cancer.

According to a large number of cancer researchers cancer is the result of basic disturbances in the blood chemistry and the cell metabolism of the body organism. Cancer does not occur in the presence of normal body fluids and normal blood chemistry. The normal vital life force is

1.   Crile, George W. - Ibid, p. 13.

disturbed, weakened or obstructed by physical or psychic agencies of an adverse nature. These adverse agencies affect primarily the autonomic nervous system which is the defensive mechanism of the whole being. Dr. Crile's conception of the change from the normal body cell to that of the malignant cell is, that it is but a change of state, preceded by a change in the electrical energy emanating from the cell, wherein the cell looses its normal bipolar activity to become positive in action, thereby changing the chemistry, the physical properties and conditions of the cell and its growth. To quote Dr. Crile again:

"Thus the development of cancer may be regarded as a phenomenon of hyper-differentiation of the cells of the host, brought about by repeated selection of types suitable for multiplication under conditions which inhibit the multiplication of cells of the host. The increase of autocatalyst due to the cells of the tumor itself must, however, render the nutrient medium even less suitable than before for nuclear synthesis in the cells of the host, so that senescence of the host should be accelerated by cancer. This effect would be most intense locally and radiate outwards from the cancer tissue, forming an autocatalyst gradient descending from within outwards."[1]

Dr. Max Gerson says cancer is not a problem of deficiencies of hormones, vitamines or enzymes. It is not a problem of allergies or viruses, of known or unknown micro-organisms. It is not a poisoning through some special intermedial metabolic substance or any other substance coming from the outside. His treatment was dietary and the elimination of toxic dead tissue. Dr. Revici noted that metabolic changes with chemical abnormalities always accompanied the pathology of cancer.

We will now proceed with the homeopathic concept of life and of its relation to health and disease. In spite of all the facts gathered by scientists and all the theories generated in the minds of men concerning life, its origin and its processes, it still remains surrounded in a maze of mystery until we are made aware of the truth that life is co-existent with God, the source and activator of all animated nature. Thus, the vital force spoken of by Hahnemann takes on a most important role in the realm of life and its relation to health and disease throughout the physical, mental and emotional bodies of each individual. The vital force, endowed with formative intelligence when flowing in harmony and unobstructed, builds bodies of beauty and power perfected to perform all the essential functions of life and to repair all tissues, parts and

---

1. Crile, George W. - Ibid, p. 245.

organs injured by disease or accident or physical violence.[1] This same vital force when vitiated and weakened by generations of inherited toxins, becomes perverted and performs its function of body defense and repair less efficiently and builds, in place of normal histological cells and tissues, pathological cells and morbid growths of various types. These disturbing toxic forces also affect the mental and emotional bodies adversely, to impair the mental processes and unbalance the emotions which produce tensions and mental incompetencies of various sorts.

The first physical signs of disease show only disturbed and malfunctioning cells and organs ramifying throughout the entire organism. If the toxic influence is not mitigated and dispered by the proper medicinal agent the organism gradually weakens and dies. It is true that Divine Providence has endowed the body organism with a wonderful and complex defensive mechanism capable of protecting the being from many evils and equipped to manufacture antibodies against infective forces and toxins and institute the auto-hemic agencies of repair. It is this same defensive mechanism that responds to the stimulus of the curative medicine suited to every individual case of sickness which promotes the miracle of cure. Thus we see sickness only as a disturbed, obstructed malfunctioning vital force and health is restored and maintained, when the disturbing influence is banished, to permit the vital force again to flow in order and to restore the power and function of the autonomic nervous system whose constant, tireless, never-sleeping vigil presides over all the numerous complex functions of the body organism during the entire life span. The inherited toxins, which are chief disturbances of health, are the chronic miasms of Hahnemann, known as Psora, Syphilis and Sycosis to which may be added the numerous drug disorders of the present time which complicate natural diseases and render treatment and cure tedious and difficult.

When the causes of sickness are ascertained, the logical step is to remove them. The most effective means yet discovered for the removal of sick-making causes is the homeopathic remedy, because it restores normal function in all of the organs and parts throughout the whole organism and it brings into harmonious play all the life forces, coordinating them as a unit to ultimate in the health of each individual case treated. These statements are not mere speculations and unproved theories, they are established facts gleaned from the observations and prac-

---

1. §9 Organon - Editor.

tice of many able, painstaking and specially trained physicians throughout the past one hundred and fifty years.

The homeopathic approach to cure is one primarily fitted to cope with all forms of chronic disease including malignancy because it corrects the causative forces controlling the functional activities of life and all the agencies of growth and repair throughout the world economy, mental, emotional, and physical.

The homeopathic remedies are carefully and scientifically prepared and attuned to facilitate their effectiveness on the subtle vital force of each patient. The attunement of the remedy depends on the prescriber's ability to fit the symptoms and nature or character of the remedy to the needs of the patient, expressed in symptoms, states and conditions related to his sickness. The wise prescriber, with his remedy, makes use of other health inducing measures such as diet, hygiene, ventilation, moderated rest and exercise. He also makes every effort to obtain for his patients peace of mind and faith in his own God-given powers for repair and regeneration. In order to obtain the best results in terms of cure, every physician regardless of cult or school, should make use of the wonderful aid to healing, that comes with the recognition from both doctor and patient of the power for good that the invoking of spiritual aid can bring. We will be able to cure many cancers when we avail ourselves of these mighty, though subtle forces coming to us by influx from the grand central power and source of all goodness, the Divine Creator. This benign aid is given only for the asking. Let us remember that spiritual law rules over, trancends and shapes all physical or natural laws in the universe. If the spiritual law should be suspended but for an instant universal chaos would ensue.

Of course the world is interested in statistics even though they can be misleading and unreliable. I know of no table of statistics concerning the percentage of cancer cures by homeopathic remedies, but I do know of many hundreds of cured cancer cases at the hands of many homeopathic physicians and the homeopathic literature is full of authentic cures of all types. In my own practice of over fifty years my records will show a high percentage of cures. These include incipient cases and advanced and terminal ones. The percentage of cures in the incipient cases is eighty percent, ten per cent in the late and terminal cases.[1]

From these observations it is easy to see the great advantage that is with the incipient cases for probable cure. But the fact that even some advanced cases are cured holds a rosy promise for the realm of cancer prevention. By the early removal of the basic inherited miasmatic toxins which are racial in scope and avoiding all the irritating or exciting causes so wide spread in the environment of modern life today, we can, not only obtain a higher rate of cure, but we can achieve heartening results in the field of cancer prevention. The homeopathic concept of healing with its logical philosophy is primarily the medicine of disease prevention. It is especially suited to the developing, growing stages of childhood and young adult life. In youth the responses to both the sick-making irritants and to curative remedies are more pronounced and effective in action. This does not imply that illness and disease coming in the older periods of life are less amenable to the curative action of homeopathic remedies, for even cases that are incurable may receive the most effective palliation and comfort with improved vitality and apparent prolonging of life through homeopathy.

We believe that with a better understanding of the homeopathic approach to the cancer problem and because of the positive results in cure that have been accomplished by its use, much of the terror and despair that grips humanity today can be removed and a more hopeful and courageous attitude established. Such an improved state in public thinking will be an asset to both research and cure. This paper is humbly offered as a meager contribution to the vast stores of cancer research now in the world.

---

1. Dr. Grimmer is extremely humble of his work. Actually from certain remarks he made once it is estimated that between 1925 and 1929 about 150 biopsy diagnosed cancers were cured by his treatment (when there was little previous allopathic treatment). Another 75 cases seen between 1925 and 1929 were palliated for many years (usually from 7 - 15 years) with excellent quality of life; these were cases where extensive allopathic treatment had been done. Dr. Grimmer probably treated several thousand cases of cancer over his 57 year practice. - Information collected from handwritten manuscripts from Grimmer and from extensive discussions with family-memberts and friends. - Editor.

CANCER CURES AND SPECIFICS[1]

For centuries traditional medicine has searched for a specific cure for cancer without avail. And seemingly the more intensified the search and effort, the greater and wider the increase of the dread scourge. Billions of dollars for research are being extracted from the American public annually by the promise of the discovery of a specific cure for cancer.

Research is a valuable and laudible force for good, if it is conducted on a broad and unprejudiced basis. But when it is pursued within the compass of one school of medical thought, especially when that line of thought has failed so dismally in the past in results of cure, it becomes a venal, impotent and worthless institution, dispensing only widespread fear for selfish gains.

If only the researchers for cancer and all other chronic aliments afflicting the race would take a little time to study the established facts of homeopathic philosophy, they would learn and know that no specific cure for cancer, arthritis, kidney or heart disease can ever exist or be found; all the diseases mentioned have a common basic soil condition.

The cause of cancer proceeds from a multiplicity of forces and irritations and the most fundamental and important are only known by the homeopath viz. the inherited miasms and toxins discovered and expounded by Samuel Hahnemann in that wonderful and priceless gem of medical literature, the *Organon*.

Homeopathy teaches that no two individuals react to irritants, medicines, or disease toxins exactly alike, and hence each requires his own specific reedy to meet the individual peculiarities of his own blood chemistry.

It is now known no two bloods are exactly identical; they may fall only into similar distinct groups.

From all the above proven facts it is evident that no one element or medical force can be specific for all cases; only individual specifics can cure.

By the most scientific and accurate method yet devised, homeopathy determines the value and place any drug or remedy can function in and its power to cure disease.

---

1. "Editorial" in THE HOMEOPATHIC RECORDER, Vol. LXVI, No. 12, June 1951, p. 357.

By provings of remedies on healthy humans, (not on dumb animals whose emotions and mental processes are difficult if not impossible to know), with the painstaking and scientific checks employed to prevent error, the homeopathic physician is enabled to know the power and limitations of each drug in the cure of sickness. Each drug or element thus proven becomes an everlasting unit in the ever growing Materia Medica of the homeopathic store house of medical research and knowledge dedicated to the good of human kind.

Homeopathy invites all researchers to avail themselves of its valuable knowledge, obtained through one hundred and fifty years of unremitting labor and human sacrifice, that the ends of true research for humanity everywhere may be more fully realized and served.

Diet for Cancer Patients[1]

In order to control the toxemia in cancer cases it is necessary to watch the diet very closely. Absolutely no meat, meat soups or gravies, fish or fowl should be used. Aluminum ware in the cooking of the patient's food must be discarded; also in cities where you get the chlorine in water, the patient must be put on pure spring water both for cooking and drinking.

I usually start the patient on the 30th potency, when that potency has outlived its usefulness, then I give the 10M and so on. Many times during the course of the treatment, patient's symptoms will change and thereby call for a change in remedy, whichever homeopathic remedy is indicated by patient's symptoms is the one given.

Besides the CADM-MET. which is most commonly used, I use CADM-I. Usually this remedy is indicated in the glandular cases; CADM-S.. in the stomach and intestinal cases. CALC-AR. is a frequent remedy used either preceeding or following cadmium remedies in cancer of the liver. CALEN. is another remedy following the exhibition of CADMIUM in stomach cases and GRAPH. in the breast cases.

---

1. This text is taken from a letter Dr. Grimmer wrote another physician, whose name we do not know. - Editor.

The Application of Homeopathic Remedies to Cancer Cases[1]

In applying homeopathic remedies to cancer cases we proceed along the usual lines taught by Hahnemann and his loyal followers as far as we can. Here, as in every case of chronic disease, we must stress the necessity for the fullest and most complete personal and family history that is possible to obtain. From the birth hour on through infancy, childhood and maturity to the time of taking the case, every change and disturbance, mentally, morally and physically in sequence should be recorded, together with the diseases contracted along the way and the remedial measures employed for same. When the pathologic change known as cancer develops and grows with symptoms that are commonly the result of such change, we have little to guide us for the selection of the homeopathic remedy from a strictly symptomatic viewpoint.

Clinical use and observation by many faithful and able followers of the homeopathic law over a long period of time has given us a comparatively small list of remedies, the nature and symptomatology of which correspond to cancer in all its evolutionary processes in the organism, beginning with the moral and mental disturbances of the mind sphere, involving various and at times seemingly contradictory symptoms and states, at other times alternating conditions obtaining, and finally after some unusual stress or some physical or chemical injury there appear the symptoms recognized as cancer. The majority of the remedies listed that have proved curative in cancer will fall into the group that Hahnemann and others observed as having in their nature the three miasms or chronic diseases that are held by homeopaths fundamentally as constitutional sick producing causes. And the minority (of the remedies) so listed may well be assumed to have, after more mature observation, these three miasms: Psora, Syphilis and Sycosis, blended in their symptomalogy.[2]

Following is the list of proven cancer remedies, the symptomalogy of which has been confirmed by curative action. This list is gathered from a search of the repertory through the various parts of the body including those of the skin (epithelioma).[3]

---

1. From handwritten manuscript. - Editor.
2. See also "Psoro-sycotico-syphilitic Remedies" on p. 703 ff. in the article "The Polarity of Remedies in Relation to the Polarity of Disease" in the section "Electronic Reactions". - Editor.

Acet-ac., *alum.*, alumn., *apis, ambr.*, **Ars.**, *ars-i., aster., aur., aur-ar., bell-p.*, bism., **Brom.**, *bufo, cadm-cy.*, cadm-f., *cadm-i.*, **Cadm-met.**, cadm-n., cadm-p., cadm-sil., *cadm-s., calc., calc-ar., calc-f., calc-s., carb-ac.*, **Carb-an.**, *carb-v.*, carbn-h., *carbn-s.*, caust., *cist., clem.*, cob., **Con.**, crot-h., cund., cupr., dulc., elaps, *graph.*, hep., **Hydr.**, kali-ar., kali-bi., *kali-cy.*, kali-i., kali-m., kali-n., *kali-s., kreos.*, lac-c., *lach., lap-a.*, **Lyc.**, merc., *merc-i-f.*, nat-m., nat-sil-f., **Nit-ac.**, orig., ph-ac., **Phos.**, *phyt., ruta, rad-br.*, sep., *sil., sulph.*, sul-ac., *thuj., toxi.*, x-ray., zinc.

Of the seventy-five remedies listed in the cancer group, forty-five are of high grade value, the others are of inferior value and less frequently indicated and used.

From this group the uterine sub-group comprises the largest number. From this fact, we may presume that these tissues are subject to a large number of different irritations and conditions, that they are more sensitive and susceptible to the cancer toxin.

There is one smaller group of remedies that correspond to conditions arising from trauma and irritations of various kinds that are highly valuable for the cancer state. Remembering that disease gets well in the inverse order of the appearance of its symptoms, we may well understand why a breast cancer whose immediate and last manifestation of cell growth following an injury would readily yeild homeopathically to such remedies as BELL-P.,CON., or PHYT. Also how easy it is for us to perceive the potent possibility of preventing any cancer change ever starting after injury with a potency of ARN.

Irritations and injuries to other parts of the body are such as those in gastro-intestinal tract from faulty foods, indiscretion in eating, adulterated food, those irritations produced by chlorine and flourine in the drinking water, alumina poisoning coming from the use of aluminum cooking utensils and from aluminum plates in the mouth sometimes used by dentists. Such irritations as these will find the best antidotal remedy among some of the CADMIUMS, but also the irritating cause must be removed with the administration of the curative remedy to make the cure certain and permanent.

Other irritations like those occurring in smokers where the pressure and heat of the pipe combined sometimes causes a lip cancer that SEP. will frequently cure, providing the irritation is discontinued. The remedies of this smaller group are likewise contained in the general group of

---

3. See also "Malignancy & All Three Miasms" on p. 708 ff. in the article "The Polarity of Remedies in Relation to the Polarity of Disease" in the section "Electronic Reactions". - Editor.

cancer remedies. They are: alum., arn., ars., bell-p., brom., cadm-s., caust., con., cund., graph., hydr., kali-bi., kali-cy., kali-i., kali-s., lach., lyc., merc-c., nit-ac., phos., phyt., ruta, sep., sil., thuj., toxi. A careful study and wide knowledge of these remedies will reward the industrious physician with a harvest of cure in cancer conditions undreamed of without such complete knowledge.

Other irritations than those mentioned above are such as arise from the wide use of the coal-tar preparations flooding the public in ever increasing variety and given for so many complaints, headaches, rheumatic pains, acute colds, grippe, fever reducers, and sleeping potions. Bombarded with these cardiac depressants, is it any wonder that heart and kidney disease lead the list of death causing diseases with cancer soon a close second? Against these irritants our CARBONS and SNAKE POISONS furnish the best antidotes.

Perhaps the most irritating of all the irritants and depressants is the one produced by the almost universal applications of serums and vaccines given for the prevention and cure of acute infectious diseases. These subtle poisons are very far reaching and deep in their effects and our best antidotes can only be found in THUJ. and several of the specific nosodes such as DIPH. and PYROG. together with the SNAKE POISONS. Is it not possible that persistant and frequent injections of these bi-products of disease shot directly into the blood stream, especially in young children, result in a state such that conditions in the body organism for natural defense against these toxins cannot obtain, and that in fact a weakening of the reticulo-endothelial system is produced thereby reducing the reactive power of the body against cancer and kindred diseases? (The reticulo-endothelial system is said by biologists to manufacture and contain all the defensive forces of the organism.) And may this not answer the observed fact why cancer is occurring in younger subjects of each succeeding generation?

Of what avail is it to try to prevent some natural expression of acute disease that may never come, if there is involved in the immunizing process a weakening of the defensive mechanism of the body against chronic manifestations of diseases like cancer, diabetes, epilepsy and mental and physical weaknesses of various sorts. Add to all this the wholesale destruction of children's tonsils, one of the most important defense units in the organism, which lessens still more the chance of body resistance and we have a gloomy outlook for the health and well-being of the future.

How much longer can the human race stand the strain of serum poisons and crude drugs and their resultant suppressions grafted on the ever increasing miasmatic causes of disease? Only Homeopathy can retard the deep decay and frightful devastation gnawing at the vital centers of the human race.

One other benefit is presented in the vast numbers that have repudiated all medicine and taken up with the so-called cults for relief against sickness. The cults, at least give nature a chance to work, unhampered by animal toxins and crude poisons in the form of irritating and enervating drugs. The pendulum has swung from the crude and clumsy attempts of the allopaths to overwhelm disease by substitution (the implanting of a drug or serum disease in place of the natural one), and by suppression (the masking of external symptoms and the numbing of sensibilities to pain without in any way relieving the internal cause of illness) to those who at least have intelligence enough to know that nature has provided wonderful means of defense against sickness.

However, in the field of chronic inherited disease, nature alone is often unable to cure.[1] This is the realm of Homeopathy and vast numbers of more intelligent cultists must necessarily swing back to her for relief of those sicknesses that are the outgrowth of chronic miasms.

There is another pernicious form of irritation that is making many carcasses. That is the practice, advocated by most of those looked up to as authorities on the treatment of cancer, of employing large doses of either x-ray or radium on every mole, wart, small ulcer, or blemish appearing on the skin. This procedure either irritates and burns the local parts (because of over dosing) setting up necrosis of surrounding cells resulting in a rapid spreading of the sore and often turning a benign and harmless growth of small dimensions into a rapidly destructive malignant cancer, or, if the dose is lighter, the sore or mole or wart may be destroyed and apparently healed with an unsightly scar remaining. If the latter result is obtained, that patient will inevitably develop, in the course of a few months or years according to his constitutional soil inheritance, a cancer in some of his vital organs. We have few remedies that can antidote this kind of mischief because the capillaries are obliterated by those destructive agents; CADM-I., FL-AC. and PHOS. are the only three remedies I have found helpful in such cases. X-RAY and RADIUM PREPARATIONS in potencies may be found useful in some cases after further study and trial. For the anemia and cachexia that often fol-

---

1.   §50 Organon and Kent LHP Lecture XVI, para. 4. - Editor.

lows radium abuse, PHOS. is the best antidote. For the ulcerating areas of necrosis that seemingly defies all healing agents, CADM-I. is the only remedy I have known to help. For the X-ray burn, FL-AC. is the remedy that yields the best clinical results.

Industries of a certain type predispose workers to cancer preferring special parts of organs, as shown in the cobalt miners' tendency to cancer of the lungs. And the workers in aniline dyes are more often affected by vesical cancer. These observations may suggest the proving and trial of these substances in potency as possible remedies of the disease localized in the parts that cobalt and the aniline dyes each affect.

No paper on the treatment of cancer, even though it be strictly remedial, would adequately impart the necessary knowledge for the most successful results without a complimentary diet as adjunct to prescribing. And the diet, like the remedy, should be selected for the individual patient, noting susceptibilities and reactions after food selection with as much concern and interest as is shown by the skilled prescriber of the homeopathic remedy. The chemistry of food and its relation to the blood chemistry of the patient is a mighty aid or a great hinderance to the action of the curative remedy, depending upon the degree of intelligence shown in food selection.

There is a great need of more experimental work in the chemistry of food and its relation to cancer. So far this work is largely empirical and far from scientific. The only near unified opinion being the baneful effects of a meat diet, at least in advanced cases of disease; other proteins may be carefully admitted only varying in amoung with individual cases.

The mental or psychic phase of cancer must not be ignored if our best success is obtained. The terror and hopelessness concerning the incurability of cancer prevailing today in the ranks of allopathy has made the problem more difficult. The public is told by these bombastic sons of egotism that there is no cure because they have failed to find it. Anyone claiming to cure cancer is branded by them with their favorite anathema, "quack". Anyone having the temerity to criticize their methods of surgery and radiation with its attendant mutilation and torture and its high death rate occurring in a shorter period than occurs to those untouched by them and left to unhampered nature, is not only a "quack" but a public menace. It is claimed by competent observers that the approved methods of the up to date modern medical scientist are dead after two years.

From its incipiency, Homeopathy has always inspired hope and courage in its practicians and patients alike, because they are taught the advantage of working in harmony with the laws of nature of which the therapeutic law of similars is but one. Because of these facts, homeopaths are better equipped to combat this sinister and implacable force that threatens to destroy the race.

To summarize, the homeopathic treatment of cancer consists first in the selection of some specific remedy found in the Hahnemannian group that includes all three of the miasms in its symptomatology (together with the group specially related to trauma in its numerous forms). Second: the removal of all irritants that may act as exciting or activating causes. Third: in the homeopathic selection of the proper diet, avoiding foods that irritate the patient and giving those that agree with and nourish him, such foods to be based on the needs of each patient rather than for a diseased condition. And last; the bouying up of the patient's moral and mental status, appealing to his intelligent cooperation in all things, inspiring courage by explaining the certain but orderly processes by which disease comes under broken law, and goes under restored law brought about with the homeopathic specific and the intelligent effort of the patient to live in harmony with these lawful processes of nature.

Armed with these forces and the knowledge that we work in unison with the restless throb of universal order inspires us to face with confidence this baffling medical problem agitating the world today.

CADMIUM CURES OF CANCER[1]

The curing of cancer cases by homeopathic remedies is nothing new or strange. Our literature is replete with many reported cures of more or less authentic and definite cancer conditions. In fact homeopathy offers the only real therapeutic hope in the world today against this dreadful scourge.

Outside of homeopathy, the only real advance and the only helpful measure that has proven useful in the cancer fight, is that of diet. Dietary measures are as important as the selection of the indicated remedy, for unless the correct dietary rules are followed, your homeopathic remedy will fail to permanently cure in the majority of cases. On the other hand correct diet alone is not sufficient to eradicate the inherited soil that engenders and sustains cancer. For anything like uniform success one must combine the selection of the homeopathic remedy, with a diet of fruits, vegetables, cereals and nuts and, later on, when improvement has reached a high point, dairy products in moderation may be allowed.

While it is true that any deep acting constitutional remedy may prove curative in a given case of cancer, we have in the CADMIUM SALTS our most valuable units against the condition now recognized as carcinosis or carcinoma (late stage).

The pathogenesis of CADM-S. has all the weakness and all the blood changes that correspond to a late cancer condition; besides practically all the particular conditions, from skin ulcers, that resist the normal healing tendencies, to breast and uterine tumors, together with the severe stomach ulcerations that readily take on blood changes of a malignant nature. It is in the late cases where symptoms are masked by drastic drugging and by pathology, the end results of disease, that a knowledge of the CADMIUM SALTS is helpful. These patients should have been cured years ago when their symptoms would have guided to the needed remedy or remedies which would have prevented the ultimates of cancer. For homeopathy in the hands of real prescribers will so change the life forces of the body or the constitutional state that cancer

---

1. This article originally appeared in THE HOMEOPATHIC RECORDER, September, 1929, page 606. The original handwritten manuscript was entitled "Cancer Cures by the Cadmium Salts". This article has been edited by Ahmed N. Currim and has some corrections to the journal article based on Dr. Grimmer's handwritten manuscript. Also case 10 does not appear in the original handwritten manuscript nor in the journal but is a case of Dr. Kent which the editor has added to show another illustration of the Cadmium remedies to cancer cases. - Editor.

and tuberculosis will not grow or develop because of the healthful soil conditions that result from careful and really scientific prescribing. The dismal failure of surgery, x-ray and radium as curative agents in cancer, renders any proven measure more acceptable to a waiting world, for victims from the cancer scourge are constantly increasing, and allopathic medicine acknowledges its inability to cope with the situation.

The actual causes of cancer are obscured in a maize of uncertainty and ignorance. Allopathy does not know, but it has proven a few interesting things that may be helpful in the future. Dr. Maude Sly of Chicago has proven the inherited soil theory of cancer in rats. She has bred cancer in and out of various rat families by selection and mating, and thereby has confirmed what the masters of homeopathy have so long announced and contended. Dr. Crile of Cleveland, and others have demonstrated that the cancer cell has lost its normal bi-polar electrical nature and taken on a positive state, with a resulting change in the nucleus of the cell. Electronic physicians have gone farther. They have proven that not only has a change taken place in the polarity, chemistry and histology of the affected cells, but that every drop of blood in the organism shows a corresponding change, at least in polarity, if not in chemistry and histology. Before any chemical changes take place in the body (not the test tube) there is a change in polarity; and chemical changes precede histologic or pathologic changes. All disease cause and departure from health is found in this fundamental change of polarity. It is the *modus operandi*, at least of the changes of state of health to disease and *vice versa*.

Our remedies, especially in potency, are catalysts that change body forces and body states, enabling normal function to be restored when broken, and perpetuating in an orderly way all the necessary reactions in the human organism to maintain life and health. The seed and the embryo contain all the necessary chemical elements in their proper proportion for the growth, development and repair of the organism, only needing the necessary food replenishment to maintain life through its allotted cycle. Hence true medicines are only catalytic in nature, they do not enter into the body cells combined with other elements, but their presence may be necessary, to bring about the normal combinations of chemicals always present in the blood stream for life's activities. All chemical change in the body is destructive, all vital change constructive. Absorption and nutrition are vital, the chemistry has been expended in digestion and elimination. These few facts are mentioned in order that we may know how and why the homeopathic remedy acts so powerfully and positively as a curative agent against the changes found in the body cells in the condition called cancer. If we know the order in which disease develops, we can know the order in which remedies act to correct abnormal changes in the organism. When we know these things our faith is sustained by absolute knowledge.

In the past four years I have treated two hundred and twenty-five[1] cases of proven cancer, of various forms and in all stages of the disease. At this time one hundred and seventy-five are still living, many of them entirely well and free of all cancer symptoms. Only one of this group now living, shows indications of an early demise. All of those who failed to respond to the homeopathic treatment had been treated surgically or with x-ray and radium in material doses. My records show one case of late intestinal and splenic cancer in an old lady sixty-three years old, who lived five years in comparative comfort, and only recently died at sixty-eight, from weakness and exhaustion, entirely free of pain. In the last two years since my study and application of the CADMIUM SALTS my losses have been greatly reduced. I believe that any advanced case of carcinoma will need CADMIUM in some form, dependent on the symptoms of the individual before a cure can be effected.

Other remedies are sometimes needed after CADMIUM to complement and complete the cure. Sometimes other remedies must precede the use of CADMIUM. I frequently find cancer of the liver yielding to CALC-AR. in every way but the tendency to relapse, when frequently a single dose of CADMIUM[2] in high potency will render the cure permanent. In the early stages of cancer, especially of the skin, when many guiding therapeutic symptoms still are present, any one of our deep constitutional remedies may be sufficient to cure. Our literature abounds in reports of hundreds of beautiful cures.

I believe a study of the CADMIUM SALTS and their use early in every case, on strictly homeopathic lines, will enable the homeopathic physician to make many more cures of cancer than are being made at the present time. Any case of cancer complicated by a weak heart or diseased kidneys can hardly get well, because the reaction to the curative remedy will kill such a patient in a comparatively short time.

I submit, briefly, the records of a few cases to illustrate the action of CADMIUM on cancer conditions.

---

1. In the original hand-written article Dr. Grimmer corrected this to two hundred and five.
2. usually CADM-S. - Editor.

CASE 1 - MRS. J. W., AGE 63

May 6, 1926. This case was diagnosed first as one of gallstones, and operation was advised by an old school man. She was jaundiced and anemic and had lost weight rapidly. The liver was enlarged and plainly nodular. CALC-AR. 45M was given with immediate and marked benefit, which continued until June 12, 1926, when CALC-AR. 45M was repeated with improvement. This continued until Oct. 7, 1926, when a slight return of jaundice and liver pain was noted. CALC-AR. CM was given with complete subsidence of all symptoms. This lasted until April 29, 1927, when a severe bronchial cold called for CARB-AC., 10M, which cleared up promptly and left the patient well until Feb. 4, 1928. Symptoms of much intentinal gas then annoyed the patient. CARB-V. 10M was given with relief until March 8, 1928, when the old liver symptoms accompanied by nausea and weakness, with extreme coldness and aggravation from exertion demanded CADM-S., which was given in 45M potency. The patient has had no more medicine since and remains in perfect health and comfort.[1]

CASE 2 - MRS. V., AGE 52

June 8th, 1927. Five months prior to this date, this woman was in robust health, weighing 168 pounds. She was now reduced to 80 pounds, more than half her body had gone, in a very short time. She was jaundiced and cachectic; spots of ecchymosis covered her limbs; she was in a constant tremor; her heart was weak and irregular in action; she could not take the slightest bit of food or drink without soon vomiting it. She had a small vascular goitre. Her liver was enlarged and nodular, and a distinct mass, indurated and tender, was palpable in the epigastric region. At this time PLB-I. 10M was given and the patient put on a diet of diluted apple juice, an ounce every two hours. There was a steady slight gain in strength and ability to retain fluids until July 11, 1927, when there was a return of the nausea and vomiting of tough, stringy, blood-streaked mucus. KALI-BI. 10M was given for this with no relief and on July 13, 1927 the patient was weaker, with sinking sensation at the epigastrium; cold sweats, and vomiting even of a teaspoonful of water. At this low ebb-tide of life forces, CADM-P. 30 was given, with a slow, but steady uninterrupted gain of strength and a gradual decrease of all alarming symptoms, so that after a few days a little strained vegetable broth was added to the apple and pear juices as nour-

---

1. This was three years later i.e. in September 1929. - Editor.

CASE 2 - MRS. V., AGE 52. ...

ishment. The gain was maintained with no further medication until January 7, 1928 when symptoms of nausea returned. The patient now weighed 100 pounds and was living on a soft diet of fruits and vegetables with a little cereal and cream. The second dose of CADM-P. 30 was given now. From this time on the patient gained rapidly in weight and strength. Whole-wheat bread and butter and cheese were added to her diet. No more medicine was given this patient until September, 1928, when a dose of CADM-P. 10M was administered, She now weighed 130 pounds, her strength and color had returned, her liver was normal in size and the abdominal mass was gone.[1] This patient remains vigorously well, attends to all her duties, administering to the needs of a large family. She has almost regained her complete body weight, now 160 pounds, and looks more like a woman of 40 than the 54 years she is.

CASE 3 - MR. B. R. C., AGE 42.

September 8, 1928. This man, two years prior to this date had gone through a six months' siege with duodenal ulcers, which had not entirely healed, as the patient was in more or less distress with inability to gain in weight or strength. Two days prior to the above date the patient had played harder at tennis than usual, and had eaten a rather hearty meal; that night he was awakened with severe epigastric pains which soon was followed by vomiting of food with some blood. He was given CADM-I. 10M, put on the usual diet of liquid fruit and vegetable juices, and improved for about ten days, when suddenly a severe intestinal hemorrhage ensued. HAM. 10M was given with only a short lasting relief, followed by ARN. 10M, because of an extensive body soreness; still no relief. Recurrent hemorrhage persisted and not even water could be taken by mouth without producing bloody vomiting and an increase of intestinal hemorrhage. This was Sept. 25, 1928. CALEN. 30 was given and all food stopped, nutrition being maintained by enemas of glucose. There was complete cessation of hemorrhage for twenty-one days, and an abdominal mass in the hepatic region began to recede. At this time, October 16, 1928, an attempt at nourishment by mouth provoked vomiting and a slight hemorrhage. CALEN. 50M was given with complete relief and the ability of the patient to take a little liquid nourishment by mouth without nausea or emesis.

---

1. At this date September 1929. - Editor.

CASE 3 - MR. B. R. C., AGE 42. ...

Nov. 3. 1928[1] CALEN. 50M was given. There was a steady gain with no more medicine required until December 15, 1928 when a slight return of symptoms called for CALEN. CM with improvement until January 18, 1929 when CADM-MET. 10M was given with immediate and permanent improvement in every way. This man now weighs 189 pounds, eats everything, contrary to orders, and is in better health than ever before in his life.

CASE 4 - MR. B., AGE 58

Sept. 21, 1928. This patient was reduced from 210 pounds to 145 pounds, was of bad color, extremely weak, with severe burning pains radiating from liver over the abdomen. His liver almost filled the abdominal cavity and was notched and nodular. He had been a heavy drinker and a recent attack of "flu" had added to his weakness and misery. At this date CALC-AR. 45M was given with steady gain on a diet of fruits and vegetables. CALC-AR. 45M was repeated Nov. 10, 1928, followed by steady gain in strength and weight and a relief of symptoms. Dec. 15, 1928, CALC-AR. CM was given. There was not the response to this prescription that followed the preceding ones and on Jan. 7, 1929, because of the burning pains, weakness and nausea, with chilliness and aggravation from exertion. CADM-S. 45M was given with wonderful relief and a gain that has been maintained to this day. The liver is almost normal in size and feel; the man now weighs 195 pounds and is deeply grateful for his release from the grave as he terms it.

CASE 5 - MRS. S., AGE 48

Sept. 15, 1928. This woman has had digestive troubles for years. X-ray diagnosed probable malignancy of the duodenum. CADM-S. 50M, two doses, two months apart, cured all symptoms and x-ray now shows normal intestines. The patient has gained in weight, strength and color.

CASE 6 - MRS. B., AGE 54

Jan. 16, 1928. CADM-I. 10M. This is a case of intestinal cancer with toxic goitre and marked cardiac disturbance. She had a quick response and steady gain in weight and strength until Aug. 14, 1928 when she overate and upset her digestion; CADM-I. 10M soon righted her until

---

1. The article in THE HOMEOPATHIC RECORDER had a few lines missing at this point which were inserted from the original handwritten manuscript. - Editor.

Case 6 - Mrs. B., age 54 ...

Oct. 15, 1928, when a severe cold upset her. Cadm-i. 10M kept her well until the last report on Feb. 7, 1929, when I dismissed her cured. She remains strong and well to this day.[1]

Case 7 - Mr. B., age 67

Aug. 6, 1927. Splenic cancer, with weakness and the usual blood findings. Calad. given with slight benefit. Oct. 7, 1928, Rad-chl. 10M. Patient became much worse, and went to another doctor, who put him in a hospital, made all the tests to confirm a certain diagnosis of cancer, and then advised a splenic operation, which was refused. On Nov. 24, 1928, I again saw the patient and gave Cadm-met. 10M, with no more medicine to the present date. A complete metamorphosis has been wrought; the blood findings are almost normal, the spleen is reduced, and the weight, color, strength and comfort of the patient are wonderfully good for a man 69 years of age.

Case 8 - Mrs. T., age 36

Jan. 15, 1929. Mrs. T. always had pain and swelling of the breasts with her menses. A lump in the right breast was removed a year ago, and pronounced cancer, after a microscopic examination. She is pale, emaciated, weak and cachectic. The left breast is now indurated and sore with retracted nipples, pains worse at period. Cadm-met. 10M has been given at intervals; single doses, Jan. 15, 1929; March 19, 1929; May 22, 1929. The breast is well and the patient much improved every way.

Case 9

Feb. 9, 1928, I was asked to prescribe for one of our eminent surgeons for a severe protracted intestinal hemorrhage. The patient was bled white and was very weak and feeble. He was in the late seventies and much reduced from a once very vigorous and powerful man. Three doses of Cadm-met., one the 30th potency, given Feb. 9, 1929, the others of the 10M given March 12, 1928 and Oct. 1, 1928, have restored this aged benefactor to a healthy happy state, enabling him to finish his life work, in the form of a valuable medical treasure of knowledge and philosophy of healing that will aid and comfort great numbers in the future.

---

1. September 1929 - Editor.

Case 10[1]

Miss X., aged twenty-seven. In the last stage of cancer of the stomach. Constant vomiting. Everything taken into the stomach, even water, vomited. Coffee-ground vomit. Burning in the stomach like fire, day and night. Emaciated to a skeleton. Had been treated with morphine, which gave no relief. Nausea and retching increased by motion. Hot things ameliorated momentarily. Cold things caused pain. Great anxiety. CADM-S. 50M. kept her comfortable until she passed away several weeks later, and enabled her to take soups and simple liquid nourishment.

Conclusion

As a summary of these case reports, I would like to bring to your attention the fact that homeopathy in the hands of its master prescribers is the greatest and most efficient force the world has today against the scourge of cancer. Yet in spite of this fact many of our men are running after will-o'-the-wisps, that float above the quagmires of materialistic pseudo-science as panaceas for the cure of cancer. Millions are raised and spent annually for research without avail, and the governments of the world are taxing their already over burdened citizens in this same endless march, always in circles.

Like lost wanderers in the wilderness they go, without compass or guide to lead them safely to their goal; yet above them, and around them shines the light of homeopathy, like the polar star to lead the way to the goal they are so arduously seeking.

If they would but cast the blinders of prejudice from their eyes, and, like the wise men of old, follow the star to the manger of physical salvation, then, at last, the prayers and hopes of an agonizing world would be answered.

---

1. Case 10 is one of Dr. J.T. Kent's cases and was taken from the JOURNAL OF HOMEOPATHICS, Vol. VI, No. 11, Feb., 103, p. 412. This case does not appear in the original article of Dr. Grimmer but has been added by the editor to illustrate additional use of CADM-S. - Editor.

FURTHER RESULTS IN THE HOMEOPATHIC TREATMENT OF CANCER[1]

Two years ago, we were privileged to read before this group of my colleagues. a paper entitled Cadmium Cures of Cancer,[2] wherein were stated the results of the treatment, up to that date, of two hundred and twenty-five cases, with a loss of fifty cases in four years. At this time, there has been added to that list twenty-two more deaths by cancer, but these last named lived six years, most of the time in comfort, performing their accustomed work, and all dying with a minimum of suffering. Many experienced no suffering, and without morphine or any other narcotic or anesthetic drug, they went quietly and peacefully to their rest. The remaining hundred and fifty - these give every promise of living many years, excepting some of those, whose advanced age at any time may intervene to end life. From these figures, we may claim a cure of two-thirds of all cases treated after a lapse of six years, by strictly homeopathic methods, because most, if not all, of the remaining patients will die from causes other than that of cancer. Remember, these were not incipient cases, they all showed the cachexia, and the clinical and laboratory evidence of the developed active cancer disease. Many had been treated surgically and by radium and x-ray with only harm resulting, before they came to homeopathy. Because of these facts, and because of new data collected under wider and more varied experience in the application of homeopathic research in cancer, I am hopeful of far greater achievement in the near future in the cure and abatement of this implacable disease. It is destined to be accomplished by all the true disciples of Hahnemannian homeopathy.

We need but correlate our remedy prescribing with dietetic and hygienic measures to accomplish even more astounding results than we have in the past (in terms of cure). We need also to discover a method of making an absolute diagnosis of the pre-cancer stage. When this desirable thing is a certainty, and it is in sight even now but not quite perfected, we shall witness the recognition of the power of the homeopathic law over man's most destructive and heretofore ineradicable foe. After a review of all modern research, and after the futile and discouraging results obtained by surgery, x-ray and radium over a long period of

---

1. Read at the I.H.A., Bureau of Clinical medicine, June, 1931. This paper appeared in THE HOMEOPATHIC RECORDER, Vol. XLVI, No. 9, September, 1931, p. 674.
2. See the article "Cadmium Cures of Cancer" on p. 800 ff. - Editor.

time, we know that Hahnemannian homeopathy holds out to the afflicted the only real hope for cure in the early cases, and amelioration of suffering and the prolonging of life in the advanced cases.

The more experience I have with the use of the CADMIUM PREPARA-TIONS, the more convinced I am of their indispensable need in cancer. Not that they always perfect the cure alone and unaided, but they are the most effective antidote I have yet found to aluminum poisoning, and that factor plays a far more important role in cancer than most of us believe in the past. Intestinal forms of the disease, especially, are undoubtedly much aggravated by the presence of that subtle poison. Aluminum is one of the most common of the irritants entering as excit-ing causes in many cases of cancer.[1] CADM-I. is the most effective anti-dote to radium and x-ray burns to be found among the homeopathic remedies, competing with PHOS. for radium poison and with FL-AC. and SIL. for the x-ray abuses. These remedies are the most effective agents yet found against the frightful results both locally and systematically, that radium and x-ray produce.

From a homeopathic view, the cancer problem presents four basic aspects, each a study in itself:

The first is the physiological phase, and this is related to both doctor and patient. The horror and depressing effects of a cancer diagnosis, right or wrong, is in itself, overwhelming in most cases. To the patient no hope remains, it is useless to try, the only concern left is to avoid as much suffering as he can and possibly prolong for a time a life already doomed. To the doctor, especially if he is scientific and imbued with the up to date ideas of the so-called authorities, it means just another fated victim for whom there is no remedy or help, only an object of experimentation of mutilation and torture, all in the name of science and progress. No attempt by intelligent effort is made to seek causes and invoke law, which is the first attribute of true philosophy and sci-ence. The patient under such mental states is permitted and left to go, to think, act, eat, and do as he chooses, unguided, unaided, as a bit of driftwood on a storm tossed sea, without compass or succor.

The second aspect is the one of irritation which comes from many sources, some very subtle and obscure. Drugs, especially the coal tar derivatives, serums, vaccines, metallic poisons; and processed, adulter-

---

1. On page 825 Dr. Grimmer points out that CADM-O. is the most effective antidote to Alumini-um poisoning or toxicity. - Editor.

ated, demineralized, devitalized, irritating foods, are found in this group.

The third aspect is that of dietetics, the removal of all irritating and harmful foods, and the careful selection of non-irritating, balanced, individualized nourishment.

The fourth aspect, is that of remedy selection. This is more difficult and complicated than that of ordinary prescribing because so many things enter in the history and cause of cancer, and because no two cases are alike. We may have to antidote some specific drug poison in one case, before anything else. Another may require the reduction of some specific basic miasm or infection, such as syphilis. A series of complimentary remedies is frequently needed to meet conditions in many cases, but all according to the homeopathic law, doses given singly, and at sufficient intervals apart, for the expression and evolution of the cases.

We may learn much from observation, relating to the nature and growth of cancer, both when left to the vital force unassisted by medicinal action, and when influenced by such action. Last year, I saw a woman, sixty-three years old, who presented a breast cancer in active stage, far advanced, but only for a short time, prior to my seeing her, had it pained. She stated that she first noticed the lump in her breast twenty-three years before and she had feared to see any doctor because of her dread of operations; she had taken no treatment, observed no rules of diet, worked hard under more or less trying circumstances, yet nature unassisted, had kept her alive, free of pain and fit for over twenty years. What work homeopathy could have done with that case in its incipiency. We all see the answer in the number of lumps and nodules that disappear under good prescribing.

This brings us to the most vital part of our subject, that of prevention; for if we can cure a large number of developed cases, and if nature, unaided, can retard the disease ravages for twenty years, what will good prescribing plus proper diet and proper living do, to prevent the development of cancer. It has long been known that constitutional homeopathic treatment will prevent cancer in the large majority of cases. In these times when this silent terror is dominating the world, especially the world of dominant medicine, it becomes our solemn duty, to give to humanity, these potent facts. Millions of dollars are wasted annually in donations for allopathic ignorance, to squander in cruel animal experimentations that ignore and pervert the laws of God and nature, and fail to bring anything save additional suffering and sacrifice to an already overburdened race. Is it wrong, to let a suffering and terrorized world, know that homeopathy is the balm of healing to check the destroying conquest of this hideous monster, conceived in violated law, born in wickedness, and nurtured in ignorance?

Some Cancer Remedies and their Indications[1]

The more I study cancer, the more I prescribe for cancer, the more I am convinced that the earlier we start prescribing for cancer the better our results would be. Sometimes it is astonishing the results we get in very late cases; but these are exceptions far from the rule. We relieve their pain and suffering and improve their general health and increase their days - there is no question about that. As for curing, it is very rare in advanced cases.

In the early cases, where there is just the state of incipiency, where you have already the beginning cachexia and pain, and in some cases quite a little pathology beginning to show - small nodules of the breast and characteristic glandular involvement - you will be astounded what careful prescribing will do in most of these cases.

Cancer is a condition, the outgrowth of very low states - to use the language of Dr. Kent - and undoubtedly made up of all the miasms plus drug, serum and other irritations. I am convinced that all those factors enter into the admitted increase of cancer. Treatment by the "old school" is just as it was twenty years ago, in spite of the fact that their losses are appalling. They have made some apparently exceptional cures. In my practice I have never seen the cure of cancer by any of these methods; I have seen a lot of harm done. I believe they shorten the life of the patient, and I believe they deprive one of the ability to prescribe successfully with a homeopathic remedy.

You will have to antidote the effects of radium and x-ray by using a potentized remedy. CADM-I., FL-AC., PHOS. and SIL. have been my best remedies for the painful effects of radium and X-ray burns. Both produce, as you know, obliteration of the capillary circulation.[2]

---

1. A talk before I.H.A., Bureau of Clinical Medicine, June 26, 1936. This article appeared in The Homeopathic Recorder, Vol. LII, No. 4, April, 1937.
   All the remdies in this article, and in fact in the whole book have been collected in a separate section: Repeertory Rubrics for Kent's Repertory from Grimmer, prepared by the Editor. All page numbers refer to Dr. Kent's Repertory third or later editions and were added by the editor. When this article was originally written by Dr. Grimmer it seems that he used the second edition of Kent's Repertory without page numbers.
   Several errors in the original article were corrected using Dr. Grimmer's manuscripts.
   Additional rubrics of cancer than those in the second edition, are found in the third edition: The cancer rubric together with subrubrics can be searched in various sections of the repertory under Cancer, Condylomalomata, Excresences, Exostosis, Fungoid Growths, Hardness, Induration, Noma, Nonosities, Polypus, Proud Flesh, Ranula, Tubercles, Tumor, Ulcers, Warts, etc. - Editor.

The great difficulty in advanced cases of cancer is the inability to obtain therapeutic individualization of symptoms. They have the pathology and all the common symptoms that go with it, but they are not sufficient to make a good homeopathic prescription. They tell you about cancer, but they tell you only in a very general way of a group of remedies.

The experiments of Crile and his bi-polar theory of living processes[1] have been very interesting to me. He states that the cancer cell has made a change from its normal bi-polar polarity to that of a positive polarity. That is exactly what we find in our electronic reactions. Not only is the cancer cell positive, but the patient's whole blood stream is electromagnetically positive where cancer predominates. We know where the mixed miasms come in and where we have sycosis and syphilis mixed with cancer other polarities may be present.

My experience has been that there is not a case of cancer without a tubercular background. It grows on a tubercular soil. It is the miasm where in the blending of all the other miasms result.

Pathology is often the only thing you can obtain. In such cases one must go back in the history of the patients as far as he can, from the beginning of life, and trace it step by step, his sicknesses, reactions to environment, the history of things that have come upon him by way of accident, and irritations - all those things, including vaccinations and serums - and better still, the history of his immediate progenitors and his immediate family. Here is another thought: if you can get the closest remedy on your first prescription and do not have to try too many remedies until the case is mixed, you are infinitely better off and there is a much better chance for the patient. That is why it is so necessary to get the indications, meager though they be.

We are all familiar with the crude animal experiments that Dr. Maude Sly of University of Chicago has been doing; she has been able to breed cancer in mice families and out of mice families simply by selective mating. These facts establish the inherited causation as a basic causation and many of our allopathic friends are willing to acknowledge that; not all of them, but many do accept these results as evidence that cancer in its incipiency or in its fundamentals is inherited, at least the cell tendency. I prefer to use the word "tendency"; I don't think a person has to die of cancer because his father and mother had it, but he

---

2. See the article "Further Results in the Homeopathic Treatment of Cancer" on p. 808 ff. - Editor.
1. Crile, George W.: A Bipolar Theory of Living Processes, The Macmillan Co., New York, 1926. - Editor.

has that tendency, and that is what you have to consider in the study of the case for a remedy.

Especially in those cases following injury where they have apparently been in fair or robust health and suddenly after the trauma a lump comes into the breast, in some cases painful and some not. We have two remedies par excellence in such conditions[1] - there are others, but these are the two outstanding remedies that are worth study and consideration. One of them is BELL-P., where there is more or less inflammation and soreness - much like ARN.; but we have the glandular involvement which is not so marked in ARN. BELL-P. is better given than ARN. The other remedy, with which I have had most success, is CON., in the case that has a shrivelled breast, with weakness and general symptoms of cachexia coming on. It is generally distinguished in the large majority of cases by *painlessness, or at least the pain doesn't come on early.* I have seen a few painful cases, but they were late cases after they started to break down. These are my two best remedies.

If you will take up our cancer group and run through the regional areas of cancer wherever our proven remedies have cured conditions, you will find CARB-AN., CARB-V. and GRAPH. running all through. Those are the most frequent remedies to run all through the various regions.

On page 1346 of Dr. Kent's repertory under CANCEROUS AFFECTIONS there are fifty-nine remedies appearing under one or the other subrubrics; but these by no means exhaust the list of our cancer remedies. If you go through Clarke's Dictionary of Practical Materia Medica you will be astonished at the number of other remedies that have more or less complete provings for ameliorating or curing some forms of cancer.[2]

In late cases where there is much pathology and breaking down of tissue, I am very careful about giving a potency too high. I prefer a low potency, say the 6x, 12x or 30x. You get better results and you do not get those terrible aggravations of the higher potency; if the case happens to be incurable then by giving a high potency, you are going to hurry that patient on to his death. If he is incurable and his remedy is similar enough and given in the lower potencies, you will restore balance and relieve pain and bring the well-being of the patient back so he is much more comfortable. If he is a case on the borderline or can be

---

1. Kent's Rep. pg. 824. - Editor.
2. See article "Homeopathic Remedies that have Cured Patients Suffering from Cancer" on p. 821 ff.. - Editor.

cured, you can easily follow the lower with the higher potency. In the earlier cases I don't hesitate to give the remedy high and expect him to live through the aggravation. The patient responds after these prolonged aggravations and you have a very good chance of curing that case.

CARB-AN. is a glandular remedy, and you may have difficulty at times in differentiating between it and CON. The pathology is very similar, but there is a little differentiation: generally the CARB-AN. *has a purplish hue*, especially around the area of the breast. There are other differentiations in the general indications if you can dig down through the past history; but it is real painstaking work to take these cases.

GRAPH. is very apt to be indicated in cases where the breast has been lanced. In the scars of these lanced breasts you frequently get a case where GRAPH. will delight you with its action. Dr. Kent thought that GRAPH. was the best remedy of all for cancer of the breast. He had great faith in the possibilities of that remedy.

SIL. was another of the remedies that he employed if the condition was not too far advanced. A number of years ago he showed me a case of an old lady, seventy-five years old, who had a breast cancer broken down, ugly looking, extremely painful, much pus. That patient was given SIL. 10M. There was a frightful aggravation; the whole breast sloughed off and healed over perfectly. Perfect surgical work done by the homeopathic remedy. The old lady lived five years and subsequently died of pneumonia.

There are a few remedies that I am mentioning that are not in the repertory as far as I can find. One is LAC-C. You will be surprised that LAC-C. will do in those cases where the breast has been amputated. Many years ago when I was a student in Hahnemann College, I attended Dr. Kent's clinic. He very frequently left the whole thing in my charge. A patient came in with a small, painful lump in one breast. There were no symptoms apparent until we got into the history, then we found this: Frequently she had been at another hospital, a few months before she came to us. Through the over-zealous acts of a surgeon of great fame who attended, her breast was amputated and all the glands taken out - a very fine operation, for which he demanded $1,500, and took her husband's little plumbing business away from him to pay that bill. The interesting thing to us is that a few months later the other breast began to get a cancerous condition much the same way - a lump appeared, with all the same symptoms. She refused to be operated, and I assured her that I did not think she would have to be. I saw

LAC-C. in the symptomatalogy and LAC-C. was given in the 1M. potency. The result was astonishing. In a few months that thing had disappeared, the woman's health was perfect, and two years later she came in periodically to show us that the cure was effective. You can imagine her emotions when she compared what we had done and what the surgeon had done. She wanted to pay us a great deal more than we asked. We insisted that she pay the small price that the clinic demanded of everybody, and assured her that as physicians, we could take nothing else.[1] She could hardly get over the fact that for a few cents she was able to receive work so much superior to that the great surgeon had done. Don't forget LAC-C. in those cases where first one breast is involved, then the other. You may have to use LYC. or LACH., of course. These are both among the list of Dr. Kent's high grade cancer remedies.

Other remedies under the rubric CANCEROUS AFFECTIONS on page 1346 of Dr. Kent's repertory are ARS., CADM-S., KALI-BI., MERC-C., PHOS. MERC-C. is also a valuable cancer remedy and should be inserted under this rubric. It appears on page 482 under Cancer of the Stomach.

KALI-BI. is more often indicated in the true stomach ulcer; I have not found it markedly indicated in the true cancer, but if related it undoubtedly would come in; but ARS. goes all through the cancer study. Wherever cancer forms in the body, you cannot ignore the pathogenesis of ARS. It has everything that goes with cancer, but it is more especially indicated, in my experience, in the gastric, intestinal and skin cases; in the gastric and intestinal cases, ARS. is a banner remedy. You all know the indications: they are better by warm drinks and worse by cold drinks, and of course they have the weakness. Warm drinks are almost the only thing they can tolerate - the very reverse of PHOS., and PHOS. is more likely to give hemorrhagic tendencies.

MERC-C. has a distinct symptomatology of its own and it is a banner remedy. I have overlooked it many times when it might have been the better remedy, and undoubtedly we would get better results if we did not so often ignore it. We all know the poisonous effect of MERC-C. and what it does to the intestinal tract and to the vital organs. You all know the coated tongue, the offensiveness and the sweating.

Another remedy that sometimes rewards the physician who uses it, is PLB. I have seen some wonderful work done with PLB. where we had the characteristic constipation, weakness and emaciation. Dr. Kent praises

---

1. May we all marvel at the great kindness and incredible honesty that Dr. Grimmer teaches us (by his actual actions) and may we strive to do likewise. - Editor.

Alum. very highly and mentions it frequently. It has much of the symptomatology of Plb. The doctors who have been telling us so much of the dangers of aluminum know what they are talking about; it is an insidious and injurious thing. It may take years for the Alum. constipation to be developed, but in a susceptible patient it will develop, and you will have the true picture of cancer - the anemias, the neuralgias the peculiar type of constipation, the semi-paralysis that goes with it. The best results, in my experience, are with Alumn. and Alum-sil., and I have frequently found them useful.

In mammary cancer we have one of the very difficult cancers. There are some unique remedies in this group. A few are not mentioned in the general group, but most of the general group run through in conjunction with some of these others. There are thirty-three remedies in italics or bold type in this group on page 824 in the repertory. We find Apis, Arg-n., Ars., Ars-i., Aster. (which is a sea remedy and is also a good breast cancer remedy if the indications are there), Aur-ar., Bad., Bell-p., Bell. - whoever thought of Bell. in cancer? But Bell. is deep enough to take care of some cancers if we have the indications; don't ignore it. We are prone to think of remedies by their depth, but Dr. Farrington has ably spoken of the chronic side of Acon. and Bell. Bell. is a remedy that may prove useful; it may not cure the case, but it will so pave the way that another remedy, probably some of the Calcarea salts, will follow. Brom., Bufo - I have had some interesting experiences with Bufo, the venom of the South American toad. I saw a late case of cancer where the breast was entirely involved. The woman was in a low state, apparently dying and under Bufo she got up around; the breast opened up, discharged and sloughed away, much as the case did for Dr. Kent under Sil. The woman lived four years, but finally died of cancer without much pain or trouble, but she was bed-ridden for quite a while. Carb-ac., Carb-an., Congo red, in black type. I have inserted a remedy here only for your consideration and study. It was one used by the late Dr. Abrams of San Francisco. Congo red is a dye, nevertheless it is a powerful remedy in breast cancer and in some of the bladder conditions. Chim., Clem., Con., Cund., Graph., Hep., Hydr., Lach., Lyc., Merc., and Merc-i-f., Nit-ac., Ox-ac. (I have found it useful in some cases where the pain is extreme), Phos., Phyt., Psor., Sang., Sep., Sil. and Sulph. There are two more I would like to add to that list: Thuj. and Sabal. Sabal., as you know, has a wealth of severe urinary symptoms. *Dr. Boger* once made the statement that it is a splendid remedy in *cancer of the prostate.*

For skin cancer we have twenty-four remedies on page 1346 under epithelioma of which eleven are in italics or bold type, but remember that that does not limit the prescriber; however, those are the remedies to be studied first. If you can get the symptoms, you can safely give any remedy that is truly indicated. Arg-n., Ars., Ars., Bufo, Con., Hydr., Kali-s., Kreos. (another carbon and when we come to take up the female genitals we find that Kreos. and the carbons, every single one of them, go through in heavy type), Lyc., Phyt., Ran-b., Sep., Sil., Sulph.

One remedy under the rubric of cancer of the sternum (page 824 of the repertory) is Sulph. A remedy that does farther than Sulph. in that condition, in my mind, is Ars-s-f.

Fungus hematodes (page 1346 of the repertory): Ars., Calc., Carb-an., Carb-v., Kreos., Lach., Lyc., Merc., Nat-m., Nit-ac., Phos., Puls., Sep., Sil., Sulph., Thuj.; and add to that, Sabal.

Now for the cases of the gastrointestinal tract (repertory page 482). We have a number of remedies there, additions to what we have in our repertories and literature, that I have proved clinically. I wish I had more symptoms, but I can only give the symptoms that we have, and some of them are very meager. Don't forget the Cadmium salts. I still get a lot of good from them and I am happy to say that I have had half a dozen men come to me at different conventions. One said, "Doctor, I want to thank you for giving me those Cadmium salts. I cured fifty cases of ulcers of the stomach and intestinal tract, and some cancer, with Cadmium since I read your article." I warned them against giving anything like that in a routine way. There are two preparations that I have found most applicable, Cadm-ar. and Cadm-p. They correspond to those cases that have the glandular involvement, and they are very good remedies. In fact, it will reward you to study most of the Cadmium salts. Cadm-i. is a remedy that will frequently right a case that has been burned to a chip with radium.

Cancer of the male genitalia (includes penis) (repertory page 693): Ars., Bell., Carb-an., Carbn-s., Con., Phos., Phyt., Sil., Spong., Thuj.

Scrotum: Carb-an., Phos.

Scirrhus: Carb-an., Alum.

Cancer of the testes: Spong. I have found Ox-ac. far superior, especially when accompanied by great pain. (Arg-n. is an addition from Kent's Materia Medica).

Cancer of the ovaries (repertory page 715): Ars., Con., Graph., Kreos., Lach., Psor.

Cancer of the uterus: There are fifty-three remedies on page 715 with the ARSENICUMS, CARBONS, CON., GRAPH., HYDR., LACH., LYC., MURX., PHOS., SEP., SIL. and THUJ. in bold type.

Cancer of the vagina: KREOS. Don't misunderstand me that that is the only remedy, but that comes from Dr. Kent.

Cancer of the larynx (repertory page 746) is interesting. There are not many remedies: ARS., NIT-AC., PHOS., SANG., THUJ.

Cancer of the axilla (page 824 of the repertory): ASTER.

Cancer of the tongue (page 398) and throat (page 448) give plenty of trouble. We certainly can do better than operate. I was surprised to find the number of remedies Dr. Kent had gathered, and of that group we find APIS, ALUMN., ARS. So it does good to write papers on such remedies: APIS, ARS., AUR., BENZ-AC., CALC., CARB-AN., CAUST., CON., CROT-H., HYDR., KALI-CHL., KALI-CY. (this remedy has quite a reputation in the literature as curing several cases, and it is a good remedy), LACH., MUR-AC., NIT-AC., PHOS., PHYT., SEP., SIL., SULPH., THUJ. To that list I have added RAD-BR. I have had more satisfying results with RAD-BR. in these conditions than with any other remedy.

Rectal cancer (page 606) and ulceration (page 633) will give you hard work too, and you really can do something in some of those cases if they are not too far gone and if they haven't had too much tinkering with and scraping by the specialists. For ulceration on page 633 we find: ALUMN., CALC., CAUST., CHAM. (a black type remedy for ulceration of the rectum); CUB., HEP., HYDR., KALI-C., KALI-I., NAT-S., PEON., PETR., PHOS., PULS., SARS., SIL., STAPH.., SYPH.. For cancer of the rectum on page 606: ALUM., NIT-AC., RUTA, SEP.

Hemorrhoidal conditions that are prone to become cancerous, that bloom out something like the flower in the rectum, a great mass of dark red, extremely sensitive hemorrhoids bordering on malignancy. I have had one case of malignancy that PEON. kept alive a long time, and kept her comfortable after she had been operated by the surgeon.

There is a nosode that I omitted here and that is CARC. I have been more or less disappointed with its action, but I have had some apparent reactions where it acted like TUB. and CANCERINUM, not curing the case entirely, but making easier the action of the subsequent remedies. I believe it should be given early to get the best results.

Cancer of the lungs: There are two remedies. Workers in cobalt are very prone to develop cancer of the lungs. COB-M. is a very active preparation worthy of a real proving.

Discussion

Dr. Stearns: Dr. Grimmer, have you ever used potencies of sugar of milk that has been x-rayed?

Dr. Grimmer: Yes.

Dr. Stearns: Have they given you good results?

Dr. Grimmer: Very fine results. I intended to put that in.

Dr. Stearns: When it is needed, it works well. Have you ever used sugar of milk that has been subjected to the energy of the Oscilloclast?

Dr. Grimmer: I have, but I have been disappointed with it. I have had no results.

Dr. Stearns: The right method must be used for affecting sugar by means of the Oscilloclast. We use cane sugar granules. Twelve vials of granules are placed on a metal plate connected with the Oscilloclast, beginning with Rate 1. The machine is started and one of the vials is taken off every five minutes, each being appropriately labeled. Twelve vials are treated on each rate in the same way. This gives 132 vials of the charged pellets. When testing, test the whole 132. Usually only one rate will come out for a given case and that only for one of the exposures, although occasionally a second rate may come. The one that the patient responds to best can be given in the unpotentised form, and he will usually respond to a set of potencies ran up from it.

Dr. Grimmer: I have never used them in that way, and I thank you for the tip.

Dr. Stearns: We have no concept as to what happens to sugar that has been radiated by this type of modality. The violet ray also affects sugar granules and we have a set of eight different exposures of 15 minute intervals, the longest exposure being two hours. These have been potentised. The Ultra Violet potencies have never come through on cancer cases but two cases of psoriasis have been cured by them. We have verified Dr. Grimmer's observation that the Cadmium salts are especially useful in cancer cases and have found that the salts of Fluorine or Silica come more frequently than any of the others.

Dr. Benthack: In the urinary tract I have found those remedies you have mentioned are good, but if I should begin, I would mention turpentine first of all, especially when there are hemorrhoids.

HOMEOPATHIC REMEDIES THAT HAVE CURED PATIENTS SUFFERING FROM CANCER[1]

ACALYPHA INDICA

Lung cancer; violent cough followed by bloody expectoration or pure blood, bright in the morning, dark and clotted in the evening. Dullness of chest on percussion, constant severe pain in chest. Progressive emaciation, sense of weight in the stomach with sense of burning, flatulence and sputtering diarrhea.

ACTEA SPICATA

Successfully used in cancer of the stomach; sour vomiting after drinking with tearing, darting pains in epigastric region; increased salivation, fetid odor from mouth. Vertigo; fear of death, especially at night in bed; furious delirium, also during fever; mental anxiety; bad effects of fatigue and from fright. Objects seem colored blue; small joints especially affected, also wrists. Right arm and wrist more often affected from motion. Fatigue and mental exertion; touch, change of temperature aggravates. This remedy has also been curative in hepatitis, pleurisy and rheumatism.

ADRENALIN

Clinically effective in Addison's Disease, neuralgia, bronzed skin, debility, hematuria, palpitation, tachycardia, hyperemia; exceedingly rapid pulse, loss of strength and wasting. May well be needed in cancer patients with adrenal disturbance.

ALUMEN

Cases of cancer of uterus and rectum with the most obstinate constipation. Constrictions and contractions of sphincters and various parts. Stools hard as stones. Indurations following inflammation. Lupus or cancer of nose. Prolapsed uterus and rectum, excruciating pains. Hemorrhages of dark blood.

---

1. Dr. Grimmer has taken almost all of the text for these remedies from Clarke's Dictionary of Practical Materia Medica. The merit of this article lies in fact that Dr. Grimmer recognized these remedies clinically in cancer patients many of which were not specifically so identified in Clarke. - Editor.

ANILINUM

Symptoms similar to ARS. Vomiting, purging, bursting headache, epiliptiform attacks, marked cyanosis, cancerous growth.

ANTIMONIUM MURIATICUM

This remedy has been used in cases of cancer in the lower lip. It has not been proved. Its poisoning symptoms show stupor, insensibility, collapse and cold clammy surface. Pupils inactive, eyes sunken, lustreless. Nausea, vomiting, burning pains in throat and stomach. Frequent abortive effects to defecate, mucous membranes destroyed.

ARANEA DIADEMA

Cancer of lungs with hemorrhage; cases based on the tubercular miasm. Very sensitive to dampness and rainy weather; the hydrogenoid constitution of Grauvogl. Marked periodicity of symptoms; clock-like regularity; annual recurrance of symptoms and conditions. Headache relieved by smoking tobacco. Violent hemoptysis of bright red blood in debilitated subjects; bathing and damp places aggravates; coldness as if the bones were made of ice. Exhaustion, must lie down. Tootache after lying down at night. Swelling of spleen after malaria suppressed by quinine; malarial attacks worse in wet rainy weather; severe attacks of neuralgia after malaria suppressed by quinine.

ARGENTUM CYANATUM

Has been helpfull in cases of cancer of the tongue and larynx as well as in cases of angina pectoris, asthma, severe spasmodic cough, cramps, spasms of the esophagus. Poisoning effects from inhaling the fumes produced sense of constriction and burning in the throat. Violent pain in the supra sternal fossa under manibrium sterni on turning to one side. Suffocative attacks; constant dry spasmodic cough; difficult articulation. Face and tongue very red. Difficult respiration.

ARGENTUM NITRICUM

Addisons's disease; lead colored pigmentation of the skin. Mental symptoms are important indications for the use of the remedy; nervous fears and restlessness with trembling hands; skin cancers.

ARSENICUM ALBUM

Cancer, epithelioma, lupus, pernicious anemia have yielded to the power of this potent medicine. Its cardinal symptoms are great fear of

Arsenicum Album ...

death, extreme restlessness, marked weakness, rapid loss of weight, coldness and lack of vital heat; nightly aggravations especially after midnight, 2 a.m. to 4 a.m.; extreme burning pains; marked tendency to ulcerations and destruction of tissues, low types of disease; malignant fevers such as typhoid; typhus and pernicious types of malaria present a fair picture of the range and character of the sicknesses this remedy has cured.

Arsenicum iodatum

Cancerous tumors of the breast epethelioma and lung cancers based on tubercular disease, affections of the blood and glands are pronounced.

Arsenicum sulphuratum flavum and rubrum

These two remedies are sulphur combinations of Arsenicum that affect the skin and mucous membranes strongly, causing in the provers and curing in the sick malignant and simple ulceraction, especially of the stomach which is the seat of severe burning pains with vomiting and diarrhea. There are symptoms of the two components; there is intense torturing anxiety and apprehension with the restlessness of Ars.

Asteria rubens

Has been successful in curing breast cancers; nightly lancinating pains. It powerfully affects the mind and the head causing severe congestion with red face. Sexual desire increased, sexual excitement. Related to Sep. and Murx.

Aurum arsenicum

Anemia, cancer, chlorosis, lupus. Cancer based on a tubercular soil or on a syphilitic constitution (acquired or inherited). Blood, glands and bones are centers frequently involved. The depression of Aur. and the anxiety of Ars. are often present in cases needing this remedy.

Aurum muriaticum

In this remedy the sycotic miasm unites with the syphilitic and psoric miasms to produce constitutions that are feeble and prone to degenerative diseases, difficult to cure. Cancerous warts on the tongue and genitals have been cured with this medicine. The patient needing this

Aurum muriaticum ...

medicine is sensitive to heat and relieved in wet weather, he is as restless as Ars. and as depressed as Aur.

Aurum muriaticum natronatum

This double salt of natrum and chloride of gold shows more of the syphilitic miasm present; carcinoma on a syphilitic base; boring pains are marked; cancerous warts on tongue; affections of the bones and glands, enormous induration of an ovary. Induration of one part, softening of another, corrosive leucorrhea, pustules on genitals. Carcinoma of breast and uterus.

Aurum sulphuratum

Symptoms of both Aur. and Sulph., indurations, ulcerations.

Bacillinum

For cases steming from a tubercular inheritence.

Badiaga

Breast cancer from bruises with extreme soreness of affected parts. Patiens of rheumatic tendencies with syphilitic taints in the bloodstream. Gerneral muscular soreness.

Baryta iodata

Breast cancer, enlarged glands, tumors of breast. Indications from the provings of the two remedies making up the compound.

Bellis perennis

Breast cancers after trauma; compare Arn., Calen. and Con. Tumors, cancers following blows or other injuries, cuts, punctured wounds, abrasions, etc.

Bismuthum

Cancer of the stomach; nausea after every meal relieved by cold drinks; water is vomited as soon as it reaches the stomach; violent risings of a putrid smell with violent retching and vomiting of bile and brownish fluid with inexpressable pain in stomach cancer. Oppressive anxiety, small pulse, vertigo and prostration. Hemorrhage of dark blood.

BROMIUM

Breast cancer, nose bleed accompanies many complaints especially those pertaining to chest and respiratory tract; vertigo with nose bleed. Vertigo with a tendency to fall backward at the sight of running water. The glands, thyroid, testes, maxillary and parotid are swollen and indurated.

BUFO

This remedy has been extensively used with marked success in epileptic conditions and is mostly identified with such convulsive states but it also has proven helpful in severe late cancer conditions. It has removed the fetor in hopeless cases of cancer. Great weakness of memory; idiotic; extremely sensitive to light and noises, the latter is intolerable.

CADMIUM METALLICUM

CADM-MET. and other chemical combinations of CADMIUM have proven curative in many cases of stomach and intestinal cancer. Many of these cases stemmed into existence by the irritative actions of alumina toxin resulting from the cooking utensils of aluminum. And recently the water supply treated with aluminum flouride in so many of our cities and villages brings upon a helpless public a potent carcinogenic agent to light up the disease in all those with inherited tendencies to this dreaded disease. CADM-MET. and CADM-O. are the most effective antidotes against the alumina toxines. The blood changes, anemias, etc. and the gastro-intestinal tracts are especially affected by the alumina poison.

CALCAREA ARSENICOSA

Cancer and cirrhosis of the liver with CALC. and ARS. symptoms.

CARBO ANIMALIS

Often indicated in the last stages of cancer of the breast. Suited to weak broken down constitutions and to the infirmities of old age, or those prematurely aged. Marked tendency to induration of glands and tissues. Indurations after inflammations, ulcerations becoming gangrenous; all the other CARBONS are closely related to this carbon thus meeting many variations of symptomatology in the array of human illnesses. It is easy to understand why carbon can play such an important role as a successful remedy for cancer when we remember that in one of

CARBO ANIMALIS ...

its sub-forms it permeates our environment by way of radio-active fall-out so abundantly coming to us since the last ten years. But before the era of the atom and hydrogen bombs the world was subjected to great carbon excess in our atmosphere in the form of soot and dust and gases stemming from the numerous factories of industry and the myriads of automotive engines everywhere operating around us. The universal intake of carbon in excess is well shown in the carbon saturated, slate colored lungs in post-mortems noted in all large centers of population and industry. Hence carbon in potentized form is the remedy of choice to antidote the crude effects of piled carbon poison.

CHELIDONIUM

CHEL. cures conditious affecting the antrum of Highmore, lungs, liver, spleen, kidneys and the gastro-intestinal tract. It has cured cancer of the stomach and liver.

The CHEL. patient presents a picture of cachexia. The skin takes on a dirty yellowish appearance. There is great debility and drowsiness with desire to lie down. Tired from the least exertion. Nausea, irritations and cutting pains in the stomach relieved by drinking milk. There is desire for milk, but aversion to cheese. Desires hot drinks. Stomach symptoms better for a while after eating. There may be constipation of clay colored stools or diarrhea or bright yellow liquid stools.

Its most striking keynote symptom is a constant severe burn-like pain at the angle of the right scapula. Jaundice may be a persistent symptom. The persistent pain under the right shoulder blade will lead one to think of this remedy.

CHIMAPHILA UMBELLATA

Atrophy of the breast; cancer and tumors; cataract; cystitis; diabetes; dropsy; fever; enlarged glands; gleet; gonorrhea; intermittent fevers; jaundice; kidney disorders; disorders of lactation; liver ailments; procti-tis; prostatitis; pterygium; ringworm; scrophula; stricture; syphilis; tootache; malignant ulcers; urinary disorders; whitlow; are some of the associated symptoms and conditions that may or may not be present in the cancer sufferers; uterine and intestinal hemorrhages may be present in the patients needing this remedy.

CHIONANTUS VIRGINICA

To be considered in liver cancer following the abuse of quinine with suppressed malaria. Chronic recurring jaundice coming every summer. Hypertrophied liver with constipation and jaundice; appetite poor and all food distresses; very severe headache worse from the jar of coughing; prostration after mental or physical exertion. One unusual symptom, great nausea and retching to vomit with weak empty feeling somewhat relieved by eating. Bitter or sour eructations with nausea and vomiting of bile; retching and vomiting with extreme weakness; gall-stone colic. Sleep disturbed and poor; hard to get to sleep. Emaciation with liver disorders.

CHOLESTERINUM

Very effective in liver cancer in relieving pain and jaundice and prolonging life. Burnett's claims for the effectiveness of this remedy in liver cancer have been substantiated by many physicians.

CICUTA VIROSA

Cancers of the skin; epithelioma; convulsive violence as in cerebrospinal meningitis; opisthotonos; strabismus; violent spasmodic jerks; paralysis, especially of the bladder; stricture of the esophagus and strange desires such as eating coal. Moans and howls with great agitation, makes gesticulations, odd motions; head turned or twisted to one side. Bad effects from falls blows and concussions. Utter prostration after the convulsions.

CISTUS CANDENSIS

Cancer of lower lip, cancer of breast in women; hardness of breasts; lupus. Scorbutic, swollen gums seperating from the teeth, easily bleeding, putrid, disgusting. Bad effects from vexation; all mental excitement aggravates. Indurated glandular swelling of the neck and throat. This patient is extremely sensitive to cold and all complaints are worse from cold exposure; caries of the lower jaw. Suppuration of the glands of the neck, coldness of the tongue, desire for acid food and fruits.

CONIUM MACULATUM

Cancer of the breast after bruises or injuries; induration and inflammations of the breasts and nipples; scirrhous tumors ulcerating and otherwise. A great deal of vertigo accompanies the complaints running through this remedy; the mental faculties and memory are profoundly

Conium maculatum ...

affected; great weakness of memory and difficult concentration; slow impaired comprehension. One particular symptom: patient sweats on closing the eyes; many eye symptoms are present.

Crotalus horridus

The symptoms and conditions found in this snake poison are fairly common to all the serpent toxins. They all have marked effect of the heart, vessels, and blood and on the autonomic nervous system. Extreme fluctuation of temperature from severe coldness and collapse to a very high degree of fever; they all have torpor and confusion of mind even sinking into states of unconsciousness. All the symptoms and conditions are worse during and after sleep; profuse debilitationg hemorrhages of dark clotted or disorganized fluid blood is found in all the snake poisons as are gangreneous ulcerations and sloughing of tissues. These remedies are helpful in the advanced stages of the cancer disease although if recognized and applied in the early stages, definite curative results can be obtained. Each SNAKE POISON has definite characterizing indications for its own specific uses, enabling the prescriber to find the most suitable remedy for each special case. The symptoms of CENCH., CROT-H. and ELAPS are mostly right sided while those of LACH. are mostly left sided. ELAPS is noted for the blackness of its hemorrhages, discharges and secretions, even the ear-wax being black. NAJA has the power to relieve the terrible pains of cancer along with the EUPHORBIUMS.

Curare

Cancer with weakness and a tendency to faint; extreme debility difficult breathing, vertigo with fainting. States of catalepsy, worse by exercise, walking, etc. worse in dampness, cold air, cold weather, worse 2 a.m. and 2 p.m. to 3 p.m.

Cundurango

Cancerous tumors of the breast, epithelioma, carcinoma of the lips; deep cracks at corner of lips; cancers originating in the epithelial tissues, excrescences are strong indications for its use.

Epiphegus

Skin cancers; headaches of severe type brought on by exertion relieved by a good sleep. A striking symptom is the constant desire to

EPIPHEGUS ...

spit; saliva viscid. Symptoms travel right to left; worse working in the open air, rising up in bed; better from a good sleep; palpitation with weakness.

EQUISETUM

This remedy has cured one case of uterine cancer. It is a deep anti-sycotic and affects the urinary tract forcefully causing severe cystitis.

ERODIUM

Uterine hemorrhage with polypus; has controlled hemorrhage after SEC. failed.

THE EUPHORBIAS

The EUPHORBIAS are strongly curative in cancer states, each variety is useful when guided by its specific symptoms.

EUPHORBIA COROLLATA

Affects more the gastro-intestinal tract, copious vomiting; rice water stools, cold sweat, prostration, wants to die; intermittent attacks.

EUPHORBIA HETERODOXA

Cancer, relieves the burning pains of cancer.

EUPHORBIA IPECACUANHAE

A more active emetic than Ip.; long continued vomiting with a sense of heat, vertigo indistinct vision and prostration.

GUM EUPHORBIUM

The resinous exudation or juice of EUPHORBIUM RESINIFERA, a cactus-like plant of the Euphorbiaceae family. This is the principal member of the group of Euphorbian drugs; is acts drastically on the skin, bones and gastro-intestinal system; burning pains in the bones and in the cancerous growth are good indications for its use. Caries; old torpid ulcers; gangrene of old persons; burning in the throat as from a hot coal; violent attacks of cough worse on lying down. Rest aggravates, motion relieves; most symptoms worse at night, prostration is marked.

Ferrum iodatum

Breast tumors; cancer; exophthalmic goiter; inflammation and enlargement of glands; symptoms and conditions based on the tubercular diathesis.

Galium

This remedy has cured a case of nodulated tumor of the tongue which was cancerous. It is a diuretic and a solvent for gravel and stone.

Graphites

Black lead, an allotropic carbon, one of the leading anti-psoric remedies; has marked action on the skin and mucus membranes, and glandular system; eruptions with sticky exudations, chronic eczema. Suffocative attacks arousing out of sleep; salivation coming on at various times; constipation with scanty menses. There are eruptions that are dry with a tendency to form cracks and fissures. Stomach pains relieved by eating. Dejection; sadness and profound melancholy; discouragement and weeping; anguish as if at the point of death; fear of some calamity; agitation and anxiety, inclined to grieve and cry in the evening. Timid and irresolute, obliged to weep on hearing music, mental effort fatigues; dread of labor; forgetfulness with misapplication of words in speaking or writing; absense of mind; easily frightened; extreme hesitation.

Hippozaeninum

The nosode of glanders. This remedy is needed in diseases affecting profoundly the skin, mucus membranes, and glands; ulceration and necrosis, suppuration and sloughing of tissues with destruction of parts are marked expressions of this remedy. Cancer of the breast has been cured with complete restoration of a breast almost destroyed by ulceration and sloughing of tissues; lupus excedens and other malignant skin diseases were also cured. Fainting with the headache. Inflammation of the membranes of the brain; purulent collections between the bones of the skull and dura mater; scattered abcesses in brain substance; tubercles may appear in periosteum of skull, in dura mater, in plexus choroides; a diffused myelitis malleosa, attributable to inflitration; bones of skull and face (frontal most) necrosed. Pupils dilated with collapse; papules on choroid coat of eye. Several nasal catarrh; nose inflamed with thick and tinged defluxion; tonsils swollen; fauces gorged. Obstinate catarrh: discharge often one sided, albuminous,

HIPPOZAENINUM ...

tough, viscous, discolored, grey, greenish, even bloody and offensive, acrid, corroding. Chronic ozaena. Nose and mouth ulcerated; cartilages of the nose become exposed and necrosed, septum, vomer and palate bone disorganized; caries of nasal bones; this remedy checks the liability of catharral affection. This is but a brief picture of the possibilities of this potent remedy corresponding to some of the most frightful sicknesses known.

HYDRASTIS CANADENSIS

Dr. John Clarke believes that more cases of cancer have been cured with this remedy than any other in our extensive Materia Medica. This belief is shared by many other homeopathic doctors including my own observations and experience of over fifty years in practice. It is in liver cancer that this medicine has proven highly effective, even in advanced cases it has been a great comfort in the relief of pain permitting the patient to retain consciousness to the end without the need of narcotics or analgesics. Dr. Clarke observes that in many cancer cases there is what has been termed a pre-cancerous stage, a period of undefined ill health without any discernible new growth. This stage is generally maked by symptoms of dyspepsia, and this frequently takes the HYDR. type, which has been well described by A. C. Clifton.

The facial expression is dull, heavy, sodden looking, yellowish white in color. The tongue is large, flabby and slimy looking, greyish white under the fur which is yellow, slimy and sticky and indented by the teeth; eructations generally sour, at times putrid. Appetite bad, poor in digesting bread and vegetables, especially weak and causing eructations. Weight in stomach with fulness, empty aching gone feeling; this is a grand characteristic of HYDR. and it is constant, not occuring at special times; worse after a meal. The action of the bowels is either infrequent and constipated or frequent with soft, light colored stools. This type of intestinal trouble with the digestive weakness often occurs in tubercular families; there is a marked relation and sequence between tuberculosis and cancer, tuberculosis often being the main causative factor.

HYDRIN-M., the alcaloid of HYDR., has been curative in cancer of the mouth. Old school practicians have employed it as an internal remedy in uterine hemorrhage.

Iodum

When indicated it cures cancer of the breast and uterus; patient is sensitive to heat; is tearful and sad; shuns persons; anxious, apprehensious, restless, agitated; must move about; irresistabe impulse to run; fells she will fall if she walks; cross, irritable, impulse to murder; excessive mental excitement; averse to all intellectual labor. Heart palpates like lightning; effects of amourousness and disappointed love. These patients emaciate rapidly while eating excessively; glands and parts become hard, atrophied and smaller; tumors take on the same characteristics. Vertigo with trobbing in the head; agitated dreams and restless sleep, vivid dreams. Nocturnal sweat. Pulse quick, small and hard.

Jequirity

Epithelioma, granular lids, lupus, ophtalmia and ulcers have been cured with this remedy. It acts chiefly on the skin and mucous membranes.

Kali arsenicosum

Bright's disease, cancer, deafness, diarrhea, dropsy, eczema, epithelioma, exophthalmos, eye affections, herpes zoster, jealousy, measles, melancholy, military rash, neuralgia, neurasthenia, psoriasis, skin affections, neuralgia of tongue, varicose veins, ulcers, make up the role of complaints this remedy has helped and cured. The Ars. symptoms predominate; much of our knowledge relating to this remedy comes up to us from the effects of over dosing and too long continued use of the medicine on patients for chronic skin and blood diseases. A number of cases while taking this remedy developed right sided herpes; in other patients the sclerotics become thick and yellow instead of clear and blue; the iris which was blue became more grey; the fair florid skin became muddy and older looking. Epithelioma has developed in a patient after prolonged treatment with Kali-ar., for psoriasis.[1] Mentally the patient needing this remedy is morose and quarrelsome, behaves like a crazy person, startled fixed look, protruding brilliant eyes, anxiety and fright. In the female cauliflower excrescences form on the os uteri. This remedy is expressed in symptoms affecting the glands, mucus membranes and the blood.

---

1. Hence this remedy cures such states when given on the totality of symptoms. - Editor.

KALI BICHROMICUM

As there is anemia and cachexia in its pathogenisis together with the fact that it has cured lupus puts this remedy in the anticancer group. It affects the skin and mucous membranes (the internal skin) markedly. Catarrhal and rheumatic states are prominent features calling for its use. Clarke mentions four outstanding keynote symptoms that expresses the whole general nature and character of the remedy as follows.

1. Discharge from mucous membranes of tough stingy mucus or mucopus which adheres to the part and can be drawn out in strings.
2. The occurrence of pains in small spots and shifting wandering pains; rheumatic pains alternate with gastric symptoms.
3. Punched out perforating ulcers occurring on skin, mucous membranes and bones such as the palate and vomer.
4. Alternating and shifting conditions, pains wander from part to part; headache alternates with blindness.

Mentally ill-humored and low in spirit; listless; aversion to mental and physical exertion; weak memory, vanishing of thoughts; anxiety arising from chest. Vertigo; with many complaints; on stooping or rising from a seat. Beer and malt liquors aggravate though he craves them, more in hot weather, autumn and spring.

KALI CYANATUM

Apoplexy, asthma, cancer, Cheyne-Stokes breathing, ciliary neuralgia, epilepsy, headache, tri-facial neuralgia, tic douloureux, rheumatism, speech lost, cancer of the tongue are conditions this remedy has been curative in. The neuralgic pains are unbearable more commonly appear in the temporal and facial regions involving the tri-geminal nerve. Disposition gentle but crossness almost uncontrolable on entering room, while cool open air produces good spirits. Inability to recollect certain words, aphasia, prolonged stupor, intense vertigo, objects seem to be moving around him; head drawn backwards, unable to tolerate any covering on head, convulsive motion of eyelids and eyeballs pupils largely dilated and insensible to light, obscuration of vision.

KALI IODATUM

Along with AUR., MERC., and NIT-AC. this remedy forms part of the most important group of the anti-syphilitics. Is has cured may types of tumors and cancers generally based on a syphilitic or tubercular ground

KALI IODATUM ...

work and often there is a combination of both these miasms present in many cases of malignancy; nightly aggravations of complaints are a strong feature of this remedy. As the pathogenisis of this remedy is too vast to incorporate in this paper I will only give the leading mental symptoms which are the most valuable for prescribing purposes.

Half-mad all night; talkative and full of jokes; sadness; anxiety; fright at every trifle; every little noise startling; apprehensive and lachrymose in the evening; irritable; irrascible especially towards his children; excited and quarrelsome; weeping from slight cause; sadness; anxiety; dreads the return of dawn and the trival details of life seem insupportable; always troubled; troublesome and unreasonable impressions easily strengthened into fixed ideas; loss of memory; cannot find words at the moment wanted, cannot write his reports, cannot play music; formication in hands. Marked weakness of lower limbs; intellectual weakness and paroxysms of dementia accompanied by headache; intoxicatied feeling; vertigo especially in the dark; worse railroad traveling. Headache at 5 a.m.; inability to find a resting place for head, relieved rising with heaviness of it; congestion; feeling as if much water were being forced into brain. Eyes surrounded by dark rings; sunken, protruding eyes; discharge of purulent mucus in the morning. Acts powerfully on heart and vessels, sticking in heart when walking. All the symptoms of endocarditis: oppression, faint-like exaustion tumultuous violent intermittent and irregular action of the heart and pulse with tensive pain across chest especially affecting the right ventricle which gradually became dilated; breasts became atrophied and small.

KREOSOTUM

The most active of the carbons, producing rapid ulcerations and destruction of tissues. The glands and mucous membranes are centers of its action; inflammatory ulcerations, cancers, epitheliomas; hemorrhages even from small wounds; cancerous ulcers of the gastro-intestinal tract and uterus have been cured with this remedy. The genitalia of both sexes are markedly affected. Coition causes pain, weakness and distress, with hemorrhagic oozing of dark blood during and following intercourse; pulsations or throbbing along the course of vessels and in various centers of the body is a strong KREOS. indication. Cancer of vagina.

LACHESIS

This remedy in common with the other Snake venoms has cured many cancerous conditions; gangrenous ulceration; hemorrhages, and extreme sensitiveness to pain with marked aggravations of complaints during and after sleep are some of the leading characteristics for prescribing this remedy.

LAPIS ALBUS

Grauvogl introduced this remedy and cured with it a case of carcinoma; he and others have cured cases of goiter and scofulous glands. The leading indications are: burning, shooting, stinging pains, in the cardia, in the pylorus, in the breasts and uterus. It has shown great power over new growth of many kinds.

LOBELIA ERINUS

Cooper is the authority concerning this remedy's curative action in cancer of the breast. Cooper also mentions interstitial kreatitis and hereditary syphilis as having been influenced by this remedy.

LYCOPODIUM

This remedy has cured cancer of the lip and epithelioma. It has a wide range of action, meeting cases of illness of every known variety of disease both acute and chronic. To profit by its wonderful power of cure it must be prescribed on the broad general symptomatology that make up its extensive pathogenesis. This remedy together with SULPH. and CALC. make up the great trio of powerful anti-psorics which are also anti-sycotics and anti-syphilitics. This trio has well been called the central core of the Homeopathic Materia Medica around which revolve all the other remedies of our vast materia medica. Many fears are noted in this remedy; of darkness, of solitude; of men; these fears affect the patient profoundly. The heart and liver functions are disturbed to end in illness mental and physical. There are a number of keynote symptoms which may lead to a study of the remedy in its application to a sickness. Persons of keen intellect but feebler muscular development often need this remedy other symptoms aggreeing. The keynote characteristics are as follows:

1. Aggravation of symptoms and complaints 4 - 8 p.m.
2. The direction symptoms take, right to left, sore throats, ovaries, breasts, limbs, etc.
3. Relief from uncovering; particularly the symptoms of the head.

LYCOPODIUM ...

4. Aggravated by cold food and drink.
5. Fan-like movement of alae nasi especially in lung and brain conditions.
6. Tongue cannot be protruded; interfering with speech.
7. Half open eyes during sleep and nodding of the head from side to side.
8. Easy satiety: a few mouth-fuls fill up and satisfy.
9. Red sand deposited on vessels containing the urine.
10. One side of body larger and more developed especially this is often noted in the breasts.
11. Complaints are brought on by fear and fright, chagrin, anger, vexation, over-lifting, anxiety, fevers, masturbation, riding in a carriage, tobacco chewing, wine.

METHYLENE BLUE

The dyes are all cancer producing agents. Injections of crude methylene blue has cured one case of cancer of the femur in a man of fifty; the remedy has not been used in homeopathic preparations to my knowledge. Cancerous ulcerations on the skin and mucus membranes of internal organs such as uterus, lungs and gastro-intestinal tract have been mitigated and cured by this remedy; the hemorrhages are mostly bright red with few clots, cough with blood streaked expectoration with difficult breathing may be cured with this remedy.

OLEUM ANIMALE

A volatile carbon prepared from stag's horns; cancer of the breast with burning or stitching pains; stitches like red hot needles; stitches and pressure may be radiating in all directions, relieved by rubbing and in the open air. A uterine tumor cured with several doses of the 1M potency given at long intervals shows its relationship to new growth. Sensation as if stomach was full of churning water is a peculiar symptoms of the remedy and found only in a few others.

OPIUM

This is a remedy of many phases and opposite extremes and alternating states, and symptoms such as diarrhea with burning pains and violent tenesmus, and involuntary stools; or there may be an invetrate constipation often ending in complete bowel obstruction and paralysis of the bowels; cancer and gangrenous ulcerations are most often pain-

OPIUM ...

less. While a strong OP. feature in may complaints is lack of pain there may be exceptions where there is unbearable pain especially in the severe menstrual cramps and the intolerable headaches. Opium acts powerfully on the sexual sphere of both sexes; in the male, increased sexual desire with frequent erections and polutions, amourous ecstasy and excesses bring on diminished sexual desire and impotence. In the female, great excitement of sexual organs with sexual desire and orgasm or may be loss of desire from lack of nutrition. General insensibility of whole nervous system. Want of sensitiveness as against the effects of remedies with want of vital re-action. Great uneasiness in limbs; trembling of limbs after fright; trembling of whole body with shocks; jerks in the limbs and general coldness relieved by motion of body and uncovering of head. Convulsive fits especially in evening towards midnight. With sleep involuntary movements of head and arms with fists closed. Pupils dilated in brain irritations, contracted and insensible to light when semi-conscious. Stertorous breathing, in apoplexy, fits of suffocation during sleep; excessive irritability of voluntary muscles; diminished irritability of all others. Complaints are brought on by fear, fright, anger, shame, sudden joy, charcoal fumes, alcohol, lead, sun. Conditions like a chronic appendicitis dating from a severe fright.

OXYGENIUM

Inhalations of oxygen have paliated some late cases of cancer, producing profuse dischares from the ulcerating mass of tumor with reduction of its growth, but no cure followed and death supervened.

PHOSPHORUS

This extensive constitutional remedy effects every tissue in the human organism and when indicated is curative in the most serious types of sickness. It has a specific affinity for the blood and vessels, for the nerves and the nervous system and the bones. Any organ in the body may be the center of trouble, but more frequently the brain and spinal cord, the lungs, the liver and gastro-intestinal tract, the kidneys and urinary system may be points of destructive disease. The sexual sphere of both sexes is activated excessively. In the male very strong desire; constant wish for coition; later from abuses and excesses; impotence. In the female nymphomania, in inflammatory conditions of the sex organs and in cases of morbid growth there is aversion to coition.

PHOSPHORUS ...

Those needing this remedy are full of fears, of death, of solitude, of darkness, of thunder storms etc. This is a strong hemorrhagic remedy, even small wounds or tiny ulcers bleed easily, usually the blood is bright red. Acute pernicious anemia and bone cancer have yielded to this medicine. Cancers that bleed profusely and persistently bright colored blood often need this medicine. MILL. must be compared here. Causation in phosphorus cases are anger, fear, grief, worry, mental exertion, strong emotions, music, strong odors, gas, thunderstorms, sexual excesses, loss of fluids (CHIN.), sprains, lifting, wounds, exposure to drenching rains, tobacco (amblyopia), washing clothes, having hair cut. Flowers cause fainting. Lightning brings on blindness. Some of therapeutic key symptoms of the remedy will aid in its selection when they are present in any case of sickness.

1. Desire for cold drinks and food, the cold water is vomitted as soon as it becomes warm in the stomach; longing for acids and spicy things; desires salt things (NAT-M.). Antidotes the effects from excess of salt in diet. Desires cold milk which agrees; hunger with great weakness and faintness relieved by eating or drinking cold things. This is one of the most efficient medicines in cases of stomach ulceration with severe burning pains, hemorrhage and persistent vomiting in advanced cases of either acute or chronic sickness. The rectum is wide open.
2. Burning pains, wherever there is inflammation internally or externally.
3. Great fear of thunder stroms and of darkness.
4. Thirst for cold things, which when they become warm in stomach are vomitted up.
5. Must eat often or he faints.
6. Small wounds bleed profusely, the blood looses its coagulability.
7. Sudden prostration from shock or malignant types disease either acute or chronic.
8. Sleep relieves most complaints.
9. Exertion physical or mental aggravate complaints.
10. Open air relieves; warm wraps relieve.
11. The Phosphorus patient lacks vital heat although many symptoms are relieved by cold and cold things internally. This is an epitome of the symptomalogy of one of the most widely used and important remedies of the Materia Medica.

Phytolacca

This remedy acts extensively on the whole glandular system but especially on the mammary glands of women which are prone to become cancerous in those of cancer constitution. Many breast cancers have been cured with this remedy as well as cancer of the uterus and rectum. It has a wide symptomatology, but a few of the cardinal symptoms will lead the prescriber to study the remedy more fully. Irritable and nervous; cannot endure pain, it is intolerable; the pains are burning in character in the ulcerations of cancer and the inflamed throats that is common to the remedy. The sore throats are more right sided, are relieved by swallowing cold drinks, worse from warm drinks and empty swallowing. Enlarged painful cervical glands accompany the inflamed sore throats. Causation: emotion, grief, bathing, injuries, blows, etc. exposure to cold damp weather. KALI-I. is its nearest analogue, especially in syphilitic rheumatism. MERC. is closely related; PHYT. has been called by some physicians "vegetable mercury"; both remedies have many symptoms and conditions in common.

Picricum acidum

This remedy's sphere of action centers is the brain, spinal cord, and the blood stream; producing in the provings a marked cachexia and pernicious anemia and these conditions in the sick have many times been cured. It acts profoundly on the sexual function of men, with increased sexual desire, lascivious thoughts in presence of any woman, long continued erections at night with emission followed by more erections and lewd dreams; priapism day and night. Exhaustion and complete prostration of mind and body from sexual excesses, mental and physical fatigue. The skin takes on a cachectic tint, a sugestion of malignancy; skin merging into a jaundice as the disease advances. This is a cold remedy, frequent severe headache are common; fig warts and gonorrhea have been cured with this remedy.

Platinum muriaticum

Has been curative in cases of the nasal and tarsus bones, chancre, condyloma, laryngismus, abuse of mercury, stricture of esophagus and cancer of the stomach. There is only a fragmentary proving, the mental symptom"thinks she has been poisoned" might be helpful as a guide in certain cases.

SANGUINARIA

This remedy has cured cancer of the breast with severe burning pains; inflammatory symptoms of the mucous membranes of the respiratory and gastro-intestinal tracts and the skin are the most frequent seats of action of this remedy. Heat flushing and redness of the skin are pronounced; burning pains (wherever pain exists) is characteristic. Violent throbbing headache with extreme nausea and vomiting; frequent fetid eructations; great salivation are common symptoms. Severe burning in stomach; vomits bitter water and sour acrid fluids, nausea not relieved by vomiting. If the patient goes without food too long he gets a bilious headache. Sweets aggravate the burning; vomiting of worms; tormenting thirst; sweets taste bitter.

SARSAPARRILA

Ulcers, cutaneous eruptions, nodes, indurated glands, caries, necroses, articular swellings and rheumatism often improve under a persistent course of this remedy. It has cured scirrhus of the breast and many cases of inverted nipples. It has drastic action on the urinary tract and kidneys causing stone formation in both kidneys and bladder with painful dysfunction of those organs; one outstanding symptom is inability to pass urine freely except in a standing position. It is both antisyphilitic and antisycotic, it has cured figwarts and those needing it have a marked tendency to emaciation; it is suited to children with faces like old men; moist eruptions about the genitals or between the scrotum and thighs; retraction of nipples in those of cancerous inheritance or constitution. Sycotic headaches beginning at the back of head coming forward and settling at root of nose with swelling of nose. Warmth in general relieves, warm diet aggravates, cold diet relieves; warm room aggravates the vertigo, washing aggravates. Bread and yawning aggravates; seminal emissions during caresses, without erections.

SCIRRHINUM

The nosode of cancer corresponds to the cancerous diathesis; cancer of the breast with enlarged glands. Many such cases have been cured with this remedy by Burnett and many other homeopathic physicians. It is a valuable intercurrent remedy to be given during the course of the broad constitutional treatment, enhancing and complementing the action of the other indicated remedies. A patient to whom Burnett had

SCIRRHINUM ...

given this remedy mentioned that it had caused the passage of an enormous number of thread worms.

SEMPERVIVIUM TECTORUM

Has cured many cases of indurations and sores on the tongue; it also has definite action on the uterus and menstrual function in cancer constitutions; it could be thought of in cases of tongue cancer.

SEPIA

This remedy has cured cancer of rectum and uterus; it acts strongly on the sexual organs of both sexes and a great many symptoms and conditions are manifested in this sphere. Young people of both sexes frequently have ailments calling for this medicine; women during the pregnant state have many symptoms calling for it; men who have been addicted to drinking and sexual excesses are often helped by this remedy. Coition aggravates both sexes. Some keynote symptoms that are good indications for the use of the remedy are as follows:

Severe bearing down pains in the uterus with prolapse of uterus and rectum; heat flushes extend upwards. Pains shoot upwards in rectum and uterus. The complexion is a dirty sallow frequently with a yellow saddle of color across the nose. This is both an anti-psoric and anti-sycotic remedy. A ring of condylomata around the anus has been cured by it. The SEP. patient is chilly and is aggravated by cold; many of his complaints are relived by vigorous exercise and walking, weakness of the genitals, increased sex desire with frequent erections and pollutions especially at night. Great aversion to washing. Sensation of a ball in inner parts more marked in the rectum is an unusual keynote. Loss of body fluids, masturbation, music, milk, fat, pork, during and after perspiring, all aggravate this patient and his complaints. Mentally there is sadness and dejection with tears, moroseness, anguish and inquietude, sometimes with flushes of heat; dread of being alone, great uneasiness regarding health or indifference and apathetic are some of the important mentals.

SILICA

Before Hahnemann's time, SIL. was not known in medicine. Only by the process of potentization (Hahnemann's discovery) could crude material substances be made to yield their inate medicinal powers. A large part of the earth's crust is composed of Silica, as the sands carpet-

SILICA ...

ing the ocean beds and shores. The stems of plants and grains receive their firmness and toughness from the organic form of this element and much of the human weaknesses that supervenes in the lives of sick humanity need the hardening regenerative force inherent in the potentized form of SIL. to restore them to a normal state of being. Clarke tells us that "want of grit, moral or physical, is a leading indication for this remedy in homeopathic practice". This is one of the most important remedies in the realm of chronic diseases, being of wide range of action and deep seated in its effects. The symptomatology of this remedy is so vast that we can give only a brief summary of its curative power. It manifests its action on every tissue of the animal organism. It affects the mental and moral states profoundly; intense sensitiveness mentally, emotionally and physically is a striking feature of this remedy. The SIL. patient is chilly lacking vital heat and deficient in energy; easily fatigued by physical by mental effort; emotional tensions aggravate his complaints. There is a marked tendency to form pus after inflammations or injuries, abcesses are very common especially in the breasts of nursing mothers, in the lungs and pleural cavities of pneumonic or tubercular patients, in the regions of the appendix, gall-bladder and pelvic cavity. The sexual sphers is affected markedly. In the male there are excoriations, ulcerations, swellings especially of the scrotum with sexual weakness and deficient desire; prior to this stage there is immoderate excitement of sexual desire, with numerous wanton ideas and strong frequent erections. Flow of prostatic fluid during urination and while straining to pass a hard stool; great weakness and back pains after coition. All symptoms of both sexes are worse after intercourse. Many menstrual symptoms afflict the female, menses feeble, protracted, acrid blood. Metrorrhagia with excoriation and bearing down in vagina; increased menses with icy coldness of the body; leucorrhea like milk but excoriating, with pains in abdomen; discharge of blood before the proper period; discharge of blood from uterus when the child takes the breast. Painful cracks in nipples, abcess of the breast, later indurations; many sufferings resulting from suppressions, especially of the perspiration by powerful lotions and metalic ointments such as alumina and zinc. The perspiration of the feet is very offensive and when suppressed and driven back into the vital centers causes severe types of sickness which finally settles into vital organs, lungs, heart, kidneys, or liver.

SILICA ...

A few cardinal keynote symptoms will help in selecting the remedy. Very offensive foot sweat. Nervous irritable persons with dry skin, profuse saliva; weakly persons, fine skin, pale face, light complexions, lax muscles, deficient nutrition due to lack of assimilating powers. The symptoms and conditions are worse at the full and new moon. Difficulty in passing a soft stool is an uncommon symptom, stool recedes back into rectum after being partly out is another peculiar and unusual symptom. The SIL. patient likes to be magnetized; mentally he is tearful and depressed, he has fixed ideas regarding pins, searches for them, counts them yet fears them, weeps when kindly spoken to. SIL. has cured recurring cheloid.

SOL

Sunlight has cured skin cancers and lupus in the hands of the Danish doctor Finsen. Our homeopathic provings are meager; mental excitement and anxiousness in all the nerves, at first with trembling of heart, finally it remained in the stomach pit. Frightened on the approach of any one coming toward her. Violent headache from vertex down to forehead with heat sensation in face. Very sensitive to sunshine. In the female menses came six to seven days too soon. Spasms coming on at sunrise and ceasing at sunset. Spasms appearing at sunset, faintness prostration and general stiffening up of the whole system; the body strength seem more equalized.

SULPHUR

The key remedy of the Materia Medica around which all other remedies revolve. Its symtomatology is so vast that it is related to and encompasses every symtom and condition, every disease acute and chronic, to which human flesh is heir. It is the king of antipsorics, hence its power to irradicate the deep constitutional states that are behind all sickness. To obtain its most effective curative power it must be prescribed on its deep constitutional symptoms. There are some cardinal symptoms peculiar to SULPH. that when found in any case of sickness will lead to the study of this remedy.

1. It is especially useful for conditions and symptoms following the suppression of skin eruptions by strong metalic ointments or by x-ray radiation or ultra-violet radiation; also after the suppression of

SULPHUR ...

discharges from any orifices of the body by powerful chemical washes or douches.

2. The typical SULPH. patient is averse to bathing and his body odors are offensive as are the discharges and eliminations he throws off, the skin symptoms eruptions etc. are worse on becoming warm in bed. Burning soles of feet at night in bed; must uncover them.
3. Weak hungry gone sensation at pit of stomach at 11 a.m. Many symptoms are worse at noon.
4. Periodicity of complaints every twelve hours.
5. Severe asthma attacks after suppression of skin eruptions by external treatment, many times asthma alternates with skin eruptions.
6. Periodical headaches often after the suppression of malaria with quinine preparations.

When well selected remedies fail to act, or act too short a time, because of the patient's feeble reactive powers, SULPH. will often build up the vital powers of the patient to effect the cure or it will clear the way by removing the psoric poison to permit other complementary remedies on their indications, to cure the patient.

SULPHURICUM ACIDUM

Patients needing this remedy are weak and exhausted, yet mentally impatient and hurried and are prone to suffer from ulcerations both externally and internally; these ulcers readily tend to become gangrenous or cancerous. Hemorrhages of dark blood from any of the orifices of the body are among the common complaints, hemorrhages from lungs, stomach, uterus, and rectum frequently occur in the sicknesses of these patients. Inflammatory ulcerations and malignancy of the stomach occuring in those who are chronic users of alcohol to excess.

SYMPHYTUM

Has a very meager proving, but its therapeutic history is rich in amazing clinical cures of round cell sarcoma of the antrum and many cases of bone cancer. It seems to have special curative action on the periosteum and boney structures, facilitating the formation of callous in fractures, bringing about union even in compound fractures and in cases of slow delayed union. It has been curative in injuries to the eyeball by blows etc. and follows ARN. in such cases; also in injuries and bruising of the testicles. Backaches after strains and from sexual

SYMPHYTUM ...

excesses. Pott's disease and psoas abcesses from a fall have found this a helpful remedy. One case of inguinal hernia has been cured with the topical application of the tincture of the root. This remedy needs an extensive proving to give us a wider knowledge of the possibilities of this wonderful remedy's therapuetic value.

SYPHILINUM

The nosode of syphilis is mainly used on the broad general symptoms of its symptomatology, together with the family and personal history of the patient. Its nightly aggravation of complaints, with extreme mental and physical restlessness together with its intense irritability are striking indications for its use regardless of the name of the afflicting disease, be it cancer, tuberculosis, severe types or neuro-arthritis, mental disturbances or various forms of paralysis.

The nosodes of cancer, tuberculosis, psora and sycosis should be studied and used along these same general lines in order to get the most good from their use. These remedies are frequently used to great advantage as intercurrent remedies in the course of treatment in chronic disease, prior to, or following the aparently indicated remedy when the patient's response to that remedy is feeble or nil.

THERIDION

The Orange Spider poison can cure when indicated on the totality of its symptoms. Caries of bones, abcesses and cancer of the liver and lungs. It acts profoundly on the nervous system producing extreme sensitiveness to noise, the vibrations penetrating to the teeth. Vertigo on turning or stooping with blindness caused by pain in eyes, with nausea increased to vomiting, worse from noise and motion, whenever she closes her eyes the nausea and vertigo is worse. Thinking of complaints aggravates them. Time passes rapidly, sensitive to the least light or the slightest noise or jar; warmth relieves and cold aggravates this patient.

THIOSINAMINUM

This remedy has been effective in curing adhesions, cicatrices, lupus, lymphatic glands enlarged, stricture of rectum, tinitus aurium, tumors of the uterus appendages. We need provings of this medicine, it has great possibilities of cure in serious conditions of disease.

THUJA

Before Hahnemann's time the medical properties of THUJ. were unknown. It stands at the head of the anti-sycotic group. The sycotic constitution grows warts and warty growths, papilloma, cauliflower excrescence, etc. these growths appear more frequently around the rectum and genital organs and have a strong tendency to become malignant from any outside irritational cause; they bleed from slight irritations or contacts. Every tissue and organ in the human economy is affected by this remedy. It antidotes the bad effects of small-pox vaccination. It has both curative and prophylaxis powers against small pox. It disturbes the mental sphere actively and deeply. Fixed ideas are notable; as if a strange person were by his side, as if the soul were seperated from the body; as if the body, especially, the limbs were made of glass and would break easily; as if a living animal were in the abdomen. Sensation as if the whole body is very thin and delicate and could not resist the least attack; as if continuity of the body would be dissolved. Insane women will not be touched or approached. Imbecility after vaccination, restless, drivelling. Mental dejection; anxious apprehension respecting the future. Music causes him to weep with trembling of the feet; hurried with ill humor, shunning everybody; aversion to life. Affections in general involve the genital organs of both sexes. Dreams of falling from a height, of the dead. Emaciation and deadness of affected parts. All manifestations excessive, their advent insidious.

CONCLUSION

This remedy completes a list of homeopathic remedies that have proven both palliative and curative in numerous cases of cancer, treated by many different physicians during the past one hundred and fifty years and in countries all over the world. This list though quite large makes up only a fraction of the Homeopathic Materia Medica, *any one of the remaining remedies could well be effective in preventing or curing cancer cases* when given on the indications of the individual remedy needed. It is agreed by all experienced physicians who have treated cancer, that the sooner treatment can be instituted the better the chances of the patient for help or recovery. This outstanding fact is one of the great advantages of homepathic practice in the treatment of cancer and other forms of intractable disease. There is so much of the precancer stage (sometimes months or years ahead) in which to institute effective preventive measures that might well be the difference between success and failure. In fact Homeopathy is pre-eminently the medicine of pre-

CONCLUSION ...

vention. Careful constitutional treatment irradicating the inherited miasims gives the vital force of the patient uninhibited action to perform its curative function by harmonizing the vital processes of the body organism that results in normal cell activity and growth.

We hope this brief review of homeopathic remedies that have cured cancer will awaken sufficient interest in the healers from all schools of medical thought to make an unbiased investigation of the principles and clinical claims of the Homeopathic Philosophy and Materia Medica for the good of suffering humanity. We believe if these principles can be extensively applied not only more cancers will be cured but many more will be prevented, thereby reducing human suffering and sorrow in a great measure by this new approach to the cancer problem.

In closing I want to dedicate this humble effort (in spreading the light of useful knowledge) to the masters of homeopahtic healing[1] who have labored so long and arduously to give the world a lasting reservoir of healing knowledge. We can only mention a few of these dedicated men as the numbers are legion, Hahnemann, Hering, Kent, Clarke, Dunham, Lippe, H.C. Allen, Farringtons, (father and son). These names will suffice as they are the vanguard. But I want to add to these illustrious ones the names of those loyal practicians of today who, despite discouragement and shrinking numbers, carry on; who practise their art for the joy of healing, who maintain their organizations that they may pass on to the future the precious heritage of medical knowledge built up by years of painstaking labor. The contributions made by these men are priceless and their works shall stand as a shining memorial of their love and devotion to a God-inspired system of healing for the nations of the world, and bring to the future of the world the promise of a better, more spiritualized race of human beings.

---

1. Dr. Grimmer was himself, undoubtedly, one of the great masters of Homeopathy. - Editor.

REMARKS ON BREAST AND PROSTATE CANCER[1]

BY FRANKLIN H. COOKINGHAN, A.B., M.D. AND DISCUSSION WITH DR. A.H. GRIMMER[2]

This subject is one that has intrigued me for many years due to the various aspects that it presents. The types are rather numerous. The age of the patient carries certain implications, e.g., the type of growth, the rapidity of metastasis, the resistance of the patient to the tumor and the type of treatment. The earlier the patient visits the physician and receives a very careful examination, the better are her chances for recovery.

There are a number of pitfalls in the diagnosis of cancer of the breast and these may be considered first as the nonmalignant tumors of the mammary gland. In the evaluation of nonmalignent cystic tumors of the breast, it is wise to avoid the term mastitis. There is no evidence to suggest that cystic disease is inflammatory. Many of these cysts do not reach the palpable stage of development and need not be considered. We are concerned solely with the later development that is found by the patients usually in the bath. At the time of the examination, the cyst may be found to be solitary, or there may be several with perhaps cystic degeneration of the entire breast. Since it is impossible to make a definite diagnosis, a biopsy is absolutely necessary, with a pathologic examination. Do not feel, if the biopsy is negative, that the patient may not develop cancer in the breast at a later time. There have been several cases in the practice of the writer where, after several biopsies a number of years apart, cancer has developed in that breast. Keep these patients under observation for years, seeing them at regular intervals. Haagensen gives 8% (in a study of 103 patients) as developing cancer after the removal of cysts from the breast. Cystic disease is found mainly in the third and fourth decades of life.

Adenosis and fibrous disease of the breast are not common but they must be diagnosed correctly. If the surgeon could be certain that either of these was nonmalignant, then he might leave them undisturbed. He must, in all fairness to the patient, biopsy them and thus rule out carcinoma. Having the lesion exposed and accessible, he had best excise it,

---

1. The HOMEOPATHIC RECORDER, Vol. LXXIII, Nos. 10 - 12, April, May, June, 1958, p. 98 ff.
2. Remember **Kali-cy.** in the metastasis of prostate cancer to bone as also in urinary obstruction from prostate cancer when digital exam reveals a stone-hard prostate (Clarke's Dictionary of Practical Materia Medica). Clinical experience. - Editor.

even after its nonmalignant nature has been proved, and in so doing relieve the patient of the worry that its continued presence would give her. Neither hormone nor irradiation therapy should be used on either of these cases.

Permit me now to mention several other nonmalignant diseases of the breast and briefly to suggest the treatment. *Mammary duct ectasia*: The importance of this condition is that it so closely resembles the clinical picture of carcinoma that it deserves very careful consideration and an early biopsy. The principal symptoms are breast tumor[1] and discharge from the nipple.[2] This is usually accompanied by pain that is different from the premenstrual type. Biopsy alone can differentiate it from malignancy. *Adenofibroma*: This deserves mention and these are tumors that are usually found any time after puberty and are the most frequent type of tumor found in young women. These tumors are very radio-resistant and should be treated by simple excision. *Intraductal papilloma:* These papillary neoplasms present the surgeon with one of the most difficult diagnostic problems. There are two main types - the benign intraductal papillomas, which are comparatively frequent, and the malignant papillary carcinomas which are rare. They both give rise to a serous or bloody discharge. Briefly, one must introduce a blunt needle into the duct and excise it for examination. Only the microscope will tell the difference. Breast infections or abscesses usually present no difficulties in diagnosis.

With the above preliminary introduction to tumors of the breast, let us now consider the great problem of cancer. Much study has been devoted to carcinoma of the female breast, but the ultimate cause is not yet known. Perhaps we are closer to it than for any of the other types of cancer. In extensive studies of the use of estrogen in both mice and dogs, it has been found that, while the administration of the estrogen did not produce carcinoma per se, it did promote the earlier development in the strains disposed to it. One may conclude from this that the administration of estrogen to a woman, when there is a history of mammary carcinoma in the family, is not advisable. There seems to be a lower percent of carcinoma of the breast in women where the breast has fulfilled its function of nursing and also the percent is lower in those who have born the greater number of children.

---

1. Kent Repertory 882L. Editor.
2. KR 829L. - Editor.

Women who develop breast cancer usually discover the disease themselves, either when bathing or dressing. In a series of 1033 ward cases, 92% found the involvement, while only 5% was found in the course of a physical examination.

Briefly, the symptoms are as follows:

1) The accidental **discovery of a lump** in the breast. The chief characteristic of the malignant lump is the hardness, which is more marked in carcinoma than in most of the other lumps that occur. Some of these lumps are as small as 5mm in diameter depending upon the accuracy of their palpation.[1]

2) **Pain.** This is probably a rather uncommon primary symptom. It may even be an unusual secondary one, the patient having only a feeling of tenderness on pressure. From the findings of many investigators one must conclude that the lump is the all important warning and that it usually is painless.[2]

3) **Retraction.** Retraction of the nipple is likewise quite uncommon and is discovered when dressing or bathing. Many patients have retraction signs but have not recognized them.[3]

4) **Redness of the skin.** This is quite rare and when found is probably diagnostic of the inflammatory type of cancer and may be considered inoperable.[4]

5) **Nipple Erosion.** Paget's type of carcinoma is manifested by erosion and itching about the nipple. This type of cancer should be the easiest for the patient and the physician to detect because of the discharge, erosion, and the itching which is quite annoying to the patient. This type is neither silent nor invisible but, nevertheless, is missed oftener than the usual type of involvement. Always regard this trilogy of symptoms (discharge, erosion and itching) with the utmost gravity.[5]

---

1. i.e sensitivity of the examiner's hands and fingers. KR 824L Cancer, Mammae etc.; 835L Induration, Mammae. - Editor.
2. KR 845R Pain, Mammae. - Editor.
3. KR 880L - Editor.
4. KR 829L Discoloration, Mammae; 836L Inflammation, Mammae. - Editor.
5. KR 829L Discharge; 831R Excoriation, Nipples; 837L Itching, Mammae and Nipples - Editor.

6) **Symptoms due to Metastases**. While most of the symptoms mentioned above originate from the primary tumor, in a small percent of cases they originate in metastases. The primary lump may be so small that it is not detected by the patient and the first lump found is an axillary metastasis.[1]

Do not be misled by the absence of the metastasis in the axilla. The first symptoms of a mammary carcinoma may be a pathological fracture or a persistent backache due to vertebral involvement. These latter cases are entitled to a very careful x-ray study of the spine and the long bones of the arm and leg.

When breast disease has been detected, either by the patient or by an examining physician, the next step is to prove its nature. In this task the physician depends on three kinds of evidence - a proper medical history, a careful physical examination of the breasts, and, when indicated, a properly conducted biopsy. Unfortunately in a paper of this character it it not possible to go into the subject of the methods of diagnosis of breast disease and the manner of making the examination of the suspected breast. The writer desires to take this opportunity of referring the listener to some excellent pamphlets on this subject as well as films that have been made for exhibition at county and state medical meetings.

The type of treatment depends on a number of factors - age of the individual; type of tumor; whether free of metastasis or not; if metastases are present, are they removable. If there is skeletal involvement, then the case is inoperable. The treatment will depend upon whether the surgeon has any preconceived ideas. Radical mastectomy is the mainly accepted method - in many quarters the operation may be preceded or followed by x-ray treatments.[2] McWhirter has treated a large number with partial mastectomy followed by intensive x-ray treatment. He reports a 42%, five-year survival rate and 25% ten-year survival rate. The scirrhus type of growth in the aged usually does not require any treatment, since it grows slowly and seldom metastasises.

"Research of the past ten years has remarkably expanded knowledge of carcinogenesis and of the diagnosis and treatment of cancer. The clinician is now able to control the growth of cancerous tissue more effectively than ever before." As a result of the investigations the control of

---

1. KR 824L, 835L, 838L. - Editor.
2. Today various radiation treatments are used. - Editor.

cancer offers a more hopeful future. The National Cancer Institute has published some very helpful articles on this subject. Marques, in a paper on "The Chemistry of Tumors" delivered at the recent meeting of the California State Homeopathic Medical Society held in May 1957, gave some very interesting statistics on the study of the damaging capacity of some plants on tumor tissues. The studies were carried out using certain strains of mice and the results were very carefully tabulated. "Materials from 12 plants produced grossly and histologically demonstrable damage on the tumors of these animals. A relatively pronounced effect was induced by **Dioscorea villosa, Oxydendron and Spirea ulmaria**. Tumor damage of lesser degree was exhibited by nine other plants - **Apocynum andros, Asparagus off.; Capsella bursa pastoris, Equisetum arvense, Equisetum hyomale, Hydrangea arborescens, Juniperus communis, Parietaria off. and Polytrychum juniperum.** All of these remedies or drugs are used homeopathically. Extracts of these were administered in physiological doses and the results studied and evaluated in the light of histological and cytological findings in the tumor tissues of implanted animals.

"Perhaps some day this type of investigation may form the basis of some homeopathic research. If one reviews in his mind the indications for these remedies, he may be surprised to find how applicable they may be in some forms of cancer manifestations - **Dioscorea villosa,** for instance with its characteristic pains, especially colic, in severe, painful affections of abdominal viscera. Mull over in your mind the symptoms of the other remedies mentioned and the writer is sure that certain indications will present themselves. Since the physiological doses of these plant extracts have already yielded demonstrable tissue changes in experimental animals, extension of such experiments in potentized attenuation may prove highly fruitful."

In the study of the cancer problem one must take into consideration the resistance of the patient to the invasion of a cancerous growth. This is entirely intangible, but from the homeopathic point of view a very definite avenue of approach for a prescription. A very careful study of the patient will afford a basis for help in the well being of the individual who is suffering from cancer. So far as is known, no proving of a drug has produced a cancerous invasion of the prover. That, however, does not preclude the search for the relief, perhaps the cure, of that large number of unfortunates that now appeal to us for help.

This paper constitutes, first, a plea for the early recognition of growths, either by the patient or the medical examiner; second, a very careful survey of the woman presenting herself for your care. Her life is very definitely in your hands and temporizing may cost her much suffering, whereas a systematic study of her case may lead either to recovery or, at least, to the prolongation of a useful life. Cancer of the breast is curable in a large percent of cases.

Dr. A.H. Grimmer (Chicago, Illinois): This problem is really a serious one, and Dr. Cookinham has discussed the surgical side.

I have had a lot of experience with cancer of the breast. In the main I have been more satisfied with homeopathic treatment than to have given them the purely surgical or radium or other treatments. I wish I could say we cured them all; we didn't by a long ways, but we did cure a good many of them. We have given a great many of them longer life with our remedies, and we have been able to control the pain in most cases.

On the other hand, I have seen some cases that came from some of our good surgeons after breast amputation and x-ray in big doses. The suffering that those poor patients went through from the terrifically swollen arms and radiation sickness was really worse than any cases that I have seen that went down to death under homeopathic treatment.

In prescribing the homeopathic remedy, one must find the exact remedy. One must pay a great deal of attention to Hahnemann's injunction to investigate the history of the family to find evidence of the basic miasms. If you wish really to cure any of these cases, your remedy should be based on the whole patient.

Another thing, we have a great many interferences with our remedies. We make a good study, and we think we have found a good remedy. For a short time we get a satisfactory reaction, and then comes along some sort of interference, either from the food or from the aluminum which is the most common poison we have nowadays. We find our remedies are very short acting, and we are puzzled. We can't understand why we don't get the action we formerly did or the older men got.

Our electro-magnetic tests are really a great help in prescribing these remedies, and in finding outside toxins that are interefering with them.

Dr. Cookinham (Closing): At least I succeeded in stirring up a bit of a hornet's nest, and I am pleased. (Laughter.)

Dr. Ames, you spoke about Dr. Crile and his work. I think I have followed the work of the Crile Clinic, not only the younger Crile, but George Crile, his father.

In a film put up by the Upjohn People, known as "Grand Rounds", Dr. Crile made the statement you have quoted which resembles, how-

ever, a great deal of McWhirter's work and probably it may have originated in or been stimulated by the work which McWhirter did.

There is no age limit to cancer. We get it in infancy as well as in old
age, and ordinarily the younger the patient, the more malignant the
growth, the more rapidly it metastasises and the earlier the demise.

In regard to treatment, I didn't wish to imply in my paper that I did
not use homeopathic remedies. I treat my patients homeopathically
insofar as I am able to do so. I have discussed the use of certain medications and stated that I was unaware definitely how to evaluate the
results of the administration of those remedies.

I am sure all of you have been confronted with a problem such as
this: A patient with an acute pain in the right lower quadrant of the
abdomen has nausea, perhaps vomiting, and slight rise of temperature.
You make a diagnosis of possible appendicitis, and prescribe BELL. or
BRY. or RHUS-T. The symptoms disappear but the patient goes right on
to develop his appendicitis with rupture and abscess unless interfered
with.

I think very frequently that our remedies will often relieve symptoms
without affecting the pathologic process underlying such symptoms.
How long should one wait for development? I don't know when one
crosses the Rubicon in these cases. But it is a very serious question to
consider. When does the tumor metastasise? I don't necessarily mean a
palpable metastasis in the axilla. It may cross over into the opposite
breast. In one case which I saw only about two years ago the first
involvement after she discovered the lump in her breast was a pathologic fracture of the right femur.

Doctor, this is an exceedingly difficult question, and it is on one's
own conscience how long he shall wait to determine whether the
growth is malignant or nonmalignant.

Dr. Bellokossy, that question of fear of biopsy has often been discussed, but I think the most recent work is that by Ogdenson of New
York. The volume came out only six or eight months ago. It is probably
the most extensive work on cancer of the breast. He brings up the question of fear of biopsy. I don't believe, Doctor, that, if a biopsy is done,
one has harmed the patient at all if the patient is prepared for a complete operation should the growth be malignant. There is no time lost
between the time of the biopsy and the subsequent operation. It is done
immediately. This is discussed with the patient prior to the anesthetic.
Now, if we find so and so, we want to do so and so, and the patient's
consent is obtained before the anesthesia is administered. So I don't

think, Doctor, that one can accept that there is much danger in the biopsy per se spreading the growth.

Now, as to pain in the breast. Certainly we encounter pain in the breast very frequently, as well as pain in the shoulder and pain in the arm. I think the majority of those are intercostal involvements. An x-ray of the spine will show in the middle-aged woman quite a bit, not necessarily a great deal, of cervical arthritis with pressure upon one or several intercostal nerves which take in the breast. And sometimes **Ranunculus bulbosus** or **sceleratus** will take care of that pain.

Now, when does one cure? This is a very dangerous word to use. I think that there are some recoveries from tumors of the breast. I am not going to use the word "cancer." I refer to tumors of the breast of the adenomatous or fibromatous type in young women. I think sometimes those do retrograde and perhaps entirely disappear. But in my opinion it is the only type of tumor of the breast that is "cured".

The question of the relation of the breast to the pelvis I think has not been solved. What is the relationship, for instance, of the premenstrual expression of pain and so forth in the breast? It must be through the blood stream or a hormone or something of that sort. I don't know whether there is a definite relationship between a pelvic malignancy and a breast malignancy. It seems at times as if they may develop concurrently or in sequence. It goes without saying, as I mentioned in the paper, that one of the three things necessary is a careful history and examination, and of course, that includes a pelvic examination.

Dr. Grimmer, it is true that certain sequelae may follow an operation of such magnitude as a radical removal of the breast. McWhirter does a simple mastectomy (he may remove a metastasis) and then follows with x-ray. Of course, there are certain sequential results that follow the use of x-ray. I sometimes wonder whether it is not preferable to die of the results of the cancer of the breast without the x-ray treatment. The latter may result in fibrosis of the lung, and you will have an invalid due to the extensive fibrosis.

I would like to mention, Dr. Grimmer, that I use **Cadm-s**. following your suggestion. You may recall that some years ago I sent you a specimen of blood following a radical mastectomy. That must be five or six years ago. That girl is perfectly well. We followed her up with **Cadm-s**. according to your suggestions.

I would like to mention, which is entirely irrelevant to cancer of the breast, the use of **Kali-cy**. in those metastases that follow carcinoma of the prostate and which are nearly always skeletal. One case our urologist, Harriman, who is in San Francisco, asked me to take care of during his absence, a case to which we were giving at that time a fourth of morphine every four hours for various pains demonstrated to be due to skeletal metastases by x-ray. I think I read, maybe in the Recorder, that our good friend, Grimmer, had said that **Kali-cy.** can be useful in those cases.

We started out with the 6x. We had to send to Philadelphia to get the drug, and within one week the pain was very much less. Within two weeks we had practically discontinued the use of the morphine. That patient died about three or four months after that without any pain. I thank you. (Applause)

Repertory Rubrics for Kent's Repertory from Grimmer

Prepared by Ahmed N. Currim M.D., Ph. D.

REPERTORY RUBRICS FOR KENT'S REPERTORY FROM GRIMMER

PREPARED BY AHMED N. CURRIM M.D., PH. D.

PAGE	MIND	
7 R	ANXIETY	**noise**: Ars.
9 L	AVERSION	**music**; to certain kinds of: Cadm-met.
9 L	AVERSION	**noise**; to: Cadm-met.
9 L	AVERSION	**persons**; to all: Cadm-met.
9 L	AVERSION	**persons**; to certain: Cadm-met.
10 L	CAPRICIOUSNESS	Caps.
13 L	CONCENTRATION	**difficult**: Cadm-met.
20 R	DELUSION	**affection** of friends; has lost: Ars.
21 L	DELUSION	**animals**; of hideous: Crot-h.
23 R	DELUSION	**dead**; that he himself was (is),
		– **arrangements** are being made for his funeral: Lach.
23 R	DELUSION	**despised**; he is: Lach.
27 L	DELUSION	**heart** hung by a thread; every heart beat would tear it off: Lach.
35 L	DELUSION	**wasting** away: Naja
35 R	DESPAIR	Cadm-met.
35 R	DESPAIR	**alternating**
		– **apathy** (indifference); with: Ars.
35 R		– **irritability**; with: Ars.
35 R		– **resentment**; with: Ars.
35 R		– **stupor**; with: Chlol.
35 R		**anxiety**; with: Ars.
36 L		**restlessness**; with: Ars.
36 L		**stupor**; before: Chlol.
36 L	DIPSOMANIA	Stroph.
44 L	FEAR	**death**; of: Lat-m.
45 R		**insects**; of: Ars.
47 L		**snakes**; of: Ars.
47 R		**waking**; on: Carb-v.
49 R	FRIGHT	**complaints**; from: Carb-v.
50 L	GESTURES	**hands**, grasping , throat: Naja

PAGE	MIND	
51 L	HATRED	Cadm-i.
54 L	IMPULSIVE	Cadm-met.
54 R	INDIFFERENCE	Cadm-met.
55 L	INDIFFERENCE	**joy**; to: Cadm-met.
59 R	IRRITABILITY	**heart disease**: Crat.
59 R		**heat**; during: Chlol.
60 L		– **typhoid**; in: Chlol.
60 R	JUMPING	**bed**; out of
		– **fever**; during:
		– **typhoid**: Chlol.
		– **fear**; with dreadful (typhoid): Chlol.
61 L	KLEPTOMANIA	Op.
61 L		**mendacity, lying disposition**; with: Op.
62 R	LOATHING	**life**: Cadm-met.
64 L	MANIA-A-POTU	Caps.
66 R	MISTAKES	**actions**; puts salt instead of sugar in his tea: Cadm-met.
66 R		**speaking**: Cadm-met.
66 R		– **wrong syllables**: Kali-c.
71 L	RAGE	**delirium**; during: Chin-s.
77 L	SADNESS	**heart disease**; in: Crat.
78 R	SENSITIVE	**external impressions**; to all: Ars., lach.
79 L		**noise**; to:
		– **pain**; causes or aggravates existing: Ars.
80 L	SHRIEKING	**die**; thinks she will: Lat-m.
		– **breath**; and looses her: Naja
80 L		**terror**; jumps out of bed: Chlol.
83 R	STARTING	**sleep**; from: Euph.
85 L	SUICIDAL,	**hanging**; by: Aur-ar.
85 R		**overworked** and worried with depressed mania: Pic-ac.
86 L	SWOONING	**fits**: Naja
87 L	TALKS	**imaginary** beings; to (delirium in typhoid): Chlol.
91 R	VIOLENT	**depression**; alternating with: Cadm-met.

PAGE	MIND	
94 R	WEEPING	**pains**; with: Kali-cy.

	VERTIGO	
98 R	DRUNKARDS	Asar.
101 R	MOVING	**pictures** (movies): Cadm-met.
101 R		– **breath** away, taking: Cadm-met.
101 R		– **objects** recede and return: Cadm-met.

	HEAD	
111 R	CONGESTION	**Brain**, in continued fever: Chlol., crot-h., hell., op., zinc.
131 R	MOTIONS	**tosses**; side to side: Naja
138 L	PAIN	**coldness** of body; with icy: Cadm-s.
138 R		**constant**; extreme: Cadm-met.
140 R		**hammering**
		– **vomitting**; followed by: Cadm-s.
140 L	PAIN	**fibroids** uterine ; with: Til.
142 R		**maddening**: Cadm-met.
		– **extending to** eyes and ears: Cadm-met.
142 R		**menses**; during: Teucr-s., til.
145 L		**periodical** headache: Teucr-s.
149 L		**sun**; in hot: Calc-ox.
153 L		**Extending** to nose: Parth.

	EYE	
235 L	ADHESIONS	**Cornea**: agroyl and atropine treatments; after: Kali-bi.
241 L	HEAVINESS	Parth.
242 R	INFLAMMATION	**gonorrheal**: Nat-m.
244 L	INJURIES	Calc-sil., con., kali-bi., thuj.
244 L	INJURIES	**lacerations**: Asar.
		– **painful**: Asar.
		– **surgical** operations: Asar.
249 L	PAIN	**air**; cold agg.: Asar.
249 R	PAIN	**light**: Asar.

Page	Eye	
269 R	Ulceration	**cornea**, syphilitic: Carbn-s.

	Ear	
286 R	Discharge	**chronic**: Cadm-met.

	Hearing	
321 R	Impaired	Cadm-met. **discharge**; return of, amel.: Cadm-met.

	Nose	
324 L	Cancer	Aur-s., eucal. (sinuses), symph. (antrum)
338 L	Epistaxis	**washing** face: Phos.
344 L	Pain	**root** of nose: Parth.
349 R	Sinusitis	**chronic**: Merc-k-i.

	Face	
355 R	Cancer	**Lips**: Ant-m., aur-s.,cund. – **lower**: Ant-m.,cist.
357 R	Convulsions	**Lips**: Naja
359 L	Discoloration	**dark** (dusky): Ant-t.
361 R		**red**; alcoholic beverages; after: Carb-v.
362 L		**dark** red: Chlol.
362 R		**flushing** from roots of hair to neck and chest, persisting under pressure of finger: Chlol.
366 R	Eruptions	**acrid**: Calc-f.
374 R	Expression	**intoxicated**: Naja **old-looking**; in children: Sars.
380 L	Pain	Kali-cy.
380 L		**morning**: Kali-cy.
380 L		– **4 a.m.**: Kali-cy.
380 L		– **awakened** with: Kali-cy.
381 L		**change** of weather: Kali-cy.
381 L		**cold exposure**: Kali-cy.
381 L		**cold weather**: Kali-cy.
382 L	Pain	**Neuralgic** – **with plugged sinuses**: Cadm-met.

PAGE	FACE	
382 L		**pressure**: Kali-cy.
382 L		**touch**: Kali-cy.

	TEETH	
431 R	EDGE	**feel** as if on: Parth.
431 R	ELONGATION	Parth.

	MOUTH	
398 R	CANCER	**Tongue**: Apis, arg-cy., aur-m-n., gali., rad-br., semp.
		– **warts**: Aur-m., aur-m-n.
398 R	CANCER	**Hard palate**: Scolo-v.
399 L	CONVULSIONS	Naja

	THROAT	
448 L	CANCER	**Esophagus**: Phos., plat-m.
458 L	NUMBNESS	Kali-cy.

	STOMACH	
479 L	APPETITE	**ravenous**
		– **wine**; with desire for: Asar.
480 R	AVERSION	**coffee**; smell of: Sul-ac.
482 L		**onions**: Lyc.
482 L		**pork**: Carb-v.
482 L		**tomatoes**: Lyc.
482 R	CANCER	Act-sp., ant-s-aur., ars-s-f., Ars-s-r., All the Cadmiums but especially Cadm-ar., cadm-met., cadm-p., cadm-s., calen. (Hemorrhage of stomach cancer with mets to liver), chel., merc-c. **Aliminium toxicity**: Cadm-met., **Cadm-o**.
484 L	DESIRE	**beer**: Caps.
484 L		**coffee**: Lyc.
484 L		**wine**: Caps.
485 R	DESIRE	**lime**, slate pencils, earth, chalk, clay etc.: Graph.

PAGE	STOMACH	
507 R	NAUSEA	**epilepsy**: Kali-c.
508 L		**heart disease** (failure): Crat.
508 R		**odors**; from: Cadm-met.
509 L		**pain**; during: Naja
513 L	PAIN	**fat food** (mutton tallow) amel.: Nit-ac.
516 R		**burning**
		– **alcoholic drinks** agg.: Carb-v.
517 L		– **wine** or alcoholic drinks agg.: Carb-v.
524 R	PULSATION	Asar.
525 R	RETCHING	**drunkards**; in: Asar.
531 L	ULCERS	Cadm-s., euph.
531 L		**radiation treatment for acne**: Phos.
532 L	VOMITING	**alternating** with heat and coldness: Cadm-met.
533 L		**drunkards**: Ant-t.
533 R		**headache**; during: Cadm-met.
535 L		**bile**: Cadm-met.
535 R		– **drunkards**: Ant-t.
536 R		**blood**
		– **drunkards**: Ant-t.
539 L		**mucus**
		– **drunkards**: Ant-t.
539 L		**sour**: Cadm-met.

	ABDOMEN	
541 R	CANCER	**Intestines**: All Cadmiums, cadm-met. (hemorrhage), euph-c., kreos., methyl., phos.
		Aluminium toxicity: Cadm-met., **Cadm-o.**
		toxic goiter and cardiac problems (arrythmias); with: Cadm-i.
		Liver: All the Cadmiums but especially Cadm-met., cadm-p., cadm-s., calc-ar., calen. (Hemorrhage of stomach cancer with mets to liver), cean., chion., chol.,

PAGE	ABDOMEN	
541 R	Cancer ...	**Liver:** ... euph., hydr., phos., ther. **Gall-bladder**: Chion. **Pancreas**: Cadm-i., calc-ar., cean. **Spleen**: Cadm-i., cadm-met., cean. **Colon, transverse**: Cadm-i.
554 L	MALFORMATION	**congenital of intestine**: Syph.
568 L	PAIN	**Liver**: Cadm-met.
569 R	PAIN	**Spleen**: Cadm-met.
	RECTUM	
606 L	CANCER	Alumn., paeon. (malignant hemorrhoids), phyt., rat., thiosin. (stricture), sol-t-ae., toxi. (sarcoma)
606 R	CONSTIPATION	Calc-f.
607 L		**anemia, neuralgias and semi-paralysis**; with: Alum., alum-sil., alumn., plb.
608 L		**inveterate**: Cadm-met.
610 L	DIARRHEA	**night**: Chlol.
	RECTUM	
619 L	HEMORRHAGE	Cadm-met.
628 R	PAIN	**stitching**: Paeon.
632 R	STRICTURE	Thiosin.
635 R	WORM	**taeniae** (tapeworm): Stry.
	STOOL	
635 R	BLACK	Cadm-met.
640 L	MUSHY	**black**: Cadm-met.
	BLADDER	
645 L	CANCER	Blatta-o., chim., congo red, equis-h., sabal., staph.
657 R	URINATION	**frequent**: Cadm-met., sabal.
660 R	URINATION	**retarded**, must wait for urine to start: Kali-sula.

PAGE	KIDNEY	
662 L	CANCER	Sars.

PROSTATE

667 L	CANCER	Chim., kali-cy. (mets to bone with severe pain or advanced cancer even without mets.)

URINE

681 L	BLOODY	Cadm-met.
681 R	BROWN	**wash off**; hard to: Cadm-met.
686 R	DIABETES	Med.

GENITALIA (MALE)

693 L	CANCER	**warts**: Aur-m., aur-m-n.
693 L		**Scrotum** (epithelioma): Aur-m.
		– **scirrhus**: Alum.
		Testes: Arg-n. (Kent), brom., ox-ac.
701 R	MASTURBATION	**children** (and adults): **Med.**

GENITALIA (FEMALE)

715 L	ADHESIONS	**Clitoris**: Kali-c.
715 L	CANCER	**Ovary**: Aur-m-n.
715 R		**Cervix**: Arg-m. (Kent), bomhenia
715 L		**Uterus**: Benzoquinone, bomhenia, cadm-i., cadm-met., cadm-s., cadm-o., calc-f., equis-h., erod., methyl., ol-an., thiosin.
		– **burning**, stinging, stitching pains: Lap-a.
		– **dark blood**: Cadm-met.
		– **rapidly growing**: Cadm-met.
730 L	METRORRHAGIA	**climacteric period**: Bomhenia
		dark blood: Bomhenia, cadm-met.
		lying: Mag-c. (Boger)
		polyps; with: Erod.
731 R	PAIN	Paeon.
734 L		**uterus**; menses, during, unbearable: **Op.**

PAGE	GENITALIA (FEMALE)	
738 R	PAIN ...	**drawing**
		– **ovary**: Naja
744 R	SWELLING:	Paeon.
745 R	TUMORS	**Uterus**
		– **cysts**: Mag-c.
745 R	ULCERS	**Cervix**: Bomhenia

LARYNX AND TRACHEA

746 L	CANCER	Arg-cy.
759 R	VOICE	**hoarseness**, continuous: Helx.

RESPIRATION

763 R	ARRESTED	**sleep**; on going to: Cadm-s.
763 R	ASTHMATIC	Aral., calc-sil., sol-int.
764 R		**cold damp weather**: Ant-t.
765 L		**mental exertion**: Kali-c.
765 R		**wet weather**: Ant-t.
766 L	CHEYNE-STOKES	Kali-cy., parth.
768 L	DIFFICULT	**ascending**: Helx.
769 L		**dark**; in the: Carb-v.
769 R		**exertion**; slightest (in heart disease): Crat.
769 L		**heart disease**: Crat.
770 L		**lying** on the side, right, amel.: Naja

COUGH

781R	NIGHT	**3 to 4 a.m.**: Rumx.
782 L	ASTHMATIC	Meph.
786 L	DRY	Helx.
790 L	EATING	**beginning** to eat: Seneg.
790 L	ERUCTATION	amel.: Ant-t.
796 R	LYING	Euph.
801 R	RATTLING	Teucr-s.
804 L	SLEEP	**preventing**: Helx.
804 R	SPASMODIC	Meph.
807 R	TICKLING	Helx.

PAGE	COUGH	
811 R	WHOOPING	**Prophylaxis**: Carb-v., cupr., dros., pert.

EXPECTORATION

813 L	BLOODY	Helx.
813 R		**bright red**, few clots: Methyl.
814 L		**streaked**: Methyl.
817 R	PRUNE JUICE:	Carb-v., dig. (Clarke)

CHEST

822 L	ABSCESS	**Mammae:** Paeon.
822 R	ANGINA	Arg-cy.,crat.
824 L	CANCER	**Heart**: Cact.

Lung: Acal., aran., arg-m., ars-i., bry., cadm-bi., cob-m., guaj., methyl., phos., ther.
  - **arthritis**; with: Guaj.
  - **hemoptysis**: Acal.,aran.

Mammae: Acon., Bar-i., Cadm-met., Congo red, Formal., Hippoz., Iod., Lap-a., Lob-e., Naja, Nat-thio-cy., Sars., Scir., Scroph-n.
  - **axillary** gland enlarged; with: Alum-sil., aur-nat-fl., *aster*.
  - **burning**, stitching pains: Lap-a., ol-an. (red hot needles)
  - **contusion**: Arn.,calen.
    - **gangrene**; with: Carb-an.
  - **hardness and swelling**: Cad-calc-fl.
  - **hardness and severe pain**: Nat-thio-cy.
  - **hemorrhage**
    - **bright** red blood: Bell.
    - **dark** thick clots: Elaps
    - **pain**; with: Durbital
    - **profuse** with serum and blood: Plb.

PAGE	CHEST	
824 L	CANCER	– **induration** and with small ulcers: Alum-sil., aur-nat-fl.
		– **last stages**: Carb-an.
		– **mastectomy** of opposite cancerous breast; after: Lac-c.
		– **old people**: Carb-an.
		– **scirrhus**: Sars.
		– **ulceration**
		– **induration**, axillary glands enlarged: Alum-sil.
		– **mastectomy** of opposite cancerous breast; after: Lac-c.
		– **pain**; with: Cadm-met., hippoz., lap-a., phyt.
		– **surgery/radiation**; after: Hippoz., streptom.
		– **tubercular**: Bell-p.
		Sternum: Ars-s-r.
824 R	CAVITIES	Teucr-s.
828 R	DILATION	**heart**; of: Carb-v.
828 R		**sensation** as if: Cadm-s.
829 L	DISCHARGE	**blood**: Kali-cy.
		bloody water: Kali-cy.
		dark brown on bathing: Kali-cy.
835 L	HYPERTROPHY	**heart**: Crat.
835 L	INDURATION	**Mammae**, ulcers over whole surface, periodic pains: Alum-sil.
835 R	INFLAMMATION	**Lungs**: Pyrog. (Kent, Austin)
		– **nephritis**; with acute: Pyrog. (Kent, Austin)
		– **pulse-temperature** disocciation: Pyrog. (Kent, Austin)
846 L	PAIN	**Mammae**, menses during: Cadm-met.
853 R		**burning**
		– **Lungs**: Caps.

PAGE	CHEST	
857 R	PAIN ...	**drawing**
		– **Heart**: Naja
874 R	PALPITATION	**audible**: Naja
879 L	PHTHISIS	**pulmonalis**: Teucr-s.
		– **florida**: Ther.
		– **hemoptysis** (hemorrhage): Helx.
		– **late**: Ant-t.
880 L	RETRACTION	**nipples**; of: Cadm-met.,scir.
882 L	ULCER	**Mammae**: abscess; at site of old: Paeon.
883 L	WEAKNESS	**Heart**: Crat., parth.
883 L		– **sensation** of: Lach.
		– **with flushes** of heat up spine and flushing of face: Lach.

	BACK	
896 R	PAIN	**mental exertion agg.**: Kali-c.

	EXTREMITIES	
954 L	BRITTLE	**Finger nails**: Calc-f.
954 R	CANCER	**Bones**: Merc-k-i., methyl., toxi.
963 R	COLDNESS	**Foot**, icy-cold, typhoid; in: Chinin-ar.
968 L	CONVULSION	Naja
970 L	CORRUGATED	**Finger nails**: Calc-f.
988 L	ERUPTIONS	**Upper Limbs**: Eczema: Bougenville
1002 R		**Foot**: Samarskite.
1038 L	NUMBNESS	**Hand**: Cadm-met., kali-cy.
1038 R		– **sitting**: Cadm-met.
1042 R		**Foot**: Cadm-met.
1043 L		– **sitting**: Cadm-met.
1045 L	PAIN	**mental exertion agg.**: Kali-c.
1047 L		**Joints**: Cadm-met.
1053 R		**Upper Arm**: Caust.
1054 R		– **motion**: Caust.
1064 L		**Lower Limbs**:
		– **sciatica**, right: Kali-cy.
1072 L		**Knee**: Calc-f.

PAGE	EXTREMITIES	
1200 L	SWELLING	**Knee**: Calc-f.
1207 L	THIN	**Nails**: Calc-f.
1220 R	ULCERS	**Hand**:

Hand:
- **back of**;
    - **oozing blood** without much pain: Cadm-met., formal., kali-thio-cy.
    - **painful**, bleeding, odorous: Formal., X-ray
    - **painful**, with general weakness: X-ray

1221 R		**Lower Limbs**: varicose: Paeon.
1222 L		**Foot**: Paeon.

- **rubbing** of the shoe: Paeon.

1223 L	VARICES	**Lower Limbs**: Paeon.
	SLEEP	
1234 L	COMATOSE	Naja
1243 L	DREAMS	**sickness**; of: Cadm-met.
	CHILL	
1267 L	EXCITEMENT	**emotions**; of: Asar.
1269 R	PERIODICITY	**clock-like**: Chinin-s.
	FEVER	
1284 R	CONTINUED	Chlol.
1288 L	INTERMITTENT	**PROPHYLAXIS**

before entering malarial district: Nat-m. 30 or 200 or 1M once a week for 6 weeks.

on getting into infected territory: Ars. 30 (or 200 or 1M - Editor) once a week for 4 weeks

if malarial symptoms appear: Chin. 30 or higher for several days after each paroxysm of fever (Hahnemann).

PAGE	FEVER	
1288 L	INTERMITTENT	**PROPHYLAXIS ...**
		if malaria symptoms persist: Nat-m. 200 (or higher - Editor) weekly.
1289 L	PERIODICITY	Chinin-s.
1292 L	UNDULANT	**(brucellosis)**: Merc-k-i.
1292 R	YELLOW	**prophylaxis**: Ars.,crot-h.
		sequelae of shots: Ars.

	PERSPIRATION	
1300 R	PROFUSE	**warm weather**: Lyc.

	SKIN	
1303 L	ANESTHESIA	Naja
1304 L	CANCER	**See Generalities epithelioma**
1304 L	CICATRICES	**Cancer**: Graph. (surgical scars)
1304 R		**ulceration**: Paeon.
1316 L	ERUPTIONS	**psoriasis**: Merc-k-i.
1317 R		**rash, bluish**: Phyt.
1317 R		**rash, rough**: Ail., phyt., rhus-t., sulph.
1319 L		**small pox**: Maland., sarr., vac.
1331 L	SORE	**becomes** (decubitis): Paeon.
1334 R	ULCERS	**chronic**, oozing blood, not much pain: Cadm-met., formal., kali-thio-cy., X-ray.
1336 L		**gangrenous**: Caps.
1337 L		**malignant**: Hippoz.
1339 L		**unhealthy**: Caps.

	GENERALITIES	
1342 R	NIGHT	**Merc-k-i.**
1344 L	AIR	**open**; amel.: Kali-cy.
1346 L	BATHING	**cold**; amel.: Kali-cy.
1344 R	ALCOHOLISM	Syph.
1344 R		**diabetes**; complicated with: Med.
1344 R	ALUMINIUM	**toxicity**: Cadm-met., **Cadm-o.**,Calc-ox.
1344 R	ANEMIA	Merc-k-i.

PAGE	GENERALITIES	
1345 L	ANTIDOTES, to	**aluminium** toxicity (ex. cooking vessels): Bar-c., cadm-met., cadm-o., calc-ox., plb.

antibiotics: Carb-v., mag-p., op.
 – **with weakness**:Carb-v.
 – **skin eruptions**: Rhus-v.
aspirin: Mag-p. (Kent/Grimmer)
camphor, menthol: Carb-v.
coal-tar drugs (analgesics, antigrippals, antipyretics, hypnotics etc.): Am-c., carb-v., lach., mag-p., op., other carbons and snakes
diphtheria shots: Diph., merc-cy.
meningitis shots: Apis
radiation therapy (for destruction of capillaries, eczema, moles etc.)
 – **subsequent illness**; with: Cadm-i., fl-ac., phos., rad-br., stront-c., X-ray.
 – **subsequent anemia** and cachexia after radium treatments: Phos.
 – **subsequent ulcerating necrosis** that defies healing: Cadm-i.
radium treatments: Cadm-met.
rapidly growing: Cadm-met.
serums or vaccines: Nosodes of same.
small pox vaccinations: Maland., thuj.
typhoid shots: Bapt.
X-ray burn or treatments: Cadm-met., fl-ac.
yellow fever shots: Ars.

| 1346 L | CANCEROUS AFFECTIONS | Aur-ar., merc-c., merc-k-i., syph., thiosin. |

advanced stage of cancer: Alum-sil., anan., ant-ar., ant-i., arg-m., bell-p., ben-zoquinone, cadm-chr., cadm-met., cadm-s., all cadmiums, calc-f., con., hydr., kali-thio-cy., lap-a., metastatic

PAGE   GENERALITIES

1346 L   CANCEROUS
AFFECTIONS

advanced stage of cancer ...
melanoma, nat-hexa-metaph., oxyg. (palliation), phos., phyt., scir., scroph-n., symph.

Blood: Aran., crot-h. (Editor)

Blood vessels: Bell-p.

Bones: Asaf., Aur-ar., aur-m-n., cadm-calc-fl., cadm-met. (sarcoma skull, upper arm), calc-f., euph. (sarcoma), hecla (jaw), hippoz. (skull bones), lap-a., merc-k-i. (sarcoma), methyl. (femur), phos., stront-c., symph. (sarcoma bone, jaw, antrum), toxi. (sarcoma tibia, fibula)

encephaloma: Hippoz. (dura mater, choroid plexus)

epithelioma: abr., ant-m., ars-s-f., ars-s-r., bufo, cadm-met., cic., cund., epiph., formal., hippoz., kali-ar., kali-bi., kali-thio-cy., methyl., sol, X-ray.

fungus hematodes: Sabal.

Glands: Arg-m., aur-ar., aur-m-n., brom. (thyroid, maxillary, parotid, testes), carb-an., cist., ferr-i., hippoz., iod., lap-a., merc-k-i. (Hodgkin), myris., nat-sil-f. (neck), sars., sil., thiosin.

hemorrhage: Mill., phos.

lupus: Alumn., Ars., Aur-ar., Hippoz., Kali-bi., Sol, Thiosin.

malodor in cancer: Bufo

Mucus membranes: Eucal.

pains of cancer: Bell. 30, bism-o. (gastric Cancer Pain), cod-p.1x to 3x (cancers rich in sentient nerves), cham.30 (morphine addict to decrease anxiety), crot-h., euph., euph-he., naja, ox-ac. (extreme pains in

PAGE	GENERALITIES	
1346 L	CANCEROUS AFFECTIONS	**pains of cancer ...** breast cancer), phyt.
		– **burning pains**: Euph-he.
		syphilitic or tubercular base; on: Kali-i.
		vibrations of cancer:Bomhenia, dulc.
1349 R	COLD	**heat and cold**: Cadm-i., merc-k-i.
1350 L		**wet weather agg.**: Ant-t.
1351 L	CONTRADICTORY and alternating states	Abrot. (K)., agar. (CSS), alum. (K), alumn. (K), arn. (K), ars. (K), aur. (CSS), bell. (H), bry. (H), camph. (H), chin. (H), cimic. (BG), crot-t. (K), kali-c. (K), med. (BG), op. (GRIMMER), podo. (K), psor., (CSS), sep. (CSS), staph. (CSS), tub. (CSS)
1352 R	CONVULSIONS	**dentition**; during: Op.
1353 L		**epileptic**: Kali-i., parth.
1355 L		**sleep**; during: Naja
1356R	DROPSY	**anemia**: Crat.
		heart Disease: Crat.
		renal failure: Oxyd.
1357 L	DRY	**weather agg.**: Aur-m.
1357 R	EMACIATION	Calc-ox., merc-k-i.
1360 L	FAINTNESS	**heart disease**: Lach.
1361 R	FANNED	**wants to be**: Carb-v., med.
1362 L	FLU	**sequelae, of**: Merc-k-i.
1365 R	HEMORRHAGE	**dark thin blood**: Sul-ac.
		punctured wounds; from: Aran.
1368 R	INFLAMMATION	**Bones**: Merc-k-i.
1377 R	PAIN	**Bones**: Merc-k-i.
		– **night**: Merc-k-i.

PAGE	GENERALITIES	

1391 R   POLIO

PROPHYLAXIS
- **children**: 1-3 years of age: **Lat-s. 30** every month during **epidemic 3 doses. Two months after** third dose of Lat-s. 30 give **Lat-s. 200** every 1 or 2 months for **2 or 3 doses. Two months after** the last dose of Lat-s. 200 give **Lat-s 1000 and** repeat Lat-s. 1000 **every 6 weeks** for a total of **4 doses** (including the first dose of Lat-s. 1M). This gives protection till the **next year.** Then give **Lat-s. 10M** every **6 months** for **5 years**; then **Lat-s. 50M** every year for **2 or 3 years** to give protection for life.
- **older children and adults**: **Lat-s. 30** once a month for **3 doses.** After the third dose of 30 give **Lat-s. 200** every two months for **2 doses.** Two months after the second dose of the 200th, give **Lat-s. 1000** every 6 months for **4 to 6 doses** (2 or 3 years), followed by **Lat-s. 10M** every 6 months - **4 to 6 doses** (2 or 3 years). Follow with **Lat-s. 50M** once a year for **2 or 3 doses** (2 or 3 years).
- **other remedies of prophylaxis**: Cocc., cur., gels., remedy of genus epidemicus

1391 R   POLIO — **bulbar form**: Ant-t.,op.

1391 R — **crippling**; after recovery of polio: Calc-p., calc-s., nat-ar.

1393 L   PULSE — **frequent**: Crat.

1397 L — **weak**: Crat.

PAGE	GENERALITIES	
1398 R	SCARLET FEVER	**PROPHYLAXIS OR DISEASE**
		– **coarse dark rash**: Ail., phyt., rhus-t., sulph.
		– **smooth rash**: Bell. 30 every week
1399 L	SEPTECEMIA	**small-pox vaccination**; following: Maland., sarr.
1402 L	SLEEP	**after agg.**: Crot-h.
1405 R	SWELLING	**Glands**: Merc-k-i.
		tubercular adenitis: Merc-k-i.
1406 L	SYPHILIS:	Merc-k-i.
		tertiary: Merc-k-i.
1413 L	WEAKNESS	Merc-k-i.

RELATIONSHIP OF REMEDIES FROM THE WORK OF DR. GRIMMER

PREPARED BY AHMED N. CURRIM PH. D., M.D.

REMEDY	COMPLEMENT	REMEDIES THAT FOLLOW WELL	INIMICIAL
CADM-I.		CALC-F.	
CADM-MET.		CALC-F.	
CALC-OX.		MAG-C.	
CARB-V.		CALC-F., KALI-C., MEPH.	
HIPPOZ.		STREPTOM.	
KALI-BI.		TUB.	
KALI-BR.		NAT-S.	
MAG-C.		SIL.	
LYC.		ARS., CARB-V.	
MAG-P.		KALI-C.	
MEPH.		SEP.	
NAJA		MAG-P.	
NAT-S.		KALI-I.	
NIT-AC.	CARB-V.		
SEP.		LYC.	
SYPH.		LYC.	
TOXI.	MERC-K-I.	MERC-K-I.	

REMEDIES

A

B

C

421, 428, 429, 439, 440, 450, 451, 459, 466, 467, 470, 477, 478, 494, 643, 754, 795, 803, 814, 818, 859, 862, 863, 864, 867, 868, 869, 873, 875, 878

Carbn-h. 795

Carbn-s. 400, 439, 440, 754, 795, 818, 862

Carc. 819

Caul. 31, 248

Caust. 11, 40, 57, 90, 169, 170, 248, 283, 291, 376, 379, 385, 438, 439, 450, 451, 490, 570, 754, 795, 796, 819, 870

Cean. 125, 864, 865

Cedr. 62, 128, 451

Cench. 167, 828

Cham. 4, 6, 31, 100, 288, 292, 451, 466, 493, 819, 874

Chel. 248, 439, 451, 466, 826, 863

Chim. 817, 826, 865, 866

China preparations 478

Chin. 18, 125, 169, 170, 248, 283, 284, 288, 289, 395, 439, 440, 451, 460, 470, 477, 478, 490, 495, 838, 871, 875

Chinin-ar. 439, 470, 478, 870

Chinin-s. 62, 451, 470, 478, 479, 860, 871, 872

Chion. 827, 864, 865

Chlf. 99, 288, 289

Chlol. 451, 470, 478, 859, 860, 861, 862, 865, 871

Chlor. 81, 470, 473

Chol. 439, 440, 827, 864

Cic. 286, 439, 490, 827, 874

Cimic. 248, 451, 875

Cina 6, 81, 451

Cinnb. 248

Cist. 124, 248, 754, 795, 827, 862, 874

Clem. 754, 795, 817

Cob. 795

Cob-m. 819, 868

Coc-c. 439, 440, 451

Coca 117, 119, 142, 283, 417, 439

Cocc. 153, 248, 285, 322, 439, 440, 470, 472, 490, 570, 876

Cod-p. 492, 874

Coff. 283, 284, 286, 287, 288, 439, 440, 451

Colch. 439, 470, 472, 477, 490

Coloc. 4, 31, 32, 284, 291, 439, 440

Con. 79, 124, 142, 248, 284, 285, 322, 382, 438, 439, 440, 465, 490, 494, 754, 768, 795, 796, 814, 815, 817, 818, 819, 824, 827, 873

Congo red 138, 142, 817, 865, 868

Cor-r. 440, 451

Crat. 163, 860, 864, 867, 868, 869, 870, 875, 876

Croc. 283, 284, 285

Crot-c. 248, 490

Crot-h. 146, 153, 439, 440, 443, 451, 460, 470, 475, 478, 490, 570, 795, 819, 828, 859, 861, 872, 874, 877

Crot-t. 384, 451, 875

Cub. 439, 819

Cund. 795, 796, 817, 828, 862, 874

Cupr. 18, 149, 153, 248, 284, 285, 288, 289, 379, 439, 451, 490, 570, 754, 795, 868

Cur. 153, 451, 490, 570, 828, 876

I

K

L

M

Q

R

S